MW00715201

PSYCHOPATHOLOGY
AND COGNITION

This is a volume in
PERSONALITY, PSYCHOPATHOLOGY, AND PSYCHOTHERAPY
A Series of Monographs, Texts, and Treatises

Under the Editorship of David T. Lykken and Philip C. Kendall

PSYCHOPATHOLOGY AND COGNITION

Edited by

Keith S. Dobson

Department of Psychology
University of Calgary
Calgary, Alberta, Canada

Philip C. Kendall

Department of Psychology
Temple University
Philadelphia, Pennsylvania

ACADEMIC PRESS, INC.
A Division of Harcourt Brace & Company
San Diego   New York   Boston   London   Sydney   Tokyo   Toronto

Copyright © 1993 by ACADEMIC PRESS, INC.

All Rights Reserved.
No part of this publication may be reproduced or transmitted in any form or by any
means, electronic or mechanical, including photocopy, recording, or any information
storage and retrieval system, without permission in writing from the publisher.

Academic Press, Inc.
1250 Sixth Avenue, San Diego, California 92101-4311

United Kingdom Edition published by
Academic Press Limited
24–28 Oval Road, London NW1 7DX

Library of Congress Cataloging-in-Publication Data

Psychopathology and cognition / edited by Keith Dobson, Philip C.
  Kendall.
         p. cm. -- (Personality, psychopathology, and psychotherapy
  series)
    Includes index.
    ISBN 0-12-404175-2 (hardcover)
    1. Psychology, Pathological. 2. Cognitive psychology.
  I. Dobson, Keith S.   II. Kendall, Philip C.   III. Series:
  Personality, psychopathology, and psychotherapy.
       [DNLM: 1. Mental Disorders. 2. Cognition. 3. Psychopathology.
  WM 204 P9737 1993]
  RC454.4.P7967 1993
  DNLM/DLC
  for Library of Congress   93-19571
                                                                CIP

PRINTED IN THE UNITED STATES OF AMERICA
93   94   95   96   97   98   MM   9   8   7   6   5   4   3   2   1

to all past, present, and future subjects
whose participation in research informs our
understanding and treatment of psychopathology

Contents

Part II SPECIFIC DISORDERS

3 Cognitive Conceptions of Anxiety
Mark J. Dombeck and Rick E. Ingram

4 The Role of Cognition in Depression
Ruby Ackermann Engel and Robert J. DeRubeis

5 Cognition and Pain Experience
Glenn Pancyr and Myles Genest

6 Cognition, Stress, and Health
Suzanne M. Miller and Ann O'Leary

12 Cognitive Deficits in Schizophrenia
Richard A. Steffy

Part III INTEGRATION AND FUTURE DIRECTIONS

13 Future Trends for Research and Theory in Cognition and Psychopathology
Keith S. Dobson and Philip C. Kendall

Contributors

Numbers in parentheses indicate the pages on which the authors' contributions begin.

Ruby Ackermann Engel (83), Department of Psychology, University of Pennsylvania, Philadelphia, Pennsylvania 19104

Donald H. Baucom (351), Department of Psychology, University of North Carolina, Chapel Hill, North Carolina 27599

Kelly Bemis Vitousek (191), Department of Psychology, University of Hawaii, Honolulu, Hawaii 96822

Marylene Cloitre (19), Department of Psychology, New School for Social Research, New York, New York 10003

Robert J. DeRubeis (83), Department of Psychology, University of Pennsylvania, Philadelphia, Pennsylvania 19104

Keith S. Dobson (3, 475), Department of Psychology, University of Calgary, Calgary, Alberta, Canada T2N 1N4

Mark J. Dombeck (53), Department of Psychology, San Diego State University, San Diego, California 92182

Norman Epstein (351), Department of Family Studies, University of Maryland, College Park, Maryland 20742

Myles Genest (121), Department of Psychology, Acadia University, Wolfville, Nova Scotia, Canada B0P 1X0

Mark S. Goldman (245), Department of Psychology, University of South Florida, Tampa, Florida 33620

Rick E. Ingram (53), Department of Psychology, San Diego State University, San Diego, California 92182

Philip C. Kendall (3, 387, 475), Department of Psychology, Temple University, Philadelphia, Pennsylvania 19122

Jennifer P. MacDonald (387), Department of Psychology, Temple University, Philadelphia, Pennsylvania 19122

Suzanne M. Miller (159), Department of Psychology, Temple University, Philadelphia, Pennsylvania 19122

Joseph P. Newman (293), Department of Psychology, University of Wisconsin, Madison, Wisconsin 53706

Ann O'Leary (159), Department of Psychology, Rutgers University, Piscataway, New Jersey 08855

Lisa Orimoto (191), Department of Psychology, University of Hawaii, Honolulu, Hawaii 96822

Glenn Pancyr (121), Department of Psychology, Royal University Hospital, Saskatoon, Saskatchewan, Canada S7N 0X0

Bruce C. Rather (246), Department of Psychology, University of South Florida, Tampa, Florida 33620

Zindel V. Segal (19), Clarke Institute of Psychiatry, and Department of Psychiatry, University of Toronto, Toronto, Ontario, Canada M5T 1R8

Richard A. Steffy (429), Department of Psychology, University of Waterloo, Waterloo, Ontario, Canada N2L 3G1

John F. Wallace (293), Department of Psychology, University of Wisconsin, Madison, Wisconsin 53706

Preface

The field of psychopathology has been influenced by understandings of clinical phenomena that are rooted in cognitive models. In some instances, models have been adapted from basic research in cognitive psychology, but in many instances they were born out of a descriptive and clinical perspective on psychopathology. In many cases, exciting new hybrid clinical–experimental models of psychopathology are developing.

This volume reflects the growth exemplified in the integration of clinical and experimental cognitive research in psychopathology and also critically evaluates the status of theoretical developments related to psychopathology and cognition. This book presents the different major forms of psychopathology and the associated cognitive research findings, formulations, and models. Each chapter surveys a particular disorder within the field of psychopathology, highlights and evaluates the major cognitive models for that type of disorder, compares and contrasts these models, and then suggests treatment and future research implications of those models. Although the consistency we have tried to create from chapter to chapter should help readers compare cognitive research and theories across chapters, each chapter stands alone as a current and critical review of cognition and psychopathology.

This volume has been prepared with the intention of serving the needs of professionals who desire a recent review of the field of psychopathology and cognition as well as the needs of graduate students of psychology. By drawing together in a single source the diverse forms of psychopathology we also hope that individual investigators and theorists working in one disorder will be informed by developments in other areas. It is too easy to become embroiled in research, methodological, and theoretical debates within a particular domain of psychopathology; sharing information across disorders and research domains has a general salutary effect on the discipline. We hope that readers find that this volume fulfills the goals we have set for it.

In closing, we would like to acknowledge the work of our contributors. Much of the integrative work represented here is novel, and we appreciate the efforts that the contributors have made to enhance the overall volume. Philip C. Kendall acknowledges the support of an NIMH grant (NIH 44042). Both of us acknowledge the support provided for the project as an abstract entity and the efforts that resulted in the production of the final volume by Academic Press.

Keith S. Dobson   Philip C. Kendall
Calgary, Alberta   Philadelphia, Pennsylvania

PART I

Conceptual and Methodological Issues

On the Nature of Cognition and Its Role in Psychopathology

Philip C. Kendall
Temple University

Keith S. Dobson
University of Calgary

CAUSAL FACTORS IN PSYCHOPATHOLOGY

One of the most important and interesting challenges for psychologists who study psychopathology is to attempt to disentangle the enigma of etiology from among all of the processes associated with disordered behavior. How can we best explain why certain individuals suffer great psychological distress while others, often in similar circumstances, may experience only modest discomfort? Why do some persons lose contact with reality, why do children display maladjustment, and yet other individuals attempt suicide? The etiology of psychopathology has concerned mental health professionals and society for centuries and, while definitive answers to questions of causality remain elusive, the field is approaching a time when there will be more specific answers to certain questions.

Assume for a moment that someone you know has recently been hospitalized for severe depression. You see a neighborhood friend who approaches you and asks, "Hey, I heard about Bob. What happened?" In your response, you describe what you know of the recent events. Your friend persists: "Yeah, I know he's depressed, but what happened?" You make a guess at the causal factors: "It must have been the breakup of his marriage."

You do not know the full array of factors that contributed to the disordered state, but you attempt to explain it by assigning it understandable causes. In this brief illustration, the depression is attributed to the termination of a close interpersonal relationship. Attributions are causal statements made to help explain the causes of actions. Our stated attributions are not always accurate (Zajonc, 1980), but it is noteworthy that people routinely provide explanations for their behavior and the behavior of others. Regarding abnormal behavior, there are many typical attributions for an individual's psychological distress.

Professionals who study psychopathology are faced with a wide array of causal factors to examine and potentially explain different forms of disordered behavior. As would be clear from even a cursory reading of the research literature, however, no one factor causes all psychopathology. Rather, a multitude of influences are involved in the development of psychological disorders, with different factors playing more or less important roles in each of the distinct types of abnormality. Stated differently, the causes of psychological maladjustment are diverse and they interact in numerous ways. The present volume selects cognitive functioning as a singular topic for in-depth investigation. Thus, while we do not intend to suggest that cognition causes all psychopathology, this volume will examine the role that cognitive functioning plays in specific psychological disorders. What follows in this introductory chapter is an overview of the domain of cognition as it is applied to the investigation of psychopathology. We begin, however, with a brief review of other factors related to abnormal behavior.

Genetic Factors

Repeated findings from a series of studies suggest that there are genetic predispositions toward certain major forms of psychopathology. Schizophrenia, for example, a severe disorder involving hallucinations, delusions, loss of contact with reality, and severe personality deterioration, occurs with greater frequency in the offspring of persons who themselves had been diagnosed as schizophrenic (e.g., Gottesman, 1991). Family links also have been found in other forms of psychopathology.

In addition to family studies, research into the genetics of human behavior employs the study of identical (monozygotic) twins and fraternal (dizygotic) twins. By comparing the similarities and differences between monozygotic and dizygotic twins, researchers have studied the contribution of hereditary factors to various forms of human behavior including psychopathology. By studying both types of twins, some of whom have an identifiable disorder, researchers can begin to estimate the contribution of genetics to psychopathology.

Research clearly documents that genetic factors contribute to the development of different forms of psychopathology, but very few disorders to date have been shown to be totally inherited. Due to the fact that genetic factors do not completely explain abnormal behavior, psychological and environmental factors are implicated in the etiology and the expression of schizophrenia and the clear majority of other disorders.

Environmental Factors

In many respects, human behavior is the product of what is learned from the environmental conditions surrounding that behavior. Interpersonal behavior patterns, such as those involved in friendships and marriages, are learned from interactions with others in the social environment. Someone with a family that has been warm and accepting of his/her friends, and supportive of his/her efforts to interact with peers will have the opportunity to develop into a socially appropriate adult. Nonacceptance or rejection by parents and/or peers can be associated with psychological distress. For instance, research reported by Cowen and colleagues (i.e., Cowen *et al.*, 1973) indicated that children who were identified by their classmates as rejected or aggressive were at risk for later psychopathology. We also know, for example, that children of depressed mothers are more likely themselves to evidence depression in their own lives (Gotlib and Hammen, 1992).

In addition to the quality of the social environment, aspects of the physical environment such as extreme crowding, excessive noise, lack of social support, and lack of shelter can contribute to maladjustment. Psychologically unhealthy environments are also detrimental to proper adjustment; that is, they interfere with or restrict personal development, limit personal choices, are not open to diversity, and do not encourage self-determination (Rappaport, 1977; Sarason, 1972). Parents and, to a degree, social institutions have to set boundaries for acceptable behavior. Excessive restrictiveness, however, can contribute to a detrimental social environment. Although not the sole cause of all psychological distress, the environment contributes its share to an individual's adjustment. Moreover, even a reasonably supportive environment can be misperceived by an at-risk individual. Cognitive functioning, such as that involved in misperceptions of the demands in the environment, can exacerbate, if not actually create, unwanted environmental influences.

The Family

The family is worthy of being singled out as a key social environment with great impact on the quality of adjustment of its members. The family is an especially potent microcosm for the development of successful strategies for coping and adjustment.

Consider the experience of interpersonal conflict in a family. Although everyone has had conflictual family experiences, families and individuals differ in the manner in which the conflict is handled. Family conflict resolution patterns have been implicated in the development of certain childhood disorders. For instance, Patterson (1982) has found that parents of aggressive children socialize their children differently than do most parents. Whereas most parents try to reduce interpersonal conflicts, parents of aggressive children allow conflicts to escalate. This approach results in emotionally charged interactions that do not dissipate quickly. In situations where the inevitable conflicts are resolved, those family members involved can confront the conflict in a problem-focused manner, thereby learning methods for coping with future conflict. In contrast, in situations where conflicts escalate and are not resolved, the participants are deprived of the opportunity to manage the experience and to learn from it.

Consider the following family situation. A mother with a new job outside the home states that she is not going to participate in cleaning the rooms of her two teenage children. She has cleaned for years, but her present work responsibilities and the fact that teenagers should be able to keep their own rooms clean have persuaded her to remove herself from the task. In a planned and considerate manner, she informs her children that she simply cannot continue to be the maid of the house. One teen processes the experience and concludes that it is evidence that "Mom is not caring, and she doesn't accept her responsibilities." The second teen sees it differently: "Mom has finally learned how to not get overextended. She's really getting good at keeping a lid on her responsibilities." The first teen's interpretation may lead to other thoughts of rejection and perhaps even to disliking the mom and resenting her career and her individual needs. The second teen, in contrast, may learn to value the mother more, and may respect her for her decision.

The family serves an important function in socializing children, and an absence of proper socialization can result in psychological disturbances in the children and other members of the family. Disturbed family relationships have been implicated, for example, in such problems as depression, eating disorders, and juvenile delinquency. Family experiences are not viewed similarly by all parties, and cognitive functioning is implicated in the contribution of family influences to individual psychopathology.

Social Life and Economic Stresses

Among the many popular attributions for someone's psychological distress is the notion of a person's inability to handle the "stress." Stress is a central psychological concept (Lazarus and Folkman, 1984; Meichenbaum, 1985) that has been used as the reason for excessive drinking, drug abuse, marital conflict, depression, and other psychological disorders. Are disturbed persons exposed to more stress than those who qualify as well adjusted, or do they somehow cope with the same kinds of stresses less effectively? Are there qualitative differences in the pressures that contribute to maladjustment?

Unwanted negative economic influences can detract from a person's ability to make an adequate adjustment. Consider the case of factory workers who are laid off when the major industry in a small town closes. With the lack of money to pay the mortgage, buy groceries, and care for the children, the ex-workers are under enormous economic pressures. Evidence suggests that as the economic stability of the head of household goes down, the incidence of child abuse, the frequency of alcohol problems, and rate of severe marital discord all increase.

Data suggest that economic distress has an influence on the incidence of psychological disorders. Dooley and Catalano (1980) documented that economic changes were associated with both increases in psychological disorders and increased utilization of mental health facilities. While it is not clear if the economic stress directly increases the frequency of disorders or if it influences the decision to seek help for a chronic or anticipated disorder, the data do support the view that economic stress influences psychological health. Further, although the literature is not yet definitive, it appears that an individual's personal interpretation of the economic conditions is active in the relationship between economic circumstances and maladjustment.

Major life events that are stressful to the individual, such as the death of a close family member, have unwanted negative effects on our adjustment. Pregnancy can also be a stressful experience, but for those couples who are actively trying to reproduce, pregnancy may be a welcomed condition. Indeed, early research (e.g., Holmes and Rahe, 1967) as well as more current investigations have documented that stressful life events disrupt the process of adjustment. One's *perspective* on the life event contributes to whether or not there is stress (see, e.g., Johnson, 1982). The same life event may be stressful or not, depending on the person's perspective. The contribution of cognitive functioning to the development of psychopathology has to do with the manner in which individuals process their stressful life experiences, as well as the way in which these experiences are stored in memory and later recalled.

In addition to economic and life stresses, there are many forms of social stress in contemporary society. It has been suggested, for example, that the traditional socialization of males to be "strong and silent" types has lead to emotional blunting and a lack of interpersonal connectedness, which is in turn associated with less than optimal psychological health. On the other hand, one of the powerful social stresses influencing women is the idea of the superwoman who can earn an advanced degree, acquire a job and develop a career, bear and raise children, maintain a household and husband, and somehow keep fit and enjoy herself at the same time (Jack, 1991). Despite the obvious irrationality of the demands of society on today's men and women, the pressures exist and affect the sense of value men and women place upon themselves.

Cognitive Functioning

A glass of water is placed in front of a dozen people. When asked to describe the contents, some say the glass is half full while others say it is half empty. This well-known water glass metaphor illustrates that different people see the same situation in different ways. The discrepancy in the description of the same object is the result of the individual differences that exist in the way people interpret situations. While it is true that there are a number of ways to view a given incident without any necessarily being described as pathological, it is also true that some forms of pathology seem to result from the distorted manner in which individuals view and process their experiences.

Stylistic variations in the way people process information can predispose persons to be vulnerable to certain disorders and/or provide certain protective coping skills. For example, research and theory has repeatedly implicated faulty information processing in the onset of anxiety and depression (Beck 1967; Gotlib and Hammen, 1992; Kendall and Ingram, 1989). Consider the person who always sees the glass as half empty. For such an individual, partly sunny days are described as partly cloudy, the exciting parts of a movie are forgotten and only the dull parts are recalled, and experiences that most people would view as reasonably successful are interpreted as inadequate. With a characteristically negative view of the self, others, and the world, this kind of person is likely to report the low self-concept, lack of enthusiasm and energy, and sadness that are associated with depression (Beck, 1976; Ingram, 1984). When faulty information processing contributes to psychological disorders we often refer to this as *distorted* thinking (Kendall, 1985) and consider it indicative of the influential role of cognitive functioning in psychological maladjustment.

As we have mentioned, distorted thinking can exacerbate the contribution to psychopathology from the other sources we have already described as genetic, environmental, family, and economic and social pressures. For instance, a learning environment may be most desirable when it contains optimal schooling opportunities, peers with adequate social skills, and an array of recreational and sports facilities. Such an environment, some might argue, should make proper socialization and successful adjustment easy. But does it? As we all know, there are persons who seem to have had the best opportunities but who nevertheless develop psychological problems. This outcome can be the result of biological processes, but it can also result from cognitive processes, where the experiences that most people would view as desirable are somehow seen by the troubled person as unwanted and painful. The social learning environment may seem fine to an outside observer, but if the person in question is processing their experiences in a distorted manner, these distortions can contribute to the onset of a psychological disorder.

PRECISION ABOUT COGNITION

Cognition is not a singular or unitary concept, but is rather a general term that refers to a complex system, which can be subdivided for increased understanding. For instance, it has been suggested that cognitive content, cognitive processes, cognitive products, and cognitive structures can be distinguished (Ingram and Kendall, 1986; Kendall and Ingram, 1987, 1989). Cognitive structures can be defined as the manner in which information is internally represented in memory. Cognitive structures, or templates, reflect an accumulation of experiences in memory that guides the filtering or screening of new experiences. Cognitive content refers to the information that is actually represented — the contents of the cognitive structures. Cognitive processes are the procedures by which the cognitive system operates — how we go about perceiving, recalling, and interpreting experiences. Cognitive products are the cognitions that result from the interaction of information, cognitive structures, content, and processes (e.g., attributions).

Psychopathology may be related to problems in any or all of the above areas of cognition, and the understanding of specific disorders benefits from consideration of each of these factors for each individual client. Anxious persons, for instance, bring a certain form of cognitive structure to events they face. A dominant cognitive structure for anxiety is threat — threat of loss, criticism, or harm (e.g., Beck and Emery, 1985). An individual who brings an anxiety-prone memory template to new experiences might see the threat of embarrassment or the risk of danger, and process the experiences accordingly. Anxious cognitive processes might include self-talk such as "What if somebody notices?" or "What if I get sick or hurt?" Cognitive structures serve to trigger automatic cognitive content and information processing about behavioral events. Attributions about the event reflect the influences of the preexisting structure, and also contribute to the schema that is brought to the next behavioral event.

Not all dysfunctional cognition is the same. One key distinction concerns the difference between *cognitive deficits* or *deficiency* and *cognitive distortion* (Kendall, 1985; see also Kendall and MacDonald, Ch. 11, this volume). Deficiencies refer to the lack of certain forms of thinking (e.g., the absence of information processing where it would be beneficial), whereas distortions refer to active but dysfunctional thinking processes. The deficiency–distortion distinction originally highlighted the differences between the forerunners of cognitive–behavioral therapy that focused on modifying distorted thinking with adults (e.g., Beck, 1976; Ellis, 1971) and early cognitive–behavioral training that dealt mostly with remediating deficiencies in thinking with children (e.g., self-instructional training; Meichenbaum and Goodman, 1971; Kendall, 1977). The distinction can be furthered with reference to different types of disorders (Kendall, 1993). Anxiety and depression, for example, are typically associated with misperceptions of the social/interpersonal environment. Active information processing is occurring, but it is distorted (e.g., Brewin, 1985). In a series of studies of depressed children, for example, depressed youngsters viewed themselves as less capable than did nondepressed children when, in fact, teachers (the source of objective outsiders' judgment) saw the two groups of children as nondistinct (Kendall *et al.*, 1990). In the teachers' eyes, the depressed children were not less competent across several dimensions. It was the depressed children who evidenced distortion through their misperception of their actual competencies.

Consider the following vignette as illustrative of the type of distorted thinking an anxious person might experience. A small group of newly acquainted adults is engaging in conversation — generally getting to know one another. Of the dozen or so people, most have said something, even if just to express agreement. One adult, however, has said nothing; despite looking at the various other speakers and seeming to follow the conversation, she has been a silent observer. Although observing itself is not troublesome, this adult is silent because of her excessive self-doubt. For instance, she is thinking to herself, "That lady seems to be so outgoing, everyone likes her. I'm never going to fit in. It's just like always. What do I have to do to fit in? What can I say? Something about the weather . . . ? No, that's dumb. No one will be interested." Her self-talk reflects her active information processing, but also belies her misappraisal of the demands in the environment. In reality, there are many opportunities for her to say a few words and, despite her self-doubt, the woman may actually be highly regarded by her friends. The truth is that she is likely to be accepted by this new set of acquaintances. Her anxiousness and tension are essentially unfounded: the woman has misperceived a demanding atmosphere in her environment, as her associates are not likely to be cruel and overjudgmental. Nevertheless, the distorted perceptions will have an effect on her, as they are linked to her feeling inadequate, at risk for rejection, and tense.

Contrast the highly self-critical and active processing style of the anxious and tense woman with the thoughtless style of an impulsive woman. Our thoughtless person bursts into the group, makes several personally intimate comments and asks publicly about someone's weight problem. At least two of the members of their group are put off by her brashness, but she does not attend to nor recognize this slight rejection. Our impulsive woman is not attentive to the social responses of others; she lacks the attention to information processing and instead acts and speaks without thinking first. Her interpersonal situation results more as a result of her failing to stop and think — a cognitive deficiency — than from active but distorted processing of information.

To further illustrate the differences between distortions and deficiencies, consider the role of cognition in other disorders. Anorexia, most often observed in females, is related to setting perfectionistic goals and demands, carrying an inaccurate view of the self (e.g., self-perception of body), and being "too good" behaviorally (see Vitousek and Orimoto, Ch. 7, this volume). These features of an overcontrolled problem reflect cognitive distortions — active processing that is dysfunctional. In contrast, psychopaths (Newman and Wallace, Ch. 9, this volume) have been found to display cognitive deficiencies, and in aggressive youth there is evidence of both cognitive deficiency and cognitive distortion (Epps & Kendall, 1993; Kendall and MacDonald, Ch. 11, this volume; Lochman and Dodge, in press). For example, there are data to suggest that aggressive youth have deficiencies in interpersonal problem solving (Deluty, 1981) and data to document that they also show distortions in their processing of information (e.g., Dodge, 1985). Limited ability to generate alternative, nonaggressive solutions to interpersonal problems is an example of their deficiencies, while misattribution of the intentionality of others' behavior (Dodge, 1985) demonstrates a tendency for distorted processing. In the instance of psychotic disorders, Steffy (Ch. 12, this volume) describes the considerable evidence concerning the nature of cognitive deficits in schizophrenia, whereas the dominant role assigned to distortions in depression is evident in Chapter 4, this volume, by Ackermann Engel and DeRubeis.

As the above begins to demonstrate, our position is that there are different types of cognitive dysfunction and that different cognitive difficulties are linked to different types of disorders. One of the primary goals of this volume is to begin to document the manifold ways in which cognitive functioning is uniquely related to different forms of disorder.

COGNITIVE CONCEPTS IN SEQUENCE: A TEMPORAL MODEL

Research continues to document the roles that expectations, attributions, self-statements, beliefs, and schemata have in the development of both adaptive and maladaptive behavior patterns. Nevertheless, the interrelationships of these and other cognitive factors have yet to be clarified. How are the functional effects of self-statements similar to or different from those of attributions? How does an individual's maladaptive schemas relate to his or her level of irrational beliefs? Do inconsistent or anxious self-statements reduce interpersonal cognitive processing and problem solving? Quite simply, we know only a modest amount about the organization and interrelations of the cognitive concepts receiving clinical and research attention.

A model with some potential utility is one built along a temporal dimension (see also Dobson, 1985; Kendall and Braswell, 1982; Kendall, 1991). Such a model reflects the fact that cognitions are associated with emotional reactions and behavior across time (e.g., cognitions occur before, during, and after behavioral events). Because events do not occur in a vacuum and because behavior is determined by multiple causes, the model must allow for the feedback that results from multiple, sequential behavioral events. That is, cognitive activity before an event will vary depending on the outcomes of previous events. The model must also allow for fluctuations in preevent cognitions associated with the different outcomes (e.g., successful, unsuccessful) attached to prior events. Moreover, because repetitions of cognition–event sequences result in some consistency in cognition, the model must highlight the development of more regularized cognitive processing (e.g., cognitive structures, cognitive styles).

Figure 1.1 illustrates a model that incorporates the flow of cognition across behavioral events of different emotional intensity. The starting point is the initial behavioral event (BE), and our discussion will move from the earliest BE point on Fig. 1.1 (at the left) to the cognitive consistency that results (at the right). In general, it should be noted that this model highlights three classes of cognitive activity: cognitions that occur after a behavioral event, cognitions that occur in anticipation of behavioral events, and stable aspects of cognitive processing.

Often events occur without warning or, if early in the life of an individual, without much predictability. Once an event has occurred, however, and particularly if it is of high emotional valence, it is likely to be cognitively processed. Attributions are the cognitive concepts often studied at the culmination of a behavioral event. Specific attributions are temporally short lived in that their occurrence is at the termination of an event, but attributional styles can develop over time. One could assess a specific attribution

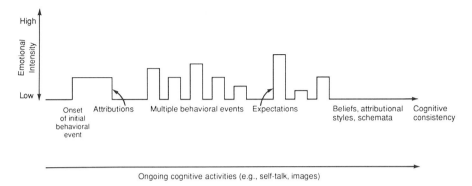

Figure 1.1.   A temporal model of the flow of cognition across behavioral events of different emotional intensity. BE represents a behavioral event. Self-statements and images occur at any point and can be studied at various points in the temporal flow. Problem-solving processes also occur at various points, at places where conflicts or BEs arise.

long after an event, although numerous factors (e.g., recall from memory) may interfere with accurate recall. How patients explain events — both the causes of the negative events they experience and the negative outcome of their behavior — is a central feature of the function of cognition that is of interest within this model.

During the accumulation of a history of behavioral events and event outcomes, the child or adolescent entertains more precise anticipatory cognitions (i.e., expectancies). Expectancies have been described, for example, as outcome expectancies and self-efficacy expectancies (Bandura, 1977; 1986). Other anticipatory cognitions include intentions, plans, and commitments. These latter variables may become more stable and consistent over time than situationally specific expectancies. The generalized expectancy associated with a developing locus of control, by its very general nature, can also be related to consistent attributional patterns. For instance, the generalized expectancy of an external locus of control could be present both before (expectancy) and after (attribution) an event. Before the event, the person's externality leads to an anticipation of having a minimal effect: "Why bother to speak up, no one listens to me." After the event, when a decision has been reached without the individual's input, the event is attributed to powerful others: "See, the big mouths always get their way."

Repeated behavioral events (multiple BEs in Fig. 1.1), and the related cognitive processing that occurs with these events, will result in some degree of consistency in both cognition and behavior. Figure 1.1 illustrates that cognitive consistency (i.e., beliefs, an attributional style, or a cognitive structure) results after experience with multiple events. Cognitive variables with consistency over time are more stable than a single attribution, and more stable cognitive variables may be more predictive in a general sense. On the other hand, stable styles may be less predictive in specific situations than are the actual cognitions at the time of a specific behavioral event.

In addition to the types of cognitive functioning mentioned thus far, other cognitive variables have been demonstrated to be important in a cognitive–behavioral analysis. Such variables include imagery, self-statements, and cognitive problem-solving skills. These factors occur at all points along the temporal flow depicted in Fig. 1.1 and assessments of these factors can prove valuable in understanding and treating individuals suffering from psychopathological states.

Emotional intensity is represented vertically in Fig. 1.1, with more emotionally intense behavioral events being depicted with higher bars. Emotional intensity contributes to the development of cognition in that more intense experiences have a greater impact on the development of cognitive structures. Thus, whereas less emotional events may have a limited influence on attributions, future expectations, and memory, an emotionally significant event has greater impact on the development of a schema and on future thinking.

COGNITIVE MODELS: IMPLICATIONS FOR THERAPY

Although the focus of the current text is upon the adequacy of cognitive models for the understanding of different forms of psychopathology, it is obviously the case that these models carry important implications regarding the treatment of these different disorders. Further, although the study of abnormal psychological conditions has value in its own right, it is also true that many researchers justify their efforts in terms of their potential benefit to individuals who require treatment. In this section we briefly consider how basic research in psychopathology can inform treatment efforts, as well as how results of treatment studies can influence basic research.

Imagine that a new form of disorder is discovered today, and that you suspect cognitive factors are implicated in its cause. If you had unlimited funds, your research strategy might be to: (1) assess the cognitive correlates of the disorder; (2) employ retrospective designs to see if the correlates were predictive; (3) conduct longitudinal studies to assess the predictive validity of cognitive variables associated with the disorder; and (4) manipulate the cognitive variables in question to assess their causal properties. Whereas the first three of these research strategies are common in psychopathology research, for ethical and logistic reasons it is rare to see true experiments in a field that is focused on the etiology of disorders. What is found, on the other hand, is use of the strategy that treats a group of people with a given disorder with a particular treatment package to ascertain whether the disorder can be successfully remediated. Assuming random assignment of subjects to treatment groups, and all other features of an appropriate randomized clinical trial, this treatment research strategy is analogous to an experimental manipulation of putatively causal variables once they have led to the disorder.

Variables that are causal for a given disorder are not necessarily the same variables that either maintain that disorder or lead to recovery. As such, successful treatment by any given method does not unequivocally establish that the variables associated with that treatment are the same variables that caused the disorder. On the other hand, if a set of variables can be identified through correlational and longitudinal research as potential causal variables, and it is then established that modification of these variables through a particular treatment regimen leads to the amelioration of the symptoms of that disorder, then that treatment success is supportive (though not proof) of a causal model. For this reason, many of the chapters in the present volume also include and integrate basic descriptive research with research on the treatment of disorder.

Precisely the above type of cross-fertilization of basic research influencing treatment strategies and successful treatment leading to the investigation of specific features of disorders is seen in the area of cognition and psychopathology. Many of the chapters in this volume detail the linkages between cognitive theory and cognitive therapies, and attempt to provide comprehensive accounts of the causal, maintenance, and treatment aspects of various forms of psychopathology. It can be argued that the integration of causal investigations and treatment outcome research is an appealing attraction of the study of cognitive models of psychopathology.

ACKNOWLEDGMENT

Preparation of this chapter was facilitated by a grant (NIMH 44042) awarded to the first author. Address requests for reprints to either Philip C. Kendall, Department of Psychology, Temple University, Philadelphia, PA 19122, or Keith Dobson, Department of Psychology, University of Calgary, Alberta, Canada, T2N 1N4.

REFERENCES

Bandura, A. (1977). Self-efficacy: Toward a unifying theory of behavioral change. *Psychological Review, 84*, 191–215.

Bandura, A. (1986). *Social foundation of thought and action: A social cognitive theory*. Englewood Cliffs, NJ: Prentice-Hall.

Beck, A. T. (1967). *Depression: Clinical, experimental, and theoretical aspects*. New York: Hoeber.

Beck, A. T. (1976). *Cognitive therapy and the emotional disorders*. New York: International Universities Press.

Beck, A. T., and Emery, G. (1985). *Anxiety disorders and phobias: A cognitive perspective*. New York: Guilford Press.

Brewin, C. R. (1985). Depression and causal attributions: What is their relation? *Psychological Bulletin, 98*, 297–309.

Cowen, E. L., Pederson, A., Babigian, H., Izzo, L. D., and Trost, M. (1973). Long term follow-up of early detected vulnerable children. *Journal of Consulting and Clinical Psychology, 41*, 438–446.

Deluty, R. H. (1981). Alternative thinking ability of aggressive, assertive, and submissive children. *Cognitive Therapy and Research, 5*, 309–312.

Dobson, K. (1985). The relationship between anxiety and depression. *Clinical Psychology Review, 5*, 307–324.

Dodge, K. (1985). Attributional bias in aggressive children. In P. C. Kendall (Ed.), pp. 73–110. *Advances in cognitive–behavioral research and therapy* (Vol. 4). New York: Academic Press.

Dooley, D., and Catalano, R. (1980). Economic change as a cause of behavioral disorder. *Psychological Bulletin, 87*, 450–468.

Ellis, A. (1971). *Growth through reason*. Palo Alto, CA: Science and Behavior Books.

Epps, J. and Kendall, P. C. (1993). Hostile attributional bias in virulent adults. Manuscript submitted for publication, Temple University, Philadelphia, Pennsylvania: 19122.

Gotlib, I., and Hammen, C. L. (1992). *Psychological aspects of depression: Toward a cognitive–interpersonal integration*. New York: Wiley.

Gottesman, I. I. (1991). *Schizophrenia genesis*. New York: Freeman.

Holmes, T. H., and Rahe, R. H. (1967). The Social Readjustment Rating Scale. *Journal of Psychosomatic Research, 11*, 213–218.

Ingram, R. E. (1984). Toward an information processing analysis of depression. *Cognitive Therapy and Research, 8*, 443–447.

Ingram, R., and Kendall, P. C. (1986). Cognitive clinical psychology: Implications of an information processing perspective. In R. Ingram (Ed.), pp. 3–22. *Information processing approaches to clinical psychology*. New York: Academic Press.

Jack, D. C. (1991). *Silencing the self: Women and depression*. Cambridge, MA: Harvard University Press.

Johnson, J. H. (1982). Life events as stressors in childhood and adolescence. In B. Lahey and A. Kazdin (Eds.), *Advances in clinical child psychology* (Vol. 5, pp. 220–254). New York: Plenum.

Kendall, P. C. (1977). On the efficacious use of verbal self-instructions with children. *Cognitive Therapy and Research, 1*, 331–341.

Kendall, P. C. (1985). Toward a cognitive–behavioral model of child psychopathology and a critique of related interventions. *Journal of Abnormal Child Psychology, 13*, 357–372.

Kendall, P. C. (1991). Guiding theory for treating children and adolescents. In P. C. Kendall (Ed.), pp. 3–24. *Child and adolescent therapy: Cognitive–behavioral procedures*. New York: Guilford Press.

Kendall, P. C. (Ed.) (1991). *Child and adolescent therapy: Cognitive–behavioral procedures*. New York: Guilford Press.

Kendall, P. C. (1992). Healthy thinking. *Behavior Therapy, 23*, 1–11.

Kendall, P. C. (1993). Cognitive–behavioral therapies with youth: Guiding theory, current status, and emerging developments. *Journal of Consulting and Clinical Psychology, 61*, 235–247.

Kendall, P. C., and Braswell, L. (1982). On cognitive–behavioral assessment: Model, measures, and madness. In C. D. Speilberger and J. N. Butcher (Eds.), pp. 35–82 *Advances in personality assessment* (Vol. 1). Hillsdale, NJ: Erlbaum.

Kendall, P. C., and Ingram, R. (1987). The future of the cognitive assessment of anxiety: Let's get specific. In L. Michelson and M. Ascher (Eds.), *Anxiety and stress disorders: Cognitive–behavioral assessment and treatment*. New York: Guilford Press.

Kendall, P. C. & Ingram, R. (1989). Cognitive-behavioral perspectives: Theory and research on depression and anxiety. In P. C. Kendall & D. Watson (Eds.), *Anxiety and depression: Distinctive and overlapping features*. New York: Academic Press.

Kendall, P. C., Stark, K. D., and Adam, T. (1990). Cognitive deficit or cognitive distortion in childhood depression. *Journal of Abnormal Child Psychology, 18*, 255–270.

Kendall, P. C., Chansky, T. E., Kane, M. T., Kim, R., Kortlander, E., Ronan, K. R., Sessa, F. M., and Siqueland, L. (1992). *Anxiety disorders in youth: Cognitive–behavioral interventions*. Needham, MA: Allyn and Bacon.

Lazarus, R. S., & Folkman, S. (1984). *Stress, appraisal, and coping*. New York: Springer Publishing Co.

Lochman, J., and Dodge, K. (in press). Social cognitive processes of severely violent, moderately aggressive, and nonaggressive boys. Revision in preparation for *Journal of Consulting and Clinical Psychology*.

Meichenbaum, D. (1985). *Stress inoculation training*. New York: Plenum.

Meichenbaum, D., and Goodman, J. (1971). Training impulsive children to talk to themselves. A means of developing self-control. *Journal of Abnormal Psychology, 77*, 115–126.

Patterson, G. R. (1982). *Coercive family process*. Eugene, OR: Castalia.

Rappaport, J. (1977). *Community psychology: Values, research and action*. New York: Holt, Rinehart and Winston.

Sarason, S. B. (1972). *The creation of settings*. San Francisco: Jossey-Bass.

Zajonc, R. B. (1980). Feeling and thinking: Preferences need no inferences. *American Psychologist, 35*, 151–175.

Methodologies for Studying Cognitive Features of Emotional Disorder

Zindel V. Segal

University of Toronto

Marylene Cloitre

New School for Social Research

Cognitive modeling of psychopathology owes no small measure of its current appeal to the recent increase in reports of the efficacy of cognitive treatments for emotional disorder. Similarly, these very treatments attribute much of their potency and distinctiveness to the incorporation of cognitive constructs and assessment methods derived from cognitive psychology. It is vital that this mutual reciprocity be recognized, since the evaluation of cognitive methodologies for the study of psychopathology cannot be performed without an appreciation of their clinical context, and the adoption of cognitive constructs in clinical work must be similarly referenced against the relative support and experimental justification for their continued usage.

This chapter will examine some of the methodologies available for the study of attention, interpretation of ambiguous stimuli, judgments, and memory processes in anxiety and depressive disorders. Its evaluative perspective will be informed by the position that while cognitive constructs pervade much clinical work and guide the everyday functioning of therapists, the actual practice of therapy offers a chance for the refinement of

19

these variables and for increasing their representativeness of clinical reality (Ingram and Kendall, 1986).

We have deliberately chosen to focus our review on anxiety and depressive disorders. Many of the methodologies we will be examining were first utilized to assess these problems, and while some of these measures have been adapted for use in other areas, we feel that it is best to describe their actual context of development. It is also important to note that there may be limits in the ability to generalize these methods, especially for forms of psychopathology that are not predicated on a bias in information processing, for example, in cases where deficits rather than distortions are causally implicated. In light of this, we draw the reader's attention to the extensive literature on cognitive assessment strategies that rely on self-report inventories, role play enactments, or think aloud procedures (see Kendall and Hollon, 1981; Merluzzi *et al.*, 1981; Segal and Shaw, 1988; Segal and Swallow, in press).

BRIEF HISTORICAL EXCURSUS

It is instructive to consider that the rationale for the development of many of the measures to be discussed in this chapter has been in existence for nearly one hundred years, originating in early work in Wilhelm Wundt's psychology laboratory in Leipzig, Germany, and even in Donders's work on the subtractive method (Bower and Clapper, 1989). It is interesting to note that at this particular point in time, the introspectionists were pursuing a similar goal, namely mapping the contents of consciousness, but were relying on markedly different methods to do so. Their guiding belief was that a theory of cognition could be developed by examining the contents of introspective reports and that these reports could be obtained through self-observation. While subsequent work in cognitive psychology has demonstrated the shortcomings of this position (because of the lack of an isomorphic correspondence between those contents accessible to self-report and the underlying processes responsible for these contents), the notion that the mind could be studied through the examination of its products continues to fascinate psychologists.

One technique commonly employed by the introspectionists was free association. An experimenter read a list of words to a subject and measured the amount of time it took the person to generate responses to these words. This methodology was guided by the underlying belief that time differences reflected the operation of different cognitive processes. This idea still holds sway in the current cognitive arena, as evidenced by the plethora of methodologies that rely on reaction time, rating time, or decision time measures. In fact, one of the more enduring ideas in experimental and cognitive psychology is that the time between a stimulus and a response is occupied by a series of processes or stages, some of which are mental operations, and many of which are arranged in such a fashion that one process does not begin until the preceding one has ended. This has led to the development of methods in which the difference between average response times for two tasks is used to estimate the duration of the process by which they differ. This work is described extensively in Sternberg (1969) and is an elaboration of earlier work by Donders.

The development of methods in cognitive psychology suffered a temporary setback when the agenda of psychology was turned away from the study of mind to the study of behavior. The reemergence of interest in cognitive psychology has been traced by Anderson (1985) to developments in three distinct areas. Human factors research received a boost in World War II when practical information on research relevant to human skills was in great need. The second development stemmed from advances in computer science, especially work that demonstrated the ability of computer programs to problem solve and communicate something meaningful about the nature of intelligence. This work helped to establish the mind-as-computer methaphor, which is still dominant today. Third, advances in the study of linguistics portrayed language acquisition and fluency as inherently complex abilities that could not be explained by prevailing behavioral theories. This pushed the agenda of cognitive science into the forefront and helped to eclipse the previously dominant behavioral emphasis in these areas.

The study of mind at the turn of the century, however, was not the sole province of experimental psychologists. Practitioners concerned with the treatment of "nervous disorders" also contributed to the burgeoning field of cognitive inquiry, setting a precedent for a complementary exploration of mind often overlooked today. It could be noted that some of the concepts described by Jung in his study of complexes are not too far removed from the current work on Stroop interference studies of anxiety or depressive disorders (Segal, 1988). Jung (1910) relied on a word association technique to uncover complexes, areas of emotional conflict, which he assumed existed in patients with neurotic disorders. Words were presented to individuals who were instructed to respond by naming the first word that came to mind. Time to response was recorded, along with other physical measures such as breathing changes. Jung believed that indications of emotional reactions to words such as flushing or longer reaction times revealed the emotional valence of the stimulus item and allowed therapists to hypothesize about their significance to the patient. The number of associations or amount of emotion elicited by stimulus words would indicate the presence of complexes, or clusters of information that attracted greater amounts of psychic energy. It is interesting to consider the conceptual resemblance between this work and current views of spreading activation theories and semantic network models (Bower and Clapper, 1989). Ironically, while Jung's experimental studies had little effect on psychoanalytic thinking at the time, they have withstood some degree of empirical scrutiny (see Carlson and Levy, 1973). The important point here seems to be that even in the formative stages of cognitive analyses of emotional disorders, experimental methods were often tied in a close fashion to a clinical reality that served to anchor or ground the assessment process. It is important to retain this perspective as we proceed with our evaluation of the tasks and measures designed to assess such cognitive processes as interpretive bias, judgment heuristics, and attentional and memory bias.

INTERPRETATION OF AMBIGUOUS STIMULI

Methodologies designed to assess the particular meanings that patients extract from situations or stimuli rendered purposely ambiguous provides an intriguing vantage point from which to view the constructive capacities or biases that patients utilize in their everyday interactions. In one sense, the methodologies described in this section are premised on a contemporary version of the projective hypothesis: they capitalize on uncertainty and the equipotentiality of meanings contained in information that has yet to be ordered. Furthermore, the process of ordering itself informs the investigator about constructive capacities or default values that exist in particular patients' ways of making sense of the world. In more concrete terms, the value of this type of work is made evident when we consider that if ambiguous events are a common occurrence, then an interpretive bias (such as favoring an anxiogenic interpretation of bodily sensations over one that is more neutrally disposed) may play a role in the provocation or maintenance of anxiety or other states of emotional dysregulation.

A study examining bias in the interpretation of threat as assessed by self-report is described by McNally and Foa (1987). Three groups of subjects (treated and untreated agoraphobics, and normals) were administered a number of questionnaires designed to test the notion that agoraphobics would be more likely than normals to interpret ambiguous bodily stimuli as threatening, as well as exaggerate the probability and cost of unpleasant events related to arousal. The Interpretation Questionnaire consisted of 14 brief, ambiguous scenarios, presented to subjects in a booklet form. Scenarios were divided evenly between those with an internal or external stimulus. Sample items asked subjects to provide an explanation for scenarios such as "You feel discomfort in your chest area. Why?" or "You wake up with a start in the middle of the night, thinking you heard a noise, but all is quiet. What do you think woke you up?" Subjects were asked to respond by writing the first explanation that came to their minds. The Subjective Cost Questionnaire assessed the negative valence of 20 potentially unpleasant events and asked subjects to rate each event on a 9-point Likert scale with respect to how bad it would be for them if this had happened. Half of the events pertained to arousal-related items, whereas the other half described events that would be generally unpleasant. A Subjective Probability Questionnaire required subjects to provide an estimate of the likelihood of these same events happening to them.

The authors report that untreated agoraphobics tended to interpret ambiguous stimuli, regardless of whether it was external or internal in nature, as threatening. While this finding was somewhat inconsistent with the prediction that such a bias should be found only for internal stimuli, data from the Subjective Cost and Probability questionnaires suggest that only events related to arousal are associated with enhanced threat in untreated agoraphobics. Agoraphobics who had undergone cognitive-behavioral treatment showed much less of this bias than subjects who had not yet been treated. In a replication and extension of McNally and Foa's (1987) study, Clark, Salkovskis, Koehler, and Gelder (cited in Clark, 1988) found that panic patients interpreted only ambiguous bodily sensations as threatening. This particular paradigm is similar to the one employed by Butler and Mathews (1983) and demonstrates the ease of self-report methods for providing estimates of danger, and meanings associated with incomplete situations or problematic scenarios. The drawbacks to this approach, however, are that the effects of concurrent mood states such as depression need to be seriously considered when interpreting the results. This is especially true, since depressive mood states have been documented to induce a negative response set, which can at times mimic the type of findings investigators may be seeking and thereby lead them to wrongly conclude that their findings describe more specific processes. Panic patients did not provide threatening interpretations for scenarios involving general events, social events, or for symptoms not having a sudden onset. Taken together, this work would seem to indicate that patients who experience panic with or without agoraphobia exhibit biases in the interpretation of ambiguous information as threatening, but that only those with agoraphobia may exhibit general threat biases.

Work by Mathews *et al.* (1989b) and Eysenck *et al.* (1987), has taken advantage of the linguistic ambiguity in words that are spelled differently and mean different things but sound the same (homophones) to test for an interpretive bias in favor of threat among patients with Generalized Anxiety Disorder. Their paradigm involves presenting lists of words to subjects auditorily and asking subjects to write down the word they heard. Practice words (pencil, shoe); neutral words (month, blanket); threat words (harm, hazard); and homophones (die, dye, slay, sleigh) comprise the stimuli used. One question raised about this methodology is whether both homophones were equally familiar to subjects (as measured by a frequency of occurrence index). While it is clear that homophones were as frequent as either unambiguous neutral or threat words in the other categories, each pair of homophones may have differed in frequency within each presentation. An examination of these pairs reveals that the threat meaning is probably more familiar than the meanings of the words in the other conditions, a factor that may need to be controlled for in future work of this nature.

The prediction arising from this work is that anxious subjects, if given the choice, will tend to interpret ambiguous information in the more threatening of two possible ways. Indeed, in the Matthews *et al.* (1989b) study, all subjects tended to be dominated by the threatening meaning for the homophone. The degree of dominance, however, was not equivalent across the three groups studied, with currently anxious controls differing significantly from normals. The recovered group of anxious subjects did not differ significantly from the other two. The implication of this work is that not only does there seem to be an intentional bias that may favor environmental sources of threatening information, but this bias may extend to interpretations of stimuli that are inherently ambiguous or empty of meaning, prior to the subject's assessment. In cases where a specific event may be interpreted in a neutral or threatening fashion (e.g., a new physical sensation or a remark from an acquaintance), it may be the case that anxious individuals would be more likely to endorse relatively alarming interpretations.

While the studies described so far have examined processes that are relatively effortful in nature, it is possible to delve into levels of processing that are somewhat more automatic or unintentional. Work in this area has been reported by Gilson (1983) and Moretti *et al.* (1993). Gilson's work has exploited the phenomenon of binocular rivalry to particular advantage in order to study the dominance of one type of image with depressive content over another type of image with neutral content in patients with depressive disorder. Binocular rivalry is a perceptual phenomenon that occurs when two different stimuli are presented, one in either eye, through a binocular viewing device. When stimulus presentations are brief enough, subjects frequently report seeing only one stimulus, and these perceptual reports have been shown to be potentially influenced by subjects' feelings, affinities, or other dispositions.

In Gilson's study depressed and nondepressed subjects were presented with a series of emotionally contrasted pairs of slides. Depressive content (example: a barren tree) was paired with nondepressive content (example: a tree in full bloom), with slides being presented simultaneously at exposure durations of 500 msec for each slide pair. The main dependent measures in this study were the nature of the perceptual report, that is, which slide did the subjects report seeing, as well as recognition of slide content following the task. For a number of patients, perceptual reports were strongly associated with mood, such that depressed subjects reported seeing more slides with depressive content than did nondepressed subjects. However, there were a number of problems with the design of this study and its interpretability because of difficulties in patient selection and insufficient attention paid to control variables. Clearly, these findings are still in need of replication, yet we feel that the procedure itself warrants scrutiny by investigators interested in assessing interpretation of ambiguous stimuli at levels that reflect a greater automaticity of response. Perhaps with more reliable materials and greater attention to design features, a replication of the Gilson study can add to our understanding of depressive perceptual regularities.

Another study along similar lines is reported by Moretti et al. (1993), which examines the ability of depressed, nondepressed, and remitted depressed subjects to identify facial emotion from slides presented at quick exposures. The process underlying identification of facial emotion may be relevant to our understanding of the speed and accuracy with which positive and negative self-referent information is handled. The paradigm utilized in this work presents subjects with two faces, one of which is emotional in nature, while the other one is neutral; this momentary ambiguity forces subjects to make a decision regarding the nature of the emotion expressed, while keeping in mind the particular constraints of the instructional set they are under. Since exposure times are relatively quick and do not allow for much deliberation, the process of judgment and interpretation is thought to reflect the type of instantaneous appraisal that commonly occurs in social situations. In the Moretti et al. (1993) study, depressed patients, remitted depressives, and controls were presented with a series of stimulus cards, each displaying two pictures of the same target individual (one with a neutral expression and one with a happy or a sad expression) for 300 msec. In the "control condition," subjects were asked to indicate which image (left or right side) featured the more emotional face. Subjects assigned to the "self-referent" condition were instructed to imagine that the faces they were seeing were responses to themselves, and to indicate which side of presentation had the face that was most informative in this regard. Dependent measures in this study reflected not only reaction times but also accuracy of judgment in comparison to the actual emotion expressed in the slide.

Results indicated that both nondepressed controls and remitted depressed subjects identified positive expressions more quickly and more
accurately than negative expressions in the control and self-referent conditions. In contrast, depressed subjects identified positive expressions
more quickly and accurately than negative expressions in the control condition only. In the self-referent condition, depressed subjects were even-
handed in the speed and accuracy with which they identified positive and
negative expressions.

Tasks employing pictorial stimuli are considered to be especially ecolog-
ically valid since the stimuli bear a closer resemblance to the types of
situations subjects tend to find themselves in than do strings of adjectives.
The evaluation of emotional expressions is an important precursor to subsequent social interaction, and any bias on the part of depressed individuals to attribute negative affectivity to the responses of others can be seen
as a potential maintaining factor in reinforcing a depressive interactional
style. Although this paradigm does not examine the continuing aspects of
decoding social interactions, such as the connection to elaborated meanings and consequences for behavior, it does begin to suggest that depressives may be more acutely aware of both positive and negative information
in their social environment, whereas normals and nondepressed or recovered individuals perhaps tend to see less of the negative input coming
their way.

JUDGMENT

The value of trying to understand the vagaries of judgment in emotional
disorders is that judgmental processes such as estimates of probability and
likelihood are often important precipitants of action. Why, for example,
should the anticipation of speaking in public increase the subjective probability of fainting or stuttering? Why should the knowledge that some
aircraft do crash lead to the experience of panic once inside an airport
terminal? One explanation is that when individuals are asked to make
judgments concerning uncertain events, systematic biases in judgments
are often found. It has also been demonstrated that when subjects cannot
directly observe the probability of a particular type of event, they try to
estimate its likelihood by utilizing various heuristics. These heuristics can
often provide efficient short cuts for reasoning, but at the same time have
been shown to reflect certain biases and can lead to serious distortions in
probability estimates (Tversky and Kahneman, 1974). An intriguing question at this point is whether emotional states are associated with systematic
distortions in judgmental processes or an overreliance on intuitive heuristic devices. Perhaps such an overreliance is influenced by specific mood

states, which heighten the salience of reasoning reflective of an earlier developmental stage in favor of the use of logical or statistical decision methods. In fact, one of Beck's (1976) assertions regarding depressive cognition is that, during a depressive episode, patients will demonstrate a type of thinking that is regressive or more primitive in nature compared to their style of thinking when they are not depressed. As a result, the likelihood of logical errors, or what he calls cognitive distortions, is increased.

The nature of judgmental processes in emotional disorders can best be examined by referring to a concrete example. In a study utilizing self-report methodology, Butler and Mathews (1987) administered a subjective probability questionnaire to 57 college undergraduates, some of whom expected to write a university examination within four weeks time and some of whom had no examinations scheduled. Their Subjective Probability Questionnaire was comprised of 48 items, which subjects were asked to rate on a 9-point scale indicating how likely it would be that one of the outcomes described would occur. Half of the items referred to positive and the other half to negative events. Within each set of items, content was divided so that the referent for the event applied to the subject or to the person sitting next to them. Measures of trait anxiety were also taken in order to examine the degree of covariation between levels of anxious mood and estimates of event likelihood. Results indicated that among examination candidates, there was a trend to rate negative events more likely to occur as the examination time approached, and risk estimates tended to decrease after the examination was over. The authors also report that individuals high in trait anxiety tended to predict positive events as less likely to occur, while negative events seemed more likely to happen to them.

How can these findings be understood in terms of what is known about judgmental heuristics? In order to answer this question we first need to consider the nature of the heuristics employed. The "availability" heuristic describes a tendency by people to be influenced in their judgments by the relative availability or accessibility from memory of events related to the judgments they are being asked to make. If a subject is asked to predict the likelihood of a future event, he/she may base his/her estimate on the speed or the ease with which similar events can be recalled. The difficulty here is that factors associated with this ease of recall, other than objective frequency (such as vividness or salience), may contribute to the utilization of the availability heuristic (Kahneman and Tversky, 1972). Another important heuristic is the tendency for people to base their judgments on the extent to which a specific event is seen to be "representative" of a larger group of events. This heuristic can be especially misleading when base rate information is ignored as a consequence of its use. For example, if an individual believes that chest constriction and/or heavy breathing are important signs of an impending cardiac problem, then the appearance of these sensations following a strenuous tennis match may be seen as a warning that the person is at risk for a heart attack, rather than the effects of rigorous exercise.

Returning to the Butler and Mathews (1987) study, we may be curious as to the interaction between anxious mood and subjects' estimates of their increasing risk as exam time approached. Could the mood state of anxiety have made certain types of failure-related information more available and therefore led subjects to be swayed in their judgments by an availability-based deliberation process? Furthermore, following the examination (when risk estimates were shown to drop), the availability of failure information during a mood state of relief or relaxation may not have been as powerful an influence on judgment. It is interesting to note that individuals high in trait anxiety, who presumably did not experience a drop in levels of anxiety following the examination's conclusion, tended to maintain their likelihood estimates.

As Williams *et al.* (1988) point out, estimates of subjective risk are bound to be influenced by factors of availability and mood state. In fact, it appears that attempts to manipulate availability by having subjects imagine different scenarios or explanations for specific outcomes are effective only in cases where individuals do not have any preformed opinions on the issue to be judged. This is rarely the case in emotional disorders, where subjects usually enter situations with fairly set expectations or anticipations. In anxiety disorders, for example, the inflated subjective judgments of risk with respect to danger, harm, or contamination often arise from preformed impressions rather than are the product of judgments freshly formulated through recall of specific examples. The extent to which judgment formation is on-line could be important for understanding why subjects persist in their beliefs in light of more logical or empirical evidence.

Andersen (1990) and Andersen and Lyon (1987) report an intriguing paradigm for the measurement of judgments regarding certainty in depression. Andersen's chief construct is the extent to which patients are certain of undesired outcomes occurring and what effect this certainty has on depressive affect. In order to assess the manner in which individuals anticipate future events, she placed subjects in a situation where they were led to believe that the likelihood of experiencing an aversive event at a later point in time was either 0, 25, 50, 75, or 100%, while holding the controllability of the event constant. Subjects were told that they were to be participating in two tasks, and that success in the first task might influence participation in the second. The first task involved solving a number of anagrams, while the second (aversive) task required subjects to generate silent rebuttals to criticism that would be leveled at them by a male graduate student. The authors reported that only absolute certainty (i.e., the 100% condition) was uniquely associated with depression, and that events with a high likelihood of occurring, but which were not certain to occur, were not predictive of changes in depressive affect. The everyday analogue for the depressive predictive certainty construct might be the type of snap judgments that depressed persons make regarding uncertain future events, and the consequent hopelessness that often follows. These results also speak to the difficulty of simply using likelihood information to counter judgments made on a more absolute or dichotomous basis.

The examination of predictions or expectancies for success made by depressed persons has relied on a number of different methodologies, with the majority of tasks being drawn from the social psychology literature. In one study, Golin *et al.* (1977) asked subjects to provide expectancies for success during a dice game in which dice were either rolled by the subjects or thrown by the experimenter. Certain dice rolls were defined as successful outcomes, thereby allowing for a probability determined on the basis of chance to be calculated. Subjects were asked to make predictions of success for future rolls, and subjective estimates were compared to objective probability estimates. A second methodology is described by Alloy and Abramson (1988), who have employed a strategy where subjects are asked to rate their expectancies of success over a series of trials, following either a prior success or failure experience in chance-determined or ostensibly skill-related tasks. The value of their paradigm is that the chance of success or failure is always 50–50 and the deviation of subjects' expectancies from this criteria can be used as an indicator of potential bias. A typical finding for this body of work is that nondepressed individuals exhibit optimistic biases in their perceptions and judgments about themselves but not in their inferences about others. In the same fashion, subjects who are depressed are sometimes less biased in their self-relevant perceptions and inferences but may at times display optimistic biases or distortions in their judgments about others.

Kuiper and colleagues (Derry and Kuiper, 1981; Macdonald and Kuiper, 1984) have capitalized on the appeal of self-descriptive adjectives to secure ratings or judgments from depressed persons regarding the extent to which these adjectives are relevant to them. Subjects are shown such words as: "purposeful," "decisive," "open," and "fortunate," and are asked to decide if these words describe them or not. The authors then use rating times for yes/no responses to determine the efficiency of processing either positive or negative material in depression. Clinically depressed subjects typically display faster reaction times for self-referent negative material than for self-referent positive material. The assessment of consistency for these types of decisions is also conducted with these data, and depressed individuals tend to be more consistent in endorsing negative adjectives as self-descriptive. Normal subjects tend to judge positive adjectives as more applicable to themselves. While these effects are related to levels of judgment, it is important to keep in mind that this research sometimes runs afoul of certain mood confounds. For example, words such as "defeated," "worthless," or "miserable" may be endorsed simply because of their congruence with the patient's mood rather than because of their congruence with the patient's self-view.

In an example of a paradigm that reflects less effortful information processing, a study by Bargh and Tota (1988) used a memory load procedure to examine the accessibility of negative self-constructs in depression. Subjects were asked to judge a series of self-descriptive adjectives that were either positive or negative in content, and rate the extent to which these adjectives were applicable to themselves or to the average person. The level of automaticity was assessed for each adjective through the use of a memory load, which asked subjects to hold six digits in working memory. In examining response latencies for the memory load manipulation it was found that depressed persons' self-referential judgments of negative adjectives were accompanied by smaller increases in reaction time than those of nondepressed subjects. One interpretation of these findings is that the memory load interfered less with depressives' judgment of negative content, since these judgments were relatively accessible, while it led to greater interference for positive-content judgments. The opposite effect seemed to hold for nondepressed subjects. This task deserves greater scrutiny, since its ability to tap relatively automatic information processes could be used to advantage in order to sidestep some of the more common mood confounds found in this area of research.

Finally, Clark (1988) has studied judgment through the use of a contextual priming paradigm. In their study, panic patients and controls were presented with sentence stems on a video screen ("If I had palpitations I could be _____") followed by a word that represented either a catastrophic ("dying") or a benign ("excited") interpretation. Subjects were asked to read out loud the word that they felt would complete the sentence, as quickly as possible. In this way, judgments concerning anticipated meanings could be derived from a short prime related to the context that was to be judged. Results showed that panic patients, but not normals, had faster reaction times for words that tended to favor catastrophic completion of the sentence stem. This, too, is an intriguing task, because of its inclusion of a priming condition to assess relatively automatic information processing.

ATTENTIONAL BIAS IN EMOTIONAL DISORDERS

Attention is typically described as a "limited capacity system" (Williams *et al.*, 1988), meaning that the ability to attend to and process information has specific limits. Furthermore, it is assumed that the vast array of information in the environment far exceeds the capacity of the attentional system. As a result, only a subset of information in the environment is selected for processing. The ordering or selection of information to be processed seems to follow a functional principle of salience: people rapidly select out or "notice" things that are relevant or important to them in some way. This type of selectivity occurs during everyday activities — if we pull out a handful of coins, we can quickly identify the coin with the particular color and size we are looking for while the other coins seem to fall to the background.

Similarly, salient emotional states may produce selectivity for cues related to information associated with that emotion. The anxious or uneasy camper may attend to the rustling sound of brush, indicating a potential intruder, rather than the sounds of conversation and a crackling campfire. Or yet again, a depressed student may pick up a fleeting critical tone in a teacher's voice and may focus on it to the exclusion of other information being conveyed. One can view attentional selectivity as a useful adaptation under the constraints of a limited capacity system. However, as the preceding two examples suggest, emotions can facilitate attentional processing of features of the environment consistent with the emotion but also produce a loss of information about other aspects of the situation.

Several studies have investigated the influence of emotional state on processing preference. It has been shown that affectively biased attention can facilitate certain kinds of processing activities. For example, anxious individuals more often detect information related to threat concerns compared to normal control subjects (e.g., Mathews and MacLeod, 1985). Alternatively, attentional bias toward emotionally salient information has also been shown to produce disruptions or interference in processing activity when the emotional stimuli are peripheral or irrelevant to the completion of a particular goal or task (e.g., McNally *et al.*, 1990).

In one of the earliest demonstrations of the facilitative effects of processing emotionally salient information, Parkinson and Rachman (1981) showed that mothers awaiting the results of surgery on their children (tonsillectomy) showed greater perceptual sensitivity to words related to surgery compared to mothers who had children of the same age who were not admitted to the hospital. In this study, the women listened to taped music within which a variety of words were embedded; some of the words were related to surgery ("bleeding," "infection") while other words were not ("newspaper," "bird"). The subjects' task was simply to repeat the words as they heard them. The words were played five times and each time the volume of the tape was increased. While the two groups of mothers did not differ on how many neutral words they were able to report, the mothers with children in surgery reported more surgery-related words during the first four presentations of the tape, while on the fifth and loudest presentation this difference disappeared. These results suggest that the "surgery mothers" had greater perceptual sensitivity, or more specifically, lower auditory thresholds for detection of words related to their current concerns. Additionally, neutral words potentially auditorily confusable with the surgery words (e.g., "breeding," "inflection") tended to be identified by the "surgery mothers" at lower volumes than those for the control mothers. The investigators do not report whether mothers reported the confusable words correctly or confused them with the surgery words.

Processing facilitation of emotionally salient information has also been studied using the dichotomous listening task (Treisman and Geffen, 1967). In this task, subjects are simultaneously presented with two different messages, one to each ear though earphones; the subjects are asked to "shadow" or repeat aloud the message they hear in one earphone (the attended channel) and ignore the information being presented through the other earphone (the unattended channel). Typically, subjects are also asked to detect critical words inserted in the passage and press a button or tap indicating when the critical word occurs. Burgess *et al.* (1981) evaluated the ability of social phobics and agoraphobics compared to normal controls to detect target words or phrases representing their feared situations ("failure," "examination," "shopping alone") compared to a neutral target word ("pick"). The subjects were told not to switch attention between the two messages but to signal whenever they heard the target words in either channel. Results indicate that while clinical subjects and controls did not differ on detection of neutral and fear-relevant critical words in the attended passage, clinical subjects recognized significantly more fear-relevant critical words in the unattended passage than controls. This suggests that the clinical subjects had heightened sensitivity in perceiving fear-related information.

This paradigm has been successfully applied to other clinical disorders. For example, bulimics but not normal controls have shown enhanced perception and larger skin conductance responses (SCRs) to the word "fat" relative to the control word "pick." In a similarly designed study, individuals with Obsessive–Compulsive Disorder (OCD) have been found to show enhanced perception and larger SCRs to words such as "urine" relative to normal controls (Foa and McNally, 1986). Notably, this perceptual and physiological sensitivity was no longer evident following successful behavioral treatment, indicating that familiarity with these concepts was not a significant contributor to the enhancement effects.

At least one study has found increased vigilance to even neutral stimuli when an individual is made anxious. Shapiro and Lim (1989) used an induction procedure to elicit an anxious state in college students. Subjects were then asked to press a button as soon as they saw a neutral stimulus appear on a computer screen. While noninduced (nonanxious) subjects attended primarily to central visual stimuli, anxious subjects showed attention to peripheral as well as central stimuli. The authors suggest that this expansion in the deployment of attentional resources may be an adaptive response that an anxious state triggers, the purpose of which is to increase the probability of locating and responding to a potential threat in the environment.

Heightened sensitivity to concern-related or emotionally laden words can act to debilitate performance, however. Several studies that have used the Stroop paradigm have shown that individuals experiencing emotional distress are more likely to be distracted from tasks by emotionally salient but task-irrelevant information. In the usual form of the task (Stroop, 1935), subjects are asked to name the ink color in which a series of letters is printed. Color naming has consistently been found to be slowed when the letters make up words that are colors antagonistic to the color of the ink than when the letters are merely a string of XXXX's. The slowed response to the color word is believed to reflect a drain on processing resources, where the subject is attending not only to the color of the ink but to the meaning of the word as well. The suggestion that subjects are attending to the meaning of the word is supported by a study that showed that priming the word meaning by requiring subjects to learn another word semantically related to the target also increases interference in color naming (Warren, 1972). Stroop tasks have been used to evaluate the reactivity of both anxious and depressed individuals to words related to their specific concerns. Gotlib and McCann (1984) presented depressive words to mildly depressed and nondepressed undergraduates (as determined by Beck Depression Inventory (BDI) scores). The depressed students showed longer latencies to the depressed words than to neutral or manic words, while the nondepressed students showed no significant differences in their responses.

Segal et al. (1988) adapted the Stroop in such a way to test whether depressed individuals organized negative traits in clusters (i.e., a negative "self-schema"). Typically, the Stroop provides a measure of reactivity to single words that might represent symptoms or major concerns. Segal et al. (1988) adapted the Stroop task to test the salience of the relation between pairs of words that were known to be self-descriptive. In this paradigm, subjects were shown a word in black and white lettering, which they were asked to name before they were presented with a Stroop task word. On certain trials both black and white words and the Stroop task words referred to traits that had earlier been identified by the subjects as negatively self-descriptive. Results showed that longer response latencies were obtained for the self-descriptor when it was preceded by a related self-descriptor than when preceded by a neutral word.

Such priming effects suggest that there is an interrelationship or structural organization among self-referent words or, at least among depressives, negative self-referent information about the self might cluster together. The presence of highly interrelated and easily primed negative information among depressives might give one explanation for the maintenance of chronic negative self-evaluation. These findings were replicated in Segal and Vella (1990).

In studies of generally anxious outpatients, Mathews and MacLeod (1985) and Mogg et al. (1989) obtained color-naming responses of words related to physical or social threat. The anxious patients showed slower response times for the threat words compared to nonthreat words, while control subjects showed no difference in response latency. Furthermore, the patients showed greater disruption to words related to their predominant fear: patients with social concerns showed interference on the social threat words while only patients with somatic concerns showed interference on the physical threat words. Hope et al. (1990) recently evaluated the specificity of anxiety-related concerns according to disorder by comparing the performance of individuals with panic disorder and social phobics on a Stroop task with both social threat and physical threat words. Disorder-specific biases were found: social phobics had longer latencies for social threat words, but not for physical threat words, while panickers showed the reverse effect.

Overall, the Stroop task has been used to identify the salient concerns associated with a wide variety of emotional disorders. These include: suicidal patients (Williams and Broadbent, 1986); panic disorder patients (Ehlers et al., 1988; McNally et al., 1990; Baptista and Figueira, 1989); individuals with posttraumatic stress disorder (Cassiday et al., 1992; Foa et al., 1991; McNally et al., 1990); and individuals with eating disorders (Channon et al., 1988).

The above studies suggest that attentional and perceptual processes are enhanced for information that is congruent with an individual's emotional state. However, another group of studies has shown that among anxious individuals, direct responses to threat stimuli can be inhibited or slowed down (i.e., Shiomi, 1977;). Cloitre et al. (1992a) assessed reaction time to disorder-related threat information compared to positive and neutral information among panic disorder subjects and matched controls (Study 1) and among social phobic subjects and their matched controls (Study 2). A consistent finding across both studies was that, compared to normal control groups, both panic and social phobic groups showed slowed reaction times to threat words in two separate tasks (lexical decision and category decision). These findings run directly counter to the mood congruence effects obtained in the above studies. This apparent contradiction can be resolved by inspection of the dependent measures used across the various studies. Facilitative effects are obtained only in tasks that use yes/no responses and measure anxious subjects' tendencies to identify relatively greater numbers of threat cues or to identify them at lower levels of perceptual intensity. Speed of response, in contrast, seems to be slowed for threat information, suggesting that while anxiety may enhance awareness of threat, responsiveness to it may be inhibited. This conclusion is consistent with ethological theories that suggest that an inhibition or "braking" of psychomotor activity tends to be the first response to short-term, immediate threat (see Gilbert, 1989). These findings also suggest that the slowed reaction time in interference tasks such as the Stroop may be attributable not only to attentional processes such as distraction but to response processes (motor inhibition) as well.

In summary, the findings described above consistently indicate that there is an attentional bias *toward* emotionally salient words. There is, however, a research tradition that is concerned with the conditions under which individuals seem to *avoid* emotionally salient or, more specifically, potentially threatening information. Initial research with this focus characterized the avoidance of threatening information as the phenomenon of "perceptual defense." In the experimental paradigm associated with this phenomenon, threatening and nonthreatening stimuli are presented from relatively short to progressively longer times until the subject can identify the word. Perceptual defense is exhibited when the recognition threshold for the threatening stimuli is higher than that for neutral or nonthreatening stimuli (see Eysenck *et al.*, 1987). An early study of this phenomenon by McGinnies (1949) showed that when college students were presented with taboo words (e.g., Kotex, penis) and neutral words (e.g., house, apple), recognition thresholds were higher for the taboo words than for the neutral words.

Several criticisms have been made concerning the interpretation of this type of effect (Erdelyi, 1974; Dixon, 1981). In particular, it has been argued that subjects may recognize the taboo and nontaboo words equally well but may delay in reporting what they have seen, perhaps because they are embarrassed to do so. The problem of a "response bias" has recently been addressed in a study by MacLeod *et al.* (1986), which uses an experimental technique that controls for such an effect. In this study, subjects are asked to detect the presence of a dot probe in one of two positions on a computer monitor. On some trials, the dot is preceded by either a threatening or nonthreatening word. By examining the impact of these words on detection latencies, it was possible to evaluate whether attention had focused toward or away from the stimuli. Because the target stimuli (dot probe) was neutral and the subject's response (button press at detection of dot) was neutral, the problem of a response bias was believed to be eliminated. Results indicate that clinically anxious subjects consistently shifted their attention toward threat words. Of equal interest, however, was the finding that normal subjects tended to shift their attention *away* from the threatening material.

In another study by MacLeod and Mathews (1988), which uses the same technique, students with high trait anxiety were found to focus their attention toward exam-related words, while students with low trait anxiety did not. Twelve weeks later, when both groups showed increasing state anxiety immediately preceding a test, high-trait subjects showed increasing attentional bias to exam words, while low-trait anxious subjects showed increasing attentional avoidance. These studies suggest that attentional bias either toward or away from emotionally salient information may be the result of an interaction between trait and mood state characteristics (see Broadbent and Broadbent, 1988). Other personality variables (see Byrne, 1961) as well as situational context (see MacLeod and Mathews, 1988) and the emotional intensity of the stimulus (Watts *et al.*, 1986b) may also ultimately be shown to determine the occurrence of attentional avoidance.

In summary, the occurrence of attentional bias in both anxiety and depressive disorders has been well documented. Nevertheless, the nature of the cognitive processes or mechanisms associated with attentional bias and avoidance has yet to be characterized. While the general phenomenon of attentional bias spans a wide range of emotional disorders, it may be that the mechanisms, functions, and consequences of these biases differ depending on the type of disorder. Some of these issues receive further discussion at later points in the chapter.

MEMORY BIAS IN EMOTIONAL DISORDERS

Our memories provide us with a relatively stable and enduring record of the totality of our experiences. They are the source of our sense of self as consisting of a unique set of personal characteristics projected through time. Memory also allows us to keep in mind information relevant to our goals and plans, thereby contributing to our motivation level for action. Finally, memory serves as a reference point for our expectations about the behavior of others. Given this tremendous influence, it is no surprise that there have been many and diverse studies evaluating the relationship between emotional state and memory processes. Negative emotion seems to elicit negative memory, and conversely, the consolidation of negative memories seems to maintain or enhance negative affect. More recent studies have suggested that emotion influences memories not only within our conscious awareness but also those memories for which we have no explicit recall.

Some of the earliest studies documenting memory bias in affective disorders concerned the biased recall among clinically depressed patients for unpleasant personal memories. Lloyd and Lishman (1975) found that when clinically depressed patients were asked to think of either a pleasant or an unpleasant memory in response to a neutral cue, they found that the more severe the depression, the faster the patient was at recalling unpleasant memories.

The possibility that the more depressed patients had simply had more unpleasant events occur to them was tested in two studies. Clark and Teasdale (1982) used a task similar to that of Lloyd and Lishman (1975) but with patients who experienced diurnal variation in their depression. It was found that when patients were more depressed, they tended to remember less pleasant memories and conversely, when the patients' depressed moods abated, they tended to remember fewer unpleasant memories. Since the same subjects were recalling the events, the change in recall bias must have been related to their change in depressive status. Teasdale and Fogarty (1979) randomly assigned nonclinical subjects to conditions in which they were induced into either an "elated" or "depressed" state. Since subjects were randomized into the two mood conditions, it was assumed that the amount of actual depressive events experienced by the subjects was equal. Results showed that subjects tended to recall events with an affective quality congruent with their mood state. Research on memory bias among clinical populations was initially influenced by Beck's suggestion that depressed subjects' negative perceptions and attitudes derive from a negatively organized self-schema. The self-schema is a cognitive construct that has been variously defined (see Segal, 1988) but that generally refers to an organized and enduring construct that includes general information about the self, such as traits and particular behavioral episodes, all of which are derived from a lifetime of experience.

One experimental method frequently used to explore the notion of the self-schema was the levels of processing paradigm (Craik and Lockhart, 1972; Craik and Tulving, 1975). Studies employing this methodology enable subjects to process information in a certain way by asking them to answer questions about words according to a special dimension or word characteristic. For example, the subject might be asked to rate the word on its phonemic characteristics ("Does this word rhyme with X?"), its graphic characteristics ("Is this word in capital letters?"), or its semantic (meaning) characteristics ("Does this word refer to a feeling?"). Researchers interested in the notion of self-schema added a new dimension of processing, designated a "self-referent" processing level ("Does this word describe you?").

Studies employing this methodology typically found that information processed on a self-referent level was recalled more frequently than was information given other types of analysis (Rogers *et al.*, 1977; Derry and Kuiper, 1981; Ingram *et al.*, 1983; Clifford and Hemsley, 1987; Sutton *et al.*, 1988). This recall pattern was assumed to be the result of the depth or elaboration of processing required. It was assumed that the analysis of information proceeds from lesser to greater elaboration or complexity (e.g., from phonemic to semantic analysis) and that greater elaboration is associated with better recall. The superiority of recall for self-referent information compared to other types of analysis was understood to indicate the "deeper" and perhaps unique nature of self-concept analysis.

There is some question, however, about the validity of using the levels of processing model to provide evidence for a level of analysis that is specific to the self. The levels of processing model attempts to describe the various qualitatively distinct dimensions by which verbal stimuli may be analyzed (perceptual, structural, semantic, etc.). The introduction of the self-schema does not seem qualitatively different from the semantic or meaningful analysis of information. Rather, assessments about the self would seem to be an aspect of highly elaborative activity at the semantic level of analysis. Indeed, a recent study by Klein and Kihlstrom (1986) showed that self-reference is no more effective in producing high recall rates than other forms of semantic encoding when controlling for the way in which the processing question is phrased. From a theoretical perspective it might be suggested that while stimuli may be analyzed along qualitatively different characteristics, the processing of information about self may best be conceptualized as an instance of semantic processing.

In any case, the comparison of self-referentially processed material to phonemically or graphemically processed material has been omitted in many studies, and the focus has more appropriately been on comparisons of self-referentially processed words ("Does this word describe you?") to other types of meaningful analyses ("Does this word fit into the following sentence?"). Some studies evaluated the processing and recall of information about the self compared to familiar others (Bradley and Mathews, 1983; Bower and Gilligan, 1979; Kuiper and Rogers, 1979), while others compared recall for positive versus negative words in relation to self (Teasdale and

Dent, 1987; Dobson and Shaw, 1987; Mathews and Bradley, 1983; Ingram and Reed, 1986). Most of these studies gave evidence for the superior recall of self-related information and for greater recall of negative versus positive attributes among depressed individuals compared to nondepressed controls.

In contrast to the large number of studies on memory bias in depression, there are only a handful of studies investigating such bias in anxious and anxiety disordered populations. Some of the studies have investigated potential self-referent recall bias for words related to threats to physical or psychological well-being (e.g., "heart attack," "humiliated") or those that refer to anxious feeling states ("nervous," "trembling," "panicky"). O'Banion and Arkowitz (1977), for example, found that students with high social anxiety showed better recognition memory for negative trait words compared to students with low social anxiety. McNally *et al.* (1989) found that individuals with panic disorder showed a memory bias for self-descriptive anxiety words ("nervous," "uptight") and that this bias was somewhat enhanced when subjects had encoded words during a time of physiological arousal (induced by a step exercise). Cloitre and Liebowitz (1991) showed that, even without a self-reference type of question, that is, asking a question that induces meaningful processing ("Is this word a feeling?"), panic disordered patients had better memory for threat-related feeling words ("dizzy," "nervous") and threat-related objects or events ("ambulance," "death") compared to nonclinical controls. Zeitlin and McNally (1991) found that Vietnam veterans with Post-Traumatic Stress Disorder (PTSD) showed memory bias for combat words (i.e., "medevac," "bodybags") relative to veterans without PTSD.

Others still have found no memory bias for threat information among anxious populations (Mathews *et al.*, 1989a; Mogg *et al.*, 1989) or even an indication of a reverse effect in which there is poorer memory for threat-related information among anxious subjects (Mogg *et al.*, 1987; Watts *et al.*, 1986b). It has been suggested (Williams *et al.*, 1988) that the failure to observe memory bias in anxious subjects may be the result of a "cognitive avoidance strategy," that is, efforts on the part of anxious subjects to avoid or minimize processing of threatening information. The purpose of such avoidance might be to reduce the experience of anxious affect and the further disruption of attention to other stimuli in the environment.

The anxiety-related attentional bias toward threat stimuli observed in many of the attention tasks (dichotic listening; Stroop) may be attributable to a bias that occurs in the early stages of processing, which is primarily concerned with the detection and identification of the stimulus. This leaves open the question of whether there is continued attention bias toward threat information with more elaborated analysis or whether subjects avoid or minimize engaging in further detailed and elaborated processing. Williams *et al.* (1988) have suggested that different types of memory tasks can identify the extent and direction of attentional bias for these different stages or aspects of processing.

Performance on tasks such as free recall, cued recall, or recognition has been shown to be determined by the extent to which there has been detailed and meaningful analysis of the stimulus (Graf and Mandler, 1984; Roediger *et al.*, 1989). Depending on the exact nature of the task, these tasks are known as tests of explicit or what has sometimes been called declarative knowledge. Other tasks are believed to tap what is sometimes called implicit memory or procedural memory. These tasks typically seem to rely on a perceptual or motor memory experience; such tasks reflect implicit memory if the subject is not explicitly aware that he/she is relying on information to which he/she has recently been exposed.

An example of such a task is the word completion task. Here, a subject is presented with a word stem (e.g., oni__) and asked to write the word that first comes to mind. Typically, subjects recently exposed to the word "onion" will be more likely to complete the stem to make the word "onion," rather than suggest other possibilities. In the word fragment task, the subject is presented with a full word with letters missing (e.g., c_a_p_g_e) and asked to fill in the blanks (e.g., champagne). Here again, the subject's capacity to solve the problem is facilitated by previous exposure to a word that fits the solution. These types of tasks differ most markedly from the explicit memory tasks in that mere previous exposure to a word that fits the solution produces a facilitative effect; the degree of elaboration that occurred during the initial exposure has no impact on consequent memory performance. This contrasts with the recall tasks where better memory performance is associated with greater elaboration during initial exposure to the stimulus.

Mathews *et al.* (1989a) conducted a study in which generally anxious patients were given a self-referent encoding task for threatening, neutral, and positive words. Subjects were then given cued recall and word completion memory tasks. Results showed that anxious and control subjects did not differ on the recall of threat words but that anxious patients produced more threat word completions. These results suggest that anxious patients may give disproportionate attention to threat stimuli at some phase of processing but that they may avoid elaborating on threatening material, as is suggested by the poorer than expected recall for these items. Nevertheless, in a similar study, Cloitre and Liebowitz (1989) found that panic disordered subjects showed both a recall and a perceptual memory bias for threat words compared to nonclinical controls. Similarly, Zeitlin and McNally (1991) found that combat veterans with PTSD exhibited both an implicit and an explicit memory bias for combat words compared to combat veterans without PTSD. The differences may be attributable to differences in processing task instructions or to the type or severity of the anxiety disorders. Panic Disorder and Post-Traumatic Stress Disorder are believed to be more severe disorders than Generalized Anxiety Disorder (GAD), as evidenced by symptom intensity and impairment in social and occupational functioning (Zeitlin and McNally, 1991). Overall, the data provide some evidence for the operation of a "cognitive avoidance" strategy among some anxious subjects under some conditions. Further research is required to determine the factors under which this effect is produced.

COMORBIDITY OF DEPRESSION AND ANXIETY

This chapter has described experimental approaches to the assessment of depression and anxiety rather than that of other types of disorders such as schizophrenia or personality disorders. The focus on mood disorders stems from the fact that during the 1980s cognitive science was primarily concerned with and relatively successful in expanding its principles and testing procedures to incorporate explanations about the mutual influences that emotion and cognition exert on one another (Bower 1981; Williams *et al.*, 1988).

One benefit of this emphasis is the presence of a new methodology that can be applied to the difficult task of identifying similarities and differences in the features of depression and anxiety. Although there has been some progress in the use of self-report or clinician-based measures (Watson and Kendall, 1989a; Beck *et al.*, 1987; Riskind *et al.*, 1987), most symptom measures of anxiety and depression are highly correlated and have poor discriminant validity (Watson and Kendall, 1989b).

Beck and his colleagues (Beck, 1976; Beck and Emery, 1985) made the clinical observation that the thought content of depressed and anxious individuals appeared to be rather distinctive, an idea that became known as the content specificity hypothesis. As a caveat, there are a few general cognitive characteristics that are shared by depressed and anxious individuals, such as self-criticism, negative self-evaluation, and low self-efficacy (Beck and Emery, 1985; Carver and Sheier, 1982; Sarason, 1985; Watson and Kendall, 1989b). However, several information processing studies have indicated that there are numerous ways in which anxiety and depression are differentiated along the cognitive dimension. Depressed individuals tend to have impaired memory functioning (Johnson, Petzel *et al.*, 1983; Cohen *et al.*, 1982), give overestimates of negative event frequencies (Kuiper and MacDonald, 1983), and show biased processing of negative-depressive information (i.e., Derry and Kuiper, 1981). In contrast, anxious individuals do not show any evidence of impaired recall relative to normal controls (i.e., Cloitre and Leibowitz, 1991), give overestimates of the presence of a potential threat (i.e., McNally and Foa, 1987), and show biased processing for threat-related information (Mathews and MacLeod, 1987).

Ingram *et al*. (1987) directly compared the processing activities of anxious and depressed individuals when presented with negative information that had either depressive or threatening content. A self-referent depth of processing task was used to assess memory for depressive, anxious, or neutral words among high-test-anxious, high-depressed, high-depressed and anxious subjects, and a control group of low-anxious–low-depressed subjects. Results indicated a mood-congruent effect where depressed subjects recalled more depressive information, anxious subjects recalled more anxious information, and subjects with both anxiety and depression showed biased recall of both types of information although at a lower level than that of the other two groups. Another interesting aspect of this study was the pattern of results obtained from a variety of self-report measures. Anxious subjects reported more task-irrelevant cognitions, while depressed subjects reported more negative self-relevant assessment. The anxious and depressed subjects, however, scored higher on both types of cognitions than either of these two groups, indicating that a combined state of anxiety and depression may produce greater impairment than either state alone.

Similar results have been obtained in studies of clinically anxious and clinically depressed subjects. As noted earlier, MacLeod *et al*. (1986) found that, compared to normal controls, individuals with generalized anxiety disorder tended to allocate greater attentional resources to threatening than to neutral words. Because the anxiety patients also had relatively high levels of depression, a group of clinically depressed subjects were presented with the same task to determine whether such effects were mediated by depression. No differences in attentional allocation were found in the depressed group, suggesting that the hypervigilance for potential threat was directly associated with anxiety.

In a recent study by Cloitre *et al*. (1992b) cued recall for threat, positive, and neutral words was assessed among individuals with panic disorder, major depression, and panic disorder with major depression. The panic disorder group showed a memory bias for threat information; the depressed group did not show such bias but did perform poorly on all word groups when compared to the panic disorder group. The combined group performed as poorly as the depressed group on positive and neutral words but recall for threat information was equal to that of the pure panic group. These results suggest that comorbidity of anxiety and depression is associated with multiple cognitive dysfunctions. This group may have greater difficulty in responding to short-term cognitive therapy, since threat information predominates their thought processes and there appears to be reduced capacity to recruit or sustain nonanxiety information that might be useful in the formulation of alternative assessments of their identified problems. The multiplicity of cognitive dysfunctions found in the group with a comorbid diagnosis is parallel to that found by Ingram *et al.* (1987) in their combined group of nonclinical depressed and anxious subjects. These data suggest that specific types of cognitive dysfunctions maintain their association with particular affective states whether the affect occurs alone or in combination with another affect, and that the cooccurrence of different types of cognitive dysfunctions happens in depressed-anxious states of greater and lesser severity.

FUTURE DIRECTIONS AND CONCLUSIONS

The studies reviewed in this paper indicate that emotions bias attention, judgment, evaluation, and recall of events. The studies use relatively simple tasks (i.e., yes/no decisions) and thus may have limited applicability to everyday life in which individuals are often involved in complex problem-solving and decision-making activities. However, because these simple tasks reflect core or fundamental cognitive functions, we may conclude that emotions are intimately involved with cognition at a relatively basic level. Future research may focus on more complex activities such as problem solving, which incorporates attentional, memorial, and judgment processes.

A second concern with current clinical research is that most results are readily explainable within the context of alternative theories or conceptualizations of cognitive processes. The notion of a self-schema, for example, has been broadly constructed by Beck and colleagues (see Beck and Emery, 1985) to explain certain clinical observations. From a cognitive theory perspective, self-schemas have been specified as either a level or type of information when viewed within a depth of processing model; self-schemas have alternatively been thought of as elaborated clusters of nodes in a representational network system. The data showing better recall for self-related information does not distinguish between the two models. As the results from self-schema research indicate, clinical research has supported the cognitive principle that the mental representation of events and their associated affect guides perceptions, attitudes, and actions. A natural next step is to attend to the specific processing and representational characteristics proposed by competing models of mental representation. Certain of these models are more likely than others to facilitate empirical investigation of relatively complex clinical phenomena. For example, a levels of processing or modular systems account of mental representation is more amenable to explaining dissociation or multiple personality disorders than is a network model. Identification and testing of particular cognitive principles in clinical research will also contribute to progress in cognitive science proper since the successful application of a particular cognitive theory to pathological as well as normal functioning strengthens the power of that theory as a general model of cognitive functioning.

The collaboration between clinical and cognitive psychology is just beginning to bear fruit. There has been some concern about the usefulness of the experimental approach in clinical psychology because the character of laboratory tasks often bears little resemblance to the behavior observed in the clinic or in the natural environment. We suggest that it is precisely the presence of this disparity that makes the collaboration between clinical and cognitive psychology productive.

Banaji and Crowder (1989) have suggested that it is only through experimental investigation that general principles of behavior can be established. The authors argue that in contrast with experimental studies, "the multiplicity of uncontrolled factors in naturalistic contexts actually prohibit generalizability to other situations with different parameters" (p. 1189). This analysis seems to suggest that laboratory studies would be of no value if they resembled everyday activities. Indeed laboratory studies do not intend to mimic the phenomenology of real life but rather, by a dismantling process, seek to identify the underlying principles that determine the rich observations of everyday life.

For example, a client often comes for treatment at a time of emotional crisis. Under these circumstances, the relative contributions of current mood state and more enduring personality traits to the presenting problem cannot be easily disentangled. Nevertheless, such information can facilitate the selection of the most efficacious treatment. Laboratory studies have begun to separate out the relative contributions of mood and personality factors by assessing memory for different kinds of information, some of which are more influenced by mood state (i.e., priming tasks), others of which are more influenced by personality (i.e., direct recall of schematic information). Ideally, this type of information, either through direct use of the tasks or, eventually, by identification of the clinical markers associated with task performance, can contribute to an informed treatment disposition.

Ultimately, the information generated from the laboratory tasks will be tested in the real world. The extent to which findings from these tasks can clarify our day-to-day observations and facilitate the discovery of solutions to practical problems will determine their worth and longevity in the research world. If doubt falls on the usefulness or accuracy of a laboratory generalization, the principle may require reevaluation. Clinical observation identifies intriguing phenomena, experimentation generates tests of specific and competing explanations, and a return to the clinical setting provides the ultimate test of the identified principle. The scientist–practitioner model of training provides a context in which this cycle of activity can be effectively completed. The scientist–practitioner or a community of scientists and practitioners thus represents a locus for potential progress in understanding of the various dimensions of psychopathology and its treatment. Awareness of the mutual interdependence between research and clinical reality should foster appreciation for the training of scientist–practitioners and facilitate dialogue between those who view themselves as primarily clinicians or primarily researchers. We hope such dialogue will clarify the fact that clinicians and researchers share the same long-term goals, which are, among others, the understanding of psychopathology and the effective treatment of emotional disorders.

ACKNOWLEDGMENT

Preparation of this chapter was supported in part by a grant awarded to the first author from the John D. and Catherine T. MacArthur Foundation, Program on Conscious and Unconscious Mental Processes.

REFERENCES

Alloy, L. B., and Abramson, L. Y. (1988). Depressive realism: Four theoretical perspectives. In L. B. Alloy (Ed.), *Cognitive processes in depression*. New York: Guilford Press.

Andersen, S. M. (1990). The inevitability of future suffering: The role of depressive predictive certainty in depression. *Social Cognition, 8*, 203–228.

Andersen, S. M., and Lyon, J. E. (1987). Anticipating undesired outcomes: The role of outcome certainty in the onset of depressive affect. *Journal of Experimental Social Psychology, 23*, 428–443.

Anderson, J. R. (1985). *Cognitive psychology and its implications* (2nd ed.). New York: Freeman.

Banaji, M. R., and Crowder, R. G. (1989). The bankruptcy of everyday memory. *American Psychologist, 44*, 1185–1193.

Baptista, A., and Figueira, M. L. (1989). *Information processing in patients with panic disorder*. Paper Presented at the World Congress of Cognitive Therapy, Oxford, England.

Bargh, J. A., and Tota, M. E. (1988). Context-dependent automatic processing in depression: Accessibility of negative constructs with regard to self but not others. *Journal of Personality and Social Psychology, 54*, 925–939.

Beck, A. T. (1976). *Cognitive therapy and the emotional disorders*. New York: International Universities Press.

Beck, A. T., and Emery, G. (1985). *Anxiety disorders and phobias: A cognitive perspective*. New York: Basic Books.

Beck, A. T., Brown, G., Steer, R. A., Eidelson, J. I., and Riskind, J. H. (1987). Differentiating anxiety and depression: A test of the cognitive specificity hypothesis. *Journal of Abnormal Psychology, 96*, 179–183.

Bower, G. H. (1981). Mood and memory. *American Psychologist, 36*, 129–148.

Bower, G. H., and Clapper, J. P. (1989). Experimental methods in cognitive science. In M. L. Posner (Ed.), *Foundations of cognitive science.* Cambridge, MA: MIT Press.

Bower, G. H., and Gilligan, S. G. (1979). Remembering information related to one's self. *Journal of Research in Personality, 13*, 420–432.

Bradley, B., and Mathews, A. (1983). Negative self-schemata in clinical depression. *British Journal of Clinical Psychology, 22*, 39–42.

Broadbent, D., and Broadbent, M. (1988). Anxiety and attention bias: State and trait. *Cognition and Emotion, 2*, 165–183.

Burgess, I. S., Jones, L. N., Robertson, S. A., Radcliffe, W. N., and Emerson, E., (1981). The degree of control exerted by phobic and non-phobic verbal stimuli over the recognition behaviour of phobic and non-phobic subjects. *Behaviour Research and Therapy, 19*, 223–234.

Butler, G., and Mathews, A. (1983). Cognitive processes in anxiety. *Advances in Behaviour Research and Therapy, 5*, 51–62.

Butler, G., and Mathews, A. (1987). Anticipatory anxiety and risk perception. *Cognitive Therapy and Research, 11*(5), 551–565.

Byrne, D. (1961). The repression–sensitization skill: Rationale, reliability, and validity. *Journal of Personality, 29*, 334–349.

Carlson, R., and Levy, N. (1973). Studies of Jungian typology: I. Memory, social perception, and social action. *Journal of Personality, 41*, 559–576.

Carver, C. S., and Sheier, M. F. (1982). Control theory: A useful conceptual framework for personality-social, clinical and health psychology. *Psychology Bulletin, 92*, 111–132.

Cassiday, K. L., McNally, R. J., & Zeitlin, S. B. (1992) Cognitive processing of trauma cues in rape victims with post-traumatic stress disorder. *Cognitive Therapy and Research, 16*, 283–295.

Channon, S., Hemsley, D., and DeSilva, P. (1988). Selective processing of food words in anorexia nervosa. *British Journal of Clinical Psychology, 27*, 656–661.

Clark, D. M. (1988). A cognitive model of panic attacks. In S. Rachman and J. D. Maser (Eds.), *Panic: Psychological perspectives.* Hillsdale, NJ: Erlbaum.

Clark, D. M., and Teasdale, J. D. (1982). Diurnal variations in clinical depression and accessibility of memories of positive and negative experiences. *Journal of Abnormal Psychology, 91*, 87–95.

Clifford, P. I., and Hemsley, D. R. (1987). The influence of depression on the processing of personal attributes. *British Journal of Psychiatry, 150*, 98–103.

Cloitre, M. R., & Leibowitz, M. (1989 July) *Processing bias in panic disorder: Semantic inhibition or elaboration?* Paper presented at the World Congress of Cognitive Therapy, Oxford, England.

Cloitre, M., and Liebowitz, M. (1991). Memory bias in panic disorder: An investigation of the cognitive avoidance hypothesis. *Cognitive Therapy and Research, 15*, 371–386.

Cloitre, M., Heimberg, R., Holt, C. S., and Liebowitz, M. R. (1992a). Reaction time to threat stimuli in panic disorder and social phobia. *Behaviour Research and Therapy, 30*, 609–617.

Cloitre, M., Shear, K. M., and Kocsis, J. (1992b). *Cued recall for threat information in individuals with Panic Disorder, Major Depression and Panic Disorder with Major Depression.* Unpublished manuscript.

Cohen, R. M., Weingartner, H., Smallberg, S. A., Pickar, D., and Murphy, D. L. (1982). Effort and cognition in depression. *Archives of General Psychiatry, 39*, 593–597.

Craik, F. I. M., and Lockhart, R. S. (1972). Levels of processing: A framework for memory research. *Journal of Verbal Learning and Verbal Behavior, 11,* 671–684.

Craik, F. I. M., and Tulving, E. (1975). Depth of processing and the retention of words in episodic memory. *Journal of Experimental Psychology: General, 104,* 268–294.

Derry, P. A., and Kuiper, N. A. (1981). Schematic processing and self-reference in clinical depression. *Journal of Abnormal Psychology, 90,* 286–297.

Dixon, N. (1981). *Preconscious processing.* Chichester, England: Wiley.

Dobson, K. S., and Shaw, B. F. (1987). Specificity and stability of self-referent encoding in clinical depression. *Journal of Abnormal Psychology, 96,* 34–40.

Ehlers, A., Margraf, J., Davies, S., and Roth, W. T. (1988). Selective processing of threat cues in subjects with panic attacks. *Cognition and Emotion, 2,* 201–219.

Erdelyi, M. H. (1974). A new look at the new look: Perceptual defense and vigilance. *Psychological Review, 81*(1), 1–25.

Eysenck, M. W., MacLeod, C., and Mathews, A. (1987). Cognitive functioning in anxiety. *Psychological Research, 49,* 189–195.

Foa, E. B., and McNally, R. J. (1986). Sensitivity to feared stimuli in obsessive–compulsives: A dichotic listening analysis. *Cognitive Therapy and Research, 10,* 477–486.

Foa, E. B., Feske, U., Murdock, T. B., Kozak, M. J., and McCarthy, P. R. (1991). Processing of threat related information in rape victims. *Journal of Abnormal Psychology, 100,* 156–162.

Gilbert, P. (1989). *Human nature and suffering.* London: Erlbaum.

Gilson, M. (1983). *Depression as measured by perceptual bias in binocular rivalry.* Unpublished doctoral dissertation, Georgia State University, Atlanta, Georgia.

Golin, S., Terrell, T., and Johnson, B. (1977). Depression and the illusion of control. *Journal of Abnormal Psychology, 86,* 440–442.

Gotlib, I. H., and McCann, C. D. (1984). Construct accessibility and depression: An examination of cognitive and affective factors. *Journal of Personality and Social Psychology, 47,* 427–439.

Graf, P., and Mandler, G. (1984). Activation makes words more accessible, but not necessarily more retrievable. *Journal of Verbal Leaning and Verbal Behavior, 23,* 553–568.

Hammen, C., Marks, T., Mayol, A., and de Mayo, R. (1985). Depressive self-schemas, life stress and vulnerability to depression. *Journal of Abnormal Psychology, 94,* 308–319.

Hammen, C., Dyck, D. G., and Miklowitz, D. J. (1986). Stability and severity parameters of depressive self-schema responding. *Journal of Social and Clinical Psychology, 4,* 23–45.

Hope, D. A., Rapee, R. M., Heimberg, R. G., and Dombeck, M. (1990). Representations of the self in social phobia: Vulnerability to social threat. *Cognitive Therapy and Research, 14,* 177–190.

Ingram, R. E., and Kendall, P. C. (1986). Cognitive clinical psychology: Implications of an information processing perspective. In R. E. Ingram (Ed.), *Information processing approaches to clinical psychology* (pp. 3–21). Orlando, FL: Academic Press.

Ingram, R., and Reed, M. (1986). Information encoding and retrieval processes in depression: Findings, issues and future directions. In R. E. Ingram (Ed.), (pp. 131–150). *Information processing approaches to clinical psychology.* Orlando, FL: Academic Press.

Ingram, R. E., Smith, T. W., and Brehm, S. S. (1983). Depression and information processing: Self-schemata and the encoding of self-referent information. *Journal of Personality and Social Psychology, 45,* 412–420.

Ingram, R. E., Kendall, P. C., Smith, T. W., Donnell, C., and Ronan, K. (1987). Cognitive specificity in emotional distress. *Journal of Personality and Social Psychology, 53,* 734–742.

Johnson, J. E., Petzel, T. P., Harney, L. M., and Morgan, R. A. (1983). Recall of importance ratings of completed and uncompleted tasks as a function of depression. *Cognitive Therapy and Research, 7,* 51–56.

Jung, C. G. (1910). The association method. *American Journal of Psychology, 21,* 219–269.

Kahneman, D., and Tversky, A. (1972). Subjective probability: A judgement of representiveness. *Cognitive Psychology, 3,* 430–454.

Kendall, P. C., and Hollon, S. D. (1981). *Assessment strategies for cognitive–behavioral interventions.* New York: Academic Press.

Klein, F. B., and Kihlstrom, J. F. (1986). Elaboration, organisation and the self-reference effect in memory. *Journal of Experimental Psychology: General, 115,* 26–38.

Kuiper, N. A., and MacDonald, M. R. (1983) Schematic processing in depression: The self-based consensus bias. *Cognitive Therapy and Research, 7,* 469–484.

Kuiper, N. A., and Rogers, T. B. (1979). Encoding of personal information: Self–other differences. *Journal of Personality and Social Psychology, 37,* 499–514.

Lloyd, G. G., and Lishman, W. A. (1975). Effect of depression on the speed of recall of pleasant and unpleasant experiences. *Psychological Medicine, 5,* 173–180.

MacDonald, M. R., and Kuiper, N. A. (1984). Self-schema decision consistency in clinical depressives. *Journal of Social and Clinical Psychology, 2,* 264–272.

MacLeod, C., and Mathews, A. (1988). Anxiety and the allocation of attention to threat. *Quarterly Journal of Experimental Psychology, 40A,* 653–670.

MacLeod, C., Mathews, A., and Tata, P. (1986). Attentional bias in emotional disorders. *Journal of Abnormal Psychology, 95,* 15–20.

Mathews, A. M. (1989). *Cognitive bias in anxiety and depression: Same or different?* Paper presented at the World Congress of Cognitive Therapy, Oxford, England.

Mathews, A. M., and Bradley, B. (1983). Mood and the self-reference bias in recall. *Behavior Research and Therapy, 21,* 233–239.

Mathews, A. M., and MacLeod, C. (1985). Selective processing of threat cues in anxiety states. *Behavior Research and Therapy, 23,* 563–569.

Mathews, A. M., and MacLeod, C. (1987). An information-processing approach to anxiety. *Journal of Cognitive Psychotherapy: An International Quarterly, 1,* 105–115.

Mathews, A. M., Mogg, K., May, J., and Eysenck, M. (1989a). Implicit and explicit memory bias in anxiety. *Journal of Abnormal Psychology, 98,* 236–240.

Mathews, A., Richards, A., and Eysenck, M. (1989b). Interpretation of homophones related to threat in anxiety states. *Journal of Abnormal Psychology, 98,* 31–34.

McGinnies, E. (1949). Emotionality and perceptual defense. *Psychological Review, 56,* 244–251.

McNally, R. J., and Foa, E. B. (1987). Cognition and agoraphobia: Bias in the interpretation of threat. *Cognition Therapy and Research, 11,* 567–581.

McNally, R. J., Foa, E. B., and Donnell, C. D. (1989). Memory bias for anxiety information in patients with panic disorder. *Cognition and Emotion, 3,* 27–44.

McNally, R. J., Kaspi, S. P., Riemann, B. C., and Zeitlin, S. (1990). Selective processing of threat cues in post-traumatic stress disorder. *Journal of Abnormal Psychology, 99,* 398–402.

McNally, R. J., Riemann, B. C., and Kim, E. (1990). Selective processing of threat cues in panic disorder. *Behavior Research and Therapy, 28,* 407–412.

Merluzzi, T. V., Glass, C. R., and Genest, M. (1981). *Cognitive assessment.* New York: Guilford Press.

Mogg, K., Mathews, A., and Weinman, J. (1987). Memory bias in clinical anxiety. *Journal of Abnormal Psychology, 96,* 94–98.

Mogg, K., Mathews, A., and Weinman, J. (1989). Selective processing of threat cues in anxiety states: A replication. *Behaviour Research and Therapy, 27,* 317–323.

Moretti, M. M., Segal, Z. V., Miller, D. T., Shaw, B. F., Vella, D. D., and McCann, C. D. (1993). *Processing information directed toward the self versus others in clinically depressed, mildly depressed and remitted depressed subjects.* Manuscript submitted for publication.

O'Banion K., and Arkowitz, H. (1977). Social anxiety and selective memory for affective information about the self. *Social Behavior and Personality, 5,* 321–328.

Parkinson, L., and Rachman, S. (1981). Intrusive thoughts: The effects of uncontrolled stress. *Advances in Behavior Research and Therapy, 3,* 111–118.

Riskind, J. H., Beck, A. T., Brown, G., and Steer, R. A. (1987). Taking the measure of anxiety and depression: Validity of the reconstructed Hamilton scales. *Journal of Nervous and Mental Disease, 175,* 474–479.

Roediger, H. L., Weldon, M. S., and Challis, B. H. (1989). Explaining dissociations between implicit and explicit measures of retention: A processing account. In H. L. Roediger and F. I. M. Craik (Eds.), *Varieties of memory and consciousness: Essays in honor of Endel Tulving* (pp. 3–1). Hillsdale, NJ: Erlbaum.

Rogers, T. B., Kuiper, N. A., and Kirker, W. S. (1977). Self-reference and the encoding of personal information. *Journal of Personality and Social Psychology, 35,* 677–688.

Sarason, I. G. (1985). Cognitive processes, anxiety and the treatment of anxiety disorders. In A. H. Tuma and J. D. Maser (Eds.), *Anxiety and the anxiety disorders* (pp. 87–107). Hillsdale, NJ: Erlbaum.

Schotte, D. E., McNally, R. J., and Turner, M. (1990). A dichotic listening analysis of body weight concern in bulimia nervosa. *Journal of Eating Disorders, 9,* 109–113.

Segal, Z. V. (1988). Appraisal of the self-schema construct in cognitive models of depression. *Psychological Bulletin, 103,* 147–162.

Segal, Z. V., Hood, J. E., Shaw, B. F., and Higgins, E. T. (1988). A structural analysis of the self-schema construct in major depression. *Cognitive Therapy and Research, 12,* 471–485.

Segal, Z. V., and Swallow, S. R. (in press). Cognitive assessment in unipolar depression: Measuring products, processes and structures. *Behavior Research and Therapy.*

Segal, Z. V., and Vella, D. D. (1990). Self-schema in major depression: Replication and extension of a priming methodology. *Cognitive Therapy and Research, 14,* 161–176.

Segal, Z. V., and Shaw, B. F. (1988). Cognitive assessment: Issues and methods. In K. S. Dobson (Ed.), *Handbook of cognitive-behavioral therapies.* New York: Guilford Press.

Shapiro, K. L., and Lim, A. (1989). The impact of anxiety on visual attention to central and peripheral events. *Behavior Research and Therapy, 27,* 345–351.

Shiomi, K. (1977). Threshold and reaction time to noxious stimulation: Their relations with scores on Manifest Anxiety Scale and Maudsley Personality Inventory. *Perceptual and Motor Skills, 44,* 429–430.

Stamps, L. E., Fehr, L. A., and Lewis, R. A. (1979). Differential effects of state and trait anxiety on heart rate response and reaction time. *Biological Psychology, 8,* 265–272.

Sternberg, S. (1969). Memory scanning processes revealed by reaction time experiments. *American Scientist, 57,* 421–457.

Stroop, J. R. (1935). Studies of interference in serial verbal reactions. *Journal of Experimental Psychology, 18,* 643–662.

Sutton, L. J., Teasdale, J. D., and Broadbent, D. E. (1988). Negative self-schema: The effects of induced depressed mood. *British Journal of Clinical Psychology, 27,* 188–90.

Teasdale, J. D., and Dent, J. (1987). Cognitive vulnerability to depression: An investigation of two hypotheses. *British Journal of Clinical Psychology, 26,* 113–126.

Teasdale, J. D., and Fogarty, S. J. (1979). Differential effects of induced mood on retrieval of pleasant and unpleasant events from episodic memory. *Journal of Abnormal Psychology, 88,* 248–257.

Treisman, A., and Geffen, G. (1967). Selective attention: Perception or response? *Quarterly Journal of Experimental Psychology, 19,* 1–16.

Tversky, A., and Kahneman, D. (1974) Judgments under uncertainty: Hueristics and biases. *Science, 185,* 1124–1131.

Warren, R. E. (1972). Stimulus encoding and memory. *Journal of Experimental Psychology, 94,* 90–100.

Watson, D., and Kendall, P. C. (1989a). Understanding anxiety and depression: Their relation to negative and positive affective states. In P. C. Kendall and D. Watson (Eds.), *Anxiety and depression: Distinctive and overlapping features* (pp. 3–26). San Diego: Academic Press.

Watson, D., and Kendall, P. C. (1989b). Common and differentiating features of anxiety and depression: Current findings and future directions. In P. C. Kendall and D. Watson (Eds.), *Anxiety and depression: Distinctive and overlapping features* (pp. 3–26). San Diego: Academic Press.

Watts, F. N., McKenna, F. P., Sharrock, R., and Trezise, L. (1986a). Colour naming of phobia related words. *British Journal of Psychology, 77,* 97–108.

Watts, F. N., Trezise, L., and Sharrock, R. (1986b). Processing of phobic stimuli. *British Journal of Clinical Psychology, 25,* 253–261.

Williams, J. M. G., and Broadbent, K. (1986). Autobiographical memory in attempted suicide patients. *Journal of Abnormal Psychology, 95,* 144–149.

Williams, J. M. G., Watts, F. N., MacLeod, C., and Mathews, A. (1988). *Cognitive psychology and emotional disorders.* Chichester, England: Wiley.

Zeitlin, S., and McNally, R. J. (1991). Implicit and explicit memory bias for threat in post-traumatic stress disorder. *Behavior Research and Therapy, 29,* 451–457.

PART II

Specific Disorders

Cognitive Conceptions of Anxiety

Mark J. Dombeck

San Diego State University and
University of California, San Diego

Rick E. Ingram

San Diego State University

The past twenty years have witnessed an upsurge of theory and re-search on anxiety. While our understanding of the etiology and course of anxiety disorders has increased substantially, so too have the differ-ent conceptions of anxiety. The generalized construct "anxiety" has be-come increasingly discussed in reference to a specific family of related but distinct anxiety disorders such as generalized anxiety disorder, post-traumatic stress disorder, panic disorder, obsessive–compulsive disorder, and the various phobias. Each of these specific anxiety disorders is pre-sumed to have a distinct etiology and symptomatic course.

This increasing specificity in the classification of anxiety disorders has been accompanied by a rich and diverse body of cognitive theory devoted to understanding anxiety. In fact, as in many areas of clinical psychology, cognitive approaches have proven useful in the conceptualization, assess-ment, and treatment of anxiety disorders. The purpose of this chapter is to examine these cognitive approaches to anxiety. It is obviously not possible to do justice to the diversity of different anxiety disorders in a single chapter. Indeed, entire chapters and in some cases volumes have been

53

written that highlight cognitive approaches to individual anxiety disorders.[1] Our strategy is instead to explore the thread that runs throughout the particular anxiety disorders. Specifically, we will examine the applications of various cognitive models to anxious affect; our hope is that by focusing on this dimension that underlies all of the anxiety disorders we can facilitate a more fundamental understanding of the different varieties of anxious psychopathology. Moreover, we hope that explication of these models will stimulate the collection of empirical data that test the models' veracity. To accomplish these goals, we start by discussing our assumptions about the construct of anxiety. We next present an overview of the major cognitive models of anxiety. In the course of our presentation we comment on the clinical implications of each approach. We next suggest commonalities and distinctions among the models that may serve to provide common ground for understanding the nature of anxiety. Finally, we suggest features we believe should be present in an integrated model of anxiety disorders.

A WORKING DEFINITION OF ANXIETY

Historically, theorists have taken extreme and opposed positions toward the problem of anxiety. The basic conflict, commonly referred to as the "mind–body problem," may be simply stated as a question of whether complex problems such as anxiety are best conceptualized as falling within the realm of the physical and tangible body or in the realm of the unobservable mind. Depending on the extremes of different positions, a problem such as anxiety might be seen as a primarily physical problem or alternatively as a primarily psychological problem. Modern theoretical approaches to anxiety are either rooted in one of these basic mind–body positions or can be seen as an attempt at integration.

Virtually all theories of anxiety share the common assumption that anxiety is fundamentally real, that is, anxiety is an entity or, at the very least, an invariant cluster of entities that exists independently of human cultural constraints, which can and does have the power to influence behavior, and is common to all human experience. Hallam (1985) proposed a

---

[1] An excellent and comprehensive starting place is Barlow's (1988) monograph. Other excellent sources (with discussion of specific disorders) are Clark (1986), Craske and Barlow (1988), Heimberg (1989), Marks (1987), McNally (1990), Michelson and Ascher (1987), Last and Hersen (1988), Litz and Keane (1989), Peterson et al. (1991), Rapee (1987; 1991), Rapee and Barlow (1991), Shaw et al. (1987), Taylor and Arnow (1988), Thyer et al. (1985), and Walker et al. (1991). This listing is offered as a starting place for further exploration and is not intended to be comprehensive.

constructivist alternative view of anxiety that does not share the assumption that anxiety has an invariant underlying organization. In his view, anxiety is a name given to a constellation of intrinsically unrelated physiological and cognitive events formed by and held together through the social and cultural experiences of the anxious person. Hallam pointed to the dangers of granting *a priori* existence and causal status to what he considers to be essentially a socially fabricated and intrinsically nonscientific lay construct. In Hallam's account of anxiety, people are taught that such a thing as anxiety exists and so come to use the term as a way of organizing their experience. Once reified, the construct of anxiety is granted causal status; people interpret selective aspects of their behavior as being caused by "anxiety," an entity independent of themselves and their surroundings.

We believe Hallam (1985) is correct in emphasizing the tremendous social contribution to any manifestation of anxiety. We also share his position that anxiety is flexible and commonly reified to an unnecessary degree. However, we reject Hallam's argument with respect to the question of anxiety's independence of physiology. Hallam's stress on the notion that anxiety is solely a derivative of human culture is at odds with our understanding of anxiety as a variation on a biological/structural theme. It seems clear that anxiety, social construct or not, is a label given to a specified range of possible emotional reactions. Although there is some variability in the behaviors and affective tones that are associated with emotional categories (i.e., people may cry because they are happy and/or because they are sad), the label "anxiety," regardless of context, is associated with a negative and unpleasant affective tone. The robustness and consistency of this association across time and place is difficult to account for were anxiety solely a social construct. Rather, anxiety appears to be a constellation of cognitive, physiological, behavioral, and affective phenomena which, while heavily influenced by social and cultural forces, is predominantly organized by biological determinants. The purpose of theory, to which we now turn, is to attempt a specification of the relationships between these various phenomena.

COGNITIVE THEORIES OF ANXIETY

In the following section we review the contributions of the major cognitive theories of anxiety. We begin with a discussion of schema theory. In turn, we consider bioinformational theory, rational–emotive approaches, self-discrepancy theory, control-process theory, and the integrated "anxious apprehension" model presented by Barlow (1988).

Schema Theory

The schema theory of anxiety is primarily associated with the work of Beck. Beck (Beck and Emery, 1985) defines fear as the cognitive appraisal of a threatening stimulus. Anxiety, on the other hand, is an unpleasant feeling state evoked when fear is stimulated. Together, fear and associated anxiety serve as a signal indicating the presence of danger. The ability to recognize and respond to danger is, of course, tremendously important for the survival of any species. Anxiety in its modern form is thought to have developed to a high degree of sensitivity because of its evolutionary value as a survival-enhancing mechanism. The structures underlying anxious arousal are ideally set up to respond to the physical threats that humans experienced during their evolutionary development. As threats in the modern world have become less tangible and physical defenses less constructive, anxiety as preparation for a physical response has become increasingly problematic and has culminated with the experience of anxiety as a disorder.

Beck (Beck and Emery, 1985) views the anxiety process as the product of converging biological, psychological, and social systems. Thus, any given experience of anxiety is seem as reflecting necessary contributions from underlying affective, physiological, behavioral, and cognitive structures. Of these multiple components, Beck singles out cognitive processes, specifically appraisal processes, as the variable most often responsible for producing pathological experiences of anxiety. The emotional reaction characterized by anxiety becomes exaggerated in pathological cases as a result of biases within cognitive processing that affect how information is appraised for danger content. The appraisal process is thought to be a relatively automatic form of information processing that takes place without need of conscious guidance. Beck understands the process of appraisal as driving emotional reactions and not the other way around. It is the interpretation of the environment and not the objective danger level that ultimately determines how much fear and consequent anxiety will be experienced by the anxious subject.

Within the process of appraisal, sensory information is interpreted by cognitive structures (known as "schemata") that consist of stored information abstracted from past experience. By providing a basis for assigning meaning to sensory perceptions as they occur schemata allow for the conservation of cognitive resources while simultaneously allowing quick application of previously learned knowledge to new situations. Information processed by schemata is selectively acted upon based on its salience and similarity to information already present. The informational product of this processing is thereby selectively modified to reflect any existing biases of the cognitive system.

According to Beck (1976; Beck and Emery, 1985) the cognitive propositions incorporated in schemata governing anxiety processes reflect the themes of *danger* or *harm* to the individual. The term "danger" is broadly defined and may include threat from attack, physical distress, or psychological injury (cf. Beck and Emery, 1985; Clark, 1986; Goldstein and Chambless, 1978). Accordingly, when information is first apprehended, an initial appraisal is made to determine whether the information represents acute danger. The formation of this impression is known as primary appraisal (Lazarus, 1966; Lazarus and Folkman, 1984). Though primary appraisal is based on incomplete data and thus is potentially based upon erroneous information, it nevertheless exerts a significant influence on later processing by setting the expectation for subsequent appraisals. The emphasis on immediate danger in primary appraisal is enhanced by a concurrent secondary appraisal in which an assessment is made of the availability of resources (physical, psychological, and social) useful for coping with the dangerous situation. Both appraisal processes are thought to take place automatically and represent an ongoing integrated process.

Beck (Beck and Emery) suggests that the content of anxiety schemata influences whether an individual will experience chronic and exaggerated pathological anxiety or more normal forms of anxiety. In the case of pathological anxiety, schemata are thought to be systematically biased so that they enhance the processing of information that is perceived as threatening and dangerous. For example, the anxious schema's operation leads to hypervigilant scanning of situations for a wide variety of potential threats and to the devaluation of objectively safe situations. Thus, people with such anxious schemata perceive objectively nondangerous situations as threatening and exaggerate the extent of danger inherent in other situations. This process is illustrated empirically by Landau (1980) who found that dog-phobic individuals had poorly articulated semantic structure for categories involving dogs. Landau's (1980) analyses suggested that two dimensions, size and ferocity (rather than the categories "breed" and "grooming," which were more emphasized in nonphobic individuals), accounted for the largest percentage of variance in dog phobics' associations. Hence, the dog phobic's cognitive structure appeared to facilitate the perception of threat.

A cognitive product of biased anxiety schemata is the production of automatic thoughts (Beck, 1967; Kendall and Ingram, 1987), a name given to the involuntary, continuous, and pressured flood of images and thoughts experienced in psychopathology. The conception of automatic thoughts was first derived in the context of Beck's (1967) theory of depression, where it described the tendency of depressed individuals to report intrusive, self-defeating self-statements. More specific to anxiety, automatic thinking has been reconceptualized by Kendall and Ingram (1987) as "automatic questioning." Ingram and Kendall (1987) describe the occurrence of the automatic questioning as a rapid and automatic process likely occurring at a subconscious level. They suggest that such automatic thinking can take place in either verbal or imaginal form. In anxiety disorders they suggest that the individual's ability to evaluate the plausibility of automatic questions and images is impaired.[2] Consequently, it is common for individuals to respond to their automatic questions as though they were true and rational reflections of the situation. However, because of the fundamentally exaggerated nature of automatic questions, their acceptance as true by the individual serves only to exacerbate the anxiety response in the initial appraisal.

Under normal circumstances, situations appraised as threatening are continuously reappraised in the light of new information that allows erroneous judgments to be corrected. This correcting reappraisal process does not occur in pathological anxiety. Pathologically anxious individuals become paralyzed in their perception of, and responses to, danger and are unable to modify their behavior in light of threat-disconfirming information drawn from the reappraisal process.

In summary then, the schema approach holds anxiety to be a natural complex of biological, psychological, and social responses to danger. The schema construct highlights the psychological aspects of anxiety as the most clinically accessible link in the chain of events that leads to a full experience of anxiety. These psychological mechanisms are twofold: first, the information-biasing characteristics of the cognitive structures receiving new information from the world; and second, the faulty appraisals of danger based upon this biased information, which lead to dysfunctional anxiety.

Clinical Implications

Therapy based on Beck's (Beck, 1976; Beck and Emery, 1985; Beck, Rush, Shaw, and Emery, 1979) conceptualization is viewed as a behaviorally based, time-limited system of intervention that involves the therapist in

---

[2]This conceptualization suggests that such thought may reflect cognitive distortion. Kendall (Kendall, 1985; Kendall and Dobson, Ch. 1, this volume; Kendall et al., 1991) has drawn an important distinction between cognitive distortions and cognitive deficiencies. Distortion refers to misinterpretation and misrepresentation of information, while deficiencies relate to an absence of cognitive activities. Throughout this chapter, when we refer to distortion or biases we refer to Kendall's conception of cognitive distortion.

the role of an educator teaching clients methods with which they may identify, evaluate, and modify their dysfunctional cognitions. In essence, the general cognitive strategy seeks to increase clients' ability to reflect upon the thoughts and images that drive their anxiety and, in so doing, gain a sense of separateness and control. The cognitive therapist has many techniques that may be employed to encourage this reflection. These methods primarily take the form of verbal interaction between the therapist and client with the therapist's goal being to logically and systematically demonstrate to clients the irrational nature of their anxiety and how this irrational material may be questioned and found wanting. The therapist may teach clients to systematically challenge thoughts and to attempt to discriminate the origins of these thoughts. The thoughts may then be seen more clearly to derive from long-established, rigid habits of thinking that do not reflect the current situational context.

Clients are taught critical thinking skills in several ways. First, clients are taught to examine their thinking for its correspondence with reality and to question their idiosyncratic beliefs. Second, clients are encouraged to view themselves from new and different perspectives in order to gain a better elaborated sense of how they are perceived by others. Finally, clients are encouraged to reflect on the worst-case scenarios of their fears and to then critically examine these fears for plausibility. In learning to reflect upon their spontaneous thinking processes, the client is helped to better discriminate between reality and distortion.

When the client has developed a sufficiently critical attitude, the therapist changes the focus toward restructuring the client's beliefs and behaviors. The therapist encourages clients to develop control over their images and behaviors with the goal of substituting more positive images and ways of behaving in their place. Clients may be asked to facilitate this process by describing things that they are afraid might happen to them. Armed with an understanding of clients' fears, the therapist is able to point out distortions and illogical conclusions. This process is illustrated by the following passage adapted from Beck and Emery (1985):

Patient: I keep getting an image of myself having a heart attack.

Therapist: What happens to you after you have the heart attack?

Patient: I see myself dying and helpless. That's all I can see. I feel it is a premonition or ESP. Something like that.

Therapist: Do you have these images and nothing happens?

Patient: Yes, I have them all the time and nothing happens.

Therapist: We've seen dozens of patients with these images, and rarely does the imagined event ever occur. I suggest you keep careful track of your images and see what happens.

Patient: But what if it does happen?

Therapist: The fantasy is consistently worse than the reality. I had an interesting situation a couple of years ago. This patient had a recurring frightening image. He owns a business. In his fantasy one of his key employees dies. He sees the business go downhill and he's forced to do things that he can't do; he then falls apart and has to be hospitalized. In the fantasy he loses his business and his freedom. Well, after about six months in treatment, believe it or not, it actually happened. One of his key managers died. And almost nothing else that he saw in his images happened. It didn't occur to him that other employees could take over tasks and that he could handle this better than he thought he could. He had overlooked in his fantasy these latent positive aspects — that is, the rescue factor. Fantasy is nearly always worse than the reality when an event occurs. The point is not to treat fantasies as real data.

Patient: So, if by some chance I did have a heart attack, that wouldn't necessarily mean I would die.

Therapist: No, it wouldn't.

Bioinformational Theory

Bioinformational theory (Lang, 1984, 1985; Foa and Kozak, 1985, 1986) is primarily a theory of emotion; it centers on and attempts to provide a clear definition of the nature of affect. Fear and anxiety are understood to be examples of kinds of affect. According to Lang's (1984, 1985) model, affective processes are best thought of as physiological processes. Specifically, emotion is identified with the activation of particular motor programs stored in memory that result in somatic arousal. Because motor programs are stored in memory, the model considers emotion to be an implicit aspect of cognitive processing involved in producing behavior. Unlike appraisal theorists (e.g., Beck, 1976; Beck and Emery, 1985) who conceptualize affect and cognition as separate processes, the bioinformational model views affect as the motor/behavioral aspect of cognitive processing.

Because of their embeddedness in motor and behavioral processes, Lang (1984, 1985) refers to emotions as "action tendencies" and to the patterns comprising these processes as "action sets" or "response sets." Each action set is, in turn, one small part of a larger associational network (Quillian, 1966) that comprises the structural architecture of memory. The network is composed of three different elemental meaning units, each stored as a "node" within the network. *Stimulus* nodes hold representations of previously apprehended stimuli. For example, a stimulus node might hold concepts such as boyfriend, guitar, house, or wrist watch. *Response* nodes hold information needed to direct physiological processes within the body. Possible examples include running, walking, playing an instrument, and shouting. What is stored in a response node is not the idea or verbalization of run, walk, play, or shout, but rather the actual motor program for carrying out these events. Finally, *meaning* nodes carry information that provides semantic interpretation of the stimulus and response information nodes. The connections between these nodes organize what otherwise would be an array of unconnected motor programs and iconic stimulus representations.

Though constructed of the same basic cognitive materials, emotion networks may be differentiated from each other based on how they are characterized on three dimensions: low versus high level of arousal, pleasant versus unpleasant affective valence, and low versus high perceived amount of control. Together, ratings on these three dimensions may be thematically interpreted to provide a description for any given network. For example, the emotion of fear could be described as pertaining to networks that produce a high degree of unpleasant arousal, and are specifically concerned with unpleasant feelings of losing control. In contrast, a "joy" network might be specifically concerned with pleasant, arousing behaviors such as laughter and smiling, and feelings of control combining to produce meanings of pleasure and contentment.

Emotion is elicited directly when a stimulus array that matches information stored in the stimulus nodes of the emotion network is perceived. When such a match is made the entire network is activated, creating both the phenomenological and behavioral experiences of the particular emotion. Moreover, a type of emotion can only be manifest when its particular arrangement of stimuli are presented. Emotional expression may thus be limited to certain contexts where the eliciting stimulation is present. For example, a woman who has no trouble speaking her mind when with friends may become fearful and silent when she is in the presence of her boss.

Lang (1984, 1985) conceptualizes the structure of fear as he does other emotional networks; information is represented in memory as a set of interrelated nodes tying motor programs directly to stimulus representations. A fear emotion network can be differentiated from other networks because its contents are specifically concerned with aiding in the identification of and escape from danger. For instance, a fear network will include response nodes containing coping behaviors designed to facilitate escape from danger and threat. The activation of this fear network results in the phenomenological experience of anxiety.

People experience danger and threat throughout their lives. Consequently, it is not unusual to find well-elaborated fear networks in normal individuals. Pathological anxiety is thought to be characterized by larger and more elaborate fear networks containing larger numbers of elements and tighter associations between these elements. The increased density and "tightness of weave" characteristic of the pathological fear network act to create a wider range of contexts that elicit the emotional fear reaction. The exaggerated associations between stimulus–response element pairings within the pathological fear network create a total elicited fear response that is out of proportion to what is called for in the actual circumstance. Once activated, the network excludes other non-fear-related processing and becomes difficult to deactivate because of the density and strength of the associations between fear elements.

Modification to the Bioinformational Theory

As developed by Lang (1984, 1985), bioinformational theory does not fully address the temporal qualities of fear development, maintenance, and possible resolution. Foa and Kozak (1985, 1986) have extended bioinformational theory to account for the process of change by further explicating the ways in which meaning (e.g., the theme of danger) is stored within the fear network. As we have seen, Lang (1984, 1985) posits the existence of "meaning" nodes, which serve an integrative function by unifying stimulus and response information stored within the network. The activation of the fear network via the presentation of relevant stimulation is thought to result in the direct instantiation of stored behavioral patterns along with an understanding of the meaning of the response (e.g., "This is dangerous! Run away as fast as you can!") via the activation of meaning nodes. Foa and Kozak (1986) suggest that, in addition to Lang's (1984, 1985) original concept of meaning nodes, the meanings of danger and threat held within the fear structure are carried implicitly within the structural relationships of the fear network. In the Foa–Kozak (1985, 1986) view, the likelihood of danger in a given feared situation is implied by the probability and strength of fearful affect and behavior associated with the feared stimulation. A strong relationship between feared stimulus and self-protective response implies that the eliciting stimulus is dangerous; the stimulus cue is defined as threatening by the relationships within the network precisely because of the strength of the response it invokes. Under normal conditions, the amount of fear and anxiety elicited by a situation is in proportion to the degree of danger present in the environment. However, in cases of pathological anxiety the correspondence between the strength of expressed fear behavior and the reality of danger breaks down. This is illustrated by considering social-phobic responding in public speaking. The stimulus of the audience is enough to elicit active fear behaviors in many social-phobic individuals though there is little objective threat. Here, the fear reaction is produced due to the hypersensitivity of the fear network as it acts to amplify and, in so doing, misinterpret the audience response.

Once established, the fear network is resistant to modification because of the strength of association between its elements and its capacity to exclude non-fear-related information. Foa and Kozak (1985, 1986) discuss two conditions they consider necessary precursors that must occur in order for new information to enter and modify a fear network. First, it is necessary for the fear network to be activated and brought up into current processing. This requires that the individual whose fear is to be modified must be exposed to a stimulus array (real or imaginary) that matches the stimulus elements embedded in the fear network. Second, it is necessary that the activated network be exposed to new information incompatible with that already in the network (e.g., information concerning the objective safety of the environment). As the new incompatible information interacts with the fear network, the structure of the network is fundamentally modified so that the implicit probabilistic representation of danger is lessened (Rachman, 1980). This is accomplished through a loosening of the associations between the stimulus and response elements within the network. A speech-phobic individual who has been exposed to unavoidable positive feedback and sincere interest from audience members will be less likely to automatically respond with anxiety to the task of speaking. It is crucial that the person whose network is to be modified be actively experiencing fearful affect during the modification. The fear network has no chance of coming in contact with new information no matter how frequently or sincerely it is presented when it is dormant in memory. It is only when the fear network is active that new information entering the system will have the chance of being incorporated into the structure of the network.

Clinical Implications

The bioinformational theory argues that fearful affect is a behavioral product of the activated fear network. In pathological anxiety the elements of the fear network are described as being too tightly woven, too interconnected, and too exclusionary of threat-disconfirming information. To effectively treat pathological anxiety it is necessary to change this network structure to more accurately reflect the true degree of danger in the environment. The treatment of choice for pathological fear is exposure to fear-eliciting stimulation. Recall Foa and Kozak's (1985, 1986) two precursors of modification: the activation of the fear network and the incorporation of fear-incompatible information into the network. To accomplish these tasks, the clinician may expose the fearful client to a set of stimuli (real or imaginary) that will provoke an anxious reaction. Exposure to fear-evoking stimuli directly precipitates anxious affect. Once fear has been activated, the therapist may help the client to see that the affect he or she is experiencing is not in proportion to the objective danger present. This difficult task may be handled in several ways. First, in a process known as flooding, or a similar process known as implosion, clients are required to confront their feared situation as fully as possible until the degree of affect they experience lessens via physiological mechanisms of habituation and/or extinction. An alternative strategy is to provide a graduated series of exposures to progressively more potent fear-provoking stimulation while allowing clients to habituate fully to each level of stimulation. At each stage of exposure the client must be held in the experience of fear until they experience a lessening of fearful affect (again, via habituation and/or extinction). Over the course of the graduated exposure protocol the client learns to tolerate progressively more of the fear-provoking stimulation without experiencing anxiety.

Rational–Emotive Therapy

Rational–Emotive Therapy (RET) is associated most closely with its founder Albert Ellis. RET is not intended as a theory of emotion or psychopathology. Rather, it is a systematic method of psychotherapy designed to overcome problems (such as dysfunctional anxiety and depression) standing in the way of human happiness (Ellis 1962; Lazarus, 1989). RET has not developed a specific accounting of various emotional states and does not differentiate etiologically between forms of psychopathology. Consequently, our discussion of RET is limited to describing how its underlying theory conceptualizes the production of generalized emotional dysfunction (such as, but not limited to, anxiety disorders).

RET holds that most emotional disturbance is the product of faulty thinking. By this, Ellis (1962) suggests that because of faulty irrational beliefs they hold about the personal significance of events, people are predisposed to misinterpret and exaggerate the significance of events occurring in the world. It should be apparent from this statement that there is a strong conceptual overlap shared by RET and schema theory. It is also important to note that RET predates the development of schema theory and is generally recognized as the first articulation of the modern cognitive therapy approach to emotional disorders (Lazarus, 1989). RET places primary responsibility for the production of dysfunctional emotion on the operation of static, biased knowledge contained within the cognitive system. Some authors (Schwartz, 1982) have interpreted this to mean that RET limits its understanding of the causal structure of dysfunctional emotion to cognitive factors. Ellis disputes this, claiming that RET (like schema theory) takes an integrationist position wherein dysfunctional emotion (such as anxiety) is understood as the product of integrated emotional–cognitive processes (Ellis, 1984). RET envisions a linear unfolding of the processes underlying emotional dysfunction systematized as the ABC model. Much like schema theory, RET hold that information from the environment (the Activating event, or A) entering the cognitive system is appraised in light of the existing information contained in the cognitive system (Beliefs, or B). When this existing information is biased, the resulting appraisal of the environment is also biased, leading to misinterpretation and emotional overreaction (emotional and behavioral Consequences, or C). Like schema theory, RET holds that individuals react to their cognitive appraisals of the environment and not to the objective environment itself.

Ellis (1962) views individuals as having a predisposition to develop errors in thinking that may lead to emotional dysfunction. This process is manifest in the tendency to overgeneralize the negative consequences of events and to make happiness contingent upon the occurrence of specific and often unrealistic outcomes. Overgeneralization as a monolithic category is broken down into four component processes, which are summarized in colorful language: the "awfulizing" tendency; "I-can't-stand-it-itis"; self-worthlessness; and unrealistic overgeneralization. The four processes are thought to be cognitive derivatives of absolute "should," "ought," and/or "must" beliefs contained in the cognitive system of individuals prone to anxiety disorders.

Clinical Implications

Volumes have been devoted to the RET method of therapy. In the interests of space we here summarize only the most salient points of traditional RET. Ellis describes two forms of RET: a general and an elegant method (Ellis, 1977). The general RET therapy method is similar to the broad-based cognitive–behavioral therapy method associated with schema theory and uses many of the techniques found in that tradition. The goal of RET is to change the irrational beliefs held by clients, replacing them with more adaptive rational beliefs. In general RET this process is accomplished primarily through the use of confrontive, Socratic-style discussion between client and therapist (although other cognitive–behavioral techniques may also be used). The therapist responds to voiced and implied irrational beliefs in the client's verbal report. These irrational beliefs often take the verbal form of "should," "must," and "ought" statements; for example, "My father never should have treated me that way," "I deserved that raise—I must have it!" The therapist then translates these beliefs into simple, concise statements and confronts the client with the irrationality of the beliefs.

Through the process of confrontation, clients are taught to recognize and replace their faulty beliefs with more functional and adaptive beliefs. To continue the example, the statement, "My father never should have treated me that way," might profitably be rethought as "It is unfortunate that my father treated me that way, but it is not awful and I can cope with the consequences." The irrational statement, "I deserved that raise—I must have it!" might be rethought as "I would have preferred to have gotten that raise, but it's not horrible that I didn't get it."

Self-Discrepancy Theory

Theorists who invoke appraisal mechanisms commonly suggest that interruption of ongoing cognitive processing leads to physiological arousal. The arousal these authors have in mind is general in nature and not tied to any one specific expression of emotion. The relationship between this nonspecific arousal and anxiety is left theoretically ambiguous. Self-discrepancy theory (Higgins, 1987) attempts to resolve this situation by describing how relationships among cognitive elements interact to produce specific affective experiences, such as anxiety, via the mechanism of appraisal. This appraisal is in the form of simple comparisons between representations of current and desired cognitive states.

Self-discrepancy theory depends on several distinctions regarding how the self is constructed. Higgins (1987) proposes two classes of self-processes: standpoints on the self and domains of the self. Standpoints on the self may be understood as "a point of view from which you can be judged that reflects a set of attitudes or values" (Higgins, 1987, p. 321). In the broadest sense there are two basic points of view that people have elaborated and may use as references from which to judge themselves: their own subjective view (e.g., "me"), and the view of the significant "other" (e.g., "not me"). The category of "other" may be further broken down to reflect the characteristics of many different significant others in a person's life (e.g., friends, family, spouse). Judgments of the worth or desirability of something may be determined only when consistent standards are available against which comparisons may be made. Higgins (1987) suggests that consistent cognitive representations comprising the standpoints on the self may be used to make such judgments and comparisons. These standpoints contain information both about other people's standards, and about the consistent set of internal standards people develop with which to judge themselves.

Higgins (1987) distinguishes three ways that people think about themselves and others. He divides these into domains or categories of thought: Actual, Ideal, and Ought domains of self. The name given to each domain refers to the type of information that is stored as a part of that domain. Actual domain characteristics are qualities that are considered to be manifest in current behavior. Ideal domain characteristics are qualities that the judging viewpoint desires the self to embody. Finally, Ought characteristics are qualities that the judging standpoint holds itself responsible for acquiring. Each articulated standpoint on the self that people may use to judge themselves has each of these three domains of standards contained within itself. It should be noted that Higgins (1987) articulation of "ought" and "should" domains is conceptually similar to Ellis's earlier (1962) description of the importance of absolutist, overgeneralized "ought," "should," and "must" beliefs. Broadly, both systems of theory recognize the role of discrepancy between "how things are" and "how things should be" in the generation of dysfunctional emotion. It should also be noted that the two theories are distinct and aim toward different ends. Where Ellis only briefly touches on the role of discrepancy in the production of emotion, Higgins's primary focus is on describing how discrepancy works to produce emotion.

As previously mentioned, Higgins's (1987) Ought domain is comprised of expectancy beliefs that the self is held accountable for meeting. Failure to meet Ought domain standards (i.e., recognition of a discrepancy between Ought and Actual domains) results in a negative outcome: the expectancy of impending punishment in retribution for failing to meet the standards. The conflict is reflected in an anxious affective tone that manifests itself in one of two ways, depending on the judging standpoint. If the failure to meet Ought domain expectations has occurred based on the judgment of the "significant other" standpoint, the individual in question should experience cognitions anticipating an impending retribution or punishment of some kind from this significant other. The anxious affect experienced will be that of apprehension, acute threat, and fear. If the standard violated is the individual's own standpoint, he or she will experience anxious affect in the form of guilt, self-contempt, and uneasiness.

Higgins (1987) recognizes that cognition is complex and that affect is the product of multiple causes. Though the potential for a domain conflict may exist, the actual recognition of conflict and the affective reaction resulting from this conflict depends on the accessibility of the involved domain elements to the appraisal process. These interdependent processes are referred to as *availability* and *accessibility*, respectively. It is possible that inconsistent domain elements may be contained within the cognitive system (and thus be available for processing), but no conflict is produced because these elements are not accessible to the evaluative process. The accessibility of domain elements for processing is influenced by many factors, including how recently and how frequently the elements have been processed, and the extent to which the conflicting elements are similar to the current environmental context. Thus, the self-discrepancy model assumes that the production of affect is determined as a function of both psychological variables (e.g., the information contained in the domains and standpoints) and situational determinants (e.g., the degree to which the current situation activates potentially conflicting elements).

Clinical Implications

The theme of perceived impending punishment and threat plays an important role in the production of anxiety. It is not a far jump to see Higgins's (1987) anxious threat of impending punishment as similar to the view of anxiety as a signal of impending danger espoused by theorists such as Beck and Emery (1985). In light of these similarities, the techniques described in the section on schema theory are applicable to self-discrepancy theory. Higgins (1987) suggests three avenues by which clinical intervention might conceivably be applied. He proposes that intervention be focused on changing either anxious clients' actual behavior, their conflicting Ought beliefs, or the ease with which they become aware of these different elements and thus experience conflict. Through the use of cognitive restructuring and reframing techniques, clinicians may attempt to modify the content of either clients' Ought beliefs or their actual current self-concept beliefs that are in conflict with the Ought beliefs. Clinicians may also encourage their clients to explore and take concrete steps toward reducing conflict by acting in ways consonant with how clients believe they "ought" to act. Finally, the therapist may attempt to change the accessibility of anxious conflict by either changing the conflict-provoking contingencies in the environment or helping the client to perceive the environment in a different manner.

Control-Process Theory

Carver and Scheier's (1988, 1990) control-process theory assumes that affective experience in general, and anxiety in particular, may be understood as the result of an interruption in an organism's ongoing behavioral processes. Anxiety is understood as a signal serving to refocus attention to the source of interruption. Specifically, Carver and Scheier (1990) propose that cognitive structures and processes responsible for behavior are hierarchically organized. Each level or strata of the hierarchy is provided with a label reflecting the level of integration characteristic of the concepts that may be found there. Higher level concepts in the hierarchical structure integrate and subsume all concepts lower in the hierarchy. The top-level "system" concepts provide guidance for all lower concepts and processes. System concepts are thought to contain the basic images of the idealized self. The next lower conceptual strata within the hierarchy contains "principles," concepts reflecting desired and actual attributes of the self (e.g., definable but abstract concepts such as honesty and responsibility). Beneath the principles are "programs" for behavior conceptualized as defined units of activity. Examples of programs are complex behaviors such as "going to the store" and "taking out the trash." Each program is actually a set of integrated simpler actions coordinated to fulfill a set goal. Programs are constructed of motor sequences or well-learned and effortlessly executed movement combinations that reside as individual units at a still lower level of cognitive organization.

According to the control-process model, behavior is best viewed as being a goal-oriented process in which individuals consistently attempt to reduce discrepancies between their current and idealized qualities. An individual's behavior is motivated by "negative" feedback processes operating at each level of the cognitive hierarchy, which act to minimize the level of discrepancy between current behavior and goal-directed, desired behavior. Discrepancies result in the production of affect and the refocusing of attention toward resolving the discrepancy. As attention is refocused to bear on discrepancy, behaviors are reorganized and modified in an attempt to reassert progress toward achieving goals. This process of continual regulatory vigilance and ongoing adjustment of behavior is referred to as monitoring.

In addition to monitoring processes, Carver and Scheier (1990) also discuss a secondary mechanism that contributes to the production of affect. Whereas the monitoring process seeks to minimize discrepancies between current actions and desired goals, a second "metamonitoring" process is described that seeks to minimize the time taken to meet goal requirements. The metamonitoring process monitors the rate of progress toward reaching goals, the quickness and efficiency with which discrepancies and blocked progress toward goals are handled. This progress information is then compared against an internal standard. Positive affect is produced when this standard is met or exceeded. If the standard is not met the individual is proposed to experience negative affect.

The control-process model offers two, non-mutually exclusive accounts of anxiety production corresponding to action within both the monitoring and metamonitoring processes. The first of these anxiety-generating processes was first described by Simon (1967). Anxiety is thought to be generated when there is conflict between two separate goals. The anxious affect generated by this conflict serves as a warning signal indicating that the course of action taken by the individual needs to be reevaluated and modified. An example may serve to illustrate. A graduate student is unhappy with a grade that she has received on a test designed by her professor. She develops a goal of confronting her professor and demanding to have her test reviewed. Acting on the basis of this goal she walks to the professor's office and prepares to knock on the door. Before doing so, she overhears the professor on the telephone to a colleague saying that she has lost patience with her students and is liable to fly off the handle if one more asks her about her test. The graduate student experiences a sudden reprioritization of her operating goals; after the first jolt of anxiety is passed she sneaks away from the door reasoning that it is better to accept her test score for now rather than risk speaking to her professor in her current, exasperated state. The secondary goal that increases in salience to reorganize behavior in this example is the threat of danger to the self that may be seen to be ultimately more personally relevant than even concern over a bad grade. The secondary goal is frequently, if not always, drawn from a higher level of the cognitive hierarchy and has more direct personal relevance for the self-concept.

Within the same example, anxiety may also be seen to result from the operation of the metamonitoring process. Simon's (1967) account of anxiety stresses the operation of the monitoring process in its action to hold individuals to the goals of the highest currently operating directive. A second, metamonitoring process, stressing the suddenness with which goal priorities shift, may also account for some of the experienced anxiety. In the process of realizing that now is not a good time to ask about the test the graduate student in our example has suddenly found herself far from meeting the goals of both her older, assertive urge and the newly emerging need to reestablish safety. Carver and Scheier (1990) hold that this experience of suddenness in of itself elicits negative affect in proportion to the rapidness of the goal shift and the discrepancy she perceives between her current state and the demands of her emerging need for safety.

Clinical Implications

Though Carver and Scheier (1988, 1990) do not specifically discuss treatment recommendations for anxiety, the implications of their model are fairly clear. Anxiety is produced when there is conflict between goals of self-expression and self-preservation, particularly when this conflict occurs without warning. Anxiety may therefore be lessened by helping anxious persons to examine what they are threatened by so they may better discriminate between apparent threats that are not objectively dangerous and actual dangers. Persons who have learned to discriminate between apparent and actual dangers may be expected to experience goal-conflict-related anxiety less frequently and in relation to more objective threats. Anxious persons may also be taught skills to allow them more effective means of coping once they are anxious. Cognitive techniques, first outlined in the treatment discussion on schema theory, may be used to help anxious clients evaluate and reorganize their understanding of the environment and to change the priorities of their goals and behaviors to better reflect this new understanding. Similar techniques should also be effective in helping clients to evaluate and modify the standards against which they judge their rate of progress toward goals. Skills-training approaches such as assertiveness training and therapist modeling of effective coping responses may be expected to aid anxious persons in dealing effectively with anxiety once it has become activated.

The Anxious Apprehension Model

The anxious apprehension model developed by Barlow (1988) views anxiety as the product of a memory network similar to that described by bioinformational theory. While anxiety networks are common to all individuals, the structure of the anxiety network differs between anxiety-disordered and nondisordered individuals. The differences are primarily due to varying levels of self-efficacy held by each group; nondisordered individuals tend to have a greater belief in their personal efficacy than anxiety-disordered individuals. The anxious apprehension model describes how differences in efficacy beliefs interact with ongoing cognitive processing to produce dysfunctional anxiety.

Central to the anxious apprehension model is the conception of physical arousal as a process capable of amplifying and focusing attention. The occurrence of arousal is proposed to have the ability to narrow attentional focus toward salient stimuli while acting to exclude other nonrelevant stimuli. Although this attention-focusing process appears superficially similar to the biased cognitive processing proposed by schema theory, the two models are distinct. According to schema theory, attentional biases are first found in the *products* of information processing and are due solely to biased anxiety schemata content. In apprehension theory, attentional biasing occurs *simultaneously* with information processing and is due to an interaction between biased cognitive content and the (unique to apprehension theory) mechanism of arousal.

Barlow (1988) argues that the contemplation of performing a task naturally results in (1) arousal, and (2) an evaluation of the demands of the task. Individuals who expect to do well at the task receive a performance benefit from their arousal in the form of a narrowed field of attention allowing them to better focus on task demands. In contrast, anxiety-disordered individuals frequently expect to fail at tasks and to feel helpless and incompetent. Instead of becoming more task focused these anxious individuals experience a spiraling increase in their focus on negative expectancies. With much of their attention locked into contemplation of negative performance, these anxious individuals have few resources available for task execution. Not surprisingly, the task performance of anxious individuals tends to suffer, strengthening their initial negative expectancy. As a method of keeping their anxiety minimized, anxious individuals may develop avoidance strategies wherein they cease to attempt tasks that they expect to fail.

Anxious individuals' negative expectancies for success are thought to develop as a result of several converging factors. First, anxiety-prone individuals tend to have a biological predisposition for intense and frequent affective responding. Individuals with such a predisposition respond with heightened affect to a wider range of situations than individuals without such a predisposition. Faced with frequent and unpredictable arousal, anxiety-prone individuals conclude that they are helpless to control their environment and emotional responding. Over time, anxious individuals form an association between arousal and their perceptions of helplessness. This association is later generalized so that many forms of arousal automatically predispose these individuals to experience self-focus and feelings of helplessness. Psychopathological anxiety structures thus begin with individuals' frequent appraisal-based focus on their situational experiences of helplessness and develop into established cognitive networks that predispose individuals to negative self-focusing as a generalized response to many forms of arousal.

Clinical Implications

Barlow (1988) suggests that three key elements of the anxiety structure must be modified in order for a clinical intervention to be successful. These are the pattern of motor activation triggered along with the physical arousal, the subjective sense of helplessness, uncontrollability, and unpredictability that occur in response to affective arousal and the process of self-focused attention.

The clinician may combat the physiological activation and defensive preparedness characteristic of anxious hypervigilance through several methods. First, an alternative set of physical activation incompatible with anxiety may be elicited by having the anxious client participate in a relaxation induction or through the inducement of laughter. The use of active techniques such as relaxation training, which provide clients with the ability to control their affective responding, may indirectly demonstrate to clients that they are not out of control, thus addressing Barlow's (1988) second element: the perception of helplessness. Clinicians may further encourage their clients' perception that they can control their affect by providing educational demonstrations, both experiential (e.g., controlled panic induction through hyperventilation) and intellectual (e.g., biblio-therapy, and/or information on the physiology of affect). Clinician-supervised, graduated exposures to feared stimulation may provide a sim-ilar effect. Finally, anxious clients may be helped to overcome their dispo-sition to self-focus through attempts to educate them about the self-focusing process and to point out the operation of this mechanism in their everyday functioning. Clients may be taught to catch themselves during or just before they begin to self-focus and to initiate more adaptive behavior such as reinvesting in the task at hand.

POINTS OF OVERLAP AND DIVERGENCE BETWEEN THE THEORIES

We have reviewed a number of different theories, each with a unique viewpoint on the problem of anxiety. We now shift our focus and concen-trate upon explicating the features that bind the various theories together. The theories may be compared on three major dimensions: the centrality of danger-related cognition, the automaticity of appraisal processes, and the role played by affect. We believe that an integrated theory of anxiety flexible enough to allow for multiple positions on each of these dimensions is necessary to adequately capture the complexity of pathological anxiety.

The Primacy of Danger

Perhaps the most common theme running throughout each theory is that anxiety is intimately and primarily connected with concern over threat and danger to the self. This danger-related cognition takes a different form for each of the theories. In *schema* theory, themes of danger and threat are implicit in the cognitive schemata that operate to produce biased informa-tion processing. In *bioinformational* theory, danger-related information is held in the meaning nodes that make up the anxious information process-ing network. Foa and Kozak's (1985, 1986) modified version of the bioinfor-mational theory also centers on the themes of danger present in anxiety. However, their work suggests that danger-related information is generated as an emergent feature of the fear network's structure in operation instead of being stored as a proposition. The idea of danger is implicit in *control-process* theory in the high priority given to protecting the self-concepts that provide guidance for the cognitive system. According to the control-process theory, ongoing lower level processing is interrupted and attention is refocused on preserving the integrity of the self-concepts when threatening information is encountered. In the view of *RET*, problems such as anxiety are caused by unrealistic expectations of negative outcomes and other faulty and irrational beliefs presupposing danger to the self. Similarly, the *anxious apprehension* model places the threat of danger in the negative expectations for success held by anxious individuals. The theme of danger is perhaps most clearly stated in *self-discrepancy* theory, which literally defines anxiety as the expectation of impending danger (e.g., punishment) brought on by a perceived failure to live up to idealized standards. In sum, all of the theories are predicated on the idea that anxious cognitive responding is designed to facilitate the perception of danger to the self.

Appraisal and Automaticity of Processing

All of the theories agree that at least some features of anxiety occur automatically without conscious prompting. However, the theories take different positions on the role of automatic cognitive processing. Primary among the distinctions in automaticity of processing is the role accorded to appraisal. Appraisal may be defined roughly as the process of placing a value upon a perception. Taken literally, appraisal implies a conscious, volitional process. However, some theories (i.e., schema theory, RET) imply automatic and unconscious forms of appraisal. Thus, conscious volitional forms of appraisal may be seen to fall at one extreme of an appraisal continuum, while unconscious forms of appraisal processes fall toward the other end. Bioinformational theory, which does not make reference to appraisal at all, is perhaps the most radical account of completely unconscious appraisal processing (if the term appraisal may be said to fit at all). Consequently, we place *bioinformational theory* nearest to the automatic end of the spectrum. *Schema theory* and the *RET* approach discuss appraisal processes that operate quite automatically. However, these theories recognize that appraisal may be turned on itself, so to speak, in that an individual's anxiety may be lessened through the therapeutic application of conscious, rational argument to the appraisal process. We place schema theory and RET squarely in the middle of the appraisal continuum, as they both appear to acknowledge both volitional and automatic forms of appraisal.

The placement of the *anxious apprehension model* presents an interesting challenge. The anxious apprehension model embraces a developmental approach to anxiety structures. It is consistent with but not identical to volitional appraisal when it discusses the etiology of anxiety in the formation of negative performance expectations. When dealing with a mature anxiety structure, the anxious apprehension model is more consistent with appraisal as an automatic process. Hence, we place the anxious apprehension model in the center of the appraisal continuum for somewhat different reasons than those for schema theory and RET. The position of self-discrepancy theory and control-process theory on the issue of automaticity of appraisal is problematic. While the theories imply the operation of automatic appraisal processes in the functioning of their discrepancy-sensing mechanisms, it is not clear from published accounts how consistent they are with the idea of volitional appraisal. We have chosen to place *self-discrepancy* and *control-process theories* in the center of the appraisal continuum largely to differentiate them from the radical automaticity of bioinformational theory, which it is clear they do not represent. It should be noted that Foa and Kozak's (1985, 1986) modifications to the bioinformational theory, with their increased emphasis on the role of meaning in mediating the anxiety response, appear to imply that an appraisal process using information from the fear network occurs prior to the onset of fear. The modified bioinformational theory would then be best placed closer to the middle of the appraisal continuum (Fig. 3.1).

The Role of Affect

Schema theory, RET, control-process theory, and *self-discrepancy theory* all share the common assumptions that: (1) affect is a fundamentally different type of process than cognition; and that (2) both cognitive and affective processes must be present for anxiety to occur. These theories view affect as a secondary process elicited by the cognitive processing underlying the perception of danger. To use an example from schema theory, the biased cognitive schema of anxiety-prone individuals prompts hypervigilant scanning of the environment and a subsequently increased chance of actually triggering anxious affect. The resulting affective arousal is then fed back into the appraisal process, resulting in further increases in the disposition to perceive threat. Though affect is phenomenologically the most disturbing aspect of anxiety and clearly plays a fundamental role in the production of anxiety, schema theory is clear that it is the mediational cognitive appraisal process and not the contribution of arousal that determines whether anxiety will be experienced. In slightly altered forms this description also applies to RET, self-discrepancy theory, and control-process theory.

Danger is central	Automatic processes: No appraisal is present	Affect and Cognition are integrated processes
Schema Theory Bioinformational Theory Rational–Emotive Therapy Self-Discrepancy Theory Control–Process Theory Anxious Apprehension	Bioinformational Theory Schema Theory Rational–Emotive Theory Self-Discrepancy Theory Control–Process Theory Anxious Apprehension	Bioinformational Theory Anxious Apprehension Schema Theory Rational–Emotive Therapy Self-Discrepancy Theory Control–Process Theory
Danger is not central	**Effortful processes: Appraisal is present**	**Affect and Cognition are separate processes**

Figure 3.1. Three dimensions reflecting different assumptive positions underlying cognitive theories of anxiety. The positions of the theories on these dimensions indicate the degree to which the underlying assumptions of each theory are similar or divergent.

Bioinformational theory and the *anxious apprehension model* break with the other theories in positing that affect and cognition are fundamentally inseparable processes. Both theories view affect as the product of directly elicited action tendencies or motor programs that are structurally integrated with other cognitive elements of the anxiety network. Affective and cognitive features of anxiety are thus elicited as a unitary response from a single network and not as separate responses with origins in fundamentally different processes. For example, the negative self-focus, expectations of helplessness, and hypervigilance characteristic of anxious apprehension are proposed to be directly elicited by generalized forms of arousal in anxiety-disordered individuals. The defensive response sets characteristic of anxiety as described by bioinformational theory are likewise directly elicited when the anxiety network is triggered by threatening stimuli in the environment. The modifications made to bioinformational theory by Foa and Kozak (1985, 1986) do not fundamentally alter this conceptualization.

PSYCHOPATHOLOGICAL ANXIETY

Psychopathological anxiety, of course, is the explicit focus of several of the models we have reviewed (e.g., schema theory, RET). Although other approaches are primarily intended to explicate anxiety within the normal range of experience, these theories are also applicable to dysfunctional anxiety states. In our discussion we start with a consideration of the developmental context of anxiety disorders. We suggest that an integration of theoretical approaches emphasizing volitional and automatic appraisal processes may best account for the temporal progression of pathological anxiety. We conclude the chapter with a description of the generalized processes occurring in the formation, maintenance, and clinical implications of anxiety disorders.

Developmental Aspects

Mature anxiety structures capable of producing a clinical disorder are marvels of organized knowledge that develop out of a complex interaction between the genetic givens of an individual's existence and the environment (Izard, 1977; Izard and Blumberg, 1985). For all their sophistication, anxiety structures begin as unelaborated structures containing little or no information about threatening stimulus. Through experience with painful events the structure builds over time to include an increasingly elaborate representation of threat. From an evolutionary perspective, survival would appear to dictate that the need for cognitive appraisal should be greatest early in the developmental process when the threatening nature of a stimulus is uncertain. The need for appraisal should lessen over time as "knowledge" about the threat becomes integrated into the network. Once threat is anticipated, the continued presence of appraisal would appear to actually hurt an individual's chances for survival, as appraisal should be expected to compete for resources vital to more constructive coping-oriented processing. That is, the cognitive resources required to appraise a situation "known" to be dangerous would better be invested in attempts at defense or retreat. Thus, evolutionary logic should favor a developmental shift from appraisal to automaticity.

Dysfunctional Anxiety

The evolutionary virtue of anxiety is its efficient and automatic mobilizing function in response to danger. Anxiety's significance lies in its ability to orient organisms to danger and provide for their responses to that danger. Anxiety is optimal only when it serves these functions efficiently. In order to be effective, anxiety processes need to be in proportion to the actual degree of threat in the environment. Pathological anxiety is precisely anxiety that is out of proportion to the environment and hence unnecessarily impairs the full range of functioning necessary for the enjoyment of life.

The theories reviewed here are consistent with the view that pathological anxiety is *too* automatic, that responses are carried out without awareness or higher level cognitive modulation. Anxiety becomes pathological when it becomes a rigid and exaggerated response, out of step with the threats of the real world and resistant to modification by new, danger-disconfirming information. For example, the cognitive structures operating in the individual with Generalized Anxiety Disorder function to ensure that virtually all situations represent danger to the self.

Anxiety-disordered individuals therefore appear characterized by schemata consisting of self-representations of vulnerability and helplessness. When anxiety is activated, anxious individuals experience a shift in their attentional focus toward a heightened perception of perceived danger cues and the exclusion of other non-threat-related information (Ingram and Kendall, 1987; Kendall and Ingram, 1987). This may be illustrated using the case of a dog phobic. When a dog phobic happens to encounter a dog, an anxiety schema is activated that focuses attention on the perceived threat, for instance, the teeth, size, and estimated speed of the animal. Once an anxiety schema is triggered, cognitive distortion in the form of automatic questioning are likely to occur (e.g., "How can I get away?," "How much damage will this dog do?"). Moreover, the memories that are more likely to be retrieved in the anxiety state will be of past anxiety-provoking encounters (Mathews and MacLeod, 1985), which serve to reinforce and perhaps exacerbate the anxiety. Task focus becomes more difficult as task-irrelevant cognitions predominate (Sarason, 1980) and the individual becomes self-absorbed (Ingram, 1990). The dysfunctional individual copes with this state by withdrawal and avoidance and thus negatively reinforces the disorder by virtue of relieving the uncomfortable state.

Although various anxiety models may differ on some of these features, the therapeutic approaches they advocate are quite consistent with this view of anxiety. For instance, by encouraging people to introspect and dispute self-statements and images, therapies based on the schema approach seek to increase the amount of cognitive modulation that occurs in response to these automatic processes. Clients are also encouraged to test out the validity of their fears in the actual environment. Bioinformationally based therapies stress a pure exposure to the threatening stimuli. The key feature that is common to both therapy strategies is that they consider the anxious client's cognitive representation of the environment to be inaccurate. The various methods we have discussed all serve to bring this anxious representation back into line with a more objectively realistic assessment of danger in the environment.

CONCLUSIONS

The most elementary function served by anxiety is to increase the organism's chances to keep itself alive so that it may reproduce. The cognitive system allows the organism to accomplish this goal by providing the basis for a sensitive, accurate, and consistent mapping of the environment. This is augmented by the presence of anxiety, which allows active recognition and responding to perceived danger. During an anxious episode, attentional processes are oriented toward the perceived threat and resources are made available for improved physical coping with the danger. The degree to which this reorientation process may automatically proceed depends on the degree of information stored about the provoking stimulus. The more that is "known" or anticipated about a feared stimulus, the more the process becomes automatic. Anxiety is an evolving set of processes that change with the organism's experience. The therapies based upon the varying perspectives we have reviewed all proceed from the assumption that pathological anxiety is due at least partially to a faulty, exaggerated, and inaccurate representation of the environment as dangerous. Each therapy attempts, in the terms of the theory from which it is derived, to modify this faulty cognitive representation to better reflect an objectively realistic appraisal of the environment.

REFERENCES

Barlow, D. H. (1988). *Anxiety and its disorders: The nature and treatment of anxiety and panic*. New York: Guilford Press.

Beck, A. T. (1967) *Depression: Clinical, experimental, and theoretical aspects*. New York: Hoeber.

Beck, A. T. (1976). *Cognitive therapy and the emotional disorders*. New York: Hoeber.

Beck, A. T., and Emery, G. (1985). *Anxiety disorders and phobias: A cognitive perspective*. New York: Basic Books.

Beck, A. T., Rush, A. J., Shaw, B. F., and Emery, G. (1979). *Cognitive Therapy of Depression*. New York: Guilford.

Carver, C. S., and Scheier, M. F. (1988). A control-process perspective on anxiety. *Anxiety Research, 1*, 17–22.

Carver, C. S., and Scheier, M. F. (1990). Origins and functions of positive and negative affect: A control process view. *Psychological Review, 97*, 19–35.

Clark, D. M. (1986). A cognitive approach to panic. *Behaviour Research and Therapy, 24*, 461–470.

Craske, M. G., and Barlow, D. H. (1988). A review of the relationship between panic and avoidance. *Clinical Psychology Review, 8 (6)*, 667–685.

Ellis, A. (1962). *Reason and emotion in psychotherapy*. New York: Lyle Stuart.

Ellis, A. (1977). Rejoinder: Elegant and inelegant RET. *Counseling Psychologist, 7*, 13–19.

Ellis, A. (1984). Is the Unified-interaction approach to cognitive–behavior modification a reinvention of the wheel? *Clinical Psychology Review, 4*, 215–218.

Foa, E. B., and Kozak, M. J. (1985). Treatment of anxiety disorders: Implications for psychopathology. In A. H. Tuma and J. D. Maser (Eds.), *Anxiety and the anxiety disorders*. Hillsdale NJ: Erlbaum.

Foa, E. B., and Kozak, M. J. (1986). Emotional processing of fear: Exposure to corrective information. *Psychological Bulletin, 99*, 20–35.

Goldstein, A. J., and Chambless, D. L. (1978). A re-analysis of agoraphobia. *Behavior Therapy, 9*, 47–59.

Hallam, R. S. (1985). *Anxiety: Psychological perspectives on panic and agoraphobia*. London: Academic Press.

Heimberg, R. G. (1989). Cognitive and behavioral treatments for social phobia: A critical analysis. *Clinical Psychology Review, 9(1)*, 107–128.

Higgins, E. T. (1987). Self-discrepancy: A theory relating self to affect. *Psychological Review, 94*, 319–340.

Ingram, R. E. (1990). Self-focused attention in clinical disorders: Review and a conceptual model. *Psychological Bulletin, 107*, 156–176.

Ingram, R. E., and Kendall, P. C. (1987). The cognitive side of anxiety. *Cognitive Therapy and Research, 11*, 523–536.

Izard, C. E. (Ed.). (1977). *Human emotions*. New York: Plenum Press.

Izard, C. E., and Blumberg, M. A. (1985). Emotion theory and the roles of emotions in anxiety in children and adults. In A. H. Tuma and J. D. Maser (Eds.), *Anxiety and the anxiety disorders*. Hillsdale, NJ: Erlbaum.

Kendall, P. C. (1985). Cognitive process and procedure in behavior therapy. In G. T. Wilson, C. M. Franks, P. C. Kendall, and J. Foreyt (Eds.), pp. 123–163. *Annual review of behavior therapy* (Vol. 10). New York: Guilford Press.

Kendall, P. C., and Ingram, R. E. (1987). The future for cognitive assessment of anxiety; Let's get specific. In L. Michelson and L. M. Ascher (Eds.), *Anxiety and stress disorders: Cognitive–behavioral assessment and treatment*. New York: Guilford Press.

Kendall, P. C., Vitousek, K. B., and Kane, M. (1991). Thought and action in behavior therapy: cognitive–behavioral intervention. In M. Hersen, A. Kazdin, and A. Bellack (Eds.), pp. 596–626. *Clinical psychology handbook* (Vol. 2). New York: Pergamon.

Landau, R. J. (1980). The role of semantic schemata in phobic word interpretation. *Cognitive Therapy and Research, 4*, 427–434.

Lang, P. J. (1984) Cognition in emotion: concept and action. In C. E. Izard, J. Kagan, and R. B. Zajonc (Eds.), pp. 192–226. *Emotions, cognition, and behavior.* Cambridge: Cambridge University Press.

Lang, P. J. (1985). The cognitive psychophysiology of emotion: Fear and anxiety. In A. H. Tuma and J. D. Maser (Eds.), *Anxiety and the anxiety disorders.* Hillsdale, NJ: Erlbaum.

Last, C. G., and Hersen, M. (Eds.). (1988). *Handbook of anxiety disorders.* New York: Pergamon.

Lazarus, R. S. (1966). *Psychological stress and the coping process.* New York: McGraw-Hill.

Lazarus, R. S. (1989). Cognition and emotion from the RET viewpoint. In M. E. Bernard and R. DiGiuseppe (Eds.), pp. 47–68 *Inside rational–emotive therapy: A critical appraisal of the theory and therapy of Albert Ellis.* San Diego: Academic Press.

Lazarus, R. S., and Folkman, S. (1984). *Stress, appraisal, and coping.* New York: Springer.

Litz, B. T., and Keane, T. M., (1989). Information processing in anxiety disorders: Application to the understanding of post-traumatic stress disorder. *Clinical Psychology Review, 9(2)*, 243–257.

Marks, I. M. (1987). *Fears, phobias, and rituals: Panic, anxiety and their disorders.* New York: Oxford University Press.

Mathews, A., and MacLeod, C. (1985). Selective processing of threat cues in anxiety states. *Behaviour Research and Therapy, 23*, 563–570.

McNally, R. J. (1990). Psychological approaches to panic disorder: A review. *Psychological Bulletin, 108(3)*, 403–419.

Michelson, L., and Ascher, L. M. (Eds.). (1987). *Anxiety and stress disorders: Cognitive behavioral assessment and treatment.* New York: Guilford Press.

Peterson, K. C., Prout, M. F., and Schwartz, R. A. (1991). *Post-traumatic stress disorder: A clinician's guide.* New York and London: Plenum Press.

Quillian, M. R. (1966). Semantic memory. In M. L. Minsky (Ed.), *Semantic information processing.* Cambridge, MA: MIT Press.

Rachman, S. (1980). Emotional processing. *Behaviour Research and Therapy, 18*, 51–60.

Rapee, R. M. (1987). The psychological treatment of panic attacks: Theoretical conceptualization and review of evidence. *Clinical Psychology Review, 7(4)*, 427–438.

Rapee, R. M. (1991). Generalized anxiety disorder: A review of clinical features and theoretical concepts. *Clinical Psychology Review, 11(4)*, 419–440.

Rapee, R. M., and Barlow, D. H. (Eds.). (1991). *Chronic anxiety: Generalized anxiety disorder and mixed anxiety-depression.* New York: Guilford Press.

Sarason, I. G. (1980). *Test anxiety: Theory, research and applications.* Hillsdale, NJ: Erlbaum.

Schwartz, R. M. (1982). Cognitive–behavior modification: A conceptual review. *Clinical Psychology Review, 2*, 267–293.

Shaw, B. F., Segal, Z. V., Vallis, T. M., and Cashman, F. E. (Eds.). (1987). *Anxiety disorders: Psychological and biological perspectives.* New York: Plenum Press.

Simon, H. A. (1967). Motivational and emotional controls of cognition. *Psychological Review, 74*, 29–39.

Taylor, C. B., and Arnow, B. (1988). *The nature and treatment of the anxiety disorders.* New York: Free Press.

Thyer, B. A., Himle, J., and Curtis, G. C., (1985). Blood-injury-illness phobia: A review. *Journal of Clinical Psychology, 41(4)*, 451–459.

Walker, J. R., Norton, G. R., and Ross, C. A. (1991). *Panic disorder and agoraphobia: A comprehensive guide for the practitioner.* Pacific Grove, CA: Brooks/Cole.

The Role of Cognition in Depression

Ruby Ackermann Engel and Robert J. DeRubeis

University of Pennsylvania

Depression is said to be a disorder of mood or affect (American Psychiatric Association, 1987), yet not all patients who receive a diagnosis of depression report sad mood. Likewise, decreased motivation and disruption of vegetative functioning are usually, but not invariably, found in depression. Although no symptom, sign, or indicator is invariant in depression, one of those most frequently observed is abnormal cognition. Even writers who have proposed biological or psychodynamic formulations of depression have recognized that as part of the symptom picture one almost always sees such cognitive pathologies as extreme pessimism, self-denigration, and self-blame (e.g., Akiskal and McKinney, 1975; Freud, 1917/1957). Aaron T. Beck, in the 1950s and 1960s, (e.g., Beck, 1967; Beck & Hurvich, 1959) brought these "cognitive" symptoms into clear focus, and first proposed that the cognitive aspects of depression are central features of the disorder, not incidental ones. Although the debate continues as to whether and in what sense these cognitive aspects play a causal role in depression, there is no question that most clinicians and theorists emphasize cognitive features of depression more since Beck's landmark work. Indeed, cognitive aspects of depression have been at the core of some of the most generative modern theories of depression, as evidenced by the

83

vast and still burgeoning literature addressing the role of cognitive processes in depression.

We should clarify that the sense of cognition we will be discussing in this chapter is what is now often referred to as "social cognition" (Fiske and Taylor, 1991). Although basic cognitive deficits such as impairment of memory and attention are observed in depression (e.g., Blaney, 1986; Colby and Gotlib, 1988; Golinkoff and Sweeney, 1989; Johnson and Magaro, 1987), it is not this category of cognitive functioning that is the topic of this chapter. Rather, we will focus on the negative tone of the *judgments, memories*, and *predictions* depressed people make, as well as on the negative *assumptions* they apply when they make these judgments. In the language of social cognition research, these have been referred to as cognitive *products* and *schemata*, respectively.

Description of Depressive Cognition

The experience of most clinicians who have dealt with depressed patients is that their judgments seem frequently to be negatively skewed. In many cases, even the obviously off-base beliefs of patients are difficult to verify or falsify. Examples are the patient who believes he is worthless, or the patient who believes that her business will decline in the coming years. However, many beliefs are falsifiable. An example is that of a woman who had raised three children and believed that she had been a bad mother, and that her children now resented her for this failing. Another example is a woman in her late twenties who could not bear children, and believed that no man could become interested in her because of this inability. In both cases, these patients were able to devise and conduct tests of their hypotheses with the help of a therapist and to disconfirm these hypotheses using the data they collected.

Depressed patients are frequently aware that their thinking is more negative than it is when they are not depressed, and that it is more negative than the thinking of friends and family. At the same time, they often are unable, on their own, to generate or formulate alternative beliefs. It is as if they have cognitive "blinders" on, so that they are prevented from "seeing" more benign interpretations of events in their lives. For some patients, simply encouraging the generation of alternative explanations for an event helps to alleviate the concern about it. In this way, these depressed patients are like Dodge's aggressive children (e.g., Dodge and Frame, 1982) who appear to have more trouble generating "normal" interpretations of possible affronts than they do choosing the "normal" answer once it is presented as an option (but see Hammen and Krantz, 1976, for an example of how depressed patients tend to choose the depressing option among many interpretations).

An example of this kind of "restricted" thinking is illustrated in the case of an attorney seen in therapy by the second author. In the middle of her course of therapy, she invited neighbors for dinner. At dinner, the neighbors mentioned that they had hired another attorney to represent them in a minor legal matter. The patient initially felt hurt, but immediately remembered to apply the cognitive therapy techniques she had been learning in therapy. Challenging her inference that the neighbors did not respect her resulted in a more benign interpretation than the one she originally entertained. However, being still depressed, she viewed the fact that she was hurt, even momentarily, as indicative of a defect in her. She did not, on her own, entertain the possibility that anyone in her shoes would have taken the news personally, if only briefly. Only when this was discussed with her could she see it. Once she considered it, she was able to see that her initial reaction was indeed quite normal.

A small subset of depressed patients appear not to be bothered by such negative thinking, at least during some periods of their depressions. There are also reports that in some cultures, negative thinking is either not prominent or is absent in depression (e.g., Kleinman, 1980). In these cases the depression consists of lethargy, sleep disturbance, and loss of interest in usual activities. There is little systematic study of the incidence of these "cognitive-pathology-free" depressive episodes, either in our own culture, or in other cultures. The syndrome exhibited by the attorney just described was at times an example of this type of depression. The cognitive symptoms of depression seemed to be absent until the episode had lasted two to three weeks. During those first few weeks, she reported early morning wakening, a loss of interest in food, a lack of interest in her work, and a lack of "spunk" generally. Only after she experienced these symptoms for a few weeks did the cognitive symptoms begin to emerge. Then she began to report concerns that she was an inferior lawyer, that her marriage was a failure, and that she was a bad mother. This kind of negative thinking then continued for the duration of the depressive episode. By her report, this was the pattern she had experienced in each of her six episodes of depression.

Thus, negative thinking may not always be present in depression, but usually it is a prominent clinical feature. In the first part of the chapter, we outline two major cognitive theories of depression, Beck's (1967, 1976, 1987) model of depression and the hopelessness theory of depression (Abramson et al., 1989). Although there are other models of depression that emphasize cognitive aspects of depression as well (e.g., Ellis, 1973; Ingram, 1984;

Pyszczynski and Greenberg, 1987; Rehm, 1977), we are focusing on Beck's model and the hopelessness theory because they are arguably the most extensively researched to date. We then review empirical studies that bear on these two theories of depression. In the last part of the chapter, we describe the role of cognition in therapy for depression, and discuss the efficacy and mechanisms of treatment based on a cognitive model of depression.

COGNITIVE MODELS OF DEPRESSION

Beck's Model of Depression

Beck's (1967) original formulation of depression grew from his observations of patients in psychoanalysis. He observed that when depressed patients spoke of themselves or their life circumstances they frequently distorted or biased these reports. In his cognitive model of depression, Beck (1967, 1976, 1987) asserts that negative cognitions are an intrinsic part of the depressive syndrome. According to Beck, depressed people are characterized by negative cognitive products. Cognitive products are the judgments and predictions that people make on an ongoing basis about themselves, others, or events in their lives. These products are accessible to the person who makes them, although they are not always "conscious" in the sense that the person is acutely aware of them as he or she makes them. Nonetheless, cognitive products are inferred from the report of the person who experiences them. The negative judgments depressed patients report are about themselves, their circumstances, and their futures. Beck (1967) has termed this the "negative cognitive triad." These negative thoughts are pervasive, and result in at least the partial exclusion of positive thoughts (Beck, 1987). They are also automatic in that the thoughts are "repetitive, persistent, and not readily controllable" (Beck, 1987, p. 7). According to the cognitive model, these negative cognitions result in the affective, behavioral, and somatic symptoms of depression.

Another central tenet of Beck's theory is that depressed people have negative cognitive schemata, also known as "basic beliefs" or "assumptions," that maintain their negative outlook, and are themselves maintained, even in the face of contradictory evidence. Cognitive schemata are defined as relatively stable knowledge structures that guide the processing of current incoming information. They are generalizations derived from past experience about a particular content domain that influence the perception, interpretation, and memory of stimuli relevant to that domain (Markus, 1977). Schema-driven processing is selective and automatic and can therefore enhance the efficiency of cognitive processing. However, one by-product of schematic processing is that cognitive distortions or errors can result.

In depression, dysfunctional schemata related to the person's self-concept and expectations are activated and produce systematic errors of thinking. Some of the distortions typically found in depressed people include: the tendency to think in extreme or absolute terms (all-or-none thinking); the tendency to draw negative conclusions in the absence of evidence to support the conclusions (arbitrary inference); the tendency to draw negative global conclusions on the basis of one fact or isolated incident (overgeneralization); the tendency to overemphasize the importance of negative events and to underemphasize the significance of positive experiences (magnification and minimization); and the tendency to focus on negative details and to base conclusions on the negative details while ignoring more important features of a situation (selective abstraction) (Beck, 1967, 1976, 1987). These cognitive distortions can produce and maintain the negative cognitive triad seen in depression.

Depressive schemata represent a stable cognitive diathesis or vulnerability to depression within the cognitive model. Schemata remain latent until the person encounters a schema-relevant stressor. For example, the dysfunctional schema "If everyone doesn't like me, I am worthless" could be activated by a romantic breakup. Likewise, the schema "If I am not successful in my work, then I am not worthwhile" could be triggered by a reprimand at work. Thus, events that impinge upon an individual's specific vulnerability are most likely to be depressive because they activate previously latent negative beliefs.

Beck (1987) has described two personality types that may predispose one to develop depression: the sociotropic type and the autonomous type. Sociotropic individuals are highly invested in their interpersonal relations, and thus value acceptance and affection. Autonomous people derive their sense of worth from acting independently and achieving meaningful goals. Thus, individuals high in sociotropy are hypothesized to be vulnerable to depression following interpersonal loss or conflict, whereas highly autonomous people are theorized to be at risk for depression following failure or setbacks in achievement-related domains, such as school or work. According to Beck's theory of depression, the depressogenic cognitive schemata comprising these personality types derive from early experiences, such as the loss of a parent or rejection by peers.

It is important to note that while Beck (1987) maintains that the negative cognitive processing observed in depression is found in all types of depression (e.g., unipolar, bipolar, melancholic, nonmelancholic), the etiological pathway outlined above is not. Specifically, the cognitive model speaks only to the etiology of nonmelancholic (or "reactive") major depression. In

addition, Beck's model asserts that the negative cognitive content characteristic of depression (e.g., themes of loss or deprivation) is specific to
depression and is not observed in other emotional disorders. Rather, each
disorder is associated with a distinct cognitive profile (e.g., Beck and
Emery, 1985).

Hopelessness Theory of Depression

The hopelessness theory of depression is a descendant of the "learned
helplessness theory" (Seligman, 1975), which was based on observations
made during animal learning experiments. Following inescapable shock,
animals subsequently placed in situations in which they could escape the
shock exhibited motivational, cognitive, and behavioral deficits. For example, they appeared unable to learn the behavior that would result in
escape from the shock and, indeed, appeared to "give up" prematurely in
their escape attempts. Since the initial documentation of these helplessness
effects, the basic finding has been replicated many times and extended to
humans as well (see Peterson and Seligman, 1984).

Noting parallels between helpless humans and animals and depressed
humans, Seligman and his colleagues began to explore the possibility that
the expectation that outcomes are noncontingent on one's behavior underlies both learned helplessness and at least some of the motivational, emotional, behavioral, and cognitive deficits seen in depression. However,
inadequacies in the original learned helplessness model of depression resulted in a reformulation of the theory. For example, if depressed people
consider themselves helpless, then why do they blame themselves for failures (Abramson and Sackeim, 1977)?

The reformulated learned helplessness model emphasized the way people explain to themselves the noncontingency between their behavior and
outcomes, rather than the perception and expectation of noncontingency
per se (Abramson et al., 1978). The revised version proposed that exhibiting an insidious attributional style predisposes a person to depression.
People prone to depression are said to: (1) attribute negative events to
internal, stable, and global factors; and (2) attribute positive outcomes to
external, unstable, and specific causes (Seligman et al., 1979).

More recently, in response to criticisms of the reformulated version of
the learned helplessness model and empirical work on attributional and
other cognitive aspects of depression, the theory has been revised once
more. The "hopelessness theory of depression" clarifies and elaborates
upon the earlier reformulation (Abramson et al., 1989). In the more recent
version of the theory, the authors propose an etiological account of the
development of "hopelessness depression," a hypothesized subtype of

depression. The concept of hopelessness, defined as "negative expectations about the occurrence of highly valued outcomes, and feelings of
helplessness about changing the likelihood of occurrence of these outcomes" (Abramson *et al.*, 1988, p. 7), figures prominently in the revised
theory.

According to the theory, hopelessness is a proximal and sufficient cause
of depression. That is, the presence of hopelessness guarantees that depressive symptoms will occur. Abramson *et al.* (1989) posit that there is a
chain of events that culminates in this proximal and sufficient cause of
depression. Each link in the chain is considered a "contributory cause" in
that it increases the probability that hopelessness depression will occur.
However, no link in the chain is necessary or sufficient. Initially, the occurrence of one or more negative life events sets the stage for the depression.
Inferences the person makes about the event affect the likelihood that the
person will become hopeless following the negative event. The critical
aspects of the inference concern: (1) the perceived cause of the event;
(2) the judged consequences of the event; and (3) the status of the self,
given that the event occurred.

More specifically, the theory predicts that when negative events are
attributed to stable and global causes and are also regarded as important,
hopelessness and hopelessness depression are more likely to occur than
when the events are attributed to unstable and specific factors or are considered unimportant. Similarly, the authors argue that the more stable and
global a person perceives the negative consequences of an event and the
negative characteristics of the self to be, the more likely the person is to
become hopeless and depressed. Moreover, for hopelessness depression to
occur, there should be a match between the particular content domain of
the individual's negative attributional style (e.g., for achievement-related
events) and the negative life event.

Thus, contrary to the 1978 reformulation of the learned helplessness
theory, whether the attributed cause is internal or external is not as important a determinant of whether hopelessness depression will occur as
whether the cause is stable and global (Abramson *et al.*, 1989). However,
Abramson and colleagues note that when the negative life events are attributed to internal, stable, and global factors, lowered self-esteem is also likely
to occur in addition to other symptoms of hopelessness depression.

According to the hopelessness theory of depression, distal factors influence whether a person makes stable and global inferences about the cause
and consequences of a negative event or about the self, thereby affecting
the likelihood that the person will become hopeless. Specifically, the authors posit that there are three cognitive diatheses for hopelessness depression: (1) the general tendency to make stable and global causal attributions

about negative life events and to consider such events important (i.e., a "hypothesized depressogenic attributional style," Abramson *et al.*, 1989, p. 362); (2) the general tendency to infer that a negative life event will have severely negative consequences; and (3) the general tendency to draw negative inferences about the self.

The hopelessness theory, then, represents an improvement over prior versions in that the central concepts and assertions are more clearly articulated. However, several key issues remain unaddressed in the present version of the theory. First, it does not delineate the relationship among the three cognitive diatheses described in the theory. For example, are people with a depressogenic attributional style especially prone to infer that negative events will have negative consequences, or to draw negative inferences about the self? Are the three cognitive styles independent of one another? The theory also fails to address what cognitive structures and processes underlie a person's attributional style. Is attributional style produced by an organized cognitive structure such as a schema?[1] The theory also does not specify the origin(s) of attributional style. Do early negative experiences promote the development of a depressogenic attributional style? Is parental attributional style an important determinant of an individual's attributional style? It is hoped that further refinements of the theory will address these important issues.

Comparison of the Models

One similarity shared by Beck's model and the hopelessness theory of depression is that they both posit the existence of a cognitive diathesis in vulnerable individuals. People with the relevant cognitive vulnerability are hypothesized to be more likely than those who lack the cognitive diathesis to develop a depressive syndrome when they encounter diathesis-relevant stress. In Beck's theory negative schemas constitute the cognitive diathesis, whereas in the hopelessness theory a negative attributional style renders people more at risk to develop depression following negative life events. A related similarity is that both theories contend that the depressogenic effect of the cognitive diatheses is especially likely to occur when a negative life event is congruent with a person's specific vulnerability, that is, when it occurs in the same content domain as the cognitive diathesis.

Another way in which the two theories are similar is that their etiological claims are restricted to nonmelancholic major depression. Also, both theories allow that biological factors may place an individual at risk for non-

---

[1] Power and Champion (1986) discuss other accounts of internal representations consistent with hopelessness theory. For example, associative network theory (Bower, 1981) or a theory of mental models (e.g., Johnson-Laird, 1983) could also accommodate findings of a depressotypic attributional style.

melancholic or other types of depression. In addition, the theories suggest that cognitive styles or structures shape the interpretation of incoming information and that these interpretations have affective, motivational, and behavioral consequences. In other words, they underscore the role of maladaptive inferences in depression. One final commonality is that both Beck's model and the hopelessness theory are virtually silent regarding the specific processes through which the cognitive diatheses develop.

An obvious difference between the two models is in their scope. Whereas Beck maintains that there are negative cognitive processes present in all depressions, irrespective of etiology, hopelessness theory addresses one hypothesized subtype of depression: hopelessness depression. Another important difference is that unlike Beck's theory, in which a negative bias in thinking is considered to be a fundamental, unique characteristic of depression, the hopelessness theory claims that both depressive and nondepressive cognition can be characterized by bias or accuracy. Further, as Abramson et al. (1989) point out, only hopelessness theory delineates protective factors for depressive symptoms (namely, the tendency to make unstable and specific attributions when explaining negative events).

However, as Coyne and Gotlib (1983) note, the differences between the two theories "are mainly matters of emphasis . . . Schematic and attributional analyses prove to be complementary in many situations" (p. 474). For example, as mentioned in the previous section, it may be that attributional style is one result of the operation of cognitive schemas. Thus, an apparent discrepancy between the two theories may actually be attributable to a difference in focus. Whereas Beck underscores the role of organized knowledge structures and their effect on information processing in his model, attributional theories highlight people's explanations of incoming information and the resultant affective, cognitive, and behavioral consequences of the explanations (Coyne and Gotlib, 1983).

EMPIRICAL STATUS OF THE COGNITIVE MODELS
OF DEPRESSION

In this section, we discuss studies relevant to Beck's cognitive model of depression and the hopelessness theory of depression. Our survey of the literature is not exhaustive; rather, our intent is to summarize the major findings relevant to the central tenets of both cognitive models of depression.[2] We will review evidence pertaining to the following issues in six

[2]Readers interested in a recent, comprehensive review of studies addressing Beck's model of depression are referred to Haaga et al. (1991). Readers are referred to Brewin (1985) and Sweeney et al. (1986) for recent reviews of the attributional style literature.

separate sections: (1) negative thinking in depression; (2) automaticity of depressive cognition; (3) schematic processing in depression; (4) cognitive biases and distortion in depression; (5) cognitive vulnerability to depression (i.e., the causal role of cognition in depression); and (6) the specificity of depressive cognition. Throughout the review we follow the recommendations of Kendall *et al.* (1987) in distinguishing between subjects who are clinically depressed and those who are dysphoric, since the generalizability of findings obtained using one type of sample to the other has yet to be established.

Negative Thinking in Depression

The assertion that depression is associated with an elevation in negative thinking, which is consistent with both Beck's model and the hopelessness theory, is strongly upheld by the available research literature. Several inventories, such as the Automatic Thoughts Questionnaire (Hollon and Kendall, 1980), the Crandell Cognitions Inventory (Crandell and Chambless, 1986), the Cognitions Checklist (Beck *et al.*, 1987), the Hopelessness Scale (HS; Beck *et al.*, 1974), and the Cognitive Style Test (Blackburn *et al.*, 1986b) have been developed to assess negative cognitions in depression. Studies using these inventories and others have found that depressed patients report: (1) more negative thoughts (e.g., Blackburn *et al.*, 1986b; Dobson and Shaw, 1986; Harrell and Ryon, 1983; Kendall *et al.*, 1989); (2) a more negative view of self (e.g., Beck *et al.*, 1990; Blackburn *et al.*, 1986b; Brown and Beck, 1989); (3) a more negative view of the world (e.g., Blackburn *et al.*, 1986b; Greenberg and Beck, 1989); and (4) a more negative view of the future (e.g., Abramson *et al.*, 1978; Blackburn *et al.*, 1986b; Dohr *et al.*, 1989; Hamilton and Abramson, 1983; Lam *et al.*, 1987; Lewinsohn *et al.*, 1981; Wilkinson and Blackburn, 1981) than do nondepressed controls.

In addition, several of these studies have found, using both between- and within-subject comparisons, that depressed patients are more negative in their thinking when they are depressed than when they are remitted (Blackburn *et al.*, 1986b; Dobson and Shaw, 1986; Dohr *et al.*, 1989; Eaves and Rush, 1984). The negative thoughts assessed by these instruments appear to be related to depressive symptoms, not only depressive disorder. Patients with depressive symptoms secondary to another psychiatric diagnosis also report such negative thinking (Hollon *et al.*, 1986; Ross *et al.*, 1986).

Automaticity of Depressive Cognition

Beck (1967) contends that not only do depressed people have negative cognitions, but that these cognitions arise automatically. Unfortunately, as

Moretti and Shaw (1989) point out, this assertion remains largely untested, especially as regards clinically depressed populations. This is because investigations of negative cognitions in depression have not, by and large, assessed the extent to which cognitive processing is unintentional or requires little attention (two hallmarks of automatic processing as traditionally defined in the cognitive psychology literature).

However, several studies using dysphoric college students do support the idea that processing of negative information is automatic in at least dysphoria (e.g., Bargh and Tota, 1988; Wenzlaff *et al.*, 1988). For example, in one study, Bargh and Tota (1988) asked dysphoric and nondepressed students to rate whether depressed- and nondepressed-content adjectives were self-descriptive. Half of the subjects were asked to remember six digits while completing the task; the remaining subjects were given no concurrent memory load. The extent to which the memory-load task increased the response latencies of the judgments was used as the index of the amount of attention the subjects needed to make the ratings. The assumption underlying the experimental manipulation is that the memory load task and the rating task both draw upon the same, limited pool of attentional resources. Self-constructs that are automatically activated do not draw heavily on the available pool of attentional resources, whereas constructs not automatically activated require more attentional resources. Thus, the memory-load task should have less impact on self-descriptiveness rating time when the rated material is automatically activated than when it is not automatically activated, because in the former case the rating task requires fewer attentional resources.

Bargh and Tota (1988) found that, among dysphoric subjects, the memory-load manipulation resulted in a *smaller* increase in self-descriptiveness rating time for the depressed-content than for the nondepressed-content words. That is, the self-rating task required less attention (i.e., appeared to be more automatic) when the material was negative than when it was positive. The reverse was true for nondepressed subjects. Among the nondepressed subjects, the concurrent load task resulted in a *larger* increase in response latencies for the depressed-content than for the nondepressed-content material. Thus, for dysphorics, fewer attentional resources are required when the self-referential material being processed is negative rather than positive; for nondepressives, on the other hand, fewer resources are required when processing positive rather than negative self-referential material. This pattern of findings is consistent with Beck's (1967) assertion that the negative self-referential thought in depression is automatic. However, conclusive evaluation of the status of this postulate must await further investigation with dysphoric and clinically depressed samples.

Schematic Processing in Depression

The concept of cognitive schemata is central to Beck's model of depression. As a consequence, there has been an abundance of research into their role in depression. In spite of this, the extent to which the idiosyncratic and biased information processing exhibited by depressives is attributable to the operation of cognitive schemata remains indeterminate. For example, paper-and-pencil measures such as the Dysfunctional Attitudes Scale (DAS; Weissman and Beck, 1978), which were developed to assess depressive schemata, have successfully distinguished between depressed patients and normal and psychiatric control subjects (e.g., Hamilton and Abramson, 1983; Hollon *et al.*, 1986; Reda, 1984). These findings and other similar ones have often been interpreted as demonstrating "the prominence of negative self-schemata in depressive states" (e.g., Clark and Beck, 1989, p. 390). However, as noted by Coyne and Gotlib (1986), this argument is circular: "Depressed persons make negative verbalizations because of the operation of hyperactive negative schemata, and we know this because they make negative verbalizations" (p. 698). Thus, without external referents, these studies must be considered weak evidence for the existence of schematic processing in depression.

Another problem impeding research in this area is the fact that while much of the evidence accumulated to date is, indeed, consistent with a schematic account, it is also compatible with alternative explanations. This is seen, for example, in studies that employ a self-referent encoding task (SRET). In this task, subjects are given a list of positive, neutral, and negative trait adjectives and are asked to make a decision about whether each adjective is self-descriptive. Subjects are later presented with an incidental recall or recognition task. The assumption in these studies is that a person's self-schema will determine, in part: (1) which adjectives are judged to be self-referent by the individual; (2) the response latencies of the judgments; and (3) memory for the trait adjectives.

In general, these studies find that depressed subjects recall more negative than positive adjectives. In contrast, nondepressed control subjects recall more positive than negative adjectives (Bradley and Mathews, 1983; Derry and Kuiper, 1981; Dunbar and Lishman, 1984; Kuiper and Mac-Donald, 1983). In addition, decision latencies are shorter for clinically depressed subjects when rating negative trait adjectives than when rating positive trait adjectives, whereas nondepressed control subjects are quicker for the positive adjectives (MacDonald and Kuiper, 1984). These findings are consistent with the notion that the processing of schema-congruent material is facilitated (Kuiper and MacDonald, 1982).

While SRET results *may* be generated by a stable cognitive self-structure or schema in which self-relevant information is organized and interrelated, there is another equally plausible interpretation of the results. It could be that subjects' mood simply renders certain constructs more accessible and that this increased accessibility accounts for the enhanced memory for and efficient processing of mood-congruent words (Segal, 1988). Since the depressed subjects are in a sad mood, they will show preferential recall for hedonically negative adjectives; conversely, the nondepressed will preferentially recall hedonically positive words. The constructs need not be organized or interrelated in a self-structure to produce these effects; there is no need to posit the activation of a cognitive structure to explain these results.

In addition, the common practice of using response latencies as an index of efficient or automatic processing is problematic. Bargh and Tota (1988) have argued that several factors may affect response times:

> One cannot tell from the latency alone how much of it was due to the (relatively automatic) construct activation stage and how much of it was due to the (relatively attentional) decision and response selection stage. . . . The contribution of the attention-demanding response selection stage varies as a function of situation-specific goals and strategies. . . . self-presentational forces within the experimental situation may well influence response times. (p. 929)

Yet another problem for schema research is the lack of consensus regarding the definition of the schema construct and the lack of precision with which the term "schema" is often used in the depression literature (Coyne and Gotlib, 1986; Power and Champion, 1986). Segal (1988) cogently argues that conceptual and methodological problems such as those just discussed have precluded the unambiguous demonstration of schematic processing. Until these conceptual and design-related issues are resolved, the role of cognitive self-schemata in depression will remain unclear.

Cognitive Bias and Distortion in Depression

A core postulate of Beck's model of depression is that what underlies the depressed person's negative self- and world-view is a tendency to distort reality in a negative manner. Much empirical evidence has accrued in support of this contention (e.g., Buchwald, 1977; DeMonbreun and Craighead, 1977; Dobson, 1989b; Dykman *et al.*, 1989, schema-discriminating condition; Gotlib, 1983). Moreover, clinical observations are consistent with this idea (e.g., Beck, 1967, 1976).

However, Alloy and Abramson (1979) have challenged this view. They presented dysphoric and nondepressed students with one of a series of contingency problems that varied in the actual degree of contingency. The subject's task was to estimate the degree of contingency between his/her responses (pressing or not pressing a button) and an environmental outcome (onset of a green light). Whereas the dysphoric students' judgments of contingency were rather accurate, the nondepressed students over- or underestimated the response–outcome contingency in several experimental conditions. For example, nondepressed subjects exhibited an "illusion of control" when they actually had no control, if the green light onset was frequent (75%–75% condition, Experiment 2) or was associated with success (winning money, Experiment 3). Also, nondepressed subjects underestimated their control when they actually had 50% control, if the absence of the green light onset was associated with failure (losing money, Experiment 4). Alloy and Abramson (1979) concluded that it is *non*depressed individuals who are biased and that depression may involve the *lack* of a *positive* bias.

Many of Alloy and Abramson's (1979) findings of "depressive realism" have since been replicated (Alloy and Abramson, 1982; Alloy *et al.*, 1985, Experiment 3; Alloy *et al.*, 1981, no mood induction condition; Benassi and Mahler, 1985, Experiment 1; Martin *et al.*, 1984, self-condition) and extended (Alloy and Abramson, 1982; Alloy and Clements, 1992; Mikulincer *et al.*, 1990, high-threat/no-mirror condition; Vazquez, 1987; but see Ackermann, 1988, and Bryson *et al.*, 1984, for failures to replicate the basic finding). In addition, evidence consistent with the notion that depressives and dysphorics are more realistic than nondepressives in their perceptions and inferences has been generated by studies that have not employed the contingency judgment paradigm (e.g., Campbell, 1986; Golin *et al.*, 1979).

Several authors have recently reviewed the depressive realism/distortion literature and suggested that, contrary to Beck's assertions, depressed people are more accurate in their perceptions and judgments than their nondepressed counterparts, who more frequently make distorted or positively biased judgments (e.g., Alloy and Abramson, 1988; Taylor and Brown, 1988). However, in a critical review of the literature, Ackermann and DeRubeis (1991) argue that such a conclusion is premature for several reasons. First, most of the studies within the depressive realism literature have used only dysphoric, not clinically depressed, individuals. The possibility that dysphoric individuals are more realistic than *both* severely depressed and nondepressed people has not been ruled out. That is, it may be that depressed moods are associated with *negative biases*, nondepressed moods are associated with *positive biases*, and dysphoric moods are associated with a relative *lack* of biases. To date, this possibility has not been adequately tested.

Second, many studies investigating depressive realism/distortion have utilized abstract laboratory tasks that seem to bear little relation to the matters clinicians believe depressed individuals distort in daily life (see Dobson and Franche, 1989, for a further discussion of this point). Third, many of the findings alleged to be in support of the depressive realism hypothesis come from studies in which the distortion (or accuracy) of subjects cannot be ascertained. This is because the procedures used in these studies lack an objective standard against which to compare subjects' judgments. For example, in one of the most frequently cited examples of depressive realism, a study conducted by Lewinsohn *et al.* (1980), depressed patients, nondepressed psychiatric patients, and nondepressed nonpsychiatric controls participated in several group discussions. Following each session, subjects were asked to provide ratings of their social skills; these ratings were compared with those made by trained observers who evaluated the subjects on the same social attributes. Whereas the control subjects evaluated themselves more positively than the observers did, the depressives' relatively lower self-ratings were not significantly discrepant from the observers' evaluations. The interpretation set forth by the investigators was that the depressives lacked the "illusory glow" exhibited by the nondepressives.

However, it is noteworthy that the subjects' task in this study was *not* to estimate how the observers would rate them; rather, subjects were asked to provide their own evaluation of their performance in the group discussions. We argue that the observers' ratings do not provide an objective standard of comparison (see also Ackermann and DeRubeis, 1991). In addition, as several authors have noted, an alternative explanation for the results obtained is that trained observers are prone to being particularly tough or critical in their evaluations of subjects (Ackermann and DeRubeis, 1991; Coyne and Gotlib, 1983). If this is the case, then in the Lewinsohn *et al.* (1980) study, the similarity between the depressives' and the observers' ratings may have been a function of the depressives' low self-ratings coinciding with the observers' harsh standards, rather than of realistic self-perceptions on the depressives' part. Indeed, there is some empirical support for this alternative view of the Lewinsohn *et al.* (1980) data (see Campbell and Fehr, 1990; Gotlib and Meltzer, 1987). In our own discussion of the depressive realism/distortion literature, we will not consider studies that do not allow for an assessment of accuracy (see also Dobson and Franche, 1989).

When one considers only those studies that do include an objective standard of comparison, one finds that the results are relatively mixed — findings from an almost equal number of studies support depressive realism and depressive distortion hypotheses. A consistent pattern emerges from the literature: the results obtained appear to vary as a function of the type of task used in the studies (Ackermann and DeRubeis, 1991). That is, different experimental methods have consistently produced different results. This pattern of findings is evident in Table 4.1, which summarizes the findings from depressive realism studies that do allow for an assessment of accuracy.

As noted earlier, the findings generated by studies using the contingency judgment paradigm, by and large, provide evidence of depressive realism (or at least, "dysphoric realism" — no contingency judgment studies have yet been reported using clinically depressed patients). In addition, experiments investigating subjects' judgments about themselves and other individuals (i.e., self–other studies) have also tended to support the notion that the inferences made by depressed and dysphoric individuals are generally more even-handed than the judgments made by nondepressed people (Alloy and Ahrens, 1987; Campbell, 1986; Golin *et al.*, 1977; Golin *et al.*, 1979; Hoehn-Hyde *et al.*, 1982; Martin *et al.*, 1984; Wenzlaff and Berman, 1988). For example, when presented with evaluative feedback, such as personality test results, that is ostensibly about themselves and with equivalent information that is purportedly about another person, nondepressed subjects tend to evaluate the "self-relevant" information in a more favorable light than the "other-relevant" information (e.g., Wenzlaff and Berman, 1988). Dysphoric subjects, on the other hand, are more even-handed in their judgments; they rate the equivalent information as being equally favorable in the self- and other-relevant conditions. Similarly, when making predictions regarding their own and other students' academic success, nondepressed students tend to be overly optimistic in their predictions about their own success, relative to their predictions for other similar students. That is, even when other students have credentials identical to the subject's (e.g., same Scholastic Aptitude Test scores and grade point average), nondepressed students tend to predict a more positive academic outcome for themselves than they do for similar others (Alloy and Ahrens, 1987).

In contrast to results from the aforementioned paradigms, studies examining subjects' recall of self-evaluative information provide evidence of depressive distortion. For example, results from several studies suggest that dysphoric and depressed subjects negatively distort their memory for self-relevant evaluative information. They misremember personality feedback as being more negative than was actually the case (Gotlib, 1983), and they recall less positive feedback than was actually received on an experimental task (Buchwald, 1977; Dennard and Hokanson, 1986, moderately dysphoric group, 25% reward condition; Dykman *et al.*, 1989, schema-

TABLE 4.1 Depressive Realism Findings from Studies That Allow for an Assessment of Accuracy[a]

Type of sample[b]	Dysphoric or depressed subjects inaccurate	Nondepressed subjects inaccurate
	Contingency judgment[c]	
Dysphoric		Alloy and Abramson (1979)
		Experiments 2, 3, and 4
		Alloy and Abramson (1982)
		Alloy et al. (1985)
		Experiment 3
		Alloy et al. (1981)
	Benassi and Mahler (1985)[d]	Benassi and Mahler (1985)
	Experiment 1, observer condition, and Experiments 2 and 3	Experiment 1, private condition
	Martin et al. (1984)	Martin et al. (1984)
	confederate condition	self-condition
	Mikulincer et al. (1990)	Mikulincer et al. (1990)
	mirror conditions	high-threat/no-mirror condition
	Vazquez (1987)	Vazquez (1987)
	Experiment 4	Experiments 2 and 3
	Self–Other[g]	
Dysphoric		Alloy and Ahrens (1987)
		Campbell (1986)
	Golin et al. (1977)	Golin et al. (1977)
	Martin et al. (1984)	Martin et al. (1984)
		Wenzlaff and Berman (1988)
Depressed		Golin et al. (1979)[h]
		Hoehn-Hyde et al. (1982)[e]
	Recall of evaluative information	
Dysphoric		
	Buchwald (1977)	
	Dennard and Hokanson (1986)	Dennard and Hokanson (1986)
	moderately dysphoric, 25% reward condition	75% reward condition
	Dykman et al. (1989)	
	schema-discriminating condition	
	Kennedy and Craighead (1988)	Kennedy and Craighead (1988)
	positive feedback condition	nondepressed-nonanxious S's, negative feedback condition
	Kuiper (1978)[e]	
	55% reward condition	
	Nelson and Craighead (1977)	Nelson and Craighead (1977)
	70% reward condition	30% punishment condition
Depressed		
	Gotlib (1981)	
	Gotlib (1983)	

(table continues)

TABLE 4.1   *Continued*

Type of sample[b]	Dysphoric or depressed subjects inaccurate	Nondepressed subjects inaccurate
	Interpersonal impact	
Dysphoric		
	Culp (1991)	
	Dobson (1989b)	
	Gotlib and Meltzer (1987)	
	Siegel and Alloy (1990)	Siegel and Alloy (1990)
	female subjects	
Depressed		
	Hokanson *et al.* (1991)	Hokanson *et al.* (1991) nondepressed pathology subjects[f]

[a]Only studies in which there is a statistically reliable difference in accuracy between the depressed or dysphoric group and the nondepressed controls are included in this table.
[b]Studies are broken down on the basis of whether dysphoric or clinically depressed subjects comprised the "depressed" sample.
[c]There are no studies of clinically depressed subjects using this paradigm.
[d]In this study, dysphoric subjects *overestimated* control; in all other experiments in the table, inaccuracy refers to a bias against the self for dysphoric or depressed subjects, or a bias for the self for nondepressed subjects.
[e]The proper statistical comparison was not reported; inaccuracy is inferred from reported means.
[f]This study also included a nondepressed nonpsychiatric control group whose estimates were not positively biased.
[g]For the self–other studies, "inaccurate" refers to discrepant self- and other judgments.
[h]Nondepressed sample comprised schizophrenics; all other nondepressed samples comprised nonpatients.

discriminating condition; Gotlib, 1981; Kennedy and Craighead, 1988; Kuiper, 1978, 55% reward condition; Nelson and Craighead, 1977, 70% reward condition). Nondepressed subjects, on the other hand, tend to be relatively accurate in their recall of self-relevant evaluative information in these same experiments.

Experiments investigating dysphoric and nondepressed subjects' self-evaluations of their interpersonal impact have also yielded evidence of dysphoric distortion and nondepressive accuracy. In these studies, dysphoric or depressed and nondepressed targets interact with nondepressed judges and are subsequently asked to estimate how well they (the targets) were liked by the judges.[3] The targets' estimates are then compared with

[3]An alternative, more naturalistic variant of this procedure involves asking dysphoric/depressed and nondepressed targets to either: (1) estimate their roommate's acceptance or rejection of them (Siegel and Alloy, 1990); or (2) recall the amount of positive/negative behaviors a roommate has emitted toward the target within a given period of time (Hokanson *et al.*, 1991).

the judges' actual ratings of the targets. In general, dysphoric and depressed targets tend to underestimate how well they were liked (Culp, 1991; Dobson, 1989b; Hokanson *et al.*, 1991; Siegel and Alloy, 1990), whereas nondepressed targets tend to be accurate in their estimates (Culp, 1991; Dobson, 1989b; Hokanson *et al.*, 1991).

In sum, evidence garnered from studies investigating cognitive biases and distortions in depression that do include an objective standard of comparison in their experimental design (i.e., that allow for an assessment of accuracy) suggest that whether depressed or nondepressed subjects are accurate varies as a function of the type of task used. Thus, Beck's contention that depression is associated with cognitive distortions has met with mixed support. When asked to evaluate their own interpersonal impact or to recall self-relevant evaluative information, dysphoric and depressed subjects display negative distortions, underestimate how well they are liked, and underrecall how well they have performed. However, when estimating control or rating themselves and other people, they appear to lack the optimistic, positive biases exhibited by their nondepressed counterparts. Unfortunately, on the basis of the available evidence, it is not clear why such a pattern would be obtained (see Ackermann and DeRubeis, 1991, for a discussion of several possible explanations).

Cognitive Vulnerability to Depression

The fact that depressed patients report more frequent negative thoughts than do nondepressed people is important, but it does not tell us whether, or in what sense, these thoughts might be causally related to depression. There has been much debate on this point (see Coyne and Gotlib, 1983, 1986; Segal and Shaw, 1986). There are at least two senses in which cognitions may play a causal role in the development of depression. First, it may be that holding certain beliefs or employing certain cognitive styles increases the probability that one will experience depression. That is, they may act as a risk factor. This is represented in Beck's model by schemata, and in the hopelessness theory by attributional style. There have been numerous attempts to identify people who hold these beliefs independent of, or prior to, depressive episodes. The cognitive measures most frequently examined as possible markers of depression proneness are the Dysfunctional Attitudes Scale (Weissman and Beck, 1978) and the Attributional Style Questionnaire (Seligman *et al.*, 1979), although the Automatic Thoughts Questionnaire (Hollon and Kendall, 1980) and the Hopelessness Scale (Beck *et al.*, 1974) are often used as well. As reviewed by Barnett and Gotlib (1988b), Haaga *et al.* (1991), and Brewin (1985), in the majority of studies these measures have behaved like concomitants of depressive symptoms rather than indicators of depression proneness (Blackburn and Bishop, 1983; Blackburn and Smyth, 1985; Cochran and Hammen, 1985; Dobson and Shaw, 1986, for dysfunctional attitudes; Dohr *et al.*, 1989; Hamilton and Abramson, 1983; Hollon *et al.*, 1986; Lewinsohn *et al.*, 1981; Manley *et al.*, 1982; O'Hara *et al.*, 1984; Rush *et al.*, 1986; Silverman *et al.*, 1984; Simons *et al.*, 1984; Wilkinson and Blackburn, 1981), although there are intriguing exceptions (e.g., Cutrona, 1983; Dobson and Shaw, 1986, for negative automatic thoughts; Metalsky *et al.*, 1982; Metalsky, Halberstadt, and Abramson, 1987; O'Hara *et al.*, 1982; Peterson *et al.*, 1981; Rholes *et al.*, 1985, for hopelessness cognitions; Zuroff *et al.*, 1990).

Several writers have recently argued that the existing research has not adequately tested the vulnerability hypotheses proposed in both Beck's model and the hopelessness theory. For example, Miranda and Persons (1988) have proposed that only under certain conditions will an otherwise latent cognitive vulnerability be observed in a person who is not in a depressive episode. They have argued that such a vulnerability can be exposed when the person is in a sad mood; when in a good mood, a vulnerable individual will not report dysfunctional beliefs. In one study they found that the scores of formerly depressed patients on the Dysfunctional Attitudes Scale were related to a measure of current mood state (Miranda *et al.*, 1990). That is, for these subjects, sadness of mood correlated with report of dysfunctional beliefs. No such relation was found among never depressed subjects. Miranda *et al.* interpreted this finding as supportive of the *mood-state hypothesis*, that is, that the endorsement of dysfunctional beliefs depends on the current mood state of the subject, but only among individuals vulnerable to depression.

Abramson *et al.* (1988) have also criticized the use of simple comparisons between depressed and nondepressed subjects on relevant cognitive variables in the absence of information regarding subjects' life stressors. They argue that this is a critical omission given that both cognitive theories are diathesis-*stress* theories. Vulnerable individuals are not predicted to develop depressive symptoms in the absence of negative life events. Rather, it is the *interaction* between cognitive vulnerability and negative life events that is expected to predict the development of depression. Studies specifically testing for the interaction between cognitive vulnerability and negative life events have provided mixed evidence regarding the cognitive-diathesis stress theories. Whereas some results have supported their assertions (e.g., Kwon and Oei, 1992; Metalsky *et al.*, 1987; Olinger *et al.*, 1987), others have not (e.g., Barnett and Gotlib, 1990; Hammen *et al.*, 1985a; Robins and Block, 1989; Robins *et al.*, 1990) or have provided mixed results (Barnett and Gotlib, 1988a; Hammen *et al.*, 1989a; Robins and Block, 1988; Wise and Barnes, 1986).

Moreover, both Beck and the hopelessness theory assert that depression is more likely to occur when there is a match between an individual's "specific vulnerability" and the negative life events that are experienced. Researchers are now beginning to attend to this issue in their tests of the diathesis-stress component of cognitive theories of depression. Several studies have produced at least partial support for the claim that the congruence between vulnerability and negative life events predicts onset or exacerbation of depressive symptoms among vulnerable individuals (e.g., Hammen *et al.*, 1989a, b; Hammen *et al.*, 1985b; Olinger *et al.*, 1987; Segal *et al.*, 1992).

There is a second sense in which cognitions may be considered causal. In addition to acting as a risk factor for depression, they are also hypothesized to be a *proximal* cause of depression or depressed mood in both Beck's model and in the hopelessness theory. That is, both theories say that depressed mood will result from the experience of negative inferences about the self, world, or future. This is a difficult hypothesis to test, of course, because thoughts cannot be manipulated directly. Perhaps the best evidence that cognition is causal in this sense are the studies that have successfully induced mood using the Velten (1968) procedure. In the Velten procedure, subjects are asked to read a series of depressing statements to themselves, and to concentrate on their content. The Velten procedure has been shown to engender negative moods (Velten, 1968), although the means through which it produces mood change is unclear. As noted by Beidel and Turner (1986), while it may be the case that the negative cognitions used in the studies cause the negative mood, subjects are instructed to concentrate on acquiring a mood, not just on the cognitions. This leaves open the possibility that subjects are using methods other than focusing on the negative statements to induce the negative mood. Thus, while the preponderance of evidence in the cognitive vulnerability to depression literature does not support the role of cognitive factors as risk factors, recent investigations using more refined methodologies have begun to generate positive findings. The evidence concerning the role of cognition as a proximal cause of depression has fared somewhat better, though interpretation of these findings remains ambiguous.

The Specificity of Depressive Cognition

The extent to which the cognitive products and processes observed in depression are specific to depression or are also found in other types of psychopathology has received considerable attention in the research literature. Many studies have used self-report measures to compare the cognitive products of clinically depressed patients, nondepressed psychiatric patients (with various diagnoses), and normal controls, and have found that the depressed patients generally score higher than the other groups on the Automatic Thoughts Questionnaire (e.g., Dobson and Shaw, 1986; Harrell and Ryon, 1983; Hollon *et al.*, 1986; Kendall *et al.*, 1989) and on the Crandell Cognitions Inventory (Crandell and Chambless, 1986). Similarly, studies using the Hopelessness Scale have found that depressed patients are more hopeless about the future than nondepressed psychiatric patients (Abramson *et al.*, 1978; Beck *et al.*, 1988; Brown and Beck, 1989; Hamilton and Abramson, 1983), anxious patients (Beck *et al.* 1988; Blackburn *et al.*, 1986b; Brown and Beck, 1989; Clark *et al.*, 1989), and normal controls (Abramson *et al.*, 1978; Hamilton and Abramson, 1983). In addition, depressed patients score higher than anxious patients on the Cognitive Style Test, which was designed to assess the negative cognitive triad as described by Beck (1967) (Blackburn *et al.*, 1986b).[4] While anxiety disorder patients receive higher scores than depressed patients on the anxiety subscale of the Cognitions Checklist, depressed patients receive higher scores on the depression subscale than anxious patients (Beck *et al.*, 1987; Clark *et al.*, 1989). The Dysfunctional Attitudes Scale, a measure designed to assess depressive schemata, does not appear to measure cognitions specific to the depressive syndrome; rather, it reflects cognitions relevant to more general psychopathology (Hollon *et al.*, 1986).

Other studies have asked subjects to indicate whether depressed-content and nondepressed-content adjectives are self-descriptive. These studies have generally found that depressed patients are less willing than nondepressed psychiatric patients (Derry and Kuiper, 1981; Dobson and Shaw, 1987; Roth and Rehm, 1980), anxious patients (Greenberg and Beck, 1989), nondepressed-nonanxious patients (Greenberg and Beck, 1989), and normal controls (Derry and Kuiper, 1981; Dobson and Shaw, 1987; Greenberg and Beck, 1989) to endorse nondepressed-content adjectives as being self-descriptive. Depressed patients are also more willing than nondepressed psychiatric patients (Derry and Kuiper, 1981; Dobson and Shaw, 1987; Greenberg and Beck, 1989), anxiety disorder patients (Greenberg and Beck, 1989), and normal controls (Derry and Kuiper, 1981; Dobson and Shaw, 1987) to endorse depressed-content adjectives as being self-descriptive. In addition, they are more likely to recall self-referent depressed-content adjectives than nondepressed psychiatric patients (Derry and Kuiper, 1981), anxious patients (Greenberg and Beck, 1989), and normal controls (Derry and Kuiper, 1981; Greenberg and Beck, 1989). Thus, studies using clinical samples generally provide evidence consistent with the notion that the cognitive products typically observed in depression are specific to the depressive syndrome.

[4]Note, however, that this finding was obtained only when age was statistically controlled (Blackburn *et al.*, 1986b).

Evidence derived from student samples provides partial support for the notion that dysphoria and anxiety are associated with distinct cognitive products. For example, compared to anxious and nondepressed-nonanxious students, dysphoric students report more negative, self-referent thoughts (Ingram *et al.*, 1987). They are also more willing to endorse negative, depression-relevant trait adjectives as being self-descriptive (Greenberg and Alloy, 1989). Dysphoric students also recall more depressed- than anxious-content trait adjectives and more depressed-content material relative to test-anxious and nondepressed-nonanxious controls (Ingram *et al.*, 1987). Analogously, test-anxious students recall more anxious- than depressed-content information and more anxious-content words than do dysphoric or nondepressed-nonanxious subjects (Ingram *et al.*, 1987).

Dysphoric students are also faster than anxious students in making self-descriptiveness judgments for negative depression-relevant trait adjectives (Greenberg and Alloy, 1989). In addition, dysphoric students display equivalent reaction times when rating negative depression- and anxiety-relevant words, whereas anxious students rate negative anxiety-relevant traits more quickly than negative depression-relevant words (Greenberg and Alloy, 1989). Also, whereas anxious and nondepressed-nonanxious students employ greater speed in rating positive words than when they rate negative adjectives, dysphorics' reaction times do not differ for positive versus negative trait words (Greenberg and Alloy, 1989). Thus, the studies of analogue populations provide evidence consistent with the content-specificity hypothesis in that the dysphoric and anxious students have shown differential patterns of trait endorsement, recall, and rating times.

However, there also appears to be some similarity between cognitions associated with dysphoria and those related to anxiety. For example, loss cognitions are related to both types of distress (Rholes *et al.*, 1985). Both dysphoric and anxious students are more likely to endorse negative, anxiety-relevant adjectives and less willing to endorse positive depression- and anxiety-relevant adjectives relative to nondepressed-nonanxious controls (Greenberg and Alloy, 1989). Dysphoric and anxious students are also equivalent in the speed with which they rate negative anxiety-relevant words for self-descriptiveness (Greenberg and Alloy, 1989). Thus, dysphoric and anxious students can sometimes, but not always, be distinguished from one another on the basis of their cognitive products and processes.

Summary of Empirical Evidence

Several conclusions may be drawn from our review of the empirical literature. First, there is ample evidence that depressed persons exhibit negative thinking relative to nondepressed individuals. Second, the negative thinking displayed by depressed people is distinguishable from the negative cognitive content observed in other psychopathological conditions such as anxiety. This finding is qualified, however, by evidence suggesting that while dysphoria and subclinical anxiety are distinguishable to a certain extent, there is some overlap between the two states as well. Third, the negative cognitive products observed in depression are related to the depressive syndrome, and not just major depressive disorder. Fourth, the automaticity of the negative thoughts in depression remains to be established. Fifth, while there is evidence consistent with the hypothesis that schematic processing plays an important role in depression, results obtained thus far have not ruled out alternative interpretations of the data, so that the status of the schema construct in depression remains equivocal. Sixth, the issue of whether depressed people distort reality also remains unresolved due to contradictory evidence. Finally, the causal role of cognitions in depression has received little support to date; however, the adequacy of many strategies that have been employed to test the vulnerability hypothesis has been questioned. More research attending to: (1) the congruence between negative life events and specific vulnerability to depression, and (2) the mood-state dependency of the endorsement of dysfunctional attitudes among vulnerable individuals is required before an adequate resolution of this issue can be obtained.

THE ROLE OF COGNITION IN TREATMENT

Cognition as the Target of Treatment

First described by Beck in 1967, and elaborated and refined in subsequent writings (Beck, 1976; Beck *et al.*, 1979), cognitive therapy of depression has become a widely taught and extensively researched treatment approach.[5] In the cognitive therapy of depression, emphasis is placed on cognitive products and processes. From the first treatment session, patients are encouraged to consider that behind every bad mood is a negative inference. Early on in treatment, patients are taught to attend to these inferences and, preferably, to record them systematically. The aim of treatment, then, is to challenge these inferences on the assumption that, if examined critically, most upsetting inferences will prove faulty in some respect. They can then be replaced with more sound ones.

Often in the course of therapy the automatic thoughts themselves seem quite valid and appropriate. For example, a patient who delivered an ill-prepared lecture found herself thinking, "They (the audience) hated my

[5]Readers interested in detailed summaries of treatment procedures used in cognitive therapy of depression are referred to Beck *et al.* (1979), Fennell (1989), Hollon and Beck (1979), or Ackermann-Engel (1992).

lecture," which was upsetting. Although this characterization seemed a bit exaggerated, it was agreed that the audience probably was not impressed by the lecture, and that anyone with high but reasonable standards would be disappointed by the performance. However, what appeared to be responsible for her extreme emotional reaction were her inferences about her lecturing abilities ("I'm a terrible lecturer") as well as her future as a lecturer ("I'll never be any good"). Only when these "hidden" inferences were discerned could they be examined and revised. And only then did she report mood improvement from the cognitive work.

In cognitive therapy, a given intervention is not considered successful unless it has resulted in mood change, or it is determined that the emotional reaction was appropriate to the circumstances. In this sense, although it might be said that the target of treatment is mood change, the cognitive therapist assumes that mood change is never achieved directly, so that it cannot be the target of intervention, per se. Instead, mood is the barometer, whereas beliefs are the target of examination and change.

Research on Cognitive Therapy for Depression

Perhaps the most critical factor in the sustained interest in cognitive models of depression has been the success of the therapy that is linked to them. Findings from numerous studies have provided evidence that cognitive therapy is an effective treatment approach for outpatient, nonbipolar depression. This literature has been reviewed recently by Dobson (1989a) and by Hollon et al. (1991).

The most compelling evidence for the effectiveness of cognitive therapy for clinically depressed patients is that its ability to reduce symptoms rapidly has compared favorably in direct tests against antidepressant medication treatment. There have been at least five well-conducted studies in which adult outpatients were randomly assigned to antidepressants versus cognitive therapy, and in four of those, cognitive therapy proved at least as powerful as the medication regime against which it was compared (Blackburn et al., 1981; Hollon et al., 1992; Murphy et al., 1984; Rush et al., 1977). In only one major study has cognitive therapy showed any sign of being less effective than the medication against which it was compared, and in that study the difference was not statistically reliable (Elkin et al., 1989). Antidepressant medications have been chosen as comparison treatments because of their status as standard, well-proven treatments for depression.

However, as Hollon et al. (1990) point out, most of the medication versus cognitive therapy comparisons have not also included a minimal treatment control group, due largely to the ethical concerns of the investigators. Instead, they have relied on the assumption that antidepressant medications are generally effective for the populations studied. When cognitive therapy has proved to be equal to medications, the inference has been made that cognitive therapy has been effective in an absolute sense in the absence of proof that the medications have themselves been effective in these studies. Nonetheless, there is sufficient evidence to conclude that, on average, cognitive therapy is as effective as antidepressant medications in the treatment of depressed outpatients.

Because depression is an episodic disorder that tends to recur even after most successful treatments, the ability of a treatment to maintain gains is especially critical. Cognitive therapy appears to have this capacity. Results from four follow-up studies of cognitive therapy versus medication suggest that cognitive therapy is better than an equivalent short-term antidepressant medication treatment for the prevention of relapse in the year or two following treatment termination (Blackburn *et al.*, 1986a; Evans *et al.*, 1992; Kovacs *et al.*, Rush, 1981; Simons *et al.*, 1986).

The clinical utility of cognitive therapy, then, has been demonstrated. But how does it work? Does it produce cognitive change that other antidepressant treatments do not? Does it achieve its symptom reduction or prevention effects through cognitive change, as is presumed? This has been an especially difficult set of questions for researchers to tackle. Some have speculated that cognitive therapy has effects on cognitive processes that are indistinguishable from those of antidepressant medications, and that cognitive change plays no special role in cognitive therapy relative to pharmacotherapy (Beck, 1984; Simons, 1984; Simons *et al.*, 1984). In fact, there is little evidence that specific cognitive changes are induced by cognitive therapy over and above what results from pharmacotherapy (but see DeRubeis *et al.*, 1989, for an exception). One explanation that has been proposed is that cognitive and physiological change are reciprocally causal, so that producing change in either system will result in change in the other system. According to this explanation, differences in cognition between cognitive therapy and pharmacotherapy would not be expected, even if the two treatments work through different causal mechanisms. Hollon *et al.* (1987) have termed this possible state of affairs "causal specificity/ consequential nonspecificity." They argue that one cannot infer from a lack of difference on cognitive variables at the end of treatment that change in cognition is not the means through which cognitive therapy uniquely achieves its clinical effects. Thus, even if cognitive-therapy-treated patients' cognitions are indistinguishable from pharmacotherapy-treated patients' cognitions at the end of therapy, it may be that cognition is a causal factor in cognitive therapy, but is only a consequence of change in pharmacotherapy.

Are cognitive therapy patients truly indistinguishable from drug-treated patients at the end of therapy? They shouldn't be, if the relapse prevention effect observed for cognitive therapy is valid. That is, if at the end of treatment, cognitive-therapy-treated patients are less vulnerable to relapse than are drug-treated patients, there must be a characteristic that makes them less vulnerable. That characteristic might not be measurable or observable, but it must exist. It need not be "cognitive," but it is difficult to imagine "noncognitive" characteristics that are changed more in cognitive therapy than in drug therapy and are responsible for the relapse prevention effect. Therefore, the research question becomes, "What is the cognitive characteristic, and how can it be measured?"

In one investigation, attributional style (as measured by the Attributional Style Questionnaire) evidenced more change in patients who remitted in cognitive therapy than in patients who were equally remitted in pharmacotherapy (DeRubeis et al., 1989). Moreover, change in attributional style was a powerful predictor of relapse in that study (Hollon et al., 1990). Thus, it performed as one would expect from a cognitive mediator of relapse prevention. There have not, as yet, been any attempts to replicate this finding. In addition, an issue that remains unclear in the current literature is what change in attributional style represents. As Barber and DeRubeis (1989) have discussed, it may reflect change in schemata, or it could instead represent the acquisition of skills taught in cognitive therapy.

In sum, cognitive therapy is an efficacious treatment of depression not only in the short term but in the long run as well. The mechanism(s) through which it achieves its antidepressive and prophylactic effects are now beginning to be elucidated.

DIRECTIONS FOR FUTURE RESEARCH

In closing, we outline several challenges facing future tests of cognitive theories of depression. Several of these follow directly from our survey of the literature. Most basic is the question of how to characterize the cognitive pathology in depression. Does it conform to definitions of the schema construct? Segal (1988) recommends using techniques such as the Stroop task (Stroop, 1935) and priming methodologies in order to uncouple the effects of mood from those of a cognitive self-structure on the dependent variables of interest (e.g., Segal et al., 1988). In addition, is depressive cognition automatic? Employing methods such as those of Bargh and Tota (1988) with clinically depressed populations should help resolve this question.

Longitudinal studies assessing the interaction and congruence between negative life events and a person's "specific vulnerability" will inform us regarding the validity of the diathesis-stress component of cognitive theories of depression. Factors affecting the development of the cognitive diatheses should be explored. For example, what kinds of early life experiences are associated with the development of a negative attributional style, sociotropic personality, or autonomous personality?

The apparent success of cognitive therapy in the treatment of depressed outpatients has raised a new set of applied and theoretical questions that should be addressed by empirical research. With which subtypes of the depressive disorders is cognitive therapy more (or less) potent than are the standard (e.g., pharmacological) treatments? Prime candidates for further study are: depression with melancholia, chronic depression, and depression comorbid with personality disorder. Though there are theoretical reasons to predict that cognitive therapy might fare worse than antidepressant medications in depression with melancholia, there are no good data to suggest this is so. As regards chronic depression and depression with personality disorder, it might be suspected that cognitive therapy alone or as an adjunct to medication would prove more useful than medication alone. Again, there are no good data on this question.

Another area that merits further study concerns the optimal form of cognitive therapy. There has been a movement within cognitive therapy circles, based on clinical experience over the last two decades, to place greater emphasis on the nature and development of maladaptive schemas (see Beck, 1991). It will be interesting to see if this shift in emphasis yields a more powerful form of the treatment than the earlier version, based on Beck *et al.* (1979), which has been employed in outcome studies to date.

There is also a host of theoretical questions about the mediation of cognitive therapy's short- and long-term effects. What is the nature of the psychological phenomena that are changed in cognitive therapy and that lead to the reduction of symptoms? Does schema change play a major role? Is change produced through the acquisition and application of compensatory skills? As discussed in Hollon *et al.* (1987), these are especially difficult questions to tackle in regard to a treatment's short-term effects. But insofar as short-term cognitive therapy exerts a relapse prevention effect, there should be measurable differences at the end of treatment between such a relapse-preventing therapy and one that does not prevent relapse, such as an equally brief antidepressant medication regimen.

More generally, it is important to view the role of cognition in depression within the broader context of other processes and factors also posited to affect the development and course of depression. It is probable that a heterogenous disorder like depression is multidetermined. For example, some writers underscore the importance of interpersonal (e.g., Coyne, 1976) and environmental (e.g., Brown and Harris, 1978) factors in both the onset and maintenance of depression; similarly, others have described biological aspects in their theorizing (e.g., Akiskal and McKinney, 1975). Ultimately, a complete theory of depression must address the complex interplay between cognition and other factors implicated in depression. We commend several recent attempts to do so (e.g., Billings and Moos, 1982; Lewinsohn *et al.*, 1985; Pyszczynski and Greenberg, 1987) and expect the next decade of depression research to be fruitful, exciting, and illuminating.

REFERENCES

Abramson, L. Y., and Sackeim, H. A. (1977). A paradox in depression: Uncontrollability and self-blame. *Psychological Bulletin, 84*, 835–851.

Abramson, L. Y., Seligman, M. E. P., and Teasdale, J. (1978). Learned helplessness in humans: Critique and reformulation. *Journal of Abnormal Psychology, 87*, 49–74.

Abramson, L. Y., Alloy, L. B., and Metalsky, G. I. (1988). The cognitive diathesis-stress theories of depression: Toward an adequate evaluation of the theories' validities. In L. B. Alloy (Ed.), *Cognitive processes in depression* (pp. 3–30). New York: Guilford Press.

Abramson, L. Y., Metalsky, G. I., and Alloy, L. B. (1989). Hopelessness depression: A theory-based subtype of depression. *Psychological Review, 96*, 358–372.

Ackermann, R. (1988). Is depressive realism real? An empirical investigation. Unpublished master's thesis, University of Pennsylvania, Philadelphia, PA.

Ackermann, R., and DeRubeis, R. J. (1991). Is depressive realism real? *Clinical Psychology Review, 11*, 565–584.

Ackermann-Engel, R. (1992). Brief cognitive therapy. In L. Bellak (Ed.), *Handbook of intensive brief and emergency psychotherapy* (2nd and rev. ed., pp. 164–229). New York: C. P. S., Inc.

Akiskal, H. S., and McKinney, W. T. (1975). Overview of recent research in depression. *Archives of General Psychiatry, 32*, 285–305.

Alloy, L. B., and Abramson, L. Y. (1979). Judgment of contingency in depressed and nondepressed college students: Sadder but wiser? *Journal of Experimental Psychology: General, 108*, 441–485.

Alloy, L. B., and Abramson, L. Y. (1982). Learned helplessness, depression, and the illusion of control. *Journal of Personality and Social Psychology, 42*, 1114–1126.

Alloy, L. B., and Abramson, L. Y. (1988). Depressive realism: Four theoretical perspectives. In L. B. Alloy (Ed.), *Cognitive processes in depression* (pp. 3–30). New York: Guilford Press.

Alloy, L. B., and Ahrens, A. H. (1987). Depression and pessimism for the future: Biased use of statistically relevant information in predictions for self versus others. *Journal of Personality and Social Psychology, 52*, 366–378.

Alloy, L. B., and Clements, C. M. (1992). Illusion of control: Invulnerability to negative affect and depressive symptoms after laboratory and natural stressors. *Journal of Abnormal Psychology, 101*, 234–245.

Alloy, L. B., Abramson, L. Y., and Viscusi, D. (1981). Induced mood and the illusion of control. *Journal of Personality and Social Psychology, 41*, 1129–1140.

Alloy, L. B., Abramson, L. Y., and Kossman, D. (1985). The judgment of predictability in depressed and nondepressed college students. In F. R. Brush and J. B. Overmeier (Eds.),

Affect, conditioning and cognition: Essays on the determinants of behavior (pp. 229–246). Hillsdale, NJ: Erlbaum.

American Psychiatric Association (1987). *Diagnostic and statistical manual of mental disorders* (3rd and rev. ed.). Washington, D.C.: American Psychiatric Association.

Barber, J. P., and DeRubeis, R. J. (1989). On second thought: Where the action is in cognitive therapy for depression. *Cognitive Therapy and Research, 13,* 441–457.

Bargh, J. A., and Tota, M. E. (1988). Context-dependent automatic processing in depression: Accessibility of negative constructs with regard to self but not others. *Journal of Personality and Social Psychology, 54,* 925–939.

Barnett, P. A., and Gotlib, I. H. (1988a). Dysfunctional attitudes and psychosocial stress: The differential prediction of subsequent depression and general psychological distress. *Motivation and Emotion, 12,* 251–270.

Barnett, P. A., and Gotlib, I. H. (1988b). Psychosocial functioning and depression: Distinguishing among antecedents, concomitants, and consequences. *Psychological Bulletin, 104,* 97–126.

Barnett, P. A., and Gotlib, I. H. (1990). Cognitive vulnerability to depressive symptoms among men and women. *Cognitive Therapy and Research, 14,* 47–51.

Beck, A. T. (1967). *Depression: Clinical, experimental, and theoretical aspects.* New York: Harper & Row.

Beck, A. T. (1976). *Cognitive therapy and the emotional disorders.* New York: International Universities Press.

Beck, A. T. (1984). Cognition and therapy. *Archives of General Psychiatry, 41,* 1112–1114.

Beck, A. T. (1987). Cognitive models of depression. *Journal of Cognitive Psychotherapy, An International Quarterly, 1,* 5–37.

Beck, A. T. (1991). Cognitive therapy: A 30-year retrospective. *Americal Psychologist, 46,* 368–375.

Beck, A. T. and Hurvich, M. S. (1959). Psychological correlates of depression: Frequency of "masochistic" dream content in a private practice sample. *Psychosomatic Medicine, 21,* 50–55.

Beck, A. T., and Emergy, G. (1985). *Anxiety disorders and phobias: A cognitive perspective.* New York: Basic Books.

Beck, A. T., Weissman, A., Lester, D., and Trexler, L. (1974). The measurement of pessimism: The Hopelessness Scale. *Journal of Consulting and Clinical Psychology, 42,* 861–865.

Beck, A. T., Rush, A. J., Shaw, B. F., and Emery, G. (1979). *Cognitive therapy of depression: A treatment manual.* New York: Guilford Press.

Beck, A. T., Brown, G., Steer, R. A., Eidelson, J. I., and Riskind, J. H. (1987). Differentiating anxiety and depression: A test of the cognitive content-specificity hypothesis. *Journal of Abnormal Psychology, 96,* 179–183.

Beck, A. T., Riskind, J. H., Brown, G., and Steer, R. A. (1988). Levels of hopelessness in DSM-III disorders: A partial test of content specificity in depression. *Cognitive Therapy and Research, 12,* 459–469.

Beck, A. T., Steer, R. A., Epstein, N., and Brown, G. (1990). Beck Self-Concept Test. *Psychological Assessment: A Journal of Consulting and Clinical Psychology, 2,* 191–197.

Beidel, D. C., and Turner, S. (1986). A critique of the theoretical bases of cognitive–behavioral theories and therapy. *Clinical Psychology Review, 6,* 177–197.

Benassi, V. A., and Mahler, H. I. M. (1985). Contingency judgments by depressed college students: Sadder but not always wiser. *Journal of Personality and Social Psychology, 49,* 1323–1329.

Billings, A. G., and Moos, R. H. (1982). Psychosocial theory and research on depression: An integrative framework and review. *Clinical Psychology Review, 2,* 213–237.

Blackburn, I. M., and Bishop, S. (1983). Changes in cognition with pharmacotherapy. *British Journal of Psychology, 143*, 609–617.

Blackburn, I. M., and Smyth, P. (1985). A test of cognitive vulnerability in individuals prone to depression. *British Journal of Clinical Psychology, 24*, 61–62.

Blackburn, I. M., Bishop, S., Glen, A. I. M., Whalley, L. J., and Christie, J. E. (1981). The efficacy of cognitive therapy in depression: A treatment trial using cognitive therapy and pharmacotherapy, each alone and in combination. *British Journal of Psychiatry, 139*, 181–189.

Blackburn, I. M., Eunson, K. M., and Bishop, S. (1986a). A two-year naturalistic follow-up of depressed patients treated with cognitive therapy, pharmacotherapy and a combination of both. *Journal of Affective Disorders, 10*, 67–75.

Blackburn, I. M., Jones, S., and Lewin, R. J. P. (1986b). Cognitive style in depression. *British Journal of Clinical Psychology, 25*, 241–251.

Blaney, P. (1986). Affect and memory: A review. *Psychological Bulletin, 99*, 229–246.

Bower, G. H. (1981). Mood and memory. *American Psychologist, 36*, 129–148.

Bradley, B., and Mathews, A. (1983). Negative self-schemata in clinical depression. *British Journal of Clinical Psychology, 22*, 173–182.

Brewin, C. R. (1985). Depression and causal attributions: What is their relation? *Psychological Bulletin, 98*, 297–309.

Brown, G., and Beck, A. T. (1989). The role of imperatives in psychopathology: A reply to Ellis. *Cognitive Therapy and Research, 13*, 315–321.

Brown, G. W., and Harris, T. O. (1978). *Social origins of depression: A study of psychiatric disorder in women.* New York: Free Press.

Bryson, S. E., Doan, B. D., and Pasquali, P. (1984). Sadder but wiser: A failure to demonstrate that mood influences judgments of control. *Canadian Journal of Behavioral Science, 16*, 107–117.

Buchwald, A. M. (1977). Depressive mood and estimates of reinforcement frequency. *Journal of Abnormal Psychology, 86*, 443–446.

Campbell, J. D. (1986). Similarity and uniqueness: The effects of attribute type, relevance, and individual differences in self-esteem and depression. *Journal of Personality and Social Psychology, 50*, 281–294.

Campbell, J. D., and Fehr, B. (1990). Self-esteem and perceptions of conveyed impressions: Is negative affectivity associated with greater realism? *Journal of Personality and Social Psychology, 58*, 122–133.

Clark, D. A., and Beck, A. T. (1989). Cognitive theory and therapy of anxiety and depression. In P. C. Kendall and D. Watson (Eds.), *Anxiety and depression: Distinction and overlapping features* (pp. 379–411). San Diego: Academic Press.

Clark, D. A., Beck, A. T., and Brown, G. (1989). Cognitive mediation in general psychiatric outpatients: A test of the content-specificity hypothesis. *Journal of Personality and Social Psychology, 56*, 958–964.

Cochran, S. D., and Hammen, C. L. (1985). Perceptions of stressful life events and depression: A test of attributional models. *Journal of Personality and Social Psychology, 48*, 1562–1571.

Colby, C. A., and Gotlib, I. (1988). Memory deficits in depression. *Cognitive Therapy and Research, 12*, 611–627.

Coyne, J. C. (1976). Toward an interactional description of depression. *Psychiatry, 39*, 28–40.

Coyne, J. C., and Gotlib, I. H. (1983). The role of cognition in depression: A critical appraisal. *Psychological Bulletin, 94*, 472–505.

Coyne, J. C., and Gotlib, I. (1986). Studying the role of cognition in depression: Well-trodden paths and cul-de-sacs. *Cognitive Therapy and Research, 10*, 695–705.

Crandell, C. J., and Chambless, D. L. (1986). The validation of an inventory for measuring depressive thoughts: The Crandell Cognitions Inventory. *Behaviour Research and Therapy, 24*, 403–411.

Culp, C. (1991). *The effects of dysphoria and social anxiety on interpersonal interactions and social cognition*. Unpublished doctoral dissertation, University of Pennsylvania, Philadelphia, PA.

Cutrona, C. E. (1983). Causal attributions and perinatal depression. *Journal of Abnormal Psychology, 92*, 161–172.

DeMonbreun, B. G., and Craighead, W. E. (1977). Selective recall of positive and neutral feedback. *Cognitive Therapy and Research, 1*, 311–329.

Dennard, D. O., and Hokanson, J. E. (1986). Performance on two cognitive tasks by dysphoric and nondysphoric students. *Cognitive Therapy and Research, 10*, 337–386.

Derry, P. A., and Kuiper, K. A. (1981). Schematic processing and self-reference in clinical depression. *Journal of Abnormal Psychology, 90*, 286–297.

DeRubeis, R. J., Hollon, S. D., Evans, M. D., Garvey, M. J., Grove, W. M., and Tuason, V. B. (1989). *Active components and mediating mechanisms in cognitive therapy, pharmacotherapy, and combined cognitive-pharmacotherapy for depression: III. Processes of change in the CPT project*. Unpublished manuscript, University of Pennsylvania, Philadelphia, PA.

Dobson, K. S. (1989a). A meta-analysis of the efficacy of cognitive therapy for depression. *Journal of Consulting and Clinical Psychology, 57*, 414–419.

Dobson, K. S. (1989b). Real and perceived interpersonal responses to subclinically anxious and depressed targets. *Cognitive Therapy and Research, 13*, 37–47.

Dobson, K. S., and Franche, R. (1989). A conceptual and empirical review of the depressive realism hypothesis. *Canadian Journal of Behavioural Science, 21*, 419–433.

Dobson, K. S., and Shaw, B. F. (1986). Cognitive assessment with major depressive disorders. *Cognitive Therapy and Research, 10*, 13–29.

Dobson, K. S., and Shaw, B. F. (1987). Specificity and stability of self-referent encoding in clinical depression. *Journal of Abnormal Psychology, 96*, 34–40.

Dodge, K. A., and Frame, C. L. (1982). Social cognitive deficits and biases in aggressive boys. *Child Development, 53*, 620–635.

Dohr, K. B., Rush, A. J., and Bernstein, I. H. (1989). Cognitive biases and depression. *Journal of Abnormal Psychology, 98*, 263–267.

Dunbar, D. C., and Lishman, W. A. (1984). Depression, recognition-memory, and hedonic tone: A signal detection analysis. *British Journal of Psychiatry, 144*, 376–382.

Dykman, B. M., Abramson, L. Y., Alloy, L. B., and Hartlage, S. (1989). Processing of ambiguous and unambiguous feedback by depressed and nondepressed college students: Schematic biases and their implications for depressive realism. *Journal of Personality and Social Psychology, 56*, 431–445.

Eaves, G., and Rush, A. J. (1984). Cognitive patterns in symptomatic and remitted unipolar major depression. *Journal of Abnormal Psychology, 93*, 31–40.

Elkin, I., Shea, M. T., Watkins, J. T., Imber, S. D., Sotsky, S. M., Collins, J. F., Glass, D. R., Pilkonis, P. A., Leer, W. R., Docherty, J. P., Fiester, S. J., and Parloff, M. B. (1989). NIMH treatment of depression collaborative research program: I. General effectiveness of treatments. *Archives of General Psychiatry, 46*, 971–982.

Ellis, A. (1973). Rational-emotive therapy. In R. Corsini (Ed.), *Current psychotherapies* (pp. 167–207). Itasca, IL: Peacock.

Evans, M. D., Hollon, S. D., DeRubeis, R. J., Piasecki, J., Grove, W. M., Garvey, M. J., and Tuason, V. B. (1992). Differential relapse following cognitive therapy and pharmacotherapy for depression. *Archives of General Psychiatry, 49*, 802–808.

Fennell, M. J. V. (1989). Depression. In K. Hawton, P. M. Salkovskis, J. Kirk, and D. M. Clark (Eds.), *Cognitive behaviour therapy for psychiatric problems: A practical guide* (pp. 169–234). New York: Oxford University Press.

Fiske, S. T., and Taylor, S. E. (1991). *Social cognition* (2nd ed.). New York: McGraw-Hill.

Freud, S. (1917/1957). Mourning and melancholia. In J. Strachey (Ed.), *The complete psychological works of Sigmund Freud*. London: Hogarth.

Golin, S., Terrel, F., and Johnson, B. (1977). Depression and the illusion of control. *Journal of Abnormal Psychology, 86,* 440–442.

Golin, S., Terrel, F., Weitz, J., and Drost, P. L. (1979). The illusion of control among depressed patients. *Journal of Abnormal Psychology, 88,* 454–457.

Golinkoff, M., and Sweeney, J. A. (1989). Cognitive impairments in depression. *Journal of Affective Disorders, 17,* 105–112.

Gotlib, I. H. (1981). Self-reinforcement and recall: Differential deficits in depressed and non-depressed psychiatric inpatients. *Journal of Abnormal Psychology, 90,* 521–530.

Gotlib, I. H. (1983). Perception and recall of interpersonal feedback: Negative bias in depression. *Cognitive Therapy and Research, 7,* 399–412.

Gotlib, I. H., and Meltzer, S. J. (1987). Depression and the perception of social skill in dyadic interaction. *Cognitive Therapy and Research, 11,* 42–54.

Greenberg, M. S., and Alloy, L. B. (1989). Depression versus anxiety: Processing of self- and other-referent information. *Cognition and Emotion, 3,* 207–223.

Greenberg, M. S., and Beck, A. T. (1989). Depression versus anxiety: A test of the content-specificity hypothesis. *Journal of Abnormal Psychology, 98,* 9–13.

Haaga, D. A. F., Dyck, M. J., and Ernst, D. (1991). Empirical status of cognitive theory of depression. *Psychological Bulletin, 110,* 215–236.

Hamilton, E. W., and Abramson, L. Y. (1983). Cognitive patterns and major depressive disorder: A longitudinal study in a hospital setting. *Journal of Abnormal Psychology, 92,* 173–184.

Hammen, C. L., and Krantz, S. (1976). Effect of success and failure on depressive cognitions. *Journal of Abnormal Psychology, 85,* 577–586.

Hammen, C. L., Marks, T., deMayo, R., and Mayol, A. (1985a). Self-schemas and risk for depression: A prospective study. *Journal of Personality and Social Psychology, 49,* 1147–1159.

Hammen, C. L., Marks, T., Mayol, A., and deMayo, R. (1985b). Depressive self-schemas, life stress, and vulnerability to depression. *Journal of Abnormal Psychology, 94,* 308–319.

Hammen, C. L., Ellicott, A., and Gitlin, M. (1989a). Vulnerability to specific life events and prediction of course of disorder in unipolar depressed patients. *Canadian Journal of Behavioural Science, 21,* 377–388.

Hammen, C. L., Ellicott, A., Gitlin, M., and Jamison, K. R. (1989b). Sociotropy/autonomy and vulnerability to specific life events in patients with unipolar depression and bipolar disorders. *Journal of Abnormal Psychology, 98,* 154–160.

Harrell, T. H., and Ryon, N. B. (1983). Cognitive–behavioral assessment of depression: Clinical validation of the Automatic Thoughts Questionnaire. *Journal of Consulting and Clinical Psychology, 51,* 721–725.

Hoehn-Hyde, D., Schlottman, R. S., and Rush, A. J. (1982). Perception of social interactions in depressed psychiatric patients. *Journal of Consulting and Clinical Psychology, 50,* 209–212.

Hokanson, J. E., Hummer, J. T., and Butler, A. C. (1991). Interpersonal perceptions by depressed college students. *Cognitive Therapy and Research, 15,* 443–457.

Hollon, S. D., and Beck, A. T. (1979). Cognitive therapy of depression. In P. C. Kendall and S. D. Hollon (Eds.), *Cognitive-behavioral interventions: Theory, research and procedures*. New York: Academic Press.

Hollon, S. D., and Kendall, P. C. (1980). Cognitive self-statements in depression: Development of an automatic thoughts questionnaire. *Cognitive Therapy and Research, 4*, 383–395.

Hollon, S. D., Kendall, P. C., and Lumry, A. (1986). Specificity of depressotypic cognitions in clinical depression. *Journal of Abnormal Psychology, 95*, 52–59.

Hollon, S. D., DeRubeis, R. J., and Evans, M. D. (1987). Causal mediation of change in treatment for depression: Discriminating between nonspecificity and noncausality. *Psychological Bulletin, 102*, 139–149.

Hollon, S. D., Evans, M. D., and DeRubeis, R. J. (1990). Cognitive mediation of relapse prevention following treatment for depression: Implications of differential risk. In R. E. Ingram (Ed.), *Psychological aspects of depression* (pp. 117–136). New York: Plenum.

Hollon, S. D., Shelton, R. C., and Loosen, P. T. (1991). Cognitive therapy and pharmacotherapy for depression. *Journal of Consulting and Clinical Psychology, 59*, 88–99.

Hollon, S. D., DeRubeis, R. J., Evans, M. D., Wiemer, M. J., Garvey, M. J., Grove, W. M., and Tuason, V. B. (1992). Cognitive therapy and pharmacotherapy for depression: Singly and in combination. *Archives of General Psychiatry, 49*, 774–781.

Ingram, R. E. (1984). Toward an information-processing analysis of depression. *Cognitive Therapy and Research, 8*, 443–478.

Ingram, R. E., Kendall, P. C., Smith, T. W., Donnell, C., and Ronan, K. (1987). Cognitive specificity in emotional disorders. *Journal of Personality and Social Psychology, 53*, 734–742.

Johnson, M. H., and Magaro, P. A. (1987). Effects of mood and severity on memory processes in depression and mania. *Psychological Bulletin, 101*, 28–40.

Johnson-Laird, P. N. (1983). *Mental models: Toward a cognitive science of language, inference and consciousness*. Cambridge: Cambridge University Press.

Kendall, P. C., Hollon, S. D., Beck, A. T., Hammen, C. L., and Ingram, R. E. (1987). Issues and recommendations regarding use of the Beck Depression Inventory. *Cognitive Therapy and Research, 11*, 289–299.

Kendall, P. C., Howard, B. L., and Hays, R. C. (1989). Self-referent speech and psychopathology: The balance of positive and negative thinking. *Cognitive* Therapy and Research, *13*, 583–598.

Kennedy, R. E., and Craighead, W. E. (1988). Differential effects of depression and anxiety on recall of feedback in a learning task. *Behavior Therapy, 19*, 437–454.

Kleinman, A. (1980). *Patients and healers in the context of culture*. Berkeley: University of California Press.

Kovacs, M., Rush, A. T., Beck, A. T., and Hollon, S. D. (1981). Depressed outpatients treated with cognitive therapy or pharmacotherapy: A one-year follow-up. *Archives of General Psychiatry, 38*, 33–39.

Kuiper, N. A. (1978). Depression and causal attributions for success and failure. *Journal of Personality and Social Psychology, 36*, 236–246.

Kuiper, N. A., and MacDonald, M. R. (1982). Self and other perception in mild depressives. *Social Cognition, 1*, 223–239.

Kuiper, N. A., and MacDonald, M. R. (1983). Schematic processing in depression: The self-based consensus bias. *Cognitive Therapy and Research, 7*, 469–484.

Kwon, S., and Oei, T. P. S. (1992). Differential causal roles of dysfunctional attitudes and automatic thoughts in depression. *Cognitive Therapy and Research, 16*, 309–328.

Lam, D. H., Brewin, C. R., Woods, R. T., and Bebbington, P. E. (1987). Cognition and social adversity in the depressed elderly. *Journal of Abnormal Psychology, 96*, 23–26.

Lewinsohn, P. M., Mischel, W., Chaplin, W., and Barton, R. (1980). Social competence and depression: The role of illusory self-perceptions. *Journal of Abnormal Psychology, 89*, 203–212.

Lewinsohn, P. M., Steinmetz, J. L., Larson, D. W., and Franklin, J. (1981). Depression-related cognitions: Antecedents or consequences? *Journal of Abnormal Psychology, 90*, 213–219.

Lewinsohn, P. M., Hoberman, H., Teri, L., and Hautzinger, M. (1985). An integrative theory of depression. In S. Reiss and R. Bootzin (Eds.), *Theoretical issues in behavior therapy* (pp. 331–359). New York: Academic Press.

MacDonald, M. R., and Kuiper, N. A. (1984). Self-schema decision consistency in clinical depressives. *Journal of Social and Clinical Psychology, 2*, 264–272.

Manley, P. C., McMahon, R. J., Bradley, C. F., and Davidson, P. O. (1982). Depressive attributional style and depression following childbirth. *Journal of Abnormal Psychology, 91*, 245–254.

Markus, H. (1977). Self-schemata and processing information about the self. *Journal of Personality and Social Psychology, 35*, 63–78.

Martin, D. J., Alloy, L. B., and Abramson, L. Y. (1984). The illusion of control for self and others in depressed and nondepressed college students. *Journal of Personality and Social Psychology, 46*, 125–136.

Metalsky, G. I., Abramson, L. Y., Seligman, M. E. P., Semmel, A., and Peterson, C. (1982). Attributional styles and life events in the classroom: Vulnerability and invulnerability to depressive mood reactions. *Journal of Personality and Social Psychology, 43*, 612–617.

Metalsky, G. I., Halberstadt, L. J., and Abramson, L. Y. (1987). Vulnerability to depressive mood reactions: Toward a more powerful test of the diathesis-stress and causal mediation components of the reformulated theory of depression. *Journal of Personality and Social Psychology, 52*, 386–393.

Mikulincer, M., Gerber, H., and Weisenberg, M. (1990). Judgment of control and depression: The role of self-esteem threat and self-focused attention. *Cognitive Therapy and Research, 14*, 589–608.

Miranda, J., and Persons, J. B. (1988). Dysfunctional attitudes are mood-state dependent. *Journal of Abnormal Psychology, 97*, 76–79.

Miranda, J., Persons, J. B., and Byers, C. N. (1990). Endorsement of dysfunctional beliefs depends on current mood state. *Journal of Abnormal Psychology, 99*, 237–241.

Moretti, M. M., and Shaw, B. F. (1989). Automatic and dysfunctional cognitive processes in depression. In J. S. Uleman and J. A. Bargh (Eds.), *Unintended thought* (pp. 383–421). New York: Guilford Press.

Murphy, G. E., Simons, A. D., Wetzel, R. D., and Lustman, P. J. (1984). Cognitive therapy and pharmacotherapy, singly and together in the treatment of depression. *Archives of General Psychiatry, 41*, 33–41.

Nelson, R. E., and Craighead, W. E. (1977). Selective recall of positive and negative feedback, self-control behaviors and depression. *Journal of Abnormal Psychology, 86*, 379–388.

O'Hara, M. W., Rehm, L. P., and Campbell, S. B. (1982). Predicting depressive symptomology: Cognitive–behavioral models and postpartum depression. *Journal of Abnormal Psychology, 91*, 457–461.

O'Hara, M. W., Neunaber, D. J., and Zekoski, E. M. (1984). Prospective study of postpartum depression: Prevalence, course, and predictive factors. *Journal of Abnormal Psychology, 93*, 158–171.

Olinger, J., Kuiper, N. A., and Shaw, B. F. (1987). Dysfunctional attitudes and stressful life events: An interactive model of depression. *Cognitive Therapy and Research, 11*, 25–40.

Peterson, C., and Seligman, M. E. P. (1984). Causal explanations as a risk factor for depression: Theory and evidence. *Psychological Review, 91*, 347–374.

Peterson, C., Schwartz, S. M., and Seligman, M. E. P. (1981). Self-blame and depressive symptoms. *Journal of Personality and Social Psychology, 91,* 253–259.

Power, M. J., and Champion, L. A. (1986). Cognitive approaches to depression: A theoretical critique. *British Journal of Clinical Psychology, 25,* 201–212.

Pyszczynski, T., and Greenberg, J. (1987). Self-regulatory perseveration and the depressive self-focusing style: A self-awareness theory of reactive depression. *Psychological Bulletin, 102,* 122–138.

Reda, M. A. (1984). Cognitive organization and antidepressants: Attitude modification during amitriptyline treatment in severely depressed individuals. In M. A. Reda and M. J. Mahoney (eds.), *Cognitive psychotherapies: Recent developments in theory, research, and practice.* Cambridge, MA: Ballinger.

Rehm, L. P. (1977). A self-control model of depression. *Behavior Therapy, 8,* 787–804.

Rholes, W. S., Riskind, J. H., and Neville, B. (1985). The relationship of cognitions and hopelessness to depression and anxiety. *Social Cognition, 3,* 36–50.

Robins, C. J., and Block, P. (1988). Personal vulnerability, life events, and depressive symptoms: A test of a specific interactional model. *Journal of Personality and Social Psychology, 54,* 847–852.

Robins, C. J., and Block, P. (1989). Cognitive theories of depression viewed from a diathesis-stress perspective: Evaluations of the models of Beck and of Abramson, Seligman, and Teasdale. *Cognitive Therapy and Research, 13,* 297–313.

Robins, C. J., Block, P., and Peselow, E. D. (1990). Cognition and life events in major depression: A test of the mediation and interaction hypotheses. *Cognitive Therapy and Research, 14,* 299–313.

Ross, S. M., Gottfredson, D. K., Christensen, P., and Weaver, R. (1986). Cognitive self-statements in depression: Findings across clinical populations. *Cognitive Therapy and Research, 10,* 159–166.

Roth, D., and Rehm, L. P. (1980). Relationships among self-monitoring processes, memory, and depression. *Cognitive Therapy and Research, 4,* 149–157.

Rush, A. J., Beck, A. T., Kovacs, M., and Hollon, S. D. (1977). Comparative efficacy of cognitive therapy and pharmacotherapy in the treatment of depressed outpatients. *Cognitive Therapy and Research, 1,* 17–37.

Rush, A. J., Weissenburger, J., and Eaves, G. (1986). Do thinking patterns predict depressive symptoms? *Cognitive Therapy and Research, 10,* 225–236.

Segal, Z. V. (1988). Appraisal of the self-schema construct in cognitive models of depression. *Psychological Bulletin, 103,* 147–162.

Segal, Z. V., and Shaw, B. F. (1986). Cognition in depression: A reappraisal of Coyne and Gotlib's critique. *Cognitive Therapy and Research, 10,* 671–693.

Segal, Z. V., Hood, J. E., Shaw, B. F., and Higgins, E. T. (1988). A structural analysis of the self-schema construct in major depression. *Cognitive Therapy and Research, 12,* 471–485.

Segal, Z. V., Shaw, B. F., Vella, D. D., and Katz, R. (1992). Cognitive and life stress predictors of relapse in remitted unipolar depressed patients: Test of the congruency hypothesis. *Journal of Abnormal Psychology, 101,* 26–36.

Seligman, M. E. P. (1975). *Helplessness: On depression, development, and death.* San Francisco: Freeman.

Seligman, M. E. P., Abramson, L. Y., Semmel, A., and von Baeyer, C. (1979). Depressive attributional style. *Journal of Abnormal Psychology, 88,* 242–247.

Siegel, S. J., and Alloy, L. B. (1990). Interpersonal perceptions and consequences of depressive–significant other relationships: A naturalistic study of college roommates. *Journal of Abnormal Psychology, 99,* 361–373.

Silverman, J. S., Silverman, J. A., and Eardley, D. A. (1984). Do maladaptive attitudes cause depression? *Archives of General Psychiatry, 41*, 28–30.

Simons, A. D. (1984). In reply. *Archives of General Psychiatry, 41*, 1114–1115.

Simons, A. D., Garfield, S. L., and Murphy, G. E. (1984). The process of change in cognitive therapy and pharmacotherapy for depression. *Archives of General Psychiatry, 41*, 45–51.

Simons, A. D., Murphy, G. E., Levine, J. L., and Wetzel, R. D. (1986). Cognitive therapy and pharmacotherapy for depression: Sustained improvement over one year. *Archives of General Psychiatry, 43*, 43–48.

Stroop, J. R. (1935). Studies of inference in serial verbal reactions. *Journal of Experimental Psychology, 18*, 643–662.

Sweeney, P. D., Anderson, K., and Bailey, S. (1986). Attributional style in depression: A meta-analytic review. *Journal of Personality and Social Psychology, 50*, 974–991.

Taylor, S. E., and Brown, J. D. (1988). Illusion and well-being: A social psychological perspective on mental health. *Psychological Bulletin, 103*, 193–210.

Vazquez, C. V. (1987). Judgment of contingency: Cognitive biases in depressed and nondepressed subjects. *Journal of Personality and Social Psychology, 52*, 419–431.

Velten, E. (1968). A laboratory task for induction of mood states. *Behaviour Research and Therapy, 6*, 473–482.

Weissman, A. N., and Beck, A. T. (1978). *Development and validation of the dysfunctional attitude scale: A preliminary investigation.* Paper presented at the meeting of the American Educational Research Association, Toronto, Canada.

Wenzlaff, R. M., and Berman, J. S. (1988). *Depression and judgments of self and others: Objectivity at the cost of self-enhancement?* Unpublished manuscript.

Wenzlaff, R. M., Wegner, D. M., and Roper, D. W. (1988). Depression and mental control: The resurgence of unwanted negative thoughts. *Journal of Personality and Social Psychology, 55*, 882–892.

Wilkinson, I. M., and Blackburn, I. M. (1981). Cognitive style in depressed and recovered depressed patients. *British Journal of Clinical Psychology, 20*, 283–292.

Wise, E. H., and Barnes, D. R. (1986). The relationship among life events, dysfunctional attitudes, and depression. *Cognitive Therapy and Research, 10*, 257–266.

Zuroff, D. C., Igreja, I., and Mongrain, M. (1990). Dysfunctional attitudes, dependency, and self-criticism as predictors of depressive mood states: A 12-month longitudinal study. *Cognitive Therapy and Research, 14*, 315–326.

Cognition and Pain Experience

Glenn Pancyr

Royal University Hospital
Saskatoon, Saskatchewan

Myles Genest

Acadia University
Wolfville
Nova Scotia, Canada

Why does a psychopathology book contain a chapter about pain? In most circumstances, pain serves an important survival function, preserving the integrity of the body by warning of imminent or actual physical damage. Nevertheless, pain has become the target of psychological theory, research, and interventions simply because, in most cases, it is unwanted. However, pain is also implicated in a host of psychopathological disorders.

The DSM-III-R (American Psychiatric Association, 1987) contains mental disorders for which pain is either

1. the primary element for the diagnosis (e.g., somatoform pain disorder, dyspareunia)
2. one of several important symptoms (e.g., sexual masochism, somatization disorder, separation anxiety) or
3. an important aspect of behavior related to the particular psychopathology (e.g., head banging in autistic disorder, self-mutilation in borderline personality disorder)

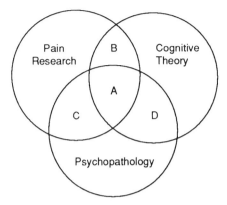

Figure 5.1. Domains of literature for the current chapter (see text).

Unfortunately, in spite of the prevalence of pain phenomena in the DSM-III-R nomenclature, the study of psychopathology associated with pain has not captured the attention of researchers or theorists. The notable exception to this rule has been the role of depression in chronic pain.

The majority of investigation and theorizing has focused on pain associated with medical/physical disorders. Psychologists have mainly examined four types of pain: (1) acute, self-limiting pain that may be benign but is sufficiently intense and severe to warrant intervention (e.g., a consequence of dental procedures); (2) chronic pain, usually associated with disease or major injury; (3) pain whose expression does not conform to medical expectations (e.g., is more severe than would be expected from tissue damage, somatoform pain disorder); (4) pain associated with psychopathology (i.e., major depression in chronic pain patients). Pain in the first category is not generally associated with psychopathology. Nevertheless, theory and research into such pain have contributed to the understanding and amelioration of all sorts of pain. As a result, rather than focus only on abnormal psychological presentations of pain, we have chosen to examine the cognitive literature concerning pain in general, with specific attention to its relevance for psychopathology.

Our Venn diagram in Fig. 5.1 depicts the literature domains that pertain to this chapter's focus. Ideally, we would only include material from A, representing the intersection between pain research, psychopathology, and cognitive theory. However, only one body of literature of any appreciable size and organization exists in area A, and that pertains to depression in chronic pain patients. Therefore, depression in chronic pain receives a great deal of attention in this chapter. Jensen *et al*. (1991) noted the difficulty of summarizing cognitive psychological literature devoted to pain. They observed that cognitive investigations of coping with pain have approached the interface between cognition and pain from several directions. Jensen *et al*. identify seven categories of such research: (1) beliefs about general locus of control; (2) beliefs about control over pain; (3) attributional style; (4) cognitive errors; (5) self-efficacy beliefs; and (6) outcome expectancies. A seventh category was reserved for "pain appraisals" that did not fit any of the categories above. These categories correspond to the major cognitive theories currently used by clinicians and researchers in the study and treatment of pain: control theory, attribution theory, cognitive theory, social learning theory, and self-efficacy theory. Because of the overlap among these theories only a few will be reviewed in this chapter.

Important work being done in areas **B** and **C** of our Venn diagram will also be reviewed (area **D** is dealt with in other chapters of this volume). For example, cognitive theory innovations arising from work in depression and anxiety have been applied to pain (area **B**), even though pain experience is not usually considered psychopathological. The application of knowledge about cognitive theory and psychopathology to problems involving pain has largely occurred through the clinical application of therapeutic techniques and strategies. Theoretical developments appear to be *following* from these clinical applications. Therefore, this chapter contains information about the application of cognitive–behavioral therapy to pain problems. But to begin, we offer some background to the use of cognitive concepts in understanding pain.

The historical context of recent cognitive developments in understanding and managing pain has been well documented (Brena, 1972; Melzack and Wall, 1983; Schneider and Karoly, 1983; Turk *et al.*, 1983). Ancient texts chronicle that before the evolution of modern medicine and the dominance of the physiological/perceptual conceptualization of pain (Brena, 1972; Schneider and Karoly, 1983), pain was considered an emotion, which generally included cognitive components. Contemporary theory has reintroduced emotion and cognition as important factors in the study of pain. Because serious psychological attention to pain is a relatively recent phenomenon, much of the research has been concurrent with the cognitive revolution.

Our presentation is divided into three sections beginning with a review of the main cognitive-theoretical influences in the study of pain. The second section is a review of the empirical literature associated with the theories outlined in the first section of the chapter. Additionally, other empirical work will also be reviewed, which is anticipated to become important to cognitive theory development in understanding pain experience, but which is not currently formalized into theory. The third and final section is devoted to implications of cognitive theory for the study and treatment of pain associated with psychopathology.

THE ORIGINS OF COGNITIVE MODELS OF PAIN

Much of the work on pain is scattered among various literatures, including those of various diseases (e.g., oncology; rheumatoid arthritis), procedures (e.g., surgery; dental procedures; invasive diagnostic tests), syndromes (e.g., cluster headache; chronic, low-back pain), and laboratory models (e.g., cold-pressor task). There have been some attempts to integrate these literatures into overall models of pain, although, for the most part, the areas remain separate.

We begin this section by introducing the psychosomatic tradition of examining pain. A major shortcoming of traditional psychosomatic theory was the failure to incorporate social and cognitive aspects of pain phenomena into a theoretical formulation. The gate-control theory is presented next, as it profoundly influenced pain research by formally including cognition as part of the experience of pain, and by validating the scientific investigation of psychological aspects of pain. Gate-control theory legitimized using cognitive theories to understand pain experience, the most prominent of these we review being self-efficacy theory and theories regarding the concept of control. This section ends with a brief review of the pain-context model because it is the most current and comprehensive model incorporating cognitive factors in the understanding of pain.

Psychosomatics

The last quarter of a century has seen a movement away from the labeling of unexplained pain as "psychogenic" and toward an examination of the specific psychological contributions to pain syndromes. The nosology nevertheless contains remnants of earlier, psychosomatic formulations, which tended to presume that many patients who experienced pain did so because they needed or wanted it. Such pain presentations are called "psychogenic pain disorder" or "hysterical pain" or "somatoform pain disorder." The basic diagnostic criteria are the presence of pain (in DSM-III-R, "preoccupation" with pain) and the absence of adequate physical findings to account for the pain or its intensity.

Failing to find sufficient organic signs to explain complaints of pain often leads to a search for psychological etiology. Unfortunately, in many instances, the absence of organic findings results not from absence of organic disturbance, but from the inadequacy of medical diagnosis or technology. Thus, patients who now are recognized as suffering from such disorders as Lupus erythematosus or Post-Polio Syndrome, could have received a few years ago a psychosomatic diagnosis simply because these syndromes were not recognized. Therefore, some pain problems currently conceptualized in psychiatric or psychological terms may eventually be shown to be primarily organic in nature.

Difficulty in providing adequate organic accounts for pain has historically led to formulations derived primarily from psychoanalytic theory (e.g., Alexander, 1950). More recently, attempts to account for puzzling pain presentations have focused on the multiple contributions to pain, including physical, psychological and social factors (e.g., Melzack and Wall, 1983; Turk *et al.*, 1983; Sternbach, 1974). Melzack and Wall's (1965) introduction of gate-control theory was the first systematic attempt to simultaneously represent the influences of emotions, past experiences, and cognitions on pain.

Gate-Control Theory

Melzack and Wall's (1965) gate-control theory proposed that pain was not, as Beecher (1959) had argued, a simple sensory event with associated physical and psychological reactions, but a perceptual experience. Gate-control theory provides a neurophysiological account of pain. Ultimately, however, it emphasizes the psychological aspects of pain as primary. Melzack and Wall's view is that there are several interacting components of pain, including sensation, emotion, and cognition, with a variety of neurophysiological mechanisms involved. The *gate* refers to the presence of central nervous system controls that influence pain-signal transmission. The gate can be opened or closed by influences quite apart from a primary sensory stimulus. In fact, chronic pain is viewed as most often controlled through what is termed the cognitive–motivational components of pain (Weisenberg, 1984) and is targeted with such interventions as hypnosis, anxiety reduction, and attentional distraction.

Although gate-control theory emphasizes the psychological experience of pain as fundamental, much of the research that it has stimulated has focused on physiological details (Genest, 1986). There has been much less psychological research or truly integrative work deriving from the model, although psychologists frequently call upon it as justification for their work. Part of the reason that gate-control theory has not generated more psychological research is that it does not lead to specific predictions concerning what effects particular emotional states or cognitive processes might have on the experience of pain (Pancyr, 1988). Other theoretical writings have been more specific in this respect, although they are generally more limited in their scope. Cognitive theories such as control theory and self-efficacy theory, that had been developed in other domains of psychopathology (e.g., depression and phobias, respectively), are now being applied to pain problems since Melzack and Wall's (1965) groundbreaking work cleared the way.

Control and Self-Efficacy

The construct of control and its relationships to pain in both laboratory and clinical contexts has received extensive attention. Precursors of current developments include Zimbardo's work with cognitive dissonance theory (Zimbardo *et al.*, 1969) and Nisbett and Schachter's (1966) work with attribution theory. This early work developed into a broad area of scientific investigation of the concept of control in pain perception and management. Work with the construct of locus of control has focused on control as a personal trait (Lefcourt, 1982). This approach has been applied to control over health outcomes (Wallston *et al.*, 1978), and more recently, specifically to pain (Toomey *et al.*, 1988).

There are a number of ways in which control may be hypothesized to influence pain. For example, Averill's (1973) categories of behavioral control, cognitive control, and decisional control are all relevant, depending on the circumstances. Perceiving oneself to be in control of a situation may have important consequences, such as by bolstering one's self-image, thus inspiring motivation to endure or to attempt to alter noxious stimulation (Thompson, 1981). Feeling out of control, on the other hand, could induce poor coping, helplessness, and intolerance of pain. Control also changes the *meaning* of an aversive situation; it conveys information about an aversive experience, enhancing predictability and permitting advanced preparation for pain (Thompson, 1981; Weisenberg, 1984), allowing otherwise unendurable pain to become endurable.

These conceptions of control and the expectation that one can produce a response that can affect the aversiveness of a painful event are related to the concept of self-efficacy as developed by Bandura (1977). Bandura described outcome expectancies as estimates of the extent to which a particular behavior is capable of producing a particular outcome, and efficacy expectancies as estimates that one can successfully execute the behavior required to produce a given outcome. Bandura's self-efficacy theory was a main element of the cognitive revolution in psychology, but it was not until the 1980s and 1990s that the concept began to attract attention in the area of pain.

The relevance of self-efficacy for the experience of pain is clear:

Judgments of personal efficacy affect what courses of action people choose to pursue, how much effort they will put forth in a given endeavour, how long they will persevere in the face of aversive experiences, whether their thought patterns help or hinder their endeavors, and how much stress they experience in coping with taxing environment demands. (Bandura *et al.*, 1987, p. 563)

Self-efficacy has been used to predict how well people will manage pain in a number of contexts, such as pain tolerance in laboratory pain studies (Dolce *et al.*, 1986) and the outcome of chronic pain treatment programs (Kores *et al.*, 1990). Recently, Bandura and his colleagues turned their attention specifically to pain, with an attempt to specify the physiological correlates of self-efficacy changes [Bandura *et al.*, 1987 (described below, with other research findings)]. Such attempts to relate psychological and physiological mechanisms are certain to become more common, as psychologists concern themselves with basic mechanisms on the one hand, and with the provision of service in health settings on the other.

The Pain Context Model

One of the most comprehensive current accounts of chronic pain is that provided by Karoly and Jensen's (1987) Pain Context Model. The model proposes four contexts or dimensional systems relevant for understanding chronic pain. Context I, the biomedical dimension, consists of traditional medical conceptualizations, assessment methods, and treatments for pain problems. Context II, the focal/experiential dimension, is the patient's reality, comprised of the sensory, affective, interpersonal, verbal, behavioral, and cognitive aspects of the patient's experience. Context III, the meaning/relational dimension, pertains to the meaning of pain as it is experienced, and is related to such factors as motivation, family interactions, mental health, and self-perception. Context IV, the conceptual/sociological dimension, refers to theories, measurement models, and health policies used by clinicians, researchers, administrators, and politicians to understand chronic pain. Each of these contexts is considered in conjunction with the conceptualization of pain as an information control/action system depicted in Fig. 5.2.

This model incorporates formulations from diverse theoretical orientations (e.g., gate-control theory, social learning theory) into a more comprehensive understanding of an individual's pain.

We might encompass many of the clinical features of chronic pain sufferers by asserting, from a control systems perspective, that (1) under the influence of reduced external stimulation and of sensory (organic) or schema-driven (acquired) processes, chronic patients tend to differentially monitor, encode, and interpret bodily activities as distressing (painful); (2) they tend to develop

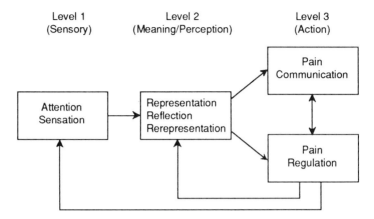

Figure 5.2 A model of recurrent pain as an information control/action system. (Adapted from *Multimethod Assessment of Chronic Pain.* Copyright © 1987, with permission of Allyn and Bacon.

self-defeating cognitive–behavioral control strategies, including the denial of responsibility/capability for pain modulation, the pursuit of incompatible goals (e.g., to display and to suppress pain signals), and the schematic anticipation and avoidance of future suffering, leading to immobility-based muscular atrophy (and more pain); and (3) self-defeating patterns and conceptual models become strengthened through contingent social and financial rewards. (Karoly and Jensen, 1987, p. 24)

Karoly and Jensen's (1987) account is comprehensive in incorporating the different areas of research in pain, and also in incorporating a collection of categories and perspectives to be considered in pain assessment and treatment. They also take a step forward by including the notion of control systems in their model. However, psychological accounts of pain — both normal and pathological presentations — still await further development before reaching the stage of integrated theory.

In his chapter in the *Textbook of Pain*, Weisenberg (1984) concludes by drawing attention to several gaps in the pain literature, including (1) a clear theoretical statement that ties the different cognitive aspects of pain together; (2) data bearing on the question of whether cognitive pain coping strategies actually provide pain relief, or whether the belief in their efficacy is the active ingredient; and (3) data bearing on whether cognitive coping strategies make the unbearable bearable, or whether these techniques actually eliminate pain. These gaps remain, though Weisenberg removed mention of them from the text of his 1989 revision of this chapter.

The research between the two versions of Weisenberg's chapter suggests that applications of cognitive theory to chronic pain problems appear to help people endure pain better and to deal better with the problems consequent to pain, but do not ameliorate the dimension of pain itself. In the next section, we examine the findings of various areas of cognitive research that bear on pain and consider their implications for the treatment of pain problems.

RESEARCH CONCERNING COGNITION AND PAIN

In this section we begin by examining the concept of control, in its varied forms, and its relation to pain problems. The contributions of self-efficacy theory, both in laboratory and clinical investigations of pain, are reviewed next. No empirical review of gate-control theory is offered because this theory does not permit making predictions about how, or in what ways, specific types of cognitions influence pain experience. The pain-context model, because of its attention to systems and its four parallel dimensions of analysis, also does not readily lend itself to empirical verification as a whole, and an empirical review of its components was not undertaken in this chapter. A large portion of this section is devoted to a review of literature related to chronic pain and depression. Although no one cognitive theory distinguishes itself above any others, the research on depression associated with pain provides the best example of how cognitive theory is being applied to pain problems. We will also briefly review research related to memory and pain. The role of memory in pain is a relatively new and exciting area of empirical research that promises to advance our understanding of both normal and abnormal pain processes. We next consider cognitive–behavioral therapies for pain, for it is within these practical applications of cognitive techniques and strategies that much cognitive theorizing about pain processes is occurring. This section ends with a comment on the significance of *meaning* in understanding pain.

Control

Perceived control has been conceptualized in various ways in the pain literature. Some researchers have referred to an individual's sense of control as a personality trait or dimension. In the first part of this section evidence is cited that suggests that individuals with a greater sense of personal control (e.g., those who rate themselves high on an internal sense of locus of control) cope with pain better than those who sense themselves as having less control in their lives. Control has also been conceptualized as a belief or expectation that arises from the environmental context in which aversive stimulation occurs. In this paradigm, researchers have manipulated individuals' perceptions of control of an aversive stimulus to determine the effects on pain experience. Research from both the trait and expectations conceptualizations of control are reviewed below.

Perceived Control as a Personality Trait

Toomey *et al.* (1991) divided 51 patients with chronic myofascial pain into low and high copers, based on their responses to the internality dimension of the Pain Locus of Control Scale. Patients reporting higher internal control reported their pain as less intense than those below the median on the dimension. The authors concluded that pain-coping strategies that relieve the frequency and intensity of pain may result in increased perceived personal control over pain. Further evidence for the association between control and pain comes from a study of headache sufferers. Courey *et al.* (1982) assessed suffering in chronic migraine and mixed migraine-muscle-tension headache sufferers with the Self-Control Schedule, the Marlowe-Crowne Social Desirability Scale, the McGill Pain Questionnaire, and other measures. Those patients with higher self-control scores were characterized by lower ratings of pain intensity, being less focused on the sensory dimensions of pain, and more likely to use certain medications. A positive relationship was also found between degree of self-control and social desirability, which might have confounded the results. Consistent with the Toomey *et al.* (1991) study, Courey *et al.* (1982) found an association between perceived self-control and low ratings of pain intensity.

Perceived control has been studied in relation to psychological disorder in chronic pain patients. McCreary and Turner (1984) assessed 59 chronic low-back pain patients with Rotter's Internal–External Locus of Control Scale and the Minnesota Multiphasic Personality Inventory (MMPI). Patients with an external locus of control tended to exhibit traits of excessive rumination and self-doubt and a general overreaction to problems.

In a similar investigation, Crisson and Keefe (1988) evaluated 62 chronic pain patients, mostly suffering low-back pain, with the Multidimensional Health Locus of Control Scale, the Coping Strategies Questionnaire, and the Symptom Checklist-90. Correlational analyses revealed that subjects who saw outcomes as occurring by chance, fate, or luck tended to use maladaptive pain-coping strategies (e.g., avoiding activity, diverting attention, praying/hoping) and rated their ability to control and decrease pain as poor. They also reported more psychological distress. Crisson and Keefe's findings of a relationship between locus of control on one hand and coping strategy utilization and psychological distress on the other held even after controlling for medical, demographic, and pain-level variables. The implication is that patients with an external locus of control may be ineffective pain copers who experience more psychological distress than other chronic pain patients. In other words, poor pain copers may exhibit psychopathology that resembles what cognitive therapists deal with in patients with other disorders (e.g., depression, anxiety).

Locus of control has also been applied to the investigation of the cultural context of pain. Tait *et al*. (1982) examined a large sample of chronic low-back pain patients from the United States and New Zealand, using the Health Locus of Control scale and various demographic and epidemiological data. Main effects were obtained for country of origin, with New Zealanders rating themselves as less dependent on physician's orders, and gender, with women endorsing less personal control over their pain conditions than men.

Perceived Control of an Aversive Stimulus or Event

In the laboratory, the issue of control has garnered a great deal of attention. It is generally accepted that pain that is personally controllable is more tolerable than pain that is not perceived as controllable (Turk, 1985; Turk and Meichenbaum, 1989). Weisenberg and his colleagues have found that personal control over pain is not always necessary for a beneficial outcome. Weisenberg *et al*. (1985) studied the impact of trait anxiety and self-efficacy, in combination with manipulated perceived control of a painful stimulus (electric shock) on reactions to a painful stimulus. The study involved five conditions, each of which manipulated perceived control in a different way. In one condition, subjects were told they could "control the situation" by having the opportunity to remove one of the shocks on each trial except the first (termed "decisional control"). Another group was told the experimenter had the opportunity to remove one of the shocks from each trial of shocks ("experimenter control"). The group allowed "behavioral control" was permitted to connect the electrodes to their own arms prior to the start of each trial. Subjects given decisional control alone yielded the largest pain reactions, while subjects given decisional plus behavioral control showed the least reaction to the painful electric current. Although self-efficacy and trait anxiety were predictive of subjects' responses to the aversive situation, experimenter control unexpectedly reduced the reaction to the painful stimulus among those with high self-efficacy and increased the reaction among those with low self-efficacy. Weisenberg *et al*. (1985) concluded that control that is perceived as inadequate may be worse than no control at all.

The relationship between pain and perceived control is complicated. A reciprocal relationship between pain and perceived control is implicated in chronic pain. Chronic pain can reduce a patient's sense of control, which in turn can lead to feelings of helplessness and depression. Conversely, coping well with chronic pain may enhance one's sense of self-control. As Weisenberg *et al.* (1985) concluded, the effect of perceived control over an aversive stimulus may depend on other factors such as one's sense of self-efficacy. In the following section we more fully examine self-efficacy theory in understanding pain experience.

Self-Efficacy

Laboratory Studies

A variety of recent laboratory investigations have demonstrated that there is a complex relationship between self-efficacy and pain, such that self-efficacy expectations appear to influence pain tolerance, but to have little impact or an indirect impact on level of distress. Vallis and Bucher (1986), for example, provided either brief skills training or a non-skill-based presentation to help eighty women cope with the induced pain of the cold-pressor task (immersion of hand and forearm in ice water). Participants provided self-efficacy strength and magnitude measures for pain tolerance. Vallis and Bucher reported that the self-efficacy of the skills training subjects significantly improved following the intervention. Further, their self-efficacy levels predicted tolerance on the posttraining cold-pressor task, across treatment conditions. The impact of self-efficacy was most significant for the group who received no skills training. Among these subjects, those who experienced relatively large increases in self-efficacy produced significantly lower discomfort scores. This was not the case, however, among the skills-training subjects, for whom self-efficacy changes were related to increases in tolerance but not reductions in discomfort. The authors note that self-efficacy is a useful moderator variable among those not trained in specific pain-coping strategies.

In a similar study, 64 college students volunteered to subject themselves to a cold-pressor pain induction (Dolce *et al.*, 1986c) to examine the association of self-efficacy expectations with pain tolerance under conditions in which tolerance quotas were used either alone or in conjunction with monetary incentives for increased pain tolerance. Self-efficacy ratings were significantly correlated with pain tolerance and were found to predict tolerance time better than ratings of subjective discomfort. Self-efficacy ratings and pain tolerance time were equally effective in predicting pain tolerance one week later. Setting quotas did improve subjects' performances, but monetary incentives did not. Although laboratory studies have found good associations between self-efficacy and pain tolerance, clinical investigations have been more equivocal.

Bandura *et al.* (1987) attempted to clarify how self-efficacy effects are related to physiological changes affecting pain. After being exposed to a pretreatment cold-pressor assessment, subjects in this study underwent cognitive-coping skills treatment, placebo treatment, or received no treatment at all. Half the subjects then received an injection of naloxone, which blocks the actions of endogenous opiates; in a double-blind procedure, the other half received a saline injection. The complex results from this well-controlled study provided evidence for both opioid and nonopioid mechanisms of cognitive pain control: "Cognitive copers administered naloxone were less able to tolerate pain stimulation than were their saline counterparts. The stronger the perceived self-efficacy to reduce pain, the greater was the opioid activation" (Bandura *et al.*, 1987, p. 563). Even when opioid mechanisms were blocked by naloxone, however, cognitive copers were able to achieve some increase in tolerance. These results suggest that subjects with the strongest levels of self-efficacy are most likely simply to *endure* pain, regardless of how intense the perceived stimulus becomes. Pain endurance leads to levels of stress that are likely to activate the CNS to release pain-blocking opioids. Thus, endurance itself may trigger pain relief because of the physiological mechanisms triggered at high intensities of pain. Bandura *et al.*'s results could not rule out the more straightforward possibility that self-efficacy expectations directly stimulate release of endogenous opioids. They noted that positing such a mechanism would be consistent with research showing that animals can learn to activate endogenous opiate systems in the presence of cues that formerly indicated painful stimulation (Watkins and Mayer, 1982).

Clinical Studies

Whereas the laboratory-pain self-efficacy literature defines self-efficacy expectations quite straightforwardly as the subject's perceived ability to cope with pain, in the case of chronic pain a more complex but more clinically relevant self-efficacy prediction may also be made: a rating of one's perceived ability to achieve desirable levels of performance relative to the desired outcomes, which are generally behaviorally anchored (Council *et al.*, 1988).

Dolce *et al.* (1986b) examined self-efficacy expectancies as outcome predictors for 63 chronic pain patients in a 4-week, multidisciplinary pain-management program. Among other measures, patients were assessed before and after treatment with the MMPI, Beck Depression Inventory, Pain Ratings, and ratings of self-efficacy expectations. Self-efficacy ratings were obtained by having subjects rate their ability to engage in daily exercise and work, and to cope without pain medications. Self-efficacy ratings improved significantly following treatment and posttreatment ratings of self-efficacy correlated positively with 6- to 12-month follow-up reports on patients' exercise, work status, and medication use. Nevertheless, in this study and a previous one (Dolce *et al.*, 1986a), these investigators found that a substantial number of patients did not display improvements in ratings of efficacy. The authors speculated that if patients attribute their improvements to external factors such as the therapist's skill, then self-efficacy expectancies may remain low despite clinical improvements.

In a study of 40 chronic low-back-pain patients, Council *et al.* (1988) measured two kinds of expectancy, self-efficacy and pain response expectancies. Pain response expectancies refer to Kirsch's (1985) response expectancy hypothesis: "Response expectancies are defined as subjective predictions of responses that occur without volitional control (e.g., pain, emotional reactions, and conversion symptoms)" (Council *et al.*, 1988, p. 324). Council *et al.* (1988) argued that a chronic pain patient might predict that he/she could perform behaviors to the extent that pain associated with the behaviors remains tolerable. Such a prediction takes into consideration the pain experience.

> It was hypothesized that perceived self-efficacy, operationalized as patients' ratings of their ability to perform movements, would bear a direct relationship to actual performance. Response expectancies for pain, operationalized as patient ratings of the degree of pain expected to accompany the movements, were predicted to bear an inverse relationship to performance. Due to their direct relationship to the experience of pain, response expectancies were hypothesized to bear a stronger relationship to avoidance behaviors (i.e., functional impairment) than self-efficacy expectancies. (Council *et al.*, 1988, p. 324)

Surprisingly, higher expected pain levels were not inversely related to performance, as had been expected. Instead, both self-efficacy *and pain response expectancies* were significantly correlated with actual performance. Although this study once again demonstrated how little is understood about the relationships among self-efficacy and pain-related outcomes, the results do show significant correspondence between average daily pain experiences and pain response expectancies for specific behaviors. The authors suggested that pain response expectancies influence performance and associated pain behavior via their effect on self-efficacy expectancies.

The investigations in this area need follow-up. It is clear that if patients' expectancies of physical impairment and pain influence actual performance, there are practical implications of better understanding these relationships. Once the relevant connections are clarified, chronic pain treatment may profitably include systematic modification of pain response expectancies. Until more consistent findings begin to emerge, it would be premature to stress a variable that, from the current state of knowledge, appears to behave unpredictably.

Pain and Depression

The role of cognition in pain has received the greatest attention in the area of chronic pain largely because of the significant advances that have been made in the cognitive treatment of clinical depression and the large proportion of chronic pain patients who are depressed. Although good epidemiological data have yet to be gathered about the prevalence of coexisting chronic pain and depression, the rate of depression in chronic pain patients is higher than that for the general population (Romano and Turner, 1985; Turner and Romano, 1984c). The percentage of chronic pain patients who are estimated also to suffer from depression ranges from 7 to 52%, according to studies reviewed by Doan and Wadden (1989). Not surprisingly, the literature suggests that as the length of suffering from chronic pain increases, so does the likelihood of suffering from depression (Doan and Wadden, 1989).

Depression Predicts Impairment

Keefe and his colleagues (Keefe *et al.*, 1986) studied the relationship of depression (assessed via the Beck Depression Inventory) to pain and pain behaviors among 207 chronic low-back-pain patients. Pain behaviors during physical examination, ratings of pain, and measures of activity level and medication intake were also recorded. Regression analyses from data gathered at a single point in time revealed that level of depression accounted for significant variation in pain and pain behaviors, independent from medical status variables.

Doan and Wadden (1989) studied 73 patients from a heterogeneous chronic pain population. Like other depressed patients, the depressed chronic pain patients exhibited cognitive distortions concerning themselves and their ability to cope. These patients seemed to have excessive hypochondriacal concern, dysphoria, and irritability, and difficulty expressing negative feelings. Among this group, depression appeared to be a better predictor of impairment than was pain severity. When the significant predictive power of depression was factored out of the relationship between pain and impairment in activity, pain failed to predict degree of impairment in activity.

These and other data emphasize the role of depression among pain patients. Clearly, depression is both significant in itself and also a major influence on adaptive behavior such as activity level and pain behaviors, which may in turn influence both adaptation to chronic pain problems and functional status.

Mediators of Depression among Pain Patients

Romano and Turner's (1985) review concluded that although some support exists for an association between chronic pain and depression, there appears to be little theory relating the two syndromes. Methodological problems exist in defining, categorizing, and reporting coexisting pain and depression. Nevertheless, there is substantial evidence that chronic pain is itself a prime cause of depression. Because not all individuals in pain become depressed, however, recent attention has turned to discovering the factors that mediate the development of depression in pain patients.

France *et al.* (1986) attempted to find mediating variables that would account for the variability in depressive disorders among 80 chronic low-back-pain (CLBP) patients. Using Research Diagnostic Criteria to assess depression, these investigators distinguished several categories of depression among the 80 patients: 21% had major depression; 54% had intermittent depression; and 20% were not depressed. They examined clinical variables (number of operations, duration of pain, and number of medications) and demographic variables (age, sex, race, marital status, education, employment status, and litigation) as possible mediators, but failed to find any of these variables helpful in predicting the presence or absence of depressive disorders in their CLBP patient sample.

Life events were examined as a mediator of depression among CLPB patients by Atkinson *et al.* (1988) in one of the few such investigations that have used both self-report and observer-rated assessments. A healthy comparison group consisted of 19 pain-free male volunteers, equated for age and socioeconomic status with the CLBP sample. Compared to nondepressed CLBP patients and the pain-free comparison group, depressed CLBP patients had experienced more stressful events. These stressful events were related to back pain, not other life problems. The investigators concluded that the association between stressful life events and chronic low-back pain is a function of both depressive symptoms and stressful life events that are specific to the pain. No differences were found between the 15 depressed and the 17 nondepressed CLBP patients on the basis of medical diagnosis, disease severity, pain history, or socioeconomic status.

Atkinson *et al.* (1988) argued that their sample of depressed CLBP patients was likely representative of a subgroup of pain patients that tend to be referred to chronic-pain-management programs. They cautiously proposed three possible casual links between chronic low-back pain, life stress, and psychopathology. First, it is possible that pain patients who are also depressed might, because of a negative cognitive bias, report more depressing events occurring in their lives than they would if they were not depressed. Second, inactivity and physical limitations imposed by the pain might directly contribute to a depressed mood. Third, persons with a physical disability and certain coping styles who are also depressed might mismanage their lives and bring on more negative events. The authors contended that the results of their study best support the third option because they found that depression and high stress were directly related to the number of stressful events occurring as a result of the back pain (e.g., hospitalization, litigation regarding the back injury, marital discord involving the back pain):

> Another possibility—and the one we favor—is that some patients with back disorders accompanied by chronic pain will suffer more if they also experience threatening life events or major life difficulties as a consequence of their back problems. Under these circumstances such patients are likely to develop depressive symptoms or mood, which might complicate their efforts to deal adaptively with the back condition. (Atkinson et al., 1988, p. 54)

Further support for this connection between chronic pain and depression comes from a study by Rudy et al. (1988). Rudy et al. found that perceived reductions in instrumental activities and a decline in perceptions of control and personal mastery were necessary prerequisites for the development of depressive symptoms in pain patients. Measures of life interference and degree of perceived self-control mediated depression secondary to chronic pain. Rudy et al. considered their study among the first to indicate some of the psychological mediators of the development of depression secondary to chronic pain.

In keeping with Rudy et al.'s (1988) finding of no strong, direct relationship between pain and depression, Smith et al. (1990) found that the relationship between severe rheumatoid arthritis and depression was mediated by degree of perceived helplessness. They concluded that both helplessness and cognitive distortion may contribute to the development of depression in rheumatoid arthritis.

Skevington (1983) studied 25 back-pain patients and 25 matched pain-free control subjects using a variety of paper-and-pencil measures. She distinguished between personal and universal helplessness. Self-blame and lowered self-esteem are generally associated with a sense of personal helplessness. In the case of universal helplessness, however, the individual believes she/he is not to blame for being unable to control certain life events; she/he also believes that no one else is capable of helping her/him. Among the CLBP patients, Skevington found that universal, not personal, helplessness was associated with depression. Because of the absence of

138 Glenn Pancyr and Myles Genest

self-blame, the universal helplessness was not associated with lowered self-esteem among these patients. The major limitation of this study was that the patients were collected from a sample of members of the Back Pain Association, and were largely nonpatients. Nevertheless, both Skevington's (1983) and Smith et al.'s (1990) work suggests depression in chronic-pain patients may be mediated by perceptions of helplessness in the face of pain.

Doan and Wadden (1989), in the study described earlier, examined a variety of possible mediators between pain and depression. They found that depressed pain patients were more preoccupied about physical problems, more irritable, and more prone to negative cognitions than were nondepressed pain patients. There also appeared to be a strong association between depression and the sensory quality of pain. This relationship, the authors ventured, might occur either because depression may alter the way we perceive and report pain, or because people sensitive to the sensory qualities of their pain may be more vulnerable to depression.

Doan and Wadden (1989) determined that 70–80% of the time, pain patients with the following characteristics will also be depressed: (1) significant impairment of social and recreational activities due to pain; (2) increasing pain throughout the day, to near-excruciating levels in late evening and bedtime; (3) endorsement of seven or more sensory pain descriptors on the McGill Pain Questionnaire.

Treatment of Depression is Important for Treatment of Pain

Although Doan and Wadden (1989) found that one-third of their sample of 73 chronic pain patients were mildly depressed and one-third were moderately to severely depressed, few of the patients exhibiting depression were receiving treatment for depression. The chronic-pain patients with depression tended to be treated more aggressively with pain medication than other pain patients. It would appear that increasing impairment in functioning was automatically viewed to be the result of pain, rather than as a result of depression that was complicating a pain problem. One of Doan and Wadden's (1989) main conclusions was that depression left untreated in chronic pain patients is associated with a poor response to pain treatment.

Dworkin et al. (1986) similarly hypothesized that prediction of treatment response of depressed and nondepressed chronic-pain patients would vary by group membership. Their study involved 454 patients with a variety of chronic-pain syndromes (e.g., cancer, CLBP, neck and head pain). Treatment modalities included nerve blocks, transcutaneous electrical nerve stimulation (TENS), analgesics, antidepressants, physical therapy, exercise, relaxation training, hypnosis, and short-term, cognitive–behavioural therapy. A positive response to pain treatment for the nondepressed patients appeared to be associated with more treatment visits, not receiving worker's compensation, fewer previous types of treatment, and having low-back pain. The depressed pain patients who responded favorably to pain treatment were more likely to be employed at the beginning of their treatment and to have pain of shorter duration. The authors conclude that activity and active involvement in pain treatment are particularly important for depressed pain patients.

Given that depression was the most important factor being assessed in the study, it is disappointing to discover that 18% (79) of the 454 pain patients were diagnosed as clinically depressed but that "these diagnoses were not based on recent standardized diagnostic criteria . . . these diagnoses were not made by psychiatrists or psychologists. . . ." (Dworkin *et al.*, 1986, p.346), but by physicians working in the pain field for many years. According to the authors, the diagnoses should be considered an assessment by pain-specialist physicians that depressed mood was present to a clinically significant degree. There were also rather serious deficiencies in the statistical presentation of the results of this study, so that it is difficult to evaluate the validity of the findings.

Ingram *et al.* (1990) have also suggested effective treatment of depression is important for the successful treatment of pain in depressed chronic-pain patients. These investigators reported that depressed chronic-pain patients exhibited significantly more negative automatic thoughts than nondepressed pain patients or healthy control subjects. Nondepressed chronic-pain patients, on the other hand, exhibited significantly more positive automatic thoughts than the chronic-pain patients or the healthy control subjects. In contrast to the findings of Doan and Wadden's (1989) review, Ingram *et al.* found that depression in pain patients was independent from pain duration; depression in their sample was also unrelated to type or intensity of pain. They also noted that the presence of cognitive distortions, operationalized as making distorted inferences about specific situational factors, was not as discriminating of depressed versus nondepressed chronic-pain patients as the differences in automatic thoughts, which were characterized as generalized self-statements that are recurrent, involuntary, and intrusive, especially if they are self-deprecatory. Ingram *et al.* recommended that cognitive–behavioural therapy for *depression* be considered the treatment of choice for depressed chronic pain patients, whereas cognitive–behavioural therapy specifically for *pain* be reserved for nondepressed chronic-pain patients. Others, however, suggest that effective psychological treatment of pain may be an effective antidepressant for chronic-pain patients.

Maruta *et al.* (1989) evaluated one hundred consecutive chronic-pain patients, without malignancy, admitted to a pain-management program, with the Research Diagnostic Criteria for depression. Forty-six patients were not depressed and the remaining patients were classified as probably or definitely depressed. Following treatment, 98 subjects were free of depression, and these gains were largely maintained at follow-up (average of 11.6 months from treatment termination) (89 patients remained non-depressed). Their treatment was a 3-week, inpatient program for pain management, which consisted of behavior modification, physical rehabilitation, medication management, education, group discussion, biofeedback and relaxation training, and family member participation. The authors concluded that pain-management programs may effectively relieve depression among chronic-pain patients.

Presentations of Depression among Pain Patients

Sprock *et al.* (1983) found that depressed pain patients exhibit deficits in abstraction, associative tightness, and speed of information processing. As with other studies reported earlier, they failed to find a correlation between cognitive deficits and pain when the contribution of depression was factored out.

Wade *et al.* (1990) used the MMPI, the Beck Depression Inventory, and seven visual analogue scales measuring degree of emotional unpleasantness, pain intensity, anxiety, frustration, fear, anger, and depression, to evaluate the emotional component of chronic pain. Sixty-nine women and 74 men who were referred by anesthesiologists for psychological evaluation comprised the chronic-pain patient sample. The authors did not indicate if these were consecutive referrals or what exclusion criteria operated during their data collection. The most frequent pain complaints were low-back pain, myofascial pain, and causalgia. Wade *et al.* found that anger was an important concomitant of depression in pain patients. They concluded that feelings of anger and frustration are such an integral part of the chronic pain experience that treatment techniques for these patients should be revised to include means to alleviate these feelings.

Turner and Romano (1984b) examined the ability of several self-report instruments to effectively screen for depression in a sample of chronic-pain patients who had also been diagnosed with the DSM-III criteria for major depression. Thirty percent of their sample of 40 chronic-pain patients met the DSM-III criteria for major depression. The Zung Depression scale and the Beck Depression Inventory (standard and short forms) were found to be equally effective screening instruments. The MMPI Depression scale, and MMPI obvious and subtle depression subscales had poorer ability to classify pain patients as depressed or nondepressed. The limits to the generalizability of the results include the small sample size investigated and the lack of cross-validation.

Using the MMPI, Smith *et al*. (1986) examined the nature of the cognitive distortion commonly found in depressed chronic low-back-pain patients. More specifically, they wished to determine if these cognitive distortions occurred more frequently in a case of general distress or in a case of somatization. They used the Cognitive Error Questionnaire, MMPI, Sickness Impact Profile, Daily Pain Diary, and a semistructured interview to assess 138 CLBP patients. Smith *et al*. contended that previous research had shown distinct MMPI profiles differentiating a somatization presentation from a general distress presentation, and that these two groups differ in how they describe their pain, the severity and course of the pain problem, and the degree of psychosocial impairment. The results from this study were correlational and based on self-reports, and cognitive distortion was measured by only one questionnaire. The authors found, however, that when subjective levels of pain and emotional distress were statistically controlled, cognitive distortion was more strongly associated with general distress, than with somatization. One might conclude that the types of cognitive distortions experienced by their sample of CLBP patients were more consistent with being generally distressed by their pain as opposed to being related to a style of thinking that is part of a tendency to focus one's attention and anxiety on health complaints.

France *et al*. (1987) found that chronic-pain patients with major depression and without major depression, and patients with primary major depression and secondary pain complaints all differed significantly in their response to the dexamethasone suppression test. As a result, they recommend the usefulness of the dexamethasone suppression test in discriminating among such groups of patients. Their findings are consistent with the view that the dexamethasone suppression test is a marker of a depressive state rather than a trait (Thase *et al.*, 1985).

Summary and Treatment Implications

Many basic questions concerning the importance of depression in chronic pain presentations have yet to be answered, such as what is the prevalence of coexisting pain and depression, what are the rates of depressive symptoms and syndromes in well-defined pain populations with matched controls, and what are the cognitive, behavioral, physiological, and sociocultural characteristics that discriminate depressed from nondepressed pain patients, and depressed patients with pain from depressed patients without pain (Romano and Turner, 1985). Prospective studies are needed to better investigate how pain or depression develop if the other is present first. And research is needed to inform clinicians about how best to treat coexisting pain and depression.

The current understanding of pain as partly affective in nature suggests that making unbearable pain bearable may be effected by such interventions as relieving the acute-pain sufferer from anxiety and the chronic-pain sufferer from depression, using standard psychotherapeutic techniques for treating these affective disorders. The emerging research that we have reviewed is consistent with this view.

Several implications for clinical assessment and treatment may be discerned from the research reviewed above. The *identification of depression* in patients with chronic pain is a crucial step in providing quality care. There is evidence to suggest that depressed pain patients will respond poorly to psychological pain treatments unless their depression is treated first. Moreover, it appears that depressed pain patients may be prone to maladaptive coping, which may aggravate their condition. The stress and life interference that depressed chronic-pain patients feel seem to be closely associated with feelings of helplessness, reduced activity levels, and reduced feelings of control, but not related to the intensity or severity of the pain itself. Therefore, some researchers have suggested that cognitive and cognitive–behavioral therapies for depression be conducted prior to admitting depressed pain patients to cognitive therapies for pain.

Memory for Pain

Research on memory for pain has begun to appear only over the past 10 years. Referring to Fig. 5.1, the research in memory falls in area B, the overlap of the domains of pain and cognitive theory. However, because this work is so new, most of the research is observational and theory generation would be somewhat premature. The gate-control theory posited the importance of past experiences in understanding individuals' pain reactions. The work that is summarized next is the first stage of documenting just what people remember about experiences with pain.

Most of the research has focused on the accuracy of memory for pain intensity (Erskine *et al.*, 1990). Some evidence exists to show that recall of acute pain is more accurate than recall of chronic pain, but as early as 1957, Jones noted that it is difficult to conjure up a vivid memory of the sensory qualities of pain. People are better at remembering verbal descriptors, or the scene or setting of the pain than the sensory experience. There are, however, several critical reasons for studying memory for pain; (1) patients' recall of pain is used in both diagnosis and assessment of treatment interventions; (2) research instruments rely on pain memories when subjects are asked to compare their present pain with a pain memory (e.g., where does your pain fall on a 1 to 10 scale); (3) memory for pain is an important aspect of theories that seek to explain how we process and react to acute pain and how chronic-pain behaviors become established.

In a review of the literature on memory for pain, Erskine *et al.* (1990) examined four types of pain: chronic continuous, acute clinical, acute procedural, and experimentally induced. It was noted that different methods used to assess recall of chronic pain can give markedly different results within the same study. The degree of relationship between actual pain experience and recall of pain was found to be about $r = .65$, but the variability of accurate recall was quite high. For example, initial data suggested that women underestimate the amount of pain they have experienced in the early stages of labor whereas chronic-pain patients may overestimate their pain. Erskine *et al.* suggested that when pain is experienced as acute and novel the accuracy of recall for its intensity is greater than when pain is either chronic or episodic. Mood and affective states also influence memory for pain, and memory for the affective quality of pain seems to be less accurate than memory for the sensory component of pain.

Linton and Melin (1982), as a test of the accuracy of pre–post measures of a pain treatment program, asked 12 chronic-pain patients to rate their pain at the beginning of treatment. At the end of treatment (3–11 weeks later), subjects were once again asked to rate what their pain *had been* prior to treatment. Eleven of the twelve patients recalled their pain at base line to have been more severe than their actual base line pain rating. Linton and Melin concluded that chronic-pain patients systematically and significantly overestimate their recollections of base line pain ratings after an intervening period of treatment lasting more than two weeks. They cautioned researchers against using subjects as their own controls to determine pre–post treatment effects because of this reporting bias. They noted, however, that their results were inconsistent with those of Hunter *et al.* (1979), who found that memory for an acute pain, measured after only a 5-day interval, was relatively good. The interrating intervals in the two studies differed considerably, however. It may be that memory for chronic pain, without any particular identifying event, is poor over an interval of several weeks.

Roche and Gijsbers (1986) conducted an investigation of the various factors thought to influence the results of memory-for-pain research, such as type of pain assessment used, duration and constancy of the pain, and circumstances for observing the pain. Twenty-three young, healthy subjects endured ischemic-induced pain and rated their pain on the McGill Pain Questionnaire. They then recalled their pain one week later, using the same pain assessment method. Another group of subjects were twice as old as the healthy subjects, and had rheumatoid arthritis for which they underwent surgery on a single joint. Pain assessments were conducted one day prior to surgery and again one week after surgery. Roche and Gijsbers reported that memory for the overall intensity of pain was better for a single experience of ischemic pain than was memory for rheumatoid pain, and that the dimension of pain most vulnerable to memory decrement was the nonsensory quality of pain. The authors further speculated that differences in mood between pre- and postsurgery might in part account for the poor recollection of pain by rheumatoid subjects. Age might have been a confound in this study.

The research of Pearce *et al*. (1990) showed that the occurrence of a state-dependent learning effect is likely operating in chronic-pain patients' memory of pain. No evidence was found, however, for mood congruity effects other than to suggest that memory for pain may be more related to the status of being a chronic-pain patient than to the state of being in pain.

These studies suggest that state-dependent effects may be present in the reporting of pain. Roche and Gijsbers (1986), in particular, indicated the importance of the mood of the subject at recall in affecting accuracy of memory. If the mood at recall is different from the mood of the subject when the pain was actually experienced, then poor memory for pain should be expected. Implications for pain assessment are that assessment of pain intensity from memory would be facilitated by using verbal scales, as opposed to visual analogue scales, and by using scales based on sensory pain descriptors instead of emotionally laden adjectives.

Another study, involving 93 chronic pain patients (Jamison *et al.*, 1989), found a tendency to overestimate pain intensity levels. Patients who reported more emotional distress, who had conflicts at home, who were less active, and who relied on medication tended to be the most inaccurate in remembering their pain. Related findings were reported by Rachman and Eyrl (1989), who found that patients with headache or menstrual pain also tended to recall the painful episodes as being more painful than they had reported at the time of the pain episode.

A limitation of research in the area is that it is atheoretical, mainly focused on gauging accuracy without attempting to incorporate the findings into any theory of pain per se. Nor have theories from memory literature played much of a role in this work. Despite the caution of Beidel and Turner (1986) that cognitive-behaviourists have failed to use the findings from basic cognitive psychology to guide clinical practice, the field has evidenced considerable enthusiasm for an emerging rapprochement between cognitive science and cognitive therapy (Tataryn *et al.*, 1989). If, as Karoly and Jensen (1987) have suggested, the next era of pain research is one in which new developments from cognitive science will be incorporated into the area of pain research, we anticipate much will be forthcoming from the study of memory.

Cognitive–Behavioral Therapy

The basic assumption of cognitive–behavioral therapy is that thoughts, attitudes, beliefs, and expectations can determine people's emotional and behavioral reactions. Because pain has recently been understood to have both cognitive and emotional components (Melzack and Wall, 1965), changing one's thoughts or attitudes might reasonably be expected to alter the subjective experience of pain. Depression is a common problem for chronic-pain patients; the application of cognitive principles to depressed pain patients has received a great deal of attention in the pain literature.

Cognitive–behavioral treatments have also been applied directly to the problem of pain. The first comprehensive clinical application of the cognitive-behavioral perspective to pain problems was proposed by Turk et al. (1983). It was still possible for reviewers in 1983 to characterize the application of social learning and cognitive–behavioral principles to the prevention and alleviation of pain as a "recent innovation" (Kerns et al., 1983). In this section we examine some empirical investigations in the area showing how cognitive–behavioral therapy has both contributed to knowledge concerning effective amelioration of acute and chronic pain and led to identification and clarification of theoretical issues. In particular, years of investigations evaluating the efficacy of specific cognitive pain-coping strategies has resulted in recognizing the importance of the idiosyncratic meaning the person ascribes to his or her pain; the importance of meaning when life is threatened by painful disease; and the importance of understanding those individuals who appear to cope with chronic pain without assistance from cognitive-behaviorists.

In 1983, Kerns et al. produced a selective review of psychological treatments for chronic pain, including biofeedback and biofeedback-assisted relaxation, operant conditioning, and cognitive–behavioral treatments. Their conclusions were discouraging. Methodological inadequacies in the studies reviewed led them to withhold unqualified acceptance of these approaches for the treatment of chronic-pain problems. Lack of adequate control groups, poor patient sample descriptions, and insufficient data on treatment follow-up were some of the main deficiencies in the studies at the time of their review.

In the ensuing years, several prominent pain researchers have published reviews of psychological treatments for pain problems, which included sections on the cognitive–behavioral perspective. Turner and

Romano (1984a) concluded from their brief survey that the evidence for a cognitive–behavioral approach to pain management merited further refinement and standardization. They recommended further study on the mechanisms of action and efficacy of cognitive–behavioral techniques and more long-term, follow-up studies. Similarly, Fernandez and Turk's (1989) meta-analytic study led them to endorse cognitive coping strategies in alleviating pain:

> Meta-analytic techniques . . . revealed that, in general, cognitive coping strategies are more effective in alleviating pain as compared to either no-treatment or expectancy controls. Each individual class of strategies significantly attenuates pain although the imagery methods are the most effective whereas pain acknowledging is the least effective. (p. 123)

Issues remain, however, concerning both the integrity of the extant research, and the links between cognitive theory and practice. Consider the following communication by Turner and Romano (1984a):

> In conclusion, we would like to encourage researchers to move toward developing knowledge accumulated from systematic soundly designed investigation, rather than continue the proliferation of unrelated studies that are virtually impossible to integrate because of methodologic deficiencies and dissimilarities. (p. 293)

Nevertheless, as the following research illustrates, there is both considerable enthusiasm for a cognitive approach to pain management and evidence that the approach — although not completely understood — is worth both clinical application and further theoretical development.

Holroyd and Andrasik (1982) conducted a 2-year follow-up study comparing the relative efficacy of cognitive therapy with biofeedback treatment for tension headache. Clients who received cognitive therapy reported that they continued to use the stress-coping training and their headaches continued to be significantly improved. A more mixed result was obtained for the biofeedback clients, both following treatment and at the 2-year follow-up. The long-term benefit of the cognitive therapy intervention was superior to that for the biofeedback intervention.

Reduction in the suffering of tension-headache patients through cognitive therapy occurs even when the interventions are largely self-administered. Tobin et al. (1988) provided headache patients with either relaxation training only or both relaxation training and cognitive therapy. Both treatments were provided primarily through self-administered audiotapes and workbooks, involving only three clinic visits during the two months of therapy. The combined treatment group reported substantially greater reductions in headache activity (e.g., 76% reduction in headache index) than did the patients who received only the relaxation training (36% reduction). Patients receiving both treatments also reported reductions in depression. High pretreatment levels of headache and daily life stress predicted a poor response to the relaxation training treatment but made no difference in the effectiveness of the combined intervention.

A bibliotherapy format was used for a treatment–control comparison group in a study of rheumatoid arthritis patients (O'Leary *et al.*, 1988). The control bibliotherapy consisted of a self-help book containing useful information about arthritis self-management. The cognitive–behavioral group received the self-help book and met weekly for 5 weeks with 2 female group leaders in groups of 5–7 people. Treatment included discussion of the biopsychosocial model of pain, training in cognitive and behavioral pain-management techniques, and personal goal setting. The pain-management techniques included relaxation with guided imagery, attentional refocusing, and relabeling. The experimenters failed to find the predicted improvement in the treatment group on activity levels and immunologic functioning. Although the results must be considered with some caution because of the high number of *t* tests performed, which raised the likelihood of making a Type I error, compared to the control group, the experimental group did obtain greater reductions in self-reported pain, depression, stress, joint inflammation, and sleep disturbance.

Although no control group was used, Skinner *et al.* (1990) obtained positive results in an evaluation of a cognitive–behavioral treatment for chronic-pain outpatients. A multidisciplinary team led the pain patients in a seven-week, one-afternoon-per-week program designed to increase patients' coping with chronic pain. Pre–post measures, and measures at one month follow-up, for mood, coping-skills acquisition, physical disability, and analgesic consumption revealed significant improvement following the course. Ratings of pain intensity, however, did not change significantly.

Spence (1989) assessed patients with chronic, occupational pain of the upper limbs as they received either individual cognitive–behavioral therapy, group cognitive–behavioral therapy, or remained on the waiting list as control subjects. Significant benefits were found for both the individual and group treatments on measures of anxiety, depression, coping strategies, impact on daily living, pain, and distress caused by pain, and these benefits were maintained at the 6-month follow-up. No clinically relevant differences were found between the two forms of treatment.

Whether the cognitive or cognitive–behavioral treatments for pain are individual or group oriented, used alone or in conjunction with other therapies, these techniques appear to be quite effective. What these studies do not yet clarify for us is the mechanism of change, or the active ingredients in these cognitive approaches. However, some general trends are becoming apparent that do begin to address these questions.

Metaconstructs in Chronic-Pain Treatments

Turk and Holzman (1986) reviewed some of the commonalities among psychological approaches in the treatment of chronic pain, looking for what they called "metaconstructs." They found several main themes shared among such treatment approaches as operant conditioning, social-skills training, hypnosis, family therapy, biofeedback, and cognitive–behavioral therapy. All of these therapies shared a requirement that the patient reconceptualize his or her pain in a way that was consistent with the treatment modality to be provided. In other words, the pain patient and the therapist must come to some mutual understandings about what the pain *means* for the client. In the cognitive–behavioral approach, reconceptualization of the patient's pain has served several main functions, for example, recasting problems in ways that are amenable to solutions, fostering hope, and promoting positive expectancy. Other metaconstructs identified by Turk and Holzman (1986) that are shared by psychological approaches to pain management included: (1) optimism and combating demoralization; (2) individualization of treatment; (3) active patient participation and responsibility; (4) skills acquisition; (5) self-efficacy; and (6) self-attribution of change. Again, we note the emphasis on the personal meaning of the pain for the patient.

The Importance of Meaning

A major theme in contemporary psychological pain research, especially from the perspective of cognitive theory, appears to be a fuller understanding of the importance of the meaning of pain. Pain measurement and assessment have gradually begun to move from an emphasis on measuring the sensory and affective qualities of pain experience (e.g., tolerance, threshold, pain intensity, and pain affect) toward self-reported pain-coping strategies, beliefs about personal control over painful experiences, and self-efficacy and outcome expectancies regarding implementation of cognitive pain-coping strategies. The continuation of this movement was predicted by Karoly and Jensen (1987):

> We anticipate also that the growing rapprochement between the cognitive and clinical science will create an atmosphere wherein the analysis of pain as it is felt or seen will be supplemented with a consideration of pain as it is understood by the patient. (p. 126)

A central component of theoretical developments in pain is likely to be that the main mediating factor in chronic pain is the meaning the pain has for the individual. Understanding pain and adjustment to chronic pain requires understanding how the patient understands the meaning of pain (and disease or injury) in his or her life.

The psychological literature commonly separates consideration of cancer pain from other types of pain without providing much in the way of justification. One reason for making a distinction between cancer pain and non–cancer pain is that cancer pain is thought to carry additional emotional and psychological considerations (e.g., fear of death), compared to the meaning of pain without cancer. Results of investigations of the cognitive aspects of pain have contributed to some researchers concluding that cancer pain is not different from other types of chronic pain.

Cancer Pain

Turk and Fernandez (1990) provide an excellent overview of the limitations of biomedical treatment of cancer pain. They also review the common assumption that cancer pain is unique. Turk and Fernandez specifically review potential psychological factors thought to influence cancer pain, such as expectancy, affective distress, symptom interpretation, perceived controllability, behavior, and cognition. Is cancer pain unique? Not according to Turk and Fernandez (1990). It is considered unique by the medical and social communities but it is not unique according to how psychological principles and treatments for pain are applicable:

> Psychological factors such as anxiety, expectancy, cognitive appraisal, self-efficacy, perceived control, along with principles of respondent conditioning, operant conditioning, and observational learning have been shown to influence reports and experience of acute pain, chronic non-malignant pain, and acute recurrent pain, but have been ignored in the cancer pain literature. (Turk and Fernandez, 1990, p. 2)

Taylor and Crisler (1988) noted that while 38% of cancer patients survive beyond 5 years from their diagnosis, this disease is dreaded more than other life-threatening conditions such as heart disease, which, at twice the mortality rate of cancer, is the leading cause of death in the United States. Some studies show that a majority of cancer patients do not report pain until after they are made aware of their disease.

In 1984, Sternbach concluded that although acute pain may promote survival, chronic pain is destructive physically, psychologically, and socially, and it disrupts thought processes. Thought process disruption may occur in the form of preoccupation with pain and the sick role, health anxiety, resistance to reassurance, abnormal illness behavior, increasing rumination, and obsession. It appears, however, that persons with malignant pain function better than other chronic-pain patients, perhaps because they go on despite their pain. In 1989, Sternbach wondered why cancer-pain patients, whose situation is life threatening, do not seem to fall prey to the chronic-pain syndrome the way others do. In his review of benign versus malignant pain, he hypothesized that perhaps the knowledge of the fatal nature of the disease makes this group's responses different from the others. Cancer patients with pain have less fear and less pain than other types of chronic-pain patients. Perhaps, unlike other chronic-pain patients, they are wrestling with issues of meaning and purpose in their life.

Life in Spite of Pain

Turk and Rudy (1990b) suggested that we may have been misdirected in our search for the best pain treatments because we have not studied the best subjects, that is those who successfully live, work, and play with chronic pain. Moreover, it appears many patients reject our treatments for chronic pain, partly because they know we do not understand their pain. In a study by Colvin et al. (1980), 237 of 300 pain patients said their pain was caused by something more serious than, or different from, what their doctors had told them. Patients will accept only a treatment whose rationale is acceptable to their understanding of their situation.

And what is the patient's goal for a pain-treatment program? Some may wish to have their pain eliminated. But the goal of most pain-treatment programs is to help the patient learn to live with the pain (Turk and Rudy, 1990b). Karoly and Jensen (1987) have captured this treatment dilemma in their summary of laboratory pain investigations:

> For the most part, laboratory investigators of pain control have given the subject nothing else to do but to try to tolerate pain for increasingly long periods of time. Although certainly not an unimportant goal, the focus on endurance, or its correlates, misses the very critical point that pain sufferers not only need to tolerate pain but also continue to engage in other life tasks — some trivial and some important, waxing and waning in their consciousness — and they are rarely free to put everything else on hold. (p. 130)

The act of looking for pain relief may in itself separate poor pain copers from those who learn to live in spite of their pain. That is, those patients who have fewer personal coping resources may be the ones most likely to have as their only goal living without pain. Learning to live with pain implies having something else to live for, which may not be true of the chronic-pain patients who have the most difficulty — who are the ones most likely to present for treatment. Turk and Rudy (1990b) articulated the other side of the issue: "If recent surveys are any indication, the vast majority of people with chronic pain are never seen in pain clinics and many may be adjusting reasonably well" (p. 9).

OUTSTANDING ISSUES AND IMPLICATIONS FOR THEORY AND TREATMENT

In the previous section we examined research from several domains of inquiry including theory-driven research, research focusing on clinical intervention studies, and research from cognitive science (i.e., memory studies). Each of these areas of inquiry have made important contributions to understanding psychological treatments for pain problems, and for psychopathology associated with pain. The memory research has sensitized investigators to the degree we rely on subjects' recall when we measure pain, which has serious implications for assessing treatment efficacy. Research on coexisting pain and depression suggests depressed pain patients should have their depression attended to first in order to maximize therapies for pain relief. Cognitive–behavioral techniques for alleviating pain have generated sufficient research with the result that several major themes are beginning to emerge. One such theme may redirect our theoretical conceptualization of pain toward a better appreciation of patients' interpretation of their pain and its relation to the treatment being offered. In this final section we consider the future of cognitive theory in understanding pain experiences. We begin by repeating the need for a more comprehensive theory of pain. We also discuss one alternative to traditional systems of classifying pain disorders and experiences, the Multiaxial Assessment of Pain (Turk and Rudy, 1990a). The section ends with comments on areas of psychopathology currently neglected in the pain literature, and on the future of cognitive theorizing about pain.

The Need for a Comprehensive Theory of Pain

What is missing in the psychological study of pain is a truly comprehensive theory of pain. Melzack and Wall's (1965) gate-control model has served a significant role in legitimizing the psychological study of pain in giving credence to the notion that a patient's internal environment has as much to due with the experience of pain as the disease process or injury affecting him or her. It now appears that current research efforts have gone beyond the point from which the gate-control model can be helpful. Having accepted that descending influences from the brain can affect pain perception, researchers are now fine-tuning their questions to ask exactly what kinds of cognitive processes will produce pain-enhancing or pain-reducing effects.

Recent developments have raised important issues for consideration. For example, with the greater understanding of the complexity of cognitive involvements in the perception, exacerbation, and amelioration of pain in adults, questions naturally arise about the cognitive development of children and their capacities for utilizing cognitive–behavioral interventions for pain control. Though gate-control theory was more comprehensive than the theories that preceded it, a new theory of pain will have to begin to incorporate new data arising from several domains of psychological inquiry, such as life-span development, psychopathology, and memory.

Classifying Pain by Psychosocial Variables

One of the outcomes of cognitive investigations of pain has been to question the standard classification systems for pain problems. Traditionally, pain has been considered a biomedical problem and pain has been classified by location (e.g., head pain, abdominal pain), by disease (arthritic pain), and by treatment response (acute pain, chronic pain). But another approach to classifying pain problems is on the basis of psychosocial variables. Turk and Rudy (1990a) empirically derived a system called the Multiaxial Assessment of Pain (MAP), which classifies chronic-pain patients according to physical, functional, psychosocial, and behavioral characteristics. Turk and Rudy's data suggest that the psychosocial and behavioral factors associated with chronic pain cut across demographically and diagnostically diverse samples of patients. Turk and Rudy (1988) identified three distinct profiles based upon coping styles: dysfunctional, interpersonally distressed, and adaptive copers. With the proposed classification system, persons with temporomandibular disorder, headache, and chronic low-back pain who are classified within the same MAP subgroup may be more similar to each other than patients with the same medical–dental diagnosis but who are classified in different MAP subgroups. Although different diagnostic groups, based on traditional classifications, may require specific medical or dental treatment, they may also benefit from different specific psychosocial interventions tailored to their MAP classification. The MAP system is a unique departure from traditional methods of conceptualizing pain problems and is deserving of further theoretical consideration.

Areas of Psychopathology Neglected in the Pain Literature

Certain areas of psychopathology, namely the anxiety and mood disorders, have received a great deal of attention in the pain literature, but other disorders have not. Pain-related behaviors such as self-mutilation by persons with severe personality or psychotic disorders, or by persons with less severe pathology who may be grieving a significant loss, have not received much attention. It would seem reasonable that we might have a great deal to learn from these individuals who induce pain in themselves, or who spontaneously appear to be able to dissociate from emotionally and physically painful experiences, or the memories of these experiences. Similarly, pain associated with sexual disorders (i.e., paraphilias such as sexual sadism and sexual masochism; sexual pain disorders such as dyspareunia) has received scant attention. A comprehensive theory of pain might include these syndromes and phenomena as well. A study of these diverse forms of pain experience may show promise in expanding the breadth of theoretical understanding of pain behaviors and subjective pain experiences.

The Future of Cognition in Pain Theorizing

Schneider and Karoly (1983) wrote,

> If investigators were to accept in common the idea that the smallest "unit" of analysis in pain is the person-in-context, and that pain as a pure sensation cannot and should not serve as the pivotal change construct, perhaps modern thinkers can recapture the essence of Hellenic reasoning. The current interest in self-regulation and systems theory in health psychology (e.g., Leventhal, Nerenz and Struas, 1980; Rodin, 1982; Schwartz, 1979) augers well for emergence of a functional and process model of pain that will minimize oversimplification in the name of disciplinary specialization. (p. 83)

Such notions are being posited for the area of psychological theorizing about health (Schwartz, 1984), coping in cancer (Cunningham, 1986), and chronic pain (Karoly and Jensen, 1987).

The growth in research concerning cognition and pain in the last decade has been dramatic. Theoretical development lags behind, though promising signs are evident in such efforts as those of Bandura and his colleagues (Bandura *et al.*, 1987) and Karoly and Jensen (1987). Continued development of the most effective interventions for patients with pain will benefit from theoretical integration of the many disparate directions of current research. Cognitive theory currently provides an auspicious possibility for theoretical synthesis.

ACKNOWLEDGMENT

The authors gratefully acknowledge the helpful comments of Carl von Baeyer in preparing this chapter.

REFERENCES

Alexander, F. (1950). *Psychosomatic medicine. Its principles and applications*. New York: Norton.

American Psychiatric Association. (1987). *Diagnostic and statistical manual of mental disorder* (3rd and rev. ed). Washington, D.C.: American Psychiatric Association.

Atkinson, J. H., Slater, M. A., Grant, I., Patterson, T. L., and Garfin, S. R. (1988). Depressed mood in chronic low back pain: Relationship with stressful life events. *Pain, 35*, 47–55.

Averill, J. R. (1973). Personal control over aversive stimuli and its relationship to stress. *Psychological Bulletin, 80*, 286–303.

Bandura, A. (1977). Self-efficacy: Toward a unifying theory of behavioural change. *Psychological Review, 84*, 191–215.

Bandura, A., O'Leary, A., Taylor, C. B., Gauthier, J., and Gossard, D. (1987). Perceived self-efficacy and pain control: Opioid and nonopioid mechanisms. *Journal of Personality and Social Psychology, 53*(3), 563–571.

Beck, A. T., and Weishaar, M. (1989). Cognitive therapy. In A. Freeman, K. M. Simon, L. E. Beutler, and H. Arkowitz (Eds.), *Comprehensive handbook of cognitive therapy* (pp. 21–36). London: Plenum.

Beck, A. T., Brown, G., Steer, R. A., Eidelson, J. I., and Riskind, J. H. (1987). Differentiating anxiety and depression: A test of the cognitive content-specificity hypothesis. *Journal of Abnormal Psychology, 96*(3), 179–183.

Beecher, H. K. (1959). *Measurement of subjective responses*. New York: Oxford University Press.

Beidel, D. C., and Turner, S. M. (1986). A critique of the theoretical bases of cognitive–behavioral theories and therapy. *Clinical Psychology Review, 6*, 177–197.

Brena, S. (1972). *Pain and religion: A psychophysiological study*. Springfield, IL: Charles C. Thomas.

Colvin, D. F., Bettinger, R., Knapp, R., Pawlicki, R., and Zimmerman, J. (1980). Characteristics of patients with chronic pain. *South Medical Journal (Bgham, AL), 73*, 1020–1023.

Council, J. R., Ahern, D. K., Follick, M. J., and Kline, C. L. (1988). Expectancies and functional impairment in chronic low back pain. *Pain, 33*, 323–331.

Courey, L., Feuerstein, M., and Bush, B. (1982). Self-control and chronic headache. *Journal of Psychosomatic Research, 26*(5), 519–526.

Crisson, J. E., and Keefe, F. J. (1988). The relationship of locus of control to pain coping strategies and psychological distress in chronic pain patients. *Pain, 35*, 147–154.

Cunningham, A. J. (1986). Information and health in the many levels of man: Toward a more comprehensive theory of health and disease. *Advances, 3*(1), 32–45.

Doan, B. D., and Wadden, N. P. (1989). Relationships between depressive symptoms and descriptions of chronic pain. *Pain, 36*, 75–84.

Dolce, J. J., Crocker, M. F., Moletteire, C., and Doleys, D. M. (1986a). Exercise quotas, anticipatory concern, and self-efficacy expectancies in chronic pain: A preliminary report. *Pain, 24*, 365–372.

Dolce, J. J., Crocker, M. F., and Doleys, D. M. (1986b). Prediction of outcome among chronic pain patients. *Behaviour Research and Therapy, 24*(3), 313–319.

Dolce, J. J., Doleys, D. M., Raczynski, J. M., Lossie, J., Poole, L., and Smith, M. (1986c). The role of self-efficacy expectancies in the prediction of pain tolerance. *Pain, 27*, 261–272.

Dworkin, R. H., Richlin, D. M., Handlin, D. S., and Brand, L. (1986). Predicting treatment response in depressed and non-depressed chronic pain patients. *Pain, 24*, 343–353.

Erskine, A., Morley, S., and Pearce, S. (1990). Memory for pain: A Review. *Pain, 41*, 255–265.

Fernandez, E., and Turk, D. C. (1989). The utility of cognitive coping strategies for altering pain perception: A meta-analysis. *Pain, 38*, 123–135.

France, R. D., Houpt, J. L., Skott, A., Krishnan, K. R. R., and Varia, I. M. (1986). Depression as a psychopathological disorder in chronic low back pain patients. *Journal of Psychosomatic Research, 30*(2), 127–133.

France, R. D., Krishnan, K. R. R., Trainor, M., and Pelton, S. (1987). Chronic pain and depression. IV.: DST as a discriminator between chronic pain and depression. *Pain, 28,* 39–44.

Genest, M. (1986). The growth of pain and the pain of growth. *Canadian Journal of Psychology, 40,* 487–490.

Holroyd, K. A., and Andrasik, F. (1982). Do the effects of cognitive therapy endure? A two-year follow-up of tension headache sufferers treated with cognitive therapy or biofeedback. *Cognitive Therapy and Research, 6*(3), 325–334.

Hunter, M., Philips, C., and Rachman, S. (1979). Memory for pain. *Pain, 6,* 35–46.

Ingram, R. E., Atkinson, J. H., Slater, M. A., Saccuzzo, D. P., and Garfin, S. R. (1990). Negative and positive cognition in depressed and nondepressed chronic-pain patients. *Health Psychology, 9*(3), 300–314.

Jamison, R. N., Sbrocco, T., and Parris, W. C. V. (1989). The influence of physical and psychosocial factors on accuracy of memory for pain in chronic pain patients. *Pain, 37,* 289–294.

Jensen, M. P., Turner, J. A., Romano, J. M., and Karoly, P. (1991). Coping with chronic pain: A critical review of the literature. *Pain, 47,* 249–283.

Jones, E. (1957). Pain. *International Journal of Psychoanalysis, 38,* 255–257.

Karoly, P., and Jensen, M. P. (1987). *Multimethod assessment of chronic pain.* New York: Pergamon.

Keefe, F. J., and Williams, D. A. (1989). New directions in pain assessment and treatment. *Clinical Psychology Review, 9,* 549–568.

Keefe, F. J., Wilkins, R. H., Cook, W. A., Jr., Crisson, J. E., and Muhlbaier, L. H. (1986). Depression, pain, and pain behaviour. *Journal of Consulting and Clinical Psychology, 54*(5), 665–669.

Kerns, R. D., Turk, D. C., and Holzman, A. D. (1983). Psychological treatment for chronic pain: A selective review. *Clinical Psychology Review, 3,* 15–26.

Kirsch, I. (1985). Response expectancy as a determinant of experience and behavior. *American Psychologist, 40,* 1189–1202.

Kores, R. C., Murphy, W. D., Rosenthal, T. L., Elias, D. B., and North, W. C. (1990). Predicting outcome of chronic pain treatment via a modified self-efficacy scale. *Behaviour Research and Therapy, 28*(2), 165–169.

Lefcourt, H. M. (1982). *Locus of control: Current trends in theory and research* (2nd ed.). Hillsdale, NJ: Erlbaum.

Linton, S. J., and Melin, L. (1982). The accuracy of remembering chronic pain. *Pain, 13,* 281–285.

Maruta, T., Vatterott, M. K., and McHardy, M. J. (1989). Pain management as an antidepressant: Long-term resolution of pain-associated depression. *Pain, 36,* 335–337.

McCreary, C., and Turner, J. (1984). Locus of control, repression–sensitization, and psychological disorder in chronic pain patients. *Journal of Clinical Psychology, 40*(4), 897–901.

Melzack, R., and Wall, P. D. (1965). Pain mechanisms: A new theory. *Science, 50,* 971–979.

Melzack, R., and Wall, P. D. (1983). *The challenge of pain.* New York: Basic Books.

Merskey, H. (1989). Psychiatry and chronic pain. *Canadian Journal of Psychiatry, 34,* 329–336.

Nisbett, R. E., and Schachter, R. S. (1966). Cognitive manipulation of pain. *Journal of Experimental Social Psychology, 2,* 227–236.

O'Leary, A., Shoor, S., Lorig, K., and Holman, H. (1988). A cognitive-behavioral treatment for rheumatoid arthritis. *Health psychology, 7*(6), 527–544.

Pancyr, G. (1988). *The effect of mood on pain: A laboratory investigation.* Unpublished doctoral dissertation, University of Saskatchewan, Saskatoon, Saskatchewan.

Pearce, S. A., Isherwood, S., Hrouda, D., Richardson, P. H., Erskine, A., and Skinner, J. (1990). Memory and pain: Tests of mood congruity and state dependent learning in experimentally induced and clinical pain. *Pain, 43,* 187–193.

Rachman, S., and Eyrl, K. (1989). Predicting and remembering recurrent pain. *Behaviour Research and Therapy, 27*(6), 621–635.

Roche, P. A., and Gijsbers, K. (1986). A comparison of memory for induced ischaemic pain and chronic rheumatoid pain. *Pain, 25,* 337–343.

Romano, J. M., and Turner, J. A. (1985). Chronic pain and depression: Does the evidence support a relationship? *Psychological Bulletin, 97*(1), 18–34.

Rudy, T. E., Kerns, R. D., and Turk, D. C. (1988). Chronic pain and depression: Toward a cognitive-behavioral mediation model. *Pain, 35,* 129–140.

Schneider, F., and Karoly, P. (1983). Conceptions of the pain experience: The emergence of multidimensional models and their implications for contemporary clinical practice. *Clinical Psychology Review, 3,* 61–86.

Schwartz, G. E. (1984). Psychobiology of health: A new synthesis. In B. C. Hammonds and C. J. Scheirer (Eds.), *Psychology and health: Master lecture series* (pp. 149–193). Washington, D.C.: American Psychological Association.

Skevington, S. M. (1983). Chronic pain and depression: Universal or personal helplessness? *Pain, 15,* 309–317.

Skinner, J. B., Erskine, A., Pearce, S., Rubenstein, I., Taylor, M., and Foster, C. (1990). The evaluation of a cognitive behavioural treatment programme in outpatients with chronic pain. *Journal of Psychosomatic Research, 34*(1), 13–19.

Smith, T. W., Aberger, E. W., Follick, M. J., and Ahern, D. K. (1986). Cognitive distortion and psychological distress in chronic low back pain. *Journal of Consulting and Clinical Psychology, 54*(4), 573–575.

Smith, T. W., Peck, J. R., and Ward, J. R. (1990). Helplessness and depression in rheumatoid arthritis. *Health Psychology, 9,* 377–389.

Spence, S. (1989). Cognitive–behavior therapy in the management of chronic, occupational pain of the upper limbs. *Behaviour Research and Therapy, 27*(4), 435–446.

Sprock, J., Braff, D. L., Saccuzzo, D. P., and Atkinson, J. H. (1983). The relationship of depression and thought disorder in pain patients. *British Journal of Medical Psychology, 56,* 351–360.

Sternbach, R. A. (1974). *Pain patients: Traits and treatment.* New York: Academic Press.

Sternbach, R. A. (1984). Acute versus chronic pain. In P. D. Wall and R. Melzack (Eds.), *Textbook of pain* (pp. 173–177). Edinburgh and New York: Churchill Livingstone.

Sternbach, R. A. (1989). Acute versus chronic pain. In P. D. Wall and R. Melzack (Eds.), *Textbook of pain: II* (pp. 242–246). Edinburgh and New York: Churchill Livingstone.

Tait, R., DeGood, D., and Carron, H. (1982). A comparison of Health Locus of Control beliefs in low-back patients from the U.S. and New Zealand. *Pain, 14,* 53–61.

Tataryn, D. J., Nadel, L., and Jacobs, W. J. (1989). Cognitive therapy and cognitive science. In A. Freeman, K. M. Simon, L. E. Beutler, and H. Arkowitz (Eds.), *Comprehensive handbook of cognitive therapy* (pp. 83–98). London: Plenum.

Taylor, C. M., and Crisler, J. R. (1988). Concerns of persons with cancer as perceived by cancer patients, physicians, and rehabilitation counselors. *Journal of Rehabilitation, January–March,* 23–28.

Thase, M. E., Frank, E., and Kupfer, D. J. (1985). Biological processes in Major Depression. In E. E. Beckham and W. R. Leber (Eds.), *Handbook of depression. Treatment, assessment, and research* (pp. 816–913). Homewood, IL: Dorsey Press.

Thompson, S. C. (1981). Will it hurt less if I can control it? A complex answer to a simple question. *Psychological Bulletin, 90*, 89–101.

Tobin, D. L., Holroyd, K. A., Baker, A., Reynolds, R. V. C., and Holm, J. E. (1988). Development and clinical trial of a minimal contact, cognitive–behavioral treatment for tension headache. *Cognitive Therapy and Research, 12*(4), 325–339.

Toomey, T. C., Lundeen, T. V., Mann, J. D., and Abashian, S. (1988). *The pain locus of control scale: A comparison of chronic pain patients and normals.* Proceedings of the Canadian Pain Society and American Pain Society, 1st Joint Annual Meeting, November.

Toomey, T. C., Mann, J. D., Abashian, S., and Thompson-Pope, S. (1991). Relationship between perceived self-control of pain, pain description and functioning. *Pain, 45,* 129–133.

Turk, D. C. (1985). Coping with pain: A review of cognitive control techniques. In M. Feuerstein, L. B. Sachs, and I. D. Turkat (Eds.), *Psychological approaches to pain control.* New York: Wiley.

Turk, D. C., and Fernandez, E. (1990). On the putative uniqueness of cancer pain: Do psychological principles apply? *Behaviour Research and Therapy, 28*(1), 1–13.

Turk, D. C., and Holzman, A. D. (1986). Commonalities among psychological approaches in the treatment of chronic pain: Specifying the meta-constructs. In A. D. Holzman and D. C. Turk (Eds.), *Pain management: A handbook of psychological treatment approaches* (pp. 257–267). New York: Pergamon.

Turk, D. C., and Meichenbaum, D. (1984). A cognitive–behavioural approach to pain management. In P. D. Wall and R. Melzack (Eds.), *Textbook of pain* (pp. 787–794). Edinburgh and New York: Churchill Livingstone.

Turk, D. C., and Meichenbaum, D. (1989). A cognitive–behavioural approach to pain management. In P. D. Wall and R. Melzack (Eds.), *Textbook of pain: II* (pp. 1001–1009). Edinburgh and New York: Churchill Livingstone.

Turk, D. C., and Rudy, T. E. (1988). Toward an empirically derived taxonomy of chronic pain patients: Integration of psychological assessment data. *Journal of Consulting and Clinical Psychology, 56,* 233–238.

Turk, D. C., and Rudy, T. E. (1990a). The robustness of an empirically derived taxonomy of chronic pain patients. *Pain, 43,* 27–35.

Turk, D. C., and Rudy, T. E. (1990b). Neglected factors in chronic pain treatment outcome studies — referral patterns, failure to enter treatment, and attrition. *Pain, 43,* 7–25.

Turk, D. C., and Rudy, T. E. (1991). Neglected topics in the treatment of chronic pain patients — relapse, noncompliance, and adherence enhancement. *Pain, 44,* 5–28.

Turk, D. C., Meichenbaum, D., and Genest, M. (1983). *Pain and behavioral medicine: A cognitive–behavioral perspective.* New York: Guilford Press.

Turner, J. A., and Chapman, C. R. (1982). Psychological interventions for chronic pain: A critical review. II. Operant conditioning, Hypnosis, and Cognitive–behavioral therapy. *Pain, 12,* 23–46.

Turner, J. A., and Romano, J. M. (1984a). Evaluating psychologic interventions for chronic pain: Issues and recent developments. In C. Benedetti, C. R. Chapman, and G. Moricca (Eds.), *Advances in pain research and therapy,* (Vol. 7, pp. 257–296). New York: Raven Press.

Turner, J. A., and Romano, J. M. (1984b). Self-report screening measures for depression in chronic pain patients. *Journal of Clinical Psychology, 40*(4), 909–913.

Turner, J. A., and Romano, J. M. (1984c). Review of prevalence of coexisting chronic pain and depression. In C. Benedetti *et al.* (Eds.), *Advances in pain research and therapy* (Vol. 7, pp. 123–130). New York: Raven Press.

Vallis, T. M., and Bucher, B. (1986). Self-efficacy as a predictor of behavior change: Interaction with type of training for pain tolerance. *Cognitive Therapy and Research, 10*(1), 79–94.

Wade, J. B., Price, D. D., Hamer, R. M., Schwartz, S. M., and Hart, R. P. (1990). An emotional component analysis of chronic pain. *Pain, 40*, 303–310.

Wallston, K. A., Wallston, B. S., and DeVellis, B. (1978). Development of the multidimensional health locus of control (MHLC) scales. *Health Education Mongraphs, 6*, 160–170.

Watkins, L. R., and Mayer, D. J. (1982). Organization of endogenous opiate and nonopiate pain control systems. *Science, 216*, 1185–1192.

Weisenberg, M. (1984). Cognitive aspects of pain. In P. D. Wall and R. Melzack (Eds.), *Textbook of pain* (pp. 162–172). Edinburgh and New York: Churchill Livingstone.

Weisenberg, M. (1989). Cognitive aspects of pain. In P. D. Wall and R. Melzack (Eds.), *Textbook of pain: II* (pp. 231–241). Edinburgh and New York: Churchill Livingstone.

Weisenberg, M., Wolf, Y., Mittwoch, T., Mikulincer, M., and Aviram, O. (1985). Subject versus experimenter control in the reaction to pain. *Pain, 23*(2), 187–200.

Zimbardo, P. G., Cohen, A. R., Weisenberg, M., Dworkin, L., and Firestone, I. (1969). The control of experimental pain. In P. G. Zimbardo (Ed.), *The cognitive control of motivation* (pp. 100). Glenview, IL: Scott Foresman.

6

Cognition, Stress, and Health

Suzanne M. Miller

Temple University

Ann O'Leary

Rutgers University

INTRODUCTION

The term "stress," while scarcely mentioned a few decades ago, has become so often used that most of us encounter it on a daily basis. Psychological abstracts reported only 50 occurrences of the term stress in the psychological literature in 1950, whereas it occurred 1711 times in 1990. Among the most important reasons for this growing attention to psychological stress is the recognition of its effects on a wide array of physical health outcomes. Research has shown that stress impacts on health through two principal pathways. One involves the physiological concomitants of stress reactions and their direct effects on the body. The other is mediated by behavioral reactions in the face of stress, such as the extensive use of tobacco or alcohol, that may themselves adversely influence health.

In this chapter, we focus on the first pathway, recognizing the necessity to take account of the second in research and practice. In particular, we describe the phenomena of stress and coping, highlighting their cognitive aspects, and illustrate these processes with examples from the health domain. Clearly, the human body and its regulation are extremely complex, and the factors that can compromise health are numerous. A cataloging of all known stress–health linkages would be beyond the scope of this

159

chapter. We therefore concentrate on integrating several cognitive theories of stress as these relate to disease states that are prevalent and health damaging, and that have been targets of active research.

Brief History of the Stress Concept

Modern stress research was given its greatest impetus by the work of Walter Cannon and Hans Selye (Appley and Trumbull, 1967). Cannon studied sympathetic nervous system activity responses to acute fear-inducing stressors in animals (Cannon, 1932); Selye described the "General Adaptation Syndrome" in terms of physiological stages of response to chronic noxious stimulation (Selye, 1956). These approaches helped to characterize and systematize how organisms respond to stressors. However, they failed to account for individual differences in human response to potentially aversive conditions, and characterized the stressed organism as a passive recipient of external forces.

Applications of psychodynamic theory to health produced the "psychosomatic medicine" movement during the 1940s and 1950s (Alexander, 1950; Dunbar, 1943). Alexander postulated that specific psychodynamic conflicts produced diseases whose symptomatology represented an unconscious expression of the conflict. For example, symptoms of asthma were thought to represent "a repressed cry for mother." A collection of diseases dubbed "psychosomatic" were identified by these investigators. These included, in addition to asthma, ulcer, rheumatoid arthritis, hypertension, ulcerative colitis, and migraine. While this approach did stimulate a focus on mind–body interactions, much of the research that was adduced to support the theory was methodologically flawed (Taylor, 1991).

The work of Richard Lazarus and his colleagues (Lazarus, 1991; Lazarus and Folkman, 1984) has provided a comprehensive framework within which to examine the "transactional" view of the stress and coping process. On this view, differences among individuals in cognitive appraisal (as well as differences across time in a single individual) are important determinants of affective and physiological responses to potentially threatening events. This approach has clarified the nature of the relationship between environmental stimuli ("stressors") and the nature, types, and timing of reactions that follow.

From the transactional perspective, stress is "a particular relationship between the person and the environment that is appraised by the person as taxing or exceeding his or her resources and endangering his or her well-being" (Lazarus and Folkman, 1984, p. 19). Other cognitive approaches to various aspects of stress and coping behaviors have also shed light on this process (e.g., Bandura, 1986; Scheier and Carver, 1992). We will attempt here to integrate these into the overarching transactional theory. Within our consideration of stress–health relations, we assume a "biopsychosocial" model (Engel, 1977) in which physiological, psychological, and social/structural factors are seen as a mutually interacting system. For the present purpose, however, we highlight the role of cognition in generating the stress response.

Stress Physiology

An important but often neglected agenda is the delineation of the biological mechanisms that might underlie presumed stress–health linkages. To date, sufficient data have begun to accumulate to permit some reasoned speculation on these underpinnings. It is useful, therefore, to outline briefly the biological components of the stress response and to distill out the implications for health outcomes.

Two major aspects of the body's response to stress are the activities of the sympathetic (SAM) and hypothalamic pituitary adrenocortical (HPAC) systems (Asterita, 1985; Cannon and De La Paz, 1911; Frankenhaeuser, 1983; Henry and Stephens, 1977; Selye, 1956). The SAM system has two arms, the sympathetic and parasympathetic systems. When the SAM system is active, it functions to sustain "effort" or "fight-or-flight" in the face of stress. SAM activity has been most strongly linked to the onset of short-lived emotional reactions, such as fear and anger. It is accompanied by the release of catecholamines, notably epinephrine and norepinephrine, into the blood stream.

The HPAC axis, on the other hand, has been identified as the part of the endocrine system that subserves "distress" or "conservation–withdrawal" responses (Frankenhaeuser, 1983; Henry and Stephens, 1977). Activation of the HPAC system results in the release of adrenocorticotropic hormones, especially the corticosteroids (cortisol in humans and other primates), and is thought to reflect feelings of being overwhelmed by threat and unable to cope. HPAC activity has been associated with chronic stress and anxiety (Baum *et al.*, 1983), social loss and disruption (Coe *et al.*, 1983), and clinical depression (Gibbons, 1964; Gitlin and Gerner, 1986).

In addition to the SAM and HPAC systems, a number of hormones, including growth hormone, prolactin, insulin, and sex hormones, play a role in the body's response to stress (see Asterita, 1985). The exact impact of the various hormones depends on their relative quantities and interactions.

More recently, researchers have identified numerous peptides that appear to modulate neuroendocrine responses. These peptides are found in both the CNS and periphery. They include the opioid peptides, cholecystokinin or CCK, and substance P, as well as other peptides previously thought to act only within traditional hormone systems, for example, insulin and angiotensin. They serve a variety of functions, depending upon the eliciting conditions. Endogenous opioids are morphinelike peptides that are released under conditions of stress, particularly when physical pain is involved (reviewed in Akil *et al.*, 1984; Olson *et al.*, 1987).

Certain diseases have been shown to be primarily immune related; these include cancer, autoimmune disorders, and infectious diseases. Further, psychological processes have been shown to affect immune function. These processes may well be mediated by neuroendocrine concomitants of negative emotional experiences, primarily through the release of such products as catecholamines or cortisol. These products have been shown to interact with immunologic agents in the blood. Further, sympathetic activity also results in direct innervation of lymphoid organs. Immune cells have also been found to have receptors for most neurotransmitters, neuromodulators, and hormones, and appear to be influenced by a variety of other hormones and numerous peptides. Indeed, immune system cells themselves secrete peptides (lymphokines), some of which are precursors of neurotransmitters (reviewed in Blalock, 1989). These mainly play a communicative role within the immune system. However, they also may affect CNS functions, as demonstrated by psychiatric effects of lymphokine treatment for cancer (Smedley *et al.*, 1983).

Cardiovascular disease (CVD) is the most common cause of death in the United States. Substantial evidence has accumulated to suggest a pathogenic role for heightened sympathetic nervous system activity in its development. The process that is primarily responsible both for myocardial infarction or MI ("heart attack") and angina pectoris (chest pain) is atherosclerosis, the build-up of scar tissue and plaque formed from hardened lipids (fats). The resultant narrowing of arterial passageways can result in insufficient oxygen supply to the heart muscle, called "ischemia," which itself is the cause of angina pectoris and, if prolonged, of heart tissue death or myocardial infarction.

Sympathetic nervous system activity, if it is excessive, frequent, and prolonged, produces a number of effects that contribute to the development of atherosclerosis (Schneiderman, 1983). One of these is tearing of the arterial wall due to blood pressure and heart-rate fluctuations. This results in scarring, which contributes to the build-up of plaque. In addition, the catecholamines that are released in connection with the sympathetic response may induce direct chemical injury to arteries. Another effect of SAM activity is the release of lipids into the blood stream where they collect and contribute to atherosclerosis.

Thus, at the risk of oversimplifying, a summary sketch of the complex relationships between the physiological stress systems outlined above and health outcomes would implicate excessive and prolonged SAM activity in the etiology of cardiovascular disease (Contrada and Krantz, 1988), and excessive HPAC activity with immunologic suppression and cancer (Contrada *et al.*, 1990; O'Leary, 1990). In addition, opioid activity has been found to influence immune activity (Morley *et al.*, 1987). However, these relationships are complex and not easily summarized. Opioid activity is also strongly connected with the experience of pain (Bolles and Fanselow, 1984), although this is not a focus of the present chapter.

THE ROLE OF COGNITION IN STRESS

Cognition is at the core of the cognitive social conceptualization of individual differences in personality (e.g., Mischel, 1973) and affects every stage of the process of coping with stress. From the moment that we are first confronted with the potential for harm, how we encode and construe the event influences our emotional reactions and coping responses. These perceptions and interpretations of the situation include how we appraise the likelihood, imminence, duration, degree of possible loss, and value of that which could be lost. Our appraisal affects the expectations and values that are primed. For example, two people experiencing the loss of a job may experience different levels of distress, depending on how they evaluate the experience. One may see it as an opportunity for development of new hobbies, interests, or a new career path, while the other may view it as a catastrophic event and be pessimistic about the chances for future employment.

Furthermore, our expectancies about the personal and external resources and coping strategies that are available for countering a threat play a significant role in our reactions and in the eventual outcome of the encounter. This category would include our perceptions of our own abilities to manage the external stimulus and our emotional responses, as well as our beliefs about the existence of tangible aids and social support to assist us in the coping process. In the example given above, the first individual might have supreme confidence in his interviewing and self-presentation skills, along with a working wife, while the second both feels unable to persuade others of his occupational skills and lacks alternative sources of income.

In fact, these two types of appraisals form the cornerstone of the transactional view (Lazarus and Folkman, 1984). In this view, there are three basic kinds of primary appraisals: (1) irrelevant, (2) benign-positive, and

(3) stressful. With regard to the latter, appraisals that construe a situation as entailing threatened or actual harm or loss to the individual have been shown to generate greater levels of stress than those that construe the stressor as a challenge to be met (Frankenhaeuser, 1983). The seminal work of Lazarus and his colleagues has demonstrated the importance of cognitive appraisals in determining levels of stress. They found that subjects exposed to a variety of frightening films evidenced greater physiological and subjective arousal when they were induced to interpret these stimuli as painful and threatening than when they were induced to interpret them as benign (Lazarus, 1966). Further, certain situational conditions moderated the formation of these appraisals, including the duration of the anticipatory interval and uncertainty about what the aversive event would involve and when it would occur.

Negative primary appraisals of the sort described above inevitably give rise to secondary appraisal processes. These entail evaluations of what might and can be done to manage the situation (Lazarus and Folkman, 1984). A wealth of research has pointed to the powerful role of control-oriented secondary appraisals in reducing stress (Steptoe and Appels, 1989). A number of studies have shown that perceptions of control help to offset physiologic and subjective arousal, even when subjects without control have equal predictability or forewarning about what might happen to them.

Beliefs that one has access to a controlling response are also stress reducing, even when subjects do not actually execute it (Miller, 1979). This may be because having the potential for control provides a guaranteed upper limit on how noxious an aversive situation can become (Miller, 1980). On the other hand, arousal may increase in situations in which the controlling response is difficult to execute or where the effectiveness of the controlling response is uncertain (Ohman and Bohlin, 1989). Under these circumstance, individuals may prefer to relinquish control to a more competent individual (Miller, 1980). Further, the lack of control may elicit stress-induced analgesia, which can undercut its negative effects (Kelly, 1986).

PERSPECTIVES ON COGNITION, STRESS, AND HEALTH

A number of cognitive processes have been found to play a role in stress. These include, among others, self-efficacy expectations, optimism, coping strategies, and the allocation of attention. While these processes all focus on how the individual encodes and retrieves information and uses this information to base predictions about the future, they vary in how globally they are presumed to operate across situations and over time. Self-efficacy is thought to reflect beliefs that are specific to particular types of behavior in particular situations. Optimism (and its inverse, hopelessness) have been conceptualized as general expectancies that are likely to be activated across a variety of situations. Coping has been approached both as situation-specific tendencies and as stylistic or dispositional tendencies that are engaged or primed as the individual interacts with threat-relevant conditions and cues. We now briefly review these constructs and relevant findings, as they have been applied to the physiological stress response and health outcomes.

Self-Efficacy

Self-efficacy expectancies play a central role in Social Cognitive Theory (SCT) (Bandura, 1986). Efficacy beliefs guide peoples' predictions regarding their abilities to perform in designated behavioral domains. Central to efficacy theory is the notion of domain specificity. Efficacy beliefs with regard to different domains are considered to be largely independent. For example, an individual may possess strong expectations of success while driving—and will therefore display minimal stress reaction in this context—but be terrified of undergoing an aversive medical diagnostic test. Long-term stress-related health outcomes for this person will depend on the extent to which she experiences the latter situation, but not the former one, over the course of her daily life. Situations that require skills similar to those required by the target behavior, such as enduring dental treatments, may also evoke low self-efficacy expectations and hence may be relevant to health status.

The focus on domain specificity is one of the distinguishing features of self-efficacy theory. From this perspective, approaches that aggregate across a variety of domain expectancies are likely to be only weakly correlated with health outcomes. On the other hand, perceived self-efficacy to cope with a particular stressor should help to buffer the immediate physiological stress response. Those who believe that they possess the capabilities required to prevent or minimize the impact of a stressor will be less anxious. Hence, they should display reduced physiological response to the stressor and, ultimately, better health outcomes.

Much of the research exploring the effects of perceived self-efficacy on the stress response has been conducted within a phobia paradigm, in which phobics are helped to confront and attain mastery over objects that they fear (usually snakes or spiders). As outlined above, phobias and related fears are most likely to be associated with SAM activity. Consistent with this, phobics have been shown to manifest peripheral signs of sympathetic nervous system arousal (particularly heightened heart rate and blood pressure) during anticipation and performance of tasks for which self-efficacy is weak (Bandura *et al.*, 1982). After successful treatment, performance of the identical tasks elicits minimal sympathetic response.

Plasma levels of the catecholamines epinephrine, norepinephrine, and dopac (providing more direct indices of SAM activity) have also been assessed. Physiological arousal has been shown to be low during the performance of tasks for which subjects feel highly efficacious, as would be expected. Arousal is also generally low in the face of tasks for which subjects feel highly inefficacious, since they have no intention of performing them. In contrast, catecholamines are highly elevated while subjects perform tasks for which they feel moderately efficacious.

Effects of perceived coping efficacy on the immune system have also been studied using the phobic stress paradigm. In one study, snake phobics were treated with a challenging guided mastery therapy (Wiedenfeld *et al.*, 1990). This type of treatment requires clients to undertake increasingly difficult tasks, following modeling by the therapist. Hence, the treatment may be considered to constitute an experimental stressor. Subjects underwent immunologic and salivary cortisol assessment at three timepoints: baseline assessment during week one, immediately following four hours of guided mastery behavioral therapy during week two, and while handling the snakes with full coping efficacy during week three. It was found that clients had substantially higher absolute numbers of several types of circulating lymphocytes during the second week stressor assessment. This result mimics the effects produced by injection of epinephrine (Crary *et al.*, 1983), and supports the findings of higher catecholamine release during phobic confrontation. Furthermore, rate of improvement in efficacy expectations during the session was positively related to degree of immune enhancement.

Another study used a naturalistic stressor, having the disease of rheumatoid arthritis (RA), to explore stress effects on local and systemic indices of immune function (O'Leary *et al.*, 1988). Female RA sufferers were randomly assigned to a cognitive–behavioral stress management condition or to a bibliotherapy control. A number of psychological and medical outcomes were assessed, including self-efficacy enhancement, self-monitored pain, psychological distress, joint impairment as rated by rheumatologists blind to subject treatment condition, and immune function (i.e., numbers of helper and suppressor T-cells and lymphocyte response to mitogens).

Overall, the treatment significantly improved perceived self-efficacy, reduced pain, and decreased joint impairment, although it had no impact on immune function. The greater the degree of self-efficacy enhancement, the greater the treatment response. These results suggest that the cognitive–behavioral intervention had an effect on local immune function (which probably underlies improvements in joint impairment), but not on systemic immune function.

Level of perceived coping efficacy also appears to affect endogenous opioid response to stress. One study explored the effectiveness of cognitive control techniques for the management of laboratory pain (Bandura *et al.*, 1987). Subjects were randomized to one of three intervention conditions: training in cognitive control of pain, administration of placebo medication, or a control. One-half of the subjects in each group were to receive either naloxone (an opiate antagonist) or a saline control injection. If cognitive control procedures are effective because they enhance central opioid activity (which dampens pain perceptions), then the administration of naloxone should undermine its effectiveness.

Before administration of the saline or naloxone, the cognitive coping condition showed enhanced pain tolerance, as well as greater self-efficacy to tolerate and reduce pain. However, following the injection, those cognitive copers who had received naloxone displayed significantly less *increase* in their ability to tolerate cold-pressor pain, particularly as the trials progressed. Furthermore, the greater the enhancement of self-efficacy to reduce pain at the end of the training period, the greater was the subject's subsequent pain tolerance, and the greater was the reduction in tolerance increase due to naloxone. Thus, it appears that since more efficacious subjects endured higher levels of painful stimulation, they were more likely to display endogenous opioid activation.

Self-efficacy expectations have also been shown to influence endogenous opioid response to a mental stressor (Bandura *et al.*, 1988). In this study, perceptions of efficacy were manipulated by administering an arithmetic task under two conditions. In the first, subjects were able to pace themselves; in the second, subjects were yoked to a randomly selected other self-paced subject. The effect of the injection was assessed by a pain tolerance test.

The manipulation was effective: self-paced subjects showed self-efficacy in their perceived mathematical ability. Other-paced subjects showed decreased self-efficacy, along with concomitant increases in heart rate. Among subjects in the low-efficacy group, those who received naloxone were significantly less able to tolerate pain than those receiving saline. This suggests that the low-efficacy manipulation led to activation of the opioid system in these subjects. Hence, perceptions of self-efficacy appear to have implications for opioid activity, even during exposure to a nonphysical stressor. In sum, perceptions of one's ability to cope with particular stressors have a substantial impact on the physiological changes that are generated in response to threat. Further, this is true across a number of response systems.

Optimism

Dispositional optimism has recently begun to receive attention as a generalized expectancy influencing stress and health. Optimists have the overarching belief that desirable outcomes will be maximized and that undesirable outcomes will be minimized. Scheier and colleagues have developed a psychometrically sound instrument for assessing optimism, the Life Orientation Test (LOT) (Scheier and Carver, 1985; See Table 6.1). In an initial study using this scale, development of physical symptoms among undergraduates during the stressful last weeks of the semester was predicted by prior scores on the LOT, controlling for symptom reports at the earlier time-point. These results have recently been replicated (Scheier and Carver, 1992; Aspinwall and Taylor, 1992). One problem, however, is that the data are limited to self-reports of symptoms and/or health.

More compelling evidence is provided by a study of patient recovery from coronary artery bypass surgery (Scheier *et al.*, 1989). Optimists were less likely to display signs of myocardial infarction [i.e., new Q waves on the electrocardiogram (EKG) and release of the enzyme-labeled aspartate amino transferase (AST)] during the surgical procedure. Patients who were more optimistic also achieved a more rapid rate of recovery and return to

---

TABLE 6.1   Items Comprising Life Orientation Test (LOT)[a]

1. In uncertain times, I usually expect the best.

2. It's easy for me to relax. (Filler item)

3. If something can go wrong for me, it will.[b]

4. I always look on the bright side of things.

5. I'm always optimistic about my future.

6. I enjoy my friends a lot. (Filler item)

7. It's important for me to keep busy. (Filler item)

8. I hardly ever expect things to go my way.[b]

9. Things never work out the way I want them to.[b]

10. I don't get upset too easily. (Filler item)

11. I'm a believer in the idea that "every cloud has a silver lining."

12. I rarely count on good things happening to me.[b]

---

[a](from Scheier and Carver, 1985)
[b]These items are reversed prior to scoring.

normal activities, controlling for relevant medical variables such as severity of surgery, extent of coronary occlusion, and status of other risk variables. As predicted, optimism proved a better predictor of an aggregate measure of 6-month recovery than did any one specific expectation regarding a single aspect of recovery.

Five-year follow-up of these patients showed that optimists were more likely to be working full-time than pessimists. Further, optimists who were experiencing some angina reported less pain associated with their symptoms than did symptomatic pessimists (Scheier *et al.*, 1989). Other work has shown that a pessimistic style at age 25 predicts poorer physical health at ages 45, 55, and 60 (with health status at age 25 taken into account) (Peterson *et al.*, 1988). Recent evidence suggests that the health-enhancing effects of an optimistic style may be mediated by its impact on immune function. Among a group of older adults, optimists were found to have better cell-mediated immunity than pessimists, even when controlling for the effects of potential confounder variables (Kamen-Siegel *et al.*, 1991; see also Bachen *et al.*, 1991). While some studies report contradictory findings (Cohen *et al.*, 1989; Chesterman *et al.*, 1990; Sieber *et al.*, 1991), the general thrust of the results suggests that an optimistic style is beneficial for health.

Coping Strategies

As defined above, individuals experience stress when they perceive that the demands of the situation severely tax or exceed their resources. Coping can be defined as the efforts that the individual makes to manage these demands (Lazarus and Folkman, 1984). Researchers generally agree that coping has two broad functions. These are the management of the problem causing the distress (problem-focused coping) and the regulation of emotion and distress (emotion-focused coping). Problem-focused coping generally consists of strategies for altering or managing the source of the problem itself. This can include making plans, standing one's ground, and seeking out information. In emotion-focused coping, individuals generally attempt to reduce or contain their level of distress. They can employ a variety of strategies to accomplish this, including self-relaxation (keeping calm), positive reappraisal (looking on the bright side), distraction (forgetting about it), and outright denial (it's not really happening).

Controllable stressors, where the individuals can do something to change the situation, typically elicit and are conducive to more problem-focused forms of coping. In contrast, uncontrollable stressors, where the individual is helpless, typically elicit more emotion-focused forms of coping, as a means of regulating affect. For example, an older woman who has just had a cancerous lump removed from her breast can console herself by feeling sorry for a younger woman in the same plight (Taylor *et al.*, 1983). Most individuals tend to use both forms of coping when they encounter different situations. Further, each form of coping is complex. Problem-focused coping comprises quite different strategies, from directly acting on the situation to simply seeking out information about it. Similarly, emotion-focused coping consists of a wide array of strategies, from ventilating one's feelings (which entails a complete focus on the situation) to reappraisal and distraction (which entail a partial focus on the situation) to outright denial (which entails blocking out awareness of the situation). Therefore, many researchers feel that it is more useful to explore the separate components of emotion- and problem-focused coping (Carver *et al.*, 1989).

To illustrate, Folkman *et al.* (1986) studied a group of married couples. They found that people used two types of problem-focused strategies in dealing with controllable outcomes, including standing one's ground and making plans. However, they also used two main types of emotion-focused strategies, including accepting responsibility and reappraising the event more positively. The use of healthy emotion-focused coping in this context may actually facilitate problem-focused coping. If a student who has failed an exam both sees herself as responsible for the situation and, at the same time, focuses on the positive aspects of the situation ("I can use this as a warning and as a goad to improve my studying skills"), she will be more likely to take steps to improve the situation (e.g., by seeking out information from the professor and organizing her time more efficiently). In contrast, when faced with uncontrollable outcomes, people generally chose emotion-focused coping strategies, in which they avoided thinking about the situation or tried to detach themselves from it.

There are a number of instruments available for assessing ongoing coping efforts (Carver *et al.*, 1989; Lazarus and Folkman, 1984; Holahan and Moos, 1986, 1987; Stone and Neale, 1984). To date, research with these scales has tended to focus more on delineating patterns of coping under threat and exploring their mental health correlates, rather than their impact on physical health outcomes. For example, a number of recent studies have conducted factor analyses to generate empirically derived overarching coping categories and have explored how these are related to aspects of emotional distress, such as depression (Dunkel-Schetter *et al.*, 1992; Folkman *et al.*, 1992).

Further, research conducted on subsets of coping strategies with less comprehensive instruments generally points to the short-term adaptive value of "avoidant" coping strategies, such as distraction. In the long run, however, more vigilantlike strategies appear to be the most beneficial for health outcomes, although the exact mechanisms underlying these relationships are not clear (Suls and Fletcher, 1985). Further, there are conditions under which avoidant strategies can be health enhancing, even with more long-term stressors, particularly in response to uncontrollable threats (Hackett and Cassem, 1973; Levine *et al.*, 1988).

Recently, investigators have begun to explore the relationship between dispositional optimism and ongoing strategies for coping with stress. In research with undergraduates, optimists (as identified by the LOT) reported greater use of problem-focused coping in the face of controllable stressors, but greater use of acceptance/resignation in the face of uncontrollable stressors (Scheier *et al.*, 1986). Optimists have also been found to be more likely to reinterpret stressful situations in a positive light and to learn from the experience (Carver *et al.*, 1989).

A study of women undergoing surgery for breast cancer showed that the overall constellation of coping strategies employed by optimists was more constructive than that of pessimists (Carver *et al.*, in press). In particular, optimists engaged in greater use of acceptance, combined with less use of denial and disengagement. The employment of these strategies, in turn, was associated with reduced psychological distress.

Among men at risk for AIDS, optimists were more likely to cope with AIDS-related intrusive ideation by maintaining a positive attitude, whereas pessimists were more likely to cope by engaging in fatalism, self-blame, and escape (Taylor *et al.*, 1991). In addition, there was evidence that coping mediated the link between optimism and both psychological and physical health outcomes in these men. Similarly, in a coronary artery bypass surgery study, optimists tended to cope differently than pessimists. They were more likely to seek out information about what lay ahead and were less likely to suppress or ignore thoughts about their situation (Scheier *et al.*, 1989). However, these coping patterns did not appear to mediate the effects of optimism on surgery outcome, although they did have an impact on quality of life.

Attention Allocation

The discussion on coping strategies suggests that it is possible to extract two important underlying dimensions: the extent to which the individual typically attends to and "monitors" the negative aspects of a stressful situation; and the extent to which the individual psychologically avoids, blocks out, and "blunts" reminders of danger (Miller, 1990). In contrast to the coping-strategy approach, where the focus tends to be on self-regulatory patterns in a given stressful encounter, the coping-style approach focuses on the individual's general disposition to seek or avoid threatening cues, while examining the interaction between this person's variable, ongoing coping efforts and specific situational features.[1]

Miller (1987) developed the Monitor–Blunter Style Scale (MBSS), which is a valid and reliable instrument for assessing coping style. Research on the monitoring–blunting dimension has shown that coping style affects how individuals respond to threats of an everyday nature (such as aversive medical procedures). In response to painful threats, monitors generally show evidence of more sustained psychophysiological and subjective arousal and less habituation than blunters, who eventually decrease in arousal (Kelly, 1986; Miller, 1979; Miller and Mangan, 1983; Phillips, 1989). Monitors also show slower recovery from acute medical problems, as well as poorer pain tolerance and greater sensitivity to internal, somatic cues (Bruehl *et al.*, 1992; Efran *et al.*, 1989; Miller *et al.*, 1988).

However, monitors do not appear to be simply more generally anxious or suffering from greater amounts of negative affectivity than blunters are (Watson and Pennebaker, 1989). Rather, they become more specifically aroused in the face of threat, which activates their tendency to scan for threatening cues. For example, when viewing a frightening film for the first time, monitors show a significantly greater increase from base line in skin conductance (i.e., sweat gland activity) across the entire film segment than do blunters (Sparks and Spirek, 1988). Moreover, the results also show a significant interaction between coping style and film segments. That is, monitors show greater physiological arousal only during periods of significant stress. Similar findings have been obtained with subjective arousal (Phipps and Zinn, 1986). Importantly, monitors can be protected from this heightened arousal under threat by receiving a high degree of predictability, or forewarning, about what they are about to experience (Sparks, 1989).

In one study, patients were undergoing an aversive diagnostic procedure for the first time (Miller and Mangan, 1983). Half of each group was then given voluminous information about the forthcoming procedure and its effects; the other half received minimal information. The only group to show a decrease in pulse rate immediately before the exam were blunters given low information, and they maintained this low pulse rate throughout. By the end of the exam, monitors who were given a large amount of information also showed reduced pulse rate, but low-information monitors and high-information blunters showed sustained higher pulse rates.

---

[1]Other dimensions, such as repression–sensitization, are relevant to attention allocation and have implications for health (e.g., Jensen, 1987). However, the repression–sensitization dimension also taps other components (such as the ability to admit to threatening information), and its use is considered to be beyond conscious awareness. Hence, this reflects a more automatized process that does not fit well with Lazarus and Folkman's (1984) notion of coping as involving ongoing cognitive and behavioral efforts to manage appraised stressors.

Similarly, among coronary patients undergoing cardiac catheterization (Watkins *et al.*, 1986), monitors receiving high levels of preparatory information showed less physiologic and self-reported arousal throughout the procedure than those receiving low levels of information. Conversely, blunters receiving low levels of information were less aroused than blunters receiving high levels of information (see also Gattuso *et al.*, 1992).

These results raise an intriguing question: Are individuals suffering from chronic disorders such as hypertension, which are characterized by prolonged, high levels of physiologic and subjective arousal, prone to exhibit a monitoring style of coping? In order to begin to explore this issue, one study looked at individuals seeking outpatient treatment at a primary care facility for various acute medical problems (e.g., upper respiratory infection and muscle strains). Hypertensives were twice as likely to be characterized by a monitoring style than a blunting style. Conversely, normotensives were two and one-half times more likely to be characterized by a blunting style than a monitoring style. Indeed, over two-thirds of the hypertensives were monitors, whereas close to three-fourths of the normotensives were blunters (Miller, Leinbach, and Brody, 1989).

Although only preliminary in nature, these results indicate that hypertensives may be characterized by an information-seeking style, which can take a physical and psychological toll. Alternatively, since hypertension is a symptomless yet life-threatening condition, information seekers may become alarmed at the emergence of even trivial symptoms, and therefore may overutilize medical services. Indeed, there is evidence that monitors are more likely than blunters to adhere to medical screening regimens, at least initially (Miller, 1992; Steptoe and O'Sullivan, 1986). The negative impact of heightened arousal on health may therefore be offset by the early detection of disease. However, the challenge is to trace the pattern of adaptation and adherence over time, as the individual selectively reconstrues and readjusts to incoming information.

INTEGRATIVE MODEL OF COGNITION, STRESS, AND HEALTH

Figure 6.1 presents an integration of the stress and coping process as described by Lazarus and colleagues, outlining the three major (and mutually interacting) stages of responses. Other cognitive approaches are placed in their appropriate contexts within the transactional model.

During the initial primary appraisal phase, the individual evaluates whether environmental conditions contain the potential for producing harm or loss. Primary appraisals are considered within Bandura's Social Cognitive Theory to be "outcome expectancies," although threatening expected outcomes comprise only a subset of all possible ones. While

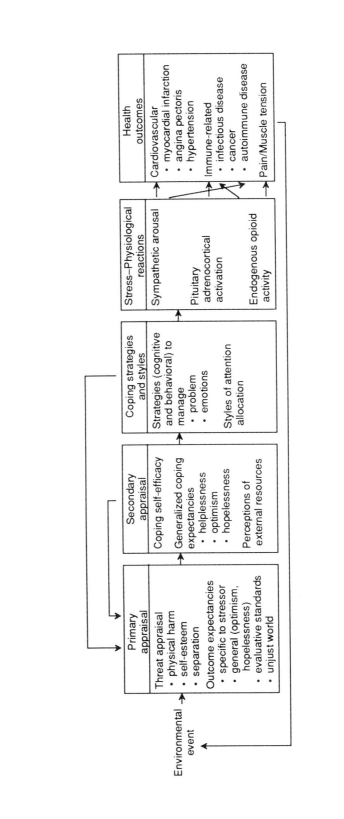

outcome expectancies in SCT are considered quite situation specific, generalized expectancies have also been studied as predictors of outcomes that
are likely to be variously determined (Scheier and Carver, 1985). For example, generalized optimism and its inverse, hopelessness, can operate as
primary appraisal variables.

During the secondary appraisal process, individuals evaluate the resources, both personal and environmental, that they may marshal to cope
with the stressor. Beliefs regarding one's own abilities for coping with
specific stressors (perceived coping self-efficacy) represent one example of
a secondary appraisal. As with outcome expectancies, stress-related self-
efficacy expectancies constitute only a subset of possible self-efficacy
beliefs. Further, they are considered to be domain specific. In addition,
generalized expectancies appear to be important. In particular, one can feel
either optimistic or hopeless about one's ability generally to obtain positive
outcomes or avoid negative ones.

Secondary appraisal processes are not only activated in response to
primary appraisals but they may also feed back to and modify them. For
instance, the threat of failure (primary appraisal) accompanying an academic examination may be considerably mitigated for someone who believes herself capable of effective preparation (secondary appraisal). It may
be exacerbated, however, for someone who has trouble with time management, concentration, and goal setting.

The third stage entails the performance of effortful coping behaviors,
which, in turn, can have a backward effect on primary and secondary
appraisal. For example, emotion-focused coping often results in a more
adaptive reappraisal of the significance of environmental conditions. Consider an individual who learns that he is HIV positive. If he is able to
consider the illness as an opportunity for personal growth and contribution to society (e.g., by giving AIDS prevention presentations, lobbying
the FDA, volunteering as a "buddy" for persons with AIDS), the appraisal
of threat will be diminished. Similarly, with respect to attention allocation,
the individual who typically distracts from and does not dwell on the
nature and consequences of a possible threat will probably construe it as
less negative than will an individual who attends to all of the terrifying
aspects of the potentially threatening encounter.

Stress is heightened when the individual perceives a serious threat (primary appraisal phase) and feels powerless to control it (secondary appraisal phase), particularly when combined with the use of less adaptive,
self-regulatory strategies and styles (coping phase). The end product of
this sequence of events, as relevant to health, is the physiological stress
reaction — SAM, HPAC, and endogenous opioid activity being three important components. These, in turn, mediate the effects of stress on health,

with SAM activity being particularly deleterious for the cardiovascular system, HPAC activity being damaging to immunity and contributing to immune-related disorders such as cancer and infectious disease, and opioid activity having the greatest relevance for pain-related disorders.

APPLICATIONS TO SPECIFIC ILLNESSES

We now review applications of the model to two specific disease states: cancer and cardiovascular disease.

Helplessness/Hopelessness and Cancer

Helplessness and hopelessness are cognitive stances toward stressful situations that may play a role in both the primary and secondary appraisal processes (Abramson, Metalsky, & Alloy, 1989). Interest in such dispositional variables as predictors of cancer has existed since ancient times: the Greek humoral pathologist Galen wrote that "melancholy" women were more likely than "sanguinous" ones to develop breast cancer. Hopelessness is a primary cognitive component of psychological distress and depression (Beck, 1983). Therefore, it makes sense that it should be associated with diseases that reflect HPAC activity and immune suppression.

In more recent years, the link of this cognitive factor to cancer has been explored more rigorously. Helplessness/hopelessness was one of several interviewer ratings found to be associated with thicker melanoma tumors in a study by Temoshok et al. (1985). In a quasi-prospective design, hopelessness assessed prior to cervical biopsy predicted which subjects would be diagnosed with cancer (Antoni and Goodkin, 1988; Schmale and Iker, 1969). A similar result has been found for breast biopsy (Wirsching et al., 1982), as well as recurrence of breast cancer (Greer et al., 1979; Jensen, 1987). Finally, hopeless reactions to life events have been reported to be predictive of the development of cancer in a large prospective study in Yugoslavia (Grossarth-Maticek et al., 1982).

Although several studies appear to converge on hopelessness as a contributor to cancer, some methodological problems with this research should be noted. Much of this research uses single interview (and interviewer) assessments and retrospective or "quasi-prospective" (assessment prior to biopsy) designs. Failures to replicate the effect have also been reported (Goodkin et al., 1986; Cassileth et al., 1985), although some of this work has been criticized on a number of grounds (see Letters to the Editor, 1985). Another problem lies in the failure of the research to identify the physiological mechanism(s) responsible for effects. While one likely pathway for effects of hopelessness on cancer outcome would be adrenocortical activity and cortisol release, possibly with consequent immune suppression, this has not received specific attention in research.

Type A Behavior Pattern and Cardiovascular Disease

A number of behavioral factors place one at risk for myocardial infarction. These include smoking, hypertension, and serum cholesterol. One additional risk factor, Type A behavior pattern, is psychological in nature and entails such processes as appraisal of threat, self-evaluation, and beliefs about control. Type A behavior pattern, originally identified by cardiologists Friedman and Rosenman (1974), is characterized by hard-driving, competitive, impatient, and, most importantly, angry and hostile reactions to the environment. It is best assessed via structured interview, in which noncontent indications of these traits (e.g., paralinguistics, voice dynamics) are rated, in addition to the manifest content obtained via self-report. The results of several large, long-term prospective studies indicate that Type A accounts for significant variance in myocardial infarcts and other cardiovascular conditions (reviewed in Contrada *et al.*, 1990).

Type A pattern has been shown to be associated with enhanced sympathetic reactivity, part of the presumed mechanism for pathogenesis, as described above. This has been demonstrated in the laboratory by performing psychophysiological assessment of peripheral indices of sympathetic arousal in response to stressful stimuli (reviewed in Contrada and Krantz, 1988). In these studies, Type A individuals become more aroused during stress than their Type B counterparts. Of greatest relevance for the present chapter is research aimed at identifying the cognitive underpinnings of this syndrome. Several have been posited, although there has been a paucity of research linking these cognitive bases to actual physiological or health outcomes.

David Glass and colleagues have speculated that a desire for increased control over the environment is the basis for Type A behavior pattern (Glass, 1977). According to this view, Type A behavior emerges under conditions of threat of loss of control and represents efforts to reexert control. In this framework, Type A behavior is identified as a set of coping efforts made in response to primary and secondary threat appraisals.

Another theoretical approach considers Type A manifestations to reflect a condition in which high self-evaluative standards for performance are combined with inadequate feedback concerning adequacy of performance (Matthews, 1982; Scherwitz *et al.*, 1978). This setup produces the driven, competitive, and achievement-striving aspects of Type A pattern. On this view, then, the perception of a threat to self-esteem (a primary appraisal) generates a set of effortful and problem-focused coping responses, which comprise the behavioral complex.

A third cognitive perspective on Type A behavior has been provided by Price (1982), who posits that a set of three core beliefs or assumptions underlie the pattern. These are: (1) the assumption that self-worth can be demonstrated only through external validation via recognized accomplishments (again, an appraisal of threat to self-esteem combined with a plan for problem-focused coping); (2) the belief that no general moral system is rewarded in our society and that injustice reigns, giving rise to hostility (a set of primary appraisals or outcome expectancies); and (3) the belief that resources are scarce and must be fought for (a secondary appraisal and plan for coping).

Unfortunately, most of the research exploring the first two models has used a paper-and-pencil self-report measure to assess Type A pattern, and this measure is known to be poor at identifying the more toxic (and less socially desirable) elements of hostility and anger. Research concerning Price's (1982) model is scant. However, it has face validity and clear relevance to the phenomena at hand, particularly the hostility component.

ILLUSTRATIVE CASE

The following case illustrates how the integrative model captures stress–cognition–health linkages in a given individual, with respect to cancer.

> Linda was terrified. She couldn't believe that what the doctor had said was true. How could she have a lump in her left breast? How could such a terrible thing have happened to her? She had visions of frightening treatments, painful procedures, and death troubling her. She barely heard the doctor when he said that the tumor appeared to be self-contained and that her prognosis was excellent. All she could think of was how she was going to get disfigured, be abandoned, and probably die anyway.
>
> Seeing how upset she was, the social worker offered to go over her case with her, to review her options, and to help get the situation in hand. But Linda didn't have the energy and she didn't think it would do any good anyway. Instead, while awaiting her operation, she stayed home and tried to forget what was happening to her, but it all came flooding back during the night in her dreams and even intruded constantly into her thoughts during the day. She avoided her friends, took a leave from her job, and spent her days fretting.
>
> By the time she was admitted to the hospital, a serious level of depression had set in. Even though her prognosis was good, the operation revealed some spread to the lymph nodes. Linda became even more disconcerted and just seemed to give up on life. Within five years she was back in the hospital, under treatment for recurrence of her breast cancer.

The above case illustrates the damaging role that appraisals of threat can play when accompanied by feelings of pessimism/hopelessness, low self-efficacy/helplessness, poor problem- and emotion-focused coping strategies, and hypervigilance. Presumably, in Linda's case, this constellation of cognitive processes activated the HPAC axis. This helped to undermine her immune system, thereby weakening her resistance to neoplastic processes. The spread of disease, in turn, negatively impacted on her cognitive state, leading to a vicious cycle.

A number of research investigations are consistent with this interpretation, (see, for example, Levy *et al.*, 1985, 1987). Nonetheless, it is important to keep in mind that evidence bearing on possible mechanisms underlying such cognition–health linkages is scant. Further, in cases like the above, it is equally possible that dysfunctional cognition and accompanying psychopathology merely reflect and arise from a more advanced, underlying disease state. More fine-grained studies are needed to tease out these effects.

INTERVENTION

Virtually all the cognitive components of the integrative model have implications for improving health outcomes. A number of stress management and cognitive–behavioral change programs have been developed, with a view to modifying dysfunctional cognition in the face of environmental threat. To the extent that altering the cognitive component of stress also alters the physiologic component, then such interventions should ultimately serve to forestall disease onset or limit disease progression.

The overarching goal of these programs is to enable individuals to process environmental events in a less stressful manner. Instead of appraising an ongoing or potential threat as overwhelmingly negative or even catastrophic, the aim is to reframe it in a more benign or positive fashion. Ultimately, the hope is that these reappraisals of specific events will generalize to alter more global outcome expectancies. For example, more pessimistically oriented individuals can learn to embrace more optimistic constructions of possible outcomes and their consequences.

A number of mutually interactive strategies can be used to accomplish this. The traditional cornerstone of stress management programs has entailed strategies such as relaxation and biofeedback, which aim to directly modify the physiological response to stress (Benson, Greenwood, and Klemshuk, 1975). The regular practice of these techniques has been shown to result in somatic effects such as reductions in blood pressure (Luborsky *et al.*, 1982) and enhanced immune function (Kiecolt-Glaser *et al.*, 1984, 1985). Above and beyond their arousal-reducing effects, these techniques may help to manage stress by increasing perceptions of efficacy, control, and coping. Individuals who learn that they have an effective strategy for managing their own somatic reactions in the face of stress will feel more confident that they can keep distress within tolerable limits. Hence the net aversiveness of the situation will be lower (Miller, 1980).

Apart from the direct arousal-reducing techniques, a critical route toward short-circuiting primary threat appraisals is by altering secondary threat appraisals. Increasing percepts of self-efficacy among low-efficacious individuals has been found to be a powerful means for achieving this end. A number of diverse interventions can be marshaled to increase self-efficacy expectations in those who are unsure of their abilities. Intervention programs can capitalize on manipulating any one of four sources of information regarding one's capabilities, in descending order of importance: (1) one's own past performance at the task or similar tasks; (2) the performance accomplishments of others who are perceived to be similar to oneself; (3) verbal persuasion by others that one is capable; and (4) perception of one's own state of physiological arousal, which is in turn partly determined by prior efficacy estimation.

Performance mastery experiences can be created by encouraging clients to undertake subtasks that are increasingly difficult or close to the desired behavioral repertoire. Similarly, modeled success by others can be presented to provide vicarious mastery experiences. A number of studies have documented the effectiveness of these approaches (Bandura, 1986). Examples of other techniques for increasing perceptions of control at the secondary appraisal level include reattribution training (to undercut feelings of helplessness; Abramson et al., 1978) and enhancing perceptions of social support (thereby undercutting loneliness and alienation; Wortman and Dunkel-Schetter, 1979).

At the level of coping, a number of stress management techniques have been designed that enhance both problem- and emotion-focused coping. These include teaching plans for coping, as well as strategies for reappraising the threat as less negative, thought stopping for controlling obsessive thinking, and so forth (Meichenbaum and Jaremko, 1983). These may also be used in a preventive fashion, to forestall the emergence of stress reactions in the face of terrifying circumstances (Auerbach, 1989).

In addition, the work on coping styles may have implications for targeting which type of strategy should be used with particular individuals. As outlined above, in the medical setting, monitors would appear to benefit from preparatory communications that impart voluminous information, while at the same time reducing anxiety, by focusing on the reassuring and positive aspects of the situation. Blunters, on the other hand, should benefit from preparatory communications that convey more circumscribed, needed information and, perhaps, that focus on the importance of adhering to relevant preventive, screening, and treatment protocols.

Monitors may also be more optimal candidates for some types of therapeutic interventions in the clinical setting than blunters are. For example, one of the most effective nonpharmacological interventions for the anxiety disorders appears to be exposure to the anxiety-inducing object or situation. Further, it has been demonstrated that increased attention to fear-inducing cues during exposure enhances the reduction of subjective and physiological indices of anxiety and promotes better therapeutic outcomes. Extrapolating from previous work, monitors should be more attentive to threatening cues during exposure treatment than blunters. This means that they should show greater initial reactivity. However, they should also show greater habituation and reduction in anxiety as they subsequently process and recode incoming information. This has been shown to be the case for phobics (Steketee *et al.*, 1989).

Blunters may thus need more intense and prolonged exposure treatments than monitors do, or they may be better suited to more avoidant stress management techniques, such as relaxation or reinterpretation. For example, among patients exposed to a stress management intervention, blunters felt the treatment had greater general appeal for them and more positive somatic effects (Avants *et al.*, 1990). Blunters undergoing chemotherapy for cancer also respond better to relaxation interventions than monitors do (Lerman *et al.*, 1990).

Some research has tested interventions designed to reduce Type A behavior pattern and its physiologic and health consequences. The most ambitious of these has been the Recurrent Coronary Prevention Project (Friedman *et al.*, 1984, 1986). In this study, over 1000 males who had suffered from myocardial infarction were randomized into two groups. The first received standard cardiac counseling concerning dietary and other behavioral aspects of cardiovascular disease management plus a cognitive–behavioral intervention for Type A pattern. This intervention focused on reassessing life priorities and assumptions concerning what constitutes "success," as well as challenging less philosophical beliefs (e.g., that shifting lanes in one's automobile saves substantial time). The second group only received the standard counseling component. At the end of four and one-half years, 35% of those exposed to the cognitive–behavioral intervention showed a decrease in Type A behavior as assessed by the structured interview, compared with 10% of the control subjects. Further, those receiving the Type A intervention had fewer repeat occurrences of MI.

We have already made mention of interventions to improve immunity. In addition, one recent study examined effects of a multifaceted cognitive–behavioral intervention in patients with malignant melanoma (Fawzy *et al.*, 1990). The intervention included enhancement of problem-solving skills, stress management techniques such as relaxation training, and group support. Significant enhancement in several cancer-related components of the immune system was obtained. However, it must be noted that differential attrition rates from the treatment and control conditions render interpretation of these findings problematic.

FUTURE DIRECTIONS

While there are a wealth of cognitive perspectives that are relevant to stress and health, exploration of their interrelations is still in its infancy. A great deal of research has assessed the role of cognitive factors in stress and coping. Much work has also been done to connect the experiential component of stress with physiological indices of arousal and dysregulation. In addition, some studies have linked stress to health outcomes. By far, however, the majority of stress studies assess mental, rather than physical, health outcomes. Further, researchers have seldom connected all the elements of the model (cognition, stress, and health) within the same investigation. There is a need for research that evaluates the proposed model, particularly focusing on the long-term development of significant health risk. This will require the use of longitudinal designs, multiple dependent measures, and well-defined disease endpoints.

It is also imperative to develop methodologically pure preventive and treatment programs, in which standardized and conceptually relevant cognitive techniques are applied across a number of health domains. A methodological challenge is to design intervention studies that will help establish the causal links between the cognitive factors under consideration with actual physiologic processes and medical outcomes. At a practical level, the information generated may enable us not only to short-circuit, but also to forestall, human suffering in the face of a variety of life crises and losses, by reducing disease risk and promoting health and adaptation.

ACKNOWLEDGMENTS

Work on this chapter was supported in part by Grants CA46591 from the National Cancer Institute and PBR-72 from the American Cancer Society to Suzanne Miller and MH45238 and MH48013 from the National Institute of Mental Health to Ann O'Leary. We thank Richard Sommers for his assistance.

REFERENCES

Abramson, L. Y., Seligman, M. E. P., and Teasdale, J. (1978). Learned helplessness in humans: Critique and reformulation. *Journal of Abnormal Psychology. 87*, 49–74.

Abramson, L. Y., Metalsky, G. I., and Alloy, L. B. (1989). Hopelessness depression: A theory-based subtype of depression. *Psychological Review, 96*, 358–372.

Akil, H., Watson, S. J., Young, E., Lewis, M. E., Khachaturian, H., and Walker, J. M. (1984). Endogenous opioids: Biology and function. *Annual Review of Neuroscience, 7*, 223–225.

Alexander, F. (1950). *Psychosomatic medicine: Its principles and applications.* New York: Norton.

Antoni, M. H., and Goodkin, K. (1988). Host moderator variables in the promotion of cervical neoplasia: I. Personality facets. *Journal of Psychosomatic Research, 32*, 327–338.

Appley, M. H., and Trumbull, R. (Eds.). (1967). *Dynamics of stress: Physiological, psychological, and social perspectives.* New York: Plenum.

Aspinwall, L. G., and Taylor, S. E. (1992). Modeling cognitive adaptation: A longitudinal investigation of the impact of individual differences and coping on college adjustment and performance. *Journal of Personality and Social Psychology, 63*, 989–1003.

Asterita, M. F. (1985). *The physiology of stress.* New York: Human Sciences Press.

Auerbach, S. M. (1989). Stress management and coping research in the health care setting: An overview and methodological commentary. *Journal of Consulting and Clinical Psychology, 57*, 388–395.

Avants, S. K., Margolin, A., and Salovey, P. (1990). Stress management techniques: Anxiety reduction, appeal, and individual differences. *Imagination, cognition, and personality, 10*, 3–23.

Bachen, E., Manuck, S., Muldoon, M., Cohen, S., and Rabin, B. (1991). *Effects of dispositional optimism on immunologic responses to laboratory stress.* Unpublished data, University of Pittsburgh.

Bandura, A. (1977). Self-efficacy: Toward a unifying theory of behavior change. *Psychological Review, 84*, 191–215.

Bandura, A. (1986). *Social foundations of thought and action: A social cognitive theory.* Englewood Cliffs, NJ: Prentice-Hall.

Bandura, A., Reese, L., and Adams, N. E. (1982). Microanalysis of action and fear arousal as a function of differential levels of perceived self-efficacy. *Journal of Personality and Social Psychology, 43*, 5–21.

Bandura, A., Taylor, C. B., Williams, S. L., Mefford, I. N., and Barchas, J. D. (1985). Catecholamine secretion as a function of perceived coping self-efficacy. *Journal of Consulting and Clinical Psychology, 53*, 406–414.

Bandura, A., O'Leary, A., Taylor, C. B., Gauthier, J., and Gossard, D. (1987). Perceived self-efficacy and pain control: Opioid and nonopioid mechanisms. *Journal of Personality and Social Psychology, 53*, 563–571.

Bandura, A., Cioffi, D., Taylor, C. B., and Brouillard, M. E. (1988). Perceived self-efficacy in coping with cognitive stressors and opioid activation. *Journal of Personality and Social Psychology, 55*, 479–488.

Baum, A., Gatchel, R. J., and Schaeffer, M. A. (1983). Emotional, behavioral, and physiological effects of chronic stress at Three Mile Island. *Journal of Consulting and Clinical Psychology, 51*, 565–572.

Beck, A. T. (1967). Cognitive therapy of depression: New perspectives. In P. J. Clayton and J. E. Barrett (Eds.), *Treatment of depression: Old controversies and new approaches* (pp. 265–290). New York: Raven Press.

Beck, A. T. (1983) Cognitive therapy of depression: New perspectives. *In Treatment of depression: Old controversies and new approaches* (P. J. Clayton & J. E. Barrett eds.), pp. 265–290. New York: Raven Press.

Benson, H., Greenwood, M. M., and Klemchuk, H. (1975). The relaxation response: Psychophysiological aspects and clinical applications. *International Journal of Psychiatry in Medicine, 6*, 87–98.

Blalock, J. E. (1989). A molecular basis for bi-directional communication between the immune and neuroendocrine systems. *Psychological Reviews, 69*, 1–32.

Bolles, R. C., and Fanselow, M. S. (1984). Endorphins and behavior. *Annual Review of Psychology, 33*, 87–101.

Bruehl, S., Carlson, C. R., and McCubbin, J. A. (1992). The relationship between pain sensitivity and blood pressure in normotensives. *Pain, 48*, 463–467.

Burgess, A. W., and Holstrom, L. L. (1976). Coping behavior of the rape victim. *American Journal of Psychiatry, 133*, 413–418.

Cannon, W. B. (1932). *The wisdom of the body*. New York: Norton.

Cannon, W. B., and De La Paz, D. (1911). Emotional stimulation of adrenal secretion. *American Journal of Physiology, 28*, 64–70.

Carver, C. S., Scheier, M. F., and Weintraub, J. K. (1989). Assessing coping strategies: A theoretically based approach. *Journal of Personality and Social Psychology, 56*, 267–283.

Carver, C. S., Pozo, C., Harris, S. D., Noriega, V., Scheier, M. F., Robinson, D. S., Ketcham, A. S., Moffat, F. L., Jr., and Clark, K. C. (in press). How coping mediates the effects of optimism on distress: A study of women with early stage breast cancer. *Journal of Personality and Social Psychology*.

Cassileth, B. R., Lusk, E. J., Miller, D. S., Brown, L. L., and Miller, C. (1985). *The New England Journal of Medicine, 312*, 1551–1555.

Chesterman, E., Cohen, F., and Adler, N. (1990). *Trait optimism as a predictor of pregnancy outcomes*, Unpublished manuscript, University of California at Los Angeles.

Coe, C. L., Weiner, S. G., and Levine, S. (1983). Psychoendocrine responses of mother and infant monkeys to disturbance and separation. In L. A. Rosenblum and H. Molts (Eds.), *Symbiosis in parent–offspring interactions* (pp. 189–214). New York: Plenum.

Cohen, R., Kearney, K. A., Kemeny, M. E., and Zegans, M. D. (1989). Acute stress, chronic stress, and immunity, and the role of optimism as a moderator. *Psychosomatic Medicine, 51*, 255.

Contrada, R., and Krantz, D. (1988). Stress, reactivity, and Type A behavior: Current status and future directions. *Annals of Behavioral Medicine, 10*, 64–70.

Contrada, R. J., Leventhal, H., and O'Leary, A. (1990). Personality and health. In L. A. Pervin (Ed.), *Handbook of personality: Theory and research* (pp. 638–669). New York: Guilford.

Crary, B., Hauser, S. L., Borysenko, M., Kutz, I., Hoban, C., Ault, K. A., Weiner, H. L., and Benson, H. (1983). Epinephrine-induced changes in the distribution of lymphocyte subsets in the peripheral blood of humans. *Journal of Immunology, 131*, 1178–1181.

Dantzer, R. (1989). Neuroendocrine correlates of control and coping. In A. Steptoe and A. Appels (Eds.), *Stress, personal control and health* (pp. 277–294). Chichester: Wiley.

Dunbar, F. (1943). *Psychosomatic diagnosis*. New York: Harper & Row.

Dunkel-Schetter, C., Feinstein, L. G., Taylor, S. E., and Falke, R. L. (1992). Patterns of coping with cancer. *Health Psychology, 11*, 79–87.

Efran, J., Chorney, R. L., Ascher, L. M., and Lukens, M. D. (1989). Coping style, paradox, and the cold pressor task. *Journal of Behavioral Medicine, 12*, 91–103.

Engel, G. L. (1977). The need for a new medical model: Challenge for biomedicine. *Science, 196*, 129–136.

Fawzy, F. I., Kemeny, M. E., Fawzy, N. W., Elashoff, R., Morton, D., Cousins, N., and Fahey, J. L. (1990). A structured psychiatric intervention for cancer patients. II. Changes over time in immunological measures. *Archives of General Psychiatry, 47*, 729–735.

Folkman, S., Lazarus, R., Dunkel-Schetter, C., DeLongis, A., and Gruen, R. (1986). The dynamics of a stressful encounter: Cognitive appraisal, coping, and encounter outcomes. *Journal of Personality and Social Psychology, 50*, 992–1003.

Folkman, S., Chesney, M., Pollack, L., and Coates, T. (1992). Stress, control, and coping and depressive mood in HIV + and HIV − gay men in San Francisco. Unpublished manuscript, University of California at San Francisco, Center for AIDS Prevention Studies.

Frankenhaeuser, M. (1983). The sympathetic-adrenal and pituitary-adrenal response to challenge: Comparison between the sexes. In T. M. Dembroski, T. H. Schmidt, and G. Blumchen (Eds.), *Biobehavioral bases of coronary heart disease* (pp. 91–105). New York: Karger.

Frankenhaeuser, M., and Johansson, G. (1982). Stress at work: Psychobiological and psychosocial aspects. Paper presented at the 20th International Congress of Applied Psychology, Edinburgh.

Friedman, M., and Rosenman, R. H. (1974). *Type A behavior and your heart.* New York: Knopf.

Friedman, M., Thoresen, C. D., Gill, J. J., Powell, L. H., Ulmer, D., Thompson, L., Price, V. A., Rabin, D. D., Breall, W. S., Dixon, T., Levy, R., and Bourg, E. (1984). Alterations of Type A behavior and reduction in cardiac recurrences in post myocardial infarction patients. *American Heart Journal, 108,* 237–248.

Friedman, M., Thoresen, C. D., Gill, J., Ulmer, D., Powell, L., Price, V., Brown, B., Thompson, L., Rabin, D., Breall, W., Bourg, E., Levy, R., and Dixon, T. (1986). Alterations of Type A behavior and its effects on cardiac recurrences in post myocardial infarction patients: Summary results of the recurrent coronary prevention project. *American Heart Journal, 112,* 653–665.

Gattuso, S. M., Litt, M. D., and Fitzgerald, T. E. (1992). Coping with gastrointestinal endoscopy: Self-efficacy enhancement and coping style. *Journal of Consulting and Clinical Psychology, 60,* 133–139.

Gibbons, J. C. (1964). Cortisol secretion rate in depressive illness. *Archives of General Psychiatry, 10,* 572–575.

Gitlin, M. J., and Gerner, R. H. (1986). The dexamethasone suppression test and response to somatic treatment: A review. *Journal of Clinical Psychiatry, 47,* 16–18.

Glass, D. C. (1977). *Behavior patterns, stress, and coronary disease.* Hillsdale, NJ: Erlbaum.

Goodkin, K., Antoni, M. H., and Blaney, P. H. (1986). Stress and hopelessness in the promotion of cervical intraepithelial neoplasia to invasive squamous cell carcinoma of the cervix. *Journal of Psychosomatic Research, 30,* 67–76.

Greer, S., Morris, T., and Pettingale, K. W. (1979). Psychological response to breast cancer. Effect on outcome. *Lancet, 13,* 785–787.

Grossarth-Maticek, R., Kanazir, D. T., Schmidt, P., and Vetter, H. (1982). Psychosomatic factors in the process of carcinogenesis. *Psychotherapy and psychosomatics, 38,* 284–302.

Hackett, T. P., and Cassem, N. H. (1973). Psychological adaption to convalescence in myocardial infarction patients. In J. P. Naughton, H. K. Hellerstein, and I. C. Mohler (Eds.), *Exercise testing and exercise training in coronary heart disease.* New York: Academic Press.

Haynes, S. G., and Matthews, K. A. (1988). Review and methodologic critique of recent studies on Type A behavior and cardiovascular disease. *Annals of Behavioral Medicine, 10,* 47–59.

Henry, J. P., and Stephens, P. M. (1977). *Stress, health, and the social environment.* New York: Springer.

Holahan, C. J., and Moos, R. H. (1986). Personality, coping, and family resources in stress resistance: A longitudinal analysis. *Journal of Personality and Social Psychology, 51,* 389–395.

Holahan, C. J., and Moos, R. H. (1987). Personal and contextual determinants of coping strategies. *Journal of Personality and Social Psychology, 52,* 946–955.

Jensen, M. R. (1987). Psychobiological factors predicting the course of breast cancer. *Journal of Personality, 55,* 317–342.

Kamen-Siegel, L., Rodin, J., Seligman, M. E. P., and Dwyer, J. (1991). Explanatory style and cell-mediated immunity in elderly men and women. *Health Psychology, 10*, 229–235.

Kelly, D. D. (1986). Stress-induced analgesia. *Annals of the New York Academy of Sciences, 467*.

Kiecolt-Glaser, J. K., Garner, W. K., Speicher, C., Penn, G. M., Holliday, J., and Glaser, R. (1984). Psychosocial modifiers of immunocompetence in medical students. *Psychosomatic Medicine, 46*, 7–14.

Kiecolt-Glaser, J. K., Stephens, R. E., Lipetz, P. D., Speicher, C. E., and Glaser, R. (1985). Distress and DNA repair in human lymphocytes. *Journal of Behavioral Medicine, 8*, 311–320.

Lazarus, R. S. (1966). *Psychological stress and the coping process*. New York: McGraw Hill.

Lazarus, R. S. (1991). *Emotion and adaptation*. New York: Oxford University Press.

Lazarus, S., and Folkman, R. S. (1984). *Stress, appraisal, and coping*. New York: Springer.

Lerman, C., Rimer, B., Blumberg, B., Cristinzio, S., Engstrom, P. F., MacElwee, N., O'Conner, K., and Seay, J. (1990). Effects of coping style and relaxation on cancer chemotherapy side-effects and emotional responses. *Cancer Nursing, 13*, 308–315.

Letters to the Editor. (1985). *New England Journal of Medicine, 312*, 1354–1359.

Levine, M. N., Guyatt, G. H., Gent, M., De Pauw, S., Goodyear, M. D., Hryniuk, W. M., Arnold, A., Findlay, B., Skillings, J. R., Bramwell, V. H., Levin, L., Bush, H., Abu-Zahra, H., and Kotalik, J. (1988). Quality of life in Stage II breast cancer: An instrument for clinical trials. *Journal of Clinical Oncology, 6*, 1798–1810.

Levy, S., Herberman, R., Maluish, A., Schlien, B., and Lippman, M. (1985). Prognostic risk assessment in primary breast cancer by behavioral and immunological parameters. *Health Psychology, 4*, 99–113.

Levy, S., Herberman, R., Lippman, M., and d'Angelo, T. (1987). Correlation of stress factors with sustained depression of natural killer cell activity and predicted prognosis in patients with breast cancer. *Journal of Clinical Oncology, 5*, 348–353.

Luborsky, L., Crits-Christoph, P., Brady, J. P., Kron, R. E., Weiss, T., Cohen, M., and Levy, L. (1982). Behavioral versus pharmacological treatment for essential hypertension — A needed comparison. *Psychosomatic Medicine, 44*, 203–213.

Matthews, K. A. (1982). Psychological perspectives on the Type A behavior pattern. *Psychological Bulletin, 91*, 293–323.

Meichenbaum, D. H., and Jaremko, M. E. (Eds.). (1983). *Stress reduction and prevention*. New York: McGraw-Hill.

Miller, S. M. (1979). Controllability and human stress: Method, evidence, and theory. *Behavior Research and Therapy, 17*, 287–304.

Miller, S. M. (1980). Why having control reduces stress: If I can stop the roller coaster I don't want to get off. In J. Garber and M. Seligman (Eds.), *Human helplessness: Theory and applications* (pp. 71–95). New York: Academic Press.

Miller, S. M. (1987). Monitoring and blunting: Validation of a questionnaire to assess styles of information-seeking under threat. *Journal of Personality and Social Psychology, 52*, 345–353.

Miller, S. M. (1990). To see or not to see: Cognitive informational styles in the coping process. In M. Rosenbaum (Ed.), *Learned resourcefulness: On coping skills, self-regulation, and adaptive behavior* (pp. 95–126). New York: Springer.

Miller, S. M. (1992). Psychosocial correlates of colposcopy. Presented at American Society of Colposcopy and Cervical Pathology, Orlando, Florida, March.

Miller, S. M., and Mangan, C. E. (1983). The interacting effects of information and coping style in adapting to gynecologic stress: Should the doctor tell all? *Journal of Personality and Social Psychology, 45*, 223–236.

Miller, S. M., Brody, D. S., and Summerton, J. (1988). Styles of coping with threat: Implications for health. *Journal of Personality and Social Psychology, 54*, 345–353.

Miller, S. M., Leinbach, A., and Brody, D. S. (1989) Coping style in hypertensives: Nature and consequences. *Journal of Consulting and Clinical Psychology, 57*, 333–337.

Mischel, W. (1973). Toward a cognitive social learning reconceptualization of personality. *Psychological Review, 80*, 252–283.

Morley, J. E., Kay, N. E., Solomon, G. F., and Plotnikoff, N. P. (1987). Neuropeptides: Conductors of the immune orchestra. *Life Sciences, 41*, 527–544.

Öhman, A., and Bohlin, G. (1989). The role of controllability in cardiovascular activation and cardiovascular disease: Help or hinderance? In A. Steptoe and A. Appels (Eds.), *Stress, personal control and health* (pp. 257–276). Chichester: Wiley.

O'Leary, A. (1990). Stress, emotion, and human immune function. *Psychological Bulletin, 108*, 363–382.

O'Leary, A. (1992). Self-efficacy and health: Behavioral and stress-physiological mediation. *Cognitive Therapy and Research, 16*, 229–245.

O'Leary, A., Shoor, S., Lorig, K., and Holman, H. R. (1988). A cognitive–behavioral treatment for rheumatoid arthritis. *Health Psychology, 7*, 527–544.

Olson, G. A., Olson, R. D., and Kastin, A. J. (1987). Endogenous opiates: 1986. *Peptides, 8*, 1135–1164.

Peterson, C., Seligman, M. E. P., and Vaillant, G. E. (1988). Pessimistic explanatory style is a risk factor for physical illness: A thirty-five-year longitudinal study. *Journal of Personality and Social Psychology, 55*, 23–27.

Phillips, K. (1989). Psychological consequences of behavioural choice in aversive situations. In A. Steptoe and A. Appels (Eds.), *Stress, personal control and health* (pp. 239–256). Chichester: Wiley.

Phipps, S., and Zinn, A. B. (1986). Psychological response to amniocentosis: II. Effects of coping. *American Journal of Medical Genetics, 25*, 143–148.

Price, V. A. (1982). *Type A behavior pattern: A model for research and practice*. New York: Academic Press.

Scheier, M. F., and Carver, C. S. (1985). Optimism, coping, and health: Assessment and implications of generalized outcome expectancies. *Health Psychology, 4*, 219–247.

Scheier, M. F., and Carver, C. S. (1987). Dispositional optimism and physical well-being: The influence of generalized outcome expectancies on health. *Journal of Personality, 55*, 169–210.

Scheier, M. F., and Carver, C. S. (1992). *Optimism, pessimism, and the process of adjustment to college life*. Unpublished manuscript, Carnegie Mellon University.

Scheier, M. F., and Carver, C. S. (1992). Effects of optimism on psychological and physical well-being: Theoretical overview and empirical update. *Cognitive Therapy and Research, 16*, 201–228.

Scheier, M. F., Weintraub, J. K., and Carver, C. S. (1986). Coping with stress: Divergent strategies of optimists and pessimists. *Journal of Personality and Social Psychology, 51*, 1257–1264.

Scheier, M. F., Matthews, K. A., Owens, J. F., Magovern, G. J., Lefebvre, R. C., Abbott, R. A., and Carver, C. S. (1989). Dispositional optimism and recovery from coronary bypass surgery: The beneficial effects on physical and psychological well-being. *Journal of Personality and Social Psychology, 57*, 1024–1040.

Scheier, M. F., Matthews, K. A., Owens, J. F., Magovern, G. J., Sr., and Carver, C. S. (1990). *Dispositional optimism and recovery after 5 years from coronary artery bypass surgery*. Unpublished manuscript, Carnegie Mellon University.

Scherwitz, L., Berton, K., and Leventhal, H. (1978). Type A behavior, self-involvement, and cardiovascular response. *Psychosomatic Medicine, 40,* 593–609.

Schmale, A., and Iker, H. (1969). The psychological setting of uterine cervical cancer. *Annals of the New York Academy of Sciences, 164,* 807–813.

Schneiderman, N. (1983). Behavior, autonomic function and animal models of cardiovascular pathology. In *Biobehavioral bases of coronary heart disease* T. M. Dembroski, T. H. Schmidt, & G. Blumchen (eds.), pp. 304–364). Basel: Karger.

Seligman, M. E. P. (1975). *Helplessness.* San Francisco: Freeman.

Selye, H. (1956). *The stress of life.* New York: McGraw-Hill.

Selye, H. (1976). *Stress in health and disease.* Woburn, MA: Butterworth.

Shavit, Y., and Martin, F. C. (1987). Opiates, stress, and immunity: Animal studies. *Annals of Behavioral Medicine, 9,* 11–20.

Sieber, W. J., Rodin, J., and Larson, L. (1991). *Time course of natural killer cell activity after exposure to uncontrollable stress in humans.* Unpublished manuscript, Yale University.

Smedley, H., Katrak, M., Sikora, K., and Wheeler, T. (1983). Neurological effects of recombinant human interferon. *British Medical Journal, 286,* 262–264.

Sparks, G. G. (1989). Understanding emotional reactions to a suspenseful movie: The interaction between forewarning and preferred coping style. *Communications Monographs, 56,* 325–340.

Sparks, G. G., and Spirek, M. M. (1988). Individual differences in coping with stressful mass media: An activation-arousal view. *Human Communications Research, 15,* 191–216.

Spiegel, D., Bloom, J. R., Kraemer, H. C., and Gottheil, E. (1989). Effect of psychosocial treatment on survival of patients with metastatic breast cancer. *Lancet, ii,* 888–891.

Steketee, G., Bransfield, S., Miller, S. M., and Foa, E. (1989). The effect of information and coping style on the reduction of phobic anxiety. *Journal of Anxiety Disorders, 3,* 69–85.

Steptoe, A., and Appels, A. (1989). *Stress, personal control and health.* Chichester: Wiley.

Steptoe, A., and O'Sullivan, J. (1986). Monitoring and blunting coping styles in women prior to surgery. *British Journal of Clinical Psychology, 25,* 143–144.

Stone, A. A., and Neale, J. M. (1984). New measure of daily coping: Development and preliminary results. *Journal of Personality and Social Psychology, 46,* 892–906.

Suls, J., and Fletcher, B. (1985). The relative efficacy of avoidant and non-avoidant coping strategies: A meta-analysis. *Health Psychology, 4,* 249–288.

Taylor, S. E. (1991). *Health psychology.* New York: McGraw-Hill.

Taylor, S. E., Wood, J. V., and Lichtman, R. R. (1983). *Life change following cancer.* Unpublished manuscript, University of California, Los Angeles.

Taylor, S. E., Kemeny, M. E., Aspinwall, L. G., Schneider, S. G., Rodriguez, R., & Herbert, M. (1991). *Optimism, coping, psychological distress, and high-risk sexual behavior among men at risk for AIDS.* Unpublished manuscript, University of California at Los Angeles.

Temoshok, L., Heller, B. W., Sagebiel, R. W., Blois, M. S., Sweet, D. M., Di Clemente, R. J., and Gold, M. L. (1985). The relationship of psychosocial factors to prognostic indicators in cutaneous malignant melanoma. *Journal of Psychosomatic Research, 29,* 139–154.

Watkins, L. O., Weaver, L., and Odegaard, V. (1986). Preparation for cardiac catheterization: Tailoring the content of instruction to coping style. *Heart and Lung, 15,* 382–389.

Watson, D., and Pennebaker, J. W. (1989). Health complaints, stress, and distress: Exploring the central role of negative affectivity. *Psychological Review, 96,* 234–254.

Wiedenfeld, S. A., O'Leary, A., Bandura, A., Brown, S., Levine, S., and Raska, K. (1990). Impact of perceived coping efficacy on components of the immune system. *Journal of Personality and Social Psychology, 59,* 1082–1094.

Wirsching, M., Stierlin, H., Hoffman, F., Weber, G., and Wirsching, B. (1982). Psychological identification of breast cancer patients before biopsy. *Journal of Psychosomatic Research, 26*, 1–10.

Wortman, C. B., and Dunkel-Schetter, C. (1979). Interpersonal relationships and cencer: A theoretical analysis. *Journal of Social Issues, 35*, 120–155.

Cognitive–Behavioral Models of Anorexia Nervosa, Bulimia Nervosa, and Obesity

Kelly Bemis Vitousek and Lisa Orimoto

University of Hawaii

This chapter will review the role of cognitive factors in the development and treatment of the major disorders of eating and weight: anorexia nervosa, bulimia nervosa, and obesity. The clustering of these three conditions under a common heading is both awkward and instructive, as it forces an examination of the complex relations among them.

First, we must recognize that the labels describing each condition convey nonequivalent amounts and kinds of information about the individuals who qualify to receive them. The diagnosis of anorexia nervosa summarizes a relatively predictable set of beliefs, emotions, and behaviors, as well as a specific weight status. The label bulimia nervosa similarly communicates information about how an affected individual is likely to think, feel, and act — at least with reference to food and weight — but implies nothing about what she will actually weigh. The statement that a third person is obese clarifies only relative weight status. Contrary to both popular and clinical stereotypes, the probable attitudes or activities of an obese individual cannot be inferred from this single descriptor of his or her physical proportions.

The decreasing level of meaningfulness across these three category labels corresponds to increasing heterogeneity in the population of people to whom each applies. Allowing a margin of error for individual differences, we can profile the "classic" anorexic as a perfectionistic, conscientious, and conforming adolescent girl. With somewhat less confidence, we can guess that the "typical" bulimic will also be a young female, but can hazard few generalizations about her personality traits. She may resemble her anorexic counterpart (and may have been anorexic herself, in a previous symptom phase), or she may represent a temperamental opposite, distinguished by impulsivity, rebelliousness, and emotional instability. The very notion of a prototypic obese individual is absurd. Such a person may be male or female, an infant or an elderly adult, and may manifest any of the normal or pathological personality variations evident in the general population.

It follows that the cognitive models devised to account for these disorders will vary widely in specificity and comprehensiveness. Cognitive theories of anorexia nervosa and bulimia nervosa provide a coherent account of the onset, persistence, and remediation of symptomatology. Cognitive variables assume a central and primary role at each of these stages, although a diverse array of familial, social, and biological elements are invoked as contributing factors. In contrast, contemporary models of obesity do not attempt to impose cognitive uniformity on fat baby boys and plump older women, emphasizing instead the primacy of biological and environmental factors. In individual cases, cognitive variables may play no role whatsoever in the production or maintenance of obesity. In others, they may exacerbate its severity, complicate its appropriate treatment, or engender secondary problems in the lives of those it affects.

While emphasizing these differences, it should be noted that a few key elements appear in cognitive models of all three conditions. Individuals in each category are profoundly affected by contemporary social values about weight and shape. The objectively overweight suffer ridicule and discrimination. Internalizing the public antipathy for their weight status, many learn to despise their bodies and to deplore the lack of self-control attributed to them. Anorexics and bulimics react to the same social contingencies, often without having experienced sanctions directly. They accept the significance of weight as a measure of personal worth, and develop symptoms in part to avoid the humiliation of real or imagined obesity.

Another common element is dieting, which can produce complex physiological and psychological consequences in individuals with any of these conditions. The effects are most pronounced in restricting anorexics, who practice abstention steadily and all too successfully, but may also be evident in the disorganized pattern of under- and overconsumption typical of bulimics, and the cyclical alternation between dieting and normal or excessive eating characteristic of many obese persons.

The categories are related in another sense, in that the boundaries between them are indistinct, and the same individual may qualify for all three over a lifetime. Anorexia and obesity cannot, by definition, occur simultaneously, but bulimia can coexist with either. The most active diagnostic controversies in the eating disorder field concern cases of symptom overlap. Should underweight anorexics who also experience bulimic episodes be given both diagnoses, or should they be classified with restricting anorexics (with whom they share the complications of starvation pathology) or with normal-weight bulimics (whom they often more closely resemble in personality and background characteristics)? Should the subgroup of overweight individuals who binge-eat without engaging in purgative tactics be designated bulimic, consigned to the residual category of "atypical eating disorder," allocated to a proposed new category of "binge eating disorder"? — or should such behavior simply be recognized as one variation along a spectrum of consummatory patterns that do not constitute discrete psychiatric conditions?

The issues that pose conceptual and diagnostic problems for the field also create technical difficulties in the organization of a chapter on the eating disorders. We have chosen to discuss anorexia nervosa and bulimia nervosa together for several reasons: the high frequency with which both syndromes affect the same individuals, either simultaneously or successively; the substantial overlap in cognitive models of their maintenance and treatment; and the existence of relevant research conducted with combined samples. The heterogeneous population of the obese will be discussed subsequently, with the binge-eating minority uneasily subsumed under a separate heading.

ANOREXIA NERVOSA AND BULIMIA NERVOSA

Cognitive–Behavioral Theory

Reduced to its essence, the cognitive model holds that anorexic and bulimic symptoms are maintained by a characteristic set of *beliefs* about weight and shape. These beliefs influence the individuals who hold them to engage in stereotypic eating-disordered behaviors, to be responsive to eccentric reinforcement contingencies, to process information in accordance with predictable cognitive biases, and, eventually, to be affected by the physiological consequences of pursuing weight control.

The existence of distorted beliefs in anorexia has been recognized throughout the scientific history of the disorder; however, early investigators tended to overlook corresponding phenomena in bulimia, presumably because their attention was compelled by the dramatic behavior and affect-regulating function of the binge–purge cycle. Cognitive theorists have consistently emphasized the close correspondence between these superficially discrepant disorders, noting that both sets of patients evaluate their self-worth in terms of weight and shape, shun weight gain and fatness, and dedicate a substantial proportion of their voluntary behavior and psychic energy to the management of eating and weight (Fairburn and Garner, 1988). Such observers were instrumental in inserting an attitudinal criterion into the DSM-III-R definition of bulimia nervosa, and refining this specification in proposed DSM-IV criteria for both disorders.

Figure 7.1 presents a conceptual model of anorexia nervosa drawn from the cognitive theory of Garner and Vitousek[1] (Garner and Bemis, 1982, 1985; Vitousek and Ewald, 1992; Vitousek and Hollon, 1990), and closely related accounts provided by Slade and Casper. Because the restricting (nonbulimic) subtype of anorexia nervosa represents the purest instance of the central psychopathology and defines the most homogeneous group of subjects, it will be used as the basis for the following discussion; issues specific to bulimia will be highlighted when relevant.

A detailed explication of the hypothesized elements and their interactions is far beyond the scope of this chapter. The comprehensive model is outlined in Garner and Bemis (1982, 1985) and Garner (1986a); for extended considerations of specific components, the reader is referred to Vitousek and Ewald (1992) on individual variables, to Garner *et al.* (1983a) on sociocultural influences, to Casper and Davis (1977) on precipitating stressors, to Slade (1982) and Bemis (1983) on positive and negative reinforcement, to Vitousek and Hollon (1990) on schematic processing, and to Garner *et al.* (1985b) on the effects of starvation. We shall provide here a brief overview before turning to a discussion of the empirical status of selected elements.

As illustrated in Fig. 7.1, the cognitive model declines to specify the precise contribution of genetic and familial factors to the etiology of anorexia nervosa, although it is assumed that the stable individual characteristics preceding symptom onset originate in the interplay between these two sets of variables. Across theoretical perspectives, the modal preanorexic personality has been described with extraordinary reliability. These young girls are depicted as insecure, perfectionistic, ascetic, and excessively compliant children who are not well prepared to become competent and independent adults. This cluster of personality traits can be recast in cognitive terms by labeling them "general self-schemas" (Vitousek and

---

[1]The former name of K. M. Vitousek is K. M. Bemis.

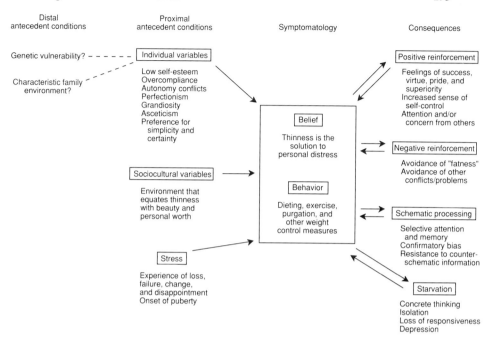

Figure 7.1. A cognitive model of anorexia nervosa.

Ewald, 1992; Vitousek and Hollon, 1990), but it is not clear that this unveri-fiable translation enhances our understanding of their contribution to symptom onset.

Shortly before the initiation of anorexic behavior, the self-concept of these individuals seems to undergo a challenge that threatens their fragile equilibrium. The apparent precipitants are rarely catastrophic events; more typically, they represent ordinary points-of-passage such as attaining men-arche, enrolling in a new school, moving away from home, or getting married (Levine and Smolak, 1989). The shift from late childhood into adolescence is often a pivotal occurrence; in most cases, its disruptive effects have less to do with the narrowly sexual implications of puberty than with the cognitive and social changes it entails — and with the rapid deposition of fat that focuses attention on body contours. Faced with the stress of transition, these young girls seem particularly susceptible to the influence of contemporary social standards for weight. They start to be-lieve that "being too fat" is an important contributor to their personal distress, and seek salvation through the pursuit of thinness.

The equation of slenderness and happiness is a delusion that eating-disordered individuals share with much of western society. Thinness has come to symbolize competence, success, control, sexual attractiveness, and a kind of androgynous independence (Bennett and Gurin, 1982), while obesity denotes laziness, self-indulgence, inferior intellect, and low social status (Frankenberg *et al.*, 1982). Thus, the anorexic notion that weight control can transform misery into joy is not statistically abnormal, however irrational, dysfunctional, and elusive it may prove for most individuals who strive to achieve it. Yet, some aspects of the exaltation of thinness and abhorrence of fatness seem to distinguish anorexics and bulimics from others who subscribe to normatively distorted views about weight. The cognitive model postulates that the meanings of weight and shape are more elaborated, overinclusive, inflexible, idiosyncratic, emotionally charged, and personally relevant for individuals who suffer from these disorders (Vitousek and Hollon, 1990).

The cognitive model does not insist on temporal precedence for eating disorder beliefs over dieting behavior. In some novice anorexics and bulimics, the idea that thinness is a solution to personal distress does seem to be formulated in advance of dieting behavior, which is then undertaken with a clear objective in mind. However, others derive the anorexic premise only after experiencing the reinforcing consequences of weight loss that was initially achieved casually, or even accidentally (Vitousek and Ewald, 1992). More desultory attempts at weight control are supplanted by a strict dietary regimen, a program of rigorous exercise, and sometimes a variety of elimination tactics such as vomiting and the abuse of laxatives and diuretics. Over time, secondary irrational beliefs about the magical properties of food and consequences of weight gain or loss start to evolve from the basic premise, and ruminations about intake and output dominate most of the individual's cognitive experience (Vitousek and Ewald, 1992).

Some anorexics seem to be responsive to external reinforcement in the form of the admiration accorded to their self-control and/or the concern elicited by their emaciation; however, the cognitive model postulates that positive *self*-reinforcement makes a much more significant and persistent contribution to the maintenance of symptomatology (Bemis, 1983; Garner and Bemis, 1982, 1985; Slade, 1982). Individuals with anorexia nervosa do not regard their disorder as an affliction but as an accomplishment, in which they feel a complete emotional and moral investment (Casper *et al.*, 1981). Every morsel of food refused, every inch in diameter reduced, every pound of flesh eliminated become occasions for self-congratulation.

The negative reinforcement of avoiding the feared state of "fatness" (i.e., normal weight) also contributes to symptom maintenance. Anorexics develop a "margin of safety" principle, believing that they must interpose greater distance between themselves and the frightening numbers on the bathroom scale that signify obesity (Crisp, 1980; Russell *et al.*, 1975). By avoiding anxiety-provoking stimuli, they insulate themselves from disconfirmatory experiences, and eventually respond mainly to idiosyncratic internal contingencies that have little basis in reality. The all-encompassing preoccupation with weight control serves as a form of avoidance behavior in another sense as well (Slade, 1982), since it enables the anorexic individual to concentrate diffuse anxieties about achievement and self-worth on a single theme.

The cognitive model also hypothesizes that organized cognitive structures develop over time around the issues of weight and its implications for the self, profoundly influencing perceptions, thoughts, affect, and behavior (Vitousek and Hollon, 1990). Weight-related self-schemata may prolong symptoms in a relatively automatic fashion by affecting the manner in which eating-disordered individuals perceive and interpret their experience. Anorexics and bulimics live in a self-created reality that has become dense with weight-related meanings. Other people are evaluated not on the basis of personal qualities but their status as thinner or fatter than the self; activities are considered not for their potential to produce pleasure or growth, but their tendency to facilitate or interfere with weight control. Views of the self are also bound inextricably to these weight-related schemata. Experiences that occasion self-evaluation or self-criticism stimulate an intensified focus on body size and shape (Striegel-Moore *et al.*, 1986), while shifts in weight dramatically influence affect and cognition. In addition to the automatic effects that schema-driven processing exerts on the maintenance of symptomatology, Vitousek and Hollon (1990) speculate that schematic principles help account for the adaptive quality of eating disorder symptoms: anorexics and bulimics may welcome the emergence of monolithic cognitive structures that reduce the confusing complexity and ambiguity of daily life.

Another variable that is both a consequence of and contributor to eating disorder symptomatology is the impairment of psychological functioning associated with starvation. Starvation produces a variety of adverse cognitive and emotional effects on normal individuals, including poor concentration, concrete thinking, rigidity, withdrawal, obsessive–compulsive behavior, and depression (Keys *et al.*, 1950). Some recent suggestive findings have linked starvation sequelae in anorexia nervosa to cognitive perseveration (Demitrack *et al.*, 1990) and to impairments in information-processing capacity and control functions (Laessle *et al.*, 1989a), all of which may serve to perpetuate the restrictive pattern from which they result.

While the emergence of binge-eating in approximately 40% of anorexics is readily explained as a consequence of semi-starvation, the development of bulimic episodes in normal-weight individuals seems more mysterious.

There is a growing recognition that similar mechanisms underlie bulimic symptomatology in both populations. Although the typical bulimic may never have attained the emaciated state of her anorexic counterpart, she shares the same beliefs about the central importance of weight and shape as measures of self-worth, and is equally dedicated to the goal of weight control (albeit less successful in its pursuit). Extreme dieting virtually always precedes the appearance of other symptoms in bulimia nervosa (Polivy and Herman, 1985; Wardle, 1988), and appears to have a host of biological, cognitive, and affective consequences that predispose to binge-eating (Wilson, 1993).

Physiologically, restrictive eaters develop an impaired sense of satiety, react more strongly to the ingestion of carbohydrates, and may become more efficient metabolically, requiring fewer and fewer calories to maintain body weight (Wilson, 1993). Some theorists suggest that although bulimics do not appear to be underweight, they are genetically programmed to be heavier than their preferred weight, and are thus in a state of deprivation even at average weight levels (Garner *et al.*, 1985a; Striegel-Moore *et al.*, 1986). Surveys confirm that bulimics have a lifetime history of greater weight variability than normal controls (Turnbull *et al.*, 1989), and may be more likely to have fathers who are overweight (Garner *et al.*, 1985a).

Prolonged dieting also interacts with a variety of cognitive and affective variables to increase the tendency to binge-eating. When food intake is restricted, food acquires potent reward value, and can be used to mitigate unpleasant mood states such as depression, anxiety, and anger (Wardle, 1988). Mood states may also mediate the cognitive appraisal of success in conforming to self-imposed dietary standards (Davis *et al.*, 1988). Distressed dieters may interpret the consumption of any unplanned food as a sign that they have already "blown it," and may as well suspend the artificial control imposed on their incessant hunger.

Once binge episodes have begun to punctuate the restricted eating behavior of the incipient bulimic, a variety of additional adaptive functions emerge. Binge-eating provides a temporary experience of "letting go" or "spacing out" (Johnson *et al.*, 1984), allowing individuals to suspend unpleasant thoughts and feelings while narrowing their attention to the immediate stimulus environment (Heatherton and Baumeister, 1991). The initiation of purgative practices such as vomiting and laxative abuse is most directly explained as a means of preventing the weight gain that would otherwise result from binge-eating, but these tactics may also acquire supplementary functions as means of tension regulation and self-punishment (Johnson *et al.*, 1984).

Since dieting is an extremely common behavior among contemporary young women and bulimia nervosa remains a relatively rare phenomenon, the former must be considered a nonsufficient, if necessary, condition in the etiology of the latter (Wilson, 1993). It is not yet clear which additional factors are required for symptom onset. As noted earlier, the bulimic population appears considerably less homogeneous than the anorexic population with respect to the personality variables that have been implicated in an obsessive concern with weight and shape. Accumulating evidence does suggest that bulimic individuals may be predisposed to general emotional instability and loss of behavioral control (Wilson, 1993); it is possible that this nonspecific vulnerability may interact with intense social pressures about weight to produce the bulimic syndrome in a subset of dieters.

In the following sections, we shall briefly review the empirical status of two of the most distinctively "cognitive" elements of the etiological model we have summarized: beliefs about weight and shape, and schematic processing of weight-related information.

Beliefs about Weight and Shape

A variety of assessment strategies have been employed to examine the distinctiveness of anorexic and bulimic beliefs about weight. Both attitudinal inventories and semistructured interview schedules confirm that clinical subjects differ from normal controls (and, typically, from obese, restrained, and dieting controls) in the stated drive for thinness and concern for body shape and weight (e.g., Cooper and Fairburn, 1987; Garner *et al.*, 1983b; Wilson and Smith, 1989). Compared to normal and psychiatric controls, anorexics and bulimics report spending more time thinking about food and weight, and react more strongly to the gain or loss of trivial amounts of weight (Bemis, 1986).

Self-statement inventories have verified that anorexics and bulimics also espouse specific irrational ideas about the magical properties of food and the implications of body weight. In the initial cognitive model of anorexia nervosa, Garner and Bemis (1982) speculated that after symptom onset a host of derivative beliefs emerge from the central anorexic premise: for example, that self-control in diverse areas is predicated on the control of eating and weight; that small increments in weight will progress inexorably to obesity; that ingested sugar will be converted instantly into stored fat; that vomiting and laxative-induced diarrhea purify the body. Other investigators have inserted these sorts of items into self-statement inventories, and have established that such measures do differentiate bulimics and/or anorexics from normal controls (e.g., Clark *et al.*, 1989; Franko *et al.*, 1988; Goldberg *et al.*, 1980; Mizes, 1990; Mizes and Klesges, 1989; Phelan, 1987; Scanlon *et al.*, 1986; Schulman *et al.*, 1986; Thompson *et al.*, 1987). Some have additionally shown that scores decrease over the course of the treatment, predict response to treatment, and correlate with other indices of eating disorder symptomatology (see Vitousek and Ewald, 1992, and Vitousek et al., 1991b, for reviews).

Numerous investigations have been conducted to examine relationships between daily events, hunger, affect, and cognition across the binge–purge cycle in bulimia nervosa. In most of these studies, subjects have been instructed to self-monitor the targeted variables in naturalistic settings, either upon occurrence, at fixed time intervals, or in response to signals from a paging device (Cooper and Bowskill, 1986; Davis et al., 1985, 1988; Elmore and de Castro, 1990; Johnson and Larson, 1982; Lingswiler et al., 1987, 1989; Schlundt et al., 1985; Zotter and Crowther, 1991). A few have collected responses during laboratory eating sessions (Kaye et al., 1986; Williamson et al., 1985). Other studies have asked subjects to characterize their episodes retrospectively (Cooper et al., 1988; Hsu, 1990; Steinberg et al., 1990).

Such investigations have confirmed that negative mood states tend to precede the binge–purge cycle; some report a decrease in anxiety and/or anger but typically not in depression following completion of the episode. Regrettably, most of these studies have emphasized affective ratings; few have collected or analyzed this potentially rich source of self-statement data in informative ways. In Hsu's (1990) questionnaire study, bulimics indicated that dichotomous self-statements such as "Now that I've done it, I might as well go all the way" frequently preceded binge episodes; other common themes included self-condemnation, bewilderment at loss of control, and resolutions to "be good" tomorrow. The self-monitoring study conducted by Lingswiler et al. (1989) also found that dichotomous cognitions were reported prior to eating episodes by both bulimic and binge-eating subjects. Using a different methodology, Zotter and Crowther (1991) obtained few instances of dichotomous thinking, but found that bulimics were more likely than normal or dieting controls to record negatively toned and distorted cognitions about food and weight.

Although recent attempts to assess cognitive content in anorexia and bulimia nervosa are encouraging, progress has been hampered by the failure to address a number of critical methodological and conceptual issues. One challenge for self-statement research concerns the vexing problem of denial and distortion in self-report. Difficulties inherent in the assessment of all private events are compounded many times over by a distinctive feature of the eating disorders: anorexics and bulimics are notoriously unsatisfactory informants about their internal experience. Crisp (1980) comments that "in no other morbid condition is the outsider more effectively and so frequently denied access to an appreciation of the relationship between behavior and manner on the one hand and inner experiences on the other."

Because anorexics are typically invested in preserving their egosyntonic symptomatology, they are prone to deliberate, instrumental distortion in self-report. Paradoxically, their tendency to overcompliance may also lead to misrepresentation, as they strive to conform to the subtly communicated biases of therapists or researchers (Bruch, 1978). Finally, anorexics' capacity to give an accurate account of their private experiences may be further restricted by poor introspective skills and by the effects of starvation, which can contribute to a diminished capacity for abstraction and general impoverishment of thought content. Bulimic subjects — at least those encountered in treatment settings — may have better access to their internal experience, and may be less likely to falsify self-report for protective purposes, but they too can be unreliable informants.

Vitousek *et al.* (1991a) have summarized a variety of strategies that could be used to reduce the effects of denial and distortion in eating-disordered subjects, including indirect questioning strategies, the use of collateral informants, and the separation of clinical and research contexts. The publication of self-report data with this population should be accompanied by extensive documentation concerning the assessment setting, the nature of the relationship between experimenter and subject, the phrasing of instructional sets, and the specific and nonspecific techniques employed in an attempt to lower defensiveness.

Another problem concerns the inadequate conceptualization of theoretical issues in most cognitive assessment research carried out within this domain. Self-statement measures are typically heterogeneous compilations of the kinds of peculiar ideas anorexic and bulimic clients verbalize in psychotherapy; rarely are inventories designed to test hypotheses about specific aspects of the cognitive model. Rather than using this scattershot approach to scale development, it might prove more informative to derive items from an organized model about the kinds of beliefs theoretically essential to the maintenance of these syndromes.

One such model suggests that the eating disorders are founded on key beliefs in a number of cognitive categories (Vitousek, 1990). In order to develop and sustain an eating disorder, it is postulated that an individual must experience the *perception* that she is fat (or, at least, is not sufficiently thin), possess the *evaluation* that it is bad to be fat (because it is unattractive, unpopular, unhealthy, and/or self-indulgent), hold the *attribution* that weight is under personal control, and develop the personal *expectation* that specific behaviors (dieting, exercise, purgation) will result in weight loss, removing the aversive consequences of perceived fatness. Our research group is currently testing an instrument composed of belief statements in each of the cognitive classes, examining whether such ideas are in fact essential to the perpetuation of symptoms, do distinguish clinical subjects from controls in the intensity and literalness of their interpretation, and can be modified over the course of therapy (perhaps differentially in clients exposed to alternative treatment modalities).

Finally, it should be noted that the assessment of self-statements about eating and weight has marked limitations as a means of testing the comprehensive cognitive model. No controversy surrounds the proposition that the thought *content* of subjects who worry about eating and weight is distinguishable from the thought content of subjects who are indifferent to such matters. Ultimately, however, we need to learn not simply what our clients think *about*, but what causes them to formulate their erroneous ideas, how such beliefs affect their experience of the world, and why they become so extraordinarily resistant to efforts to persuade them to think anything else.

Schematic Processing

In the past several years, researchers have begun to apply the methods and analyses of cognitive science to the study of many forms of psychopathology (see discussions in Dalgleish and Watts, 1990; Markus, 1990; Mathews and MacLeod, 1987; Safran *et al.*, 1990; Segal, 1988). Cognitive processing paradigms offer distinct advantages in the study of the eating disorders. Because they often employ test strategies that subjects are unable to decode and use dependent variables that are difficult to falsify, they can minimize or eliminate the dependency on self-report. They also move beyond cognitive content to explore the processes through which eating disorder beliefs develop, proliferate, and become autonomous.

Vitousek and Hollon (1990) recently outlined ten general strategies for the investigation of information processing in the eating disorders. They suggested that individuals with these conditions may differ from others in the following ways: (1) the ease and speed with which food- and weight-related stimuli are processed; (2) the elaboration of meaning around the construct of weight; (3) the intrusion of weight-related content into unrelated or ambiguous situations; (4) the possession of differentiated knowledge structures in connected domains; (5) an enhanced memory for schema-consistent information; (6) the ability to retrieve schema-relevant behavioral evidence; (7) the degree of confidence in judgments and predictions about food and weight; (8) the specific relevance of weight concerns for the self; (9) the level of cognitive and affective involvement in weight-related events; and (10) the resistance to counterschematic information.

A variety of information-processing studies bearing on these hypotheses are currently under way, and some relevant studies have already appeared in the literature. Schotte *et al.* (1990) used a dichotic listening paradigm to determine that bulimics exhibit increased perceptual sensitivity and physiological responsiveness to information about body weight. Laberg *et al.* (1991) reported that bulimics in whom negative mood had been induced showed more heart rate deceleration when viewing slides of forbidden foods, an effect that was not obtained with restrained eating controls. King *et al.* (1991) determined that anorexic, obese, and restrained subjects remembered food- and weight-related information preferentially after reading descriptive passages. Vitousek *et al.* (1992) found that anorexics and bulimics were more likely than normal or subclinical control subjects to attend to the food and weight meanings of homophones (such as "weight/wait") and homographs (such as "pound" and "light"); however, the inclusion of an additional normal control group "primed" with the knowledge that the study concerned eating disorders suggested that this effect was partially attributable to the influence of contextual cues.

A number of investigators have modified a familiar technique from cognitive science in an attempt to measure the interference in information processing caused by schema-based conflict or anxiety. The basic Stroop effect was first reported more than fifty years ago (Stroop, 1935). The task initially presented to subjects is straightforward: they are shown a card on which symbols or letters have been printed in different ink colors, and are instructed simply to identify the colors as rapidly as possible. On the next card, the symbols are replaced with the *names* of colors; the color names and the colors of the ink in which they are printed do not match, so that the word "blue" may be printed in yellow ink, and the word "red" in blue, and so on. The subject must again identify the colors of the inks in which the words have been printed. Because of the interference between ink color and the meaning of color names, processing time is slowed; subjects take substantially longer to complete this "conflict" card compared to the initial "control" card.

The Stroop paradigm has been adapted for the study of cognitive processing and psychopathology. It has been determined that if cards are prepared with words relevant to individual subjects' concerns, processing time is also delayed. Thus, socially phobic individuals perform the color-naming task more slowly when words like "foolish" or "boring" are used, although not when physical threat words such as "hospital" or "fatal" are presented (Hope *et al.*, 1990). Individuals with post-traumatic stress disorder respond slowly to words related to combat (McNally *et al.*, 1990) or to rape (Foa *et al.*, 1991), while control subjects also exposed to combat or to rape who did not develop PTSD fail to show longer latencies on the relevant Stroop cards.

Because of its considerable popularity in the wider cognitive psychopathology field, the Stroop test is one of the few cognitive experimental paradigms that has been used extensively with eating disorder subjects. Three groups of investigators have published studies using variants of the Stroop task, and many additional reports are now in press or under review. The results of these studies will be surveyed more extensively to illustrate the potential advantages and pitfalls of research on cognitive processing.

The specific stimuli used in these investigations have varied; most employ lists of both food- and weight-related words, sometimes segregated on separate cards and sometimes mixed together to form a single "eating-disorder-relevant" stimulus array. The conflict cards concerning food include items such as "candy," "chocolate," and "cake"; each stimulus is matched for graphomorphemic features and frequency of word use to a neutral word ("coats," "catalogue," "chat") that appears on a corresponding control card. Target cards concerning weight and shape include items such as "flabby," "plump," and "fat," which are paired with neutral words presented on a separate control card.

All published studies have reported that anorexic and/or bulimic subjects do manifest delayed response times to food- and/or weight-related word sets relative to normal subjects and relative to their own response times when neutral stimuli are presented (Ben-Tovim et al., 1989; Ben-Tovim and Walker, 1991; Channon et al., 1988; Cooper et al., 1992; Fairburn et al., 1991a). The results appear to be strongest for food-related stimuli, with more equivocal results obtained when weight-related words are presented. Neither familiarity with the procedure (Walker et al., 1992) nor variations in the order of card presentation (Cooper et al., 1992) appear to affect the magnitude of interference.

The theoretically preferred explanation of this effect would be that eating disorder subjects are manifesting an attentional bias toward threatening stimuli — perhaps, that the more elaborated fear structures associated with focal concerns require more cognitive processing capacity, and thus compete with the cognitive resources available for color naming (Foa et al., 1991). It has been hoped that this effect might also prove useful for several clinical and research purposes. Since the absolute differences between pathological and control groups appear to be fairly modest and the overlap in distributions considerable, the test is unlikely to have diagnostic utility (Ben-Tovim et al., 1989); however, it might be valuable as an uncontaminated index of the degree of food/weight preoccupation. Certainly, it would be desirable if it were possible to determine how obsessed an anorexic patient "really" is with eating and weight concerns at the time of intake, when she may be denying her symptomatology in the hope of evading treatment. Again, at the time of treatment termination or follow-up, when a subject may be minimizing residual symptoms for the benefit of her therapist or herself, it would be extremely convenient if an evaluator could simply pull out a stack of multicolored cards and a stopwatch, and administer the Stroop test to ascertain the truth. There is some evidence that disruptions in processing disappear with clinical recovery (Ben-Tovim *et al.*, 1989). It is also possible that the measure could provide a means of examining the mechanisms of treatment, if alternative modalities produce differential effects on Stroop times at posttest.

Important clinical questions rarely yield such simple answers, no matter how ingeniously they have been operationalized, and the Stroop task may provide another illustration of that unfortunate principle. None of the studies with clinical samples reported to date has ruled out the possibility that *hunger* is the most parsimonious explanation for observed disruptions in processing. As noted above, the interference effect is most marked for food-related stimuli, when weight and food words are separated on different cards; in studies combining food and weight stimuli on the same card, it is of course impossible to determine which item subsets are responsible for any increased latency.

Several research groups have recently investigated the possibility that the modified Stroop measures the transient effects of hunger on attention to food items, rather than more enduring and important features of psychopathology. Channon and Hayward (1990) confirmed that normal subjects also show delayed processing times when the food Stroop is administered after a 24-hour period of fasting. Our own research group is presently completing a study of the effect of shorter intervals of food deprivation, comparing hungry and full normal, weight-preoccupied, and bulimic subjects.

Another relevant investigation has been described by Schmidt and Telch (1991). A nonclinical sample of restrained eaters (see section on restraint, under cognitive theories of obesity) produced slower response times to food and body shape stimuli compared to unrestrained eaters; however, the use of a dietary preload yielded effects opposite to those hypothesized. It had been anticipated that the consumption of a milkshake by restrained subjects would result in an even greater delay in processing because of the increased salience of food and weight concerns. In fact, there was a trend toward *reduced* interference for both restrained and unrestrained subjects who received a preload. The investigators concluded that food consumption may have decreased response times for food items by alleviating hunger, noting that "from an evolutionary perspective, it makes sense for sated individuals to spend less of their attentional resources on dietary stimuli."

The results of these studies suggest that, in the eating disorders, the Stroop task may indeed be assessing statelike salient concerns instead of or in addition to more stable attentional biases, just as temporary concerns about health evoked by the imminent prospect of surgery can produce Stroop response patterns similar to those obtained with anxiety disorder samples (Cook *et al.*, 1989).

Can the Stroop still be employed as a means of penetrating the defenses of denying clients? — perhaps, at least if what they are denying is a hunger-induced concern with food. Can the Stroop be useful as a measure of therapeutic progress? Once more, we may find it informative in gauging food preoccupation secondary to dietary restriction, although it is not clear that we can interpret results as a measure of the resolution of fundamental psychopathology. However, the Stroop seems unlikely to help us identify modality-specific treatment mechanisms, since it probably assesses fairly superficial symptoms that will covary with changes in clinical status.

Can the Stroop illuminate theoretical issues about cognitive processing in the eating disorders? — again, perhaps, but only if the technique is employed and interpreted in more sophisticated ways. To tease apart statelike concerns from the more stable underlying schematic differences in which we are truly interested, appropriate control groups of chronically dieting or temporarily fasting individuals must always be used, and subjects should be tested in a variety of hungry/satiated conditions. We should also experiment with different stimulus *materials* that may yield more theoretically interesting results. For example, in addition to food and negative shape ("fat") stimuli, our research group is examining response times with *positive* shape words, such as "slender," "firm," and "thin." If these stimuli also yield increased latencies, it would suggest that the interference effect is not merely a product of fear-related distraction, but could be related to the richness of meaning associated with weight. We are also incorporating theoretically conflictual stimulus words concerning achievement and sexuality in the Stroop materials, in the hope of extending conclusions beyond an affirmation of the obvious salience of food and weight concerns through less transparent means.

Whether they would be disposed to view our naïveté with indulgence or with contempt, cognitive researchers who have struggled to understand the *basic* Stroop color–word interference effect for fifty years might caution us against our enthusiastic and often unthinking application of this methodology to our different set of questions. The original Stroop task has yielded 18 major empirical effects that must be explained by any satisfactory theoretical account of the processes producing interference (MacLeod, 1991). In applying modified Stroop-like tasks to the study of psychopathology, clinical researchers have sometimes been content to conclude that any obtained interference on disorder-relevant stimulus sets shows "something important" about information processing, without attempting to clarify what cognitive processes are implicated in this effect. The eating disorder field lags consistently behind research in the affective and anxiety disorders in the maturity of our questions and techniques. For example, Stroop studies in depression have employed a priming strategy to examine whether target stimuli not only produce disruptions in processing but are represented within cognitive structures in an organized fashion (Segal, 1988). Anxiety researchers have attempted to separate automatic attentional bias from postattentional ruminations as an explanation for delayed responding by using randomized computer screen presentations of single items to replace the card format in which responses to lists of words from the same set are timed collectively (McNally *et al.*, 1990). Novel paradigms have also been devised to examine whether Stroop findings in the anxiety disorders are better explained by perceptual processes or response bias (Dalgleish and Watts, 1990; MacLeod *et al.*, 1986).

Cognitive–Behavioral Therapy for Anorexia and Bulimia

Therapeutic Strategies

For detailed descriptions of cognitive–behavioral therapy in anorexia nervosa and bulimia nervosa, the interested reader is referred to Garner and Bemis (1982, 1985), Garner (1986a,b), and Fairburn (1985). The correspondence that cognitive theorists perceive between these disorders is again evident in the extensive overlap in recommended treatment techniques.

All of the elements specified in Fig. 7.1 become explicit targets of therapy. In general, the treatment sequence addresses these in reverse order, although some issues related to each category are dealt with at every stage (Vitousek and Ewald, 1992). Thus, the restoration of normal food intake and weight is the first order of therapeutic business, followed by attention to internal contingencies for symptomatic behavior, to cognitive processing errors, to social influences, and, finally, to stable aspects of the self such as perfectionism and poor self-esteem.

A prerequisite to work on any of these levels is the engagement of the eating-disordered individual as an active participant in the therapeutic enterprise. The guiding principle of collaborative empiricism may make the cognitive–behavioral approach particularly suitable for the crucial early stage of intervention with this resistant population. Clients are not required to surrender their tenuous sense of control to the authoritative judgments of an expert; rather, they are encouraged to join in an experimental process of discovering how their own beliefs and behaviors actually affect their experience. They are not asked to concede the irrationality of cherished values, but simply to take a closer look at the means they have chosen to secure them, and the full range of consequences that result.

A substantial proportion of the first few sessions of therapy may be devoted to helping the client develop an exhaustive list of both the "pros" and the "cons" of her eating disorder, phrased in her own terms (see Table 7.1). The construction of this list is intended to serve a number of purposes. First, the inclusion of the perceived *advantages* of symptomatology is often disarming to clients, who have heretofore been subjected to nothing but warnings about the dangers of their behavior by family members and physicians. The cognitive therapist explicitly acknowledges that weight loss must confer some significant benefits that would be missed if normal weight status were restored, and emphasizes that since the aim of therapy is to make the *client* feel better, it will be unsuccessful if she is not fully compensated for these losses.

Second, the exercise provides an opportunity for education about the etiology and implications of those symptoms that the patient does find distressing. Experiences such as depression, irritability, impaired concentration, and food preoccupation are linked to the common cause of starvation pathology. The therapist begins to articulate a theme that will recur throughout treatment: such symptoms are inextricably connected to restrictive dieting and suboptimal weight, and it is not within the client's power to eliminate them selectively while retaining the benefits she associates with the attainment of her thin ideal.

Third, the identification of pros and cons can serve an important assessment function, providing a great deal of information about an individual client's motivational system and experience of her disorder.

Finally, the technique allows the therapist to start introducing the change strategies of cognitive–behavioral therapy. Each claimed advantage and disadvantage is cast as a hypothesis that can be examined for its validity and adaptiveness, or used as the basis for prospective data collection. The *functional* emphasis inherent in this exercise reflects one of the most distinctive features of cognitive–behavioral therapy for the eating disorders, which remains evident during the entire course of treatment.

Another focus during the early phases of cognitive–behavioral treatment is the provision of psychoeducational information (Garner *et al.*, 1985b). Some treatment programs have found it both efficient and clinically advantageous to impart such didactic information in a group format (Connors *et al.*, 1984; Wolchik *et al.*, 1986). Our own specialty clinic includes a five-session psychoeducational group intended to supplement rather than replace individual cognitive–behavioral therapy. This highly structured

TABLE 7.1   Perceived Advantages and Disadvantages of Anorexia Nervosa

Perceived advantages of anorexic behavior
    I just like the way I feel when I am thin.
    I get more respect and more compliments.
    What everyone else tries to do, I am showing that I can do better.
    I like the attention.
    I like the clothes that I can wear.
    I look better this way.
    Having fat on my body is really disgusting — I refuse to put up with it.
    My family and my doctor worry about me.
    I can keep people at a distance.
    I don't have any menstrual periods.
    I feel like I am in touch with the sufferings of the world.
    I feel healthier and more energetic when I'm low in weight.
    I feel more confident and capable when I am thin — it gives me the courage to do other
      things.
    I like the feeling of self-control.
    I feel powerful when I don't eat.
    When I'm thin, I feel everything more keenly — I'm more awake and alive.
    I feel special.

Perceived disadvantages of anorexic behavior
    Being thin takes up so much time and energy.
    I think it is immoral to worry so much about how I look.
    People hassle me a lot about it.
    I can't eat a lot of the things I like.
    I am so tired of being hungry.
    There is so much pressure to eat in social settings — so I can't go to parties or restau-
      rants very often.
    I can't go on vacations — it is too hard to plan eating.
    My mood is so variable.
    Sometimes I have trouble concentrating.
    I don't like being cold all the time.
    My hair is falling out.
    I'm worried about whether or not I will be able to have children.
    I hate being a cliché.

Perceived advantages of bulimic behavior
    I can eat anything I want without worrying about it making me fat.
    I simply can't stay on diets — so without this, I would get fat in no time.
    I can eat out at restaurants without worrying about whether something is "on my
      diet" — *everything* is on my diet, when I can vomit afterwards.
    I love to cook — but I can't cook without lots of tasting, so I need to vomit or spit out
      food.
    Fullness gives me a sense of security.
    I can numb out everything that's bothering me.
    It's one time I can focus only on myself.
    It's a way of putting off things I don't want to do.
    It relieves boredom.

(Continues)

TABLE 7.1 *Continued*

I don't know any other ways to cope with depression or anxiety.

It is the only way I can relax and get to sleep.

I'm sort of stuck on the whole ritual—I look forward to it all day long. I don't know how I would get through the day without it.

If something else isn't going well—at least I can control *this* part of my life.

I like the feeling of "getting away" with something (eating a lot) that most people can't.

It's exciting—kind of thrilling, in a way.

Vomiting makes me *feel* thin when I'm feeling fat.

I feel cleansed after vomiting—like I can make a fresh start.

Vomiting gives me a quick emotional release.

Having this problem gives me an explanation and an excuse if things don't go well.

Perceived disadvantages of bulimic behavior

It is a disgusting habit.

It costs a lot of money.

It takes up a lot of time.

I'm afraid of getting caught.

Vomiting clogs the drain in my sink.

It doesn't really eliminate *all* the food that I have eaten.

It promotes a constant focus on food.

I don't really enjoy what I eat anyway. The pleasure just lasts for the first bite or two, then I feel guilty for hours.

I have no pride or self-respect.

I will always feel intimidated by my family as long as I do this.

My relationships are suffering—I can't really give to anyone else as long as I am so wrapped up in this.

I'm scared to become too close to anyone, because then I won't have the privacy I require for the behavior.

My preoccupation with food keeps me from thinking about or working on other more important things.

It leads me to do things I'm very ashamed of—lying, cheating, stealing.

My weight keeps going up and down.

I feel tired all the time.

I'm worried about losing all my teeth.

I'm scared about what this may do to my health.

series is organized around the cognitive categories outlined in the assessment section of this chapter. For example, one session addresses the *attribution* that weight is under personal control, providing contrary data about set-point theory, the heritability of weight and shape, and the ineffectiveness of dieting. A second examines the *evaluation* that thinness is desirable, reviewing information about the relative health risks of leanness and obesity, and analyzing the sociocultural basis for the modern preference for thinness.

In cognitive–behavioral therapy for both anorexia nervosa and bulimia nervosa, the normalization of eating and weight is viewed as a prerequisite to the conduct of effective psychotherapy as well as to eventual successful outcome. Patients who are starving or engaging in chaotic eating behavior are unable to participate actively in the therapeutic process; therefore, efforts to improve nutritional and weight status are an integral part of the clinical agenda from the inception of treatment. "Forbidden foods" that have been avoided because of fears that they will cause weight gain or precipitate binge-eating episodes are gradually reintroduced into the daily diet. Extensive self-monitoring of food intake and associated affect and cognition is a foundation of cognitive–behavioral interventions. Such records are used to identify binge precipitants and, in the later stages of therapy, serve as the basis for more elaborate analyses of dysfunctional beliefs.

The processes of dietary rehabilitation and weight restoration or stabilization are *not* carried out in isolation from the "real work" of cognitive–behavioral therapy; rather, they are closely integrated with the ongoing examination of core beliefs. Much as the elicitation of physical sensations cuing panic serves as the basis for restructuring catastrophic misinterpretations in the cognitive treatment of panic disorder (Clark, 1986), exposure to the experiences of eating differently and weighing more provides a wealth of material for cognitive therapy of anorexia and bulimia. Garner and Bemis (1982, 1985) and Fairburn (1983, 1985) have described a wide range of cognitive and behavioral techniques that can be used toward the modification of distorted beliefs about food, weight, and shape. These include: the evaluation of automatic thoughts and cognitive processing errors on dysfunctional thought records; decentering and reattribution techniques; prospective hypothesis testing; the analysis of cues and chains supporting the binge–purge cycle; coping and self-control strategies for high-risk situations; *in vivo* exercises; role playing; the development of alternative bases for self-evaluation and self-reinforcement; and relapse prevention techniques.

The usual course of cognitive–behavioral therapy for bulimia nervosa, at least in treatment outcome trials, is 16–20 sessions over a 4- to 6-month period. The recommended duration of therapy for anorexia nervosa is considerably longer—often 1 to 2 years of weekly sessions, with more intensive treatment in the first several months. This extended course is necessary in part to accommodate the greater resistance of anorexic clients to the change process, as well as to accomplish weight restoration in the early phase of intervention. In addition, cognitive–behavioral therapy for bulimia nervosa is typically restricted to the focal symptomatology of eating and weight concerns, dealing principally with disorder-specific behaviors and self-statements; the later stages of treatment in anorexia nervosa shift the emphasis to general problems such as perfectionism and interpersonal concerns, making more extensive use of cognitive restructuring techniques for the modification of higher order beliefs. It is not clear whether these disparities in the recommended depth and breadth of cognitive–behavioral therapy address fundamental distinctions between the two disorders, or simply reflect the slightly different theoretical orientations of the specialists who developed the respective treatment approaches.

Empirical Findings

Although the cognitive–behavioral method appears to be fairly widely used in the treatment of anorexia nervosa, particularly in university-affiliated specialty clinics, there is little compelling evidence for its efficacy. The persistent lack of data is certainly embarrassing for an approach with a commitment to empiricism, but it is, at least, nothing singular for the field. Astonishingly, there are only three controlled studies of psychotherapy of any kind for anorexia nervosa. All commentators agree that the early weight-restoration phase of treatment, which usually occurs in hospital, is vital but in some senses trivial; all concur that the real therapeutic challenge comes during the prolonged second phase, typically individual and/or family therapy on an outpatient basis. Yet, while the former has been extensively studied, the latter remains almost unexamined.

A few systematic case studies of cognitive–behavioral therapy for anorexia nervosa have been reported (Cooper and Fairburn, 1984; Garner, 1988; Peveler and Fairburn, 1989). The only controlled study published to date yielded equivocal evidence for the relative efficacy of the approach (Channon et al., 1989). In this investigation, behavioral and cognitive–behavioral therapy conditions were compared with an unspecified treatment-as-usual cell. After 6 months of active treatment and at 6- and 12-month follow-up, all groups were significantly improved; few differences were obtained between conditions. No group could be considered clinically recovered by the end of the study period. The cognitive modality appeared more acceptable to clients and was associated with higher rates of compliance, a finding that the authors noted was of some interest because of the notorious difficulty of engaging anorexics in treatment.

Unfortunately, a number of methodological problems make it difficult to draw clear conclusions from the Channon et al. (1989) trial. Sample size was small (8 per cell); as subject availability is a predictable problem with this population, it would have been preferable to increase power by reducing the comparison to two rather than three alternative modalities. The restricted number of subjects also led to some apparent inequalities in cell composition, although significant pretreatment differences could not be detected with this sample size; for example, 12% of the behaviorally treated versus 50% of the cognitively treated subjects had been hospitalized previously, and the mean age of onset was 21 and 16 years, respectively. The duration of treatment was limited (18 sessions followed by 6 booster sessions), and was markedly discrepant from that recommended by Garner and Bemis (1982, 1985). Means on dependent measures were provided only for the pretest assessment point; at posttest and follow-up, only significant differences were reported — of which there were, unsurprisingly, very few due to the low power of analyses. The first author served as the sole therapist for both behavioral and cognitive conditions, and the sole evaluator of clinical status. Finally, while the investigators stated that the cognitive condition was patterned after the model of Garner and Bemis (1982, 1985) it is not clear how closely it did conform to specified procedures. It appears that the primary focus in the cognitive–behavioral cell was the disputation of specific beliefs about weight and shape, which represents only a portion of the complex treatment package recommended for anorexia nervosa.

The state of knowledge concerning the efficacy of cognitive–behavioral therapy for bulimia nervosa is dramatically more advanced, and the evidence favoring this approach increasingly compelling. More than a dozen comparative trials have been reported; in each instance, the cognitive–behavioral condition has proven equal or superior to every modality with which it has been compared (for reviews, see Cox and Merkel, 1989; Craighead and Agras, 1991; Fairburn, 1988; Fairburn et al., 1992; Freeman and Munro, 1988; Garner, 1987; Garner et al., 1987a; Laessle et al., 1987; Rosen, 1987; Wilson, 1989, 1993). Despite considerable variability across studies, the method typically yields an 80% reduction in the frequency of binging and purging, with approximately half of treated clients reporting the elimination of bulimic episodes. Although many published trials include limited follow-up data, those that have examined subjects 1–4 years after intervention generally find excellent maintenance of treatment gains. In view of these impressive findings, several reviewers have concluded that cognitive–behavioral therapy must be regarded as the current treatment of choice for bulimia nervosa (Craighead and Agras, 1991; Fairburn, 1988; Wilson, 1989).

Perhaps the most sophisticated treatment trial in the literature was recently described in a pair of reports by Fairburn and his colleagues (Fairburn et al. 1991b, in press, b). A total pool of 75 subjects were randomly assigned to receive 19 sessions of behavioral therapy, cognitive–behavioral therapy, or interpersonal psychotherapy. The comparison between behavioral and cognitive–behavioral therapies represented a dismantling study intended to examine the effectiveness of techniques such as self-monitoring, stimulus control, and dietary planning in isolation from attention to attitudes about food, weight, and shape. The interpersonal therapy condition was included to compare the influence of a nonspecific treatment whose efficacy has been documented with a different psychiatric population (unipolar depression) to an established modality specifically tailored to the symptoms of bulimia nervosa. Interpersonal therapy is a short-term, directive, psychodynamically oriented approach focusing on contemporaneous problems in interpersonal relationships. As implemented in the Fairburn study, interpersonal therapy did not include direct focus on attitudes about weight and shape, and did not attempt to change eating behavior.

All three treatments were equally effective in reducing binge episodes and alleviating symptoms of general psychiatric distress; however, cognitive–behavioral therapy appeared superior on some indices. The full treatment package had significantly greater effects on concerns about weight and shape than the simplified behavioral intervention. Compared to interpersonal therapy, it again proved more effective in modifying weight concerns, and produced greater reductions in the frequency of vomiting.

Data collected after a 1-year closed follow-up period revealed some surprising trends (Fairburn *et al.*, in press, b). Subjects in the behavioral condition were doing so poorly that nearly half had dropped out or had been withdrawn from the study by the 12-month assessment. The high attrition rate precluded a formal analysis of the relative efficacy of this modality, but contributes to the impression that this dismantled subset of techniques is markedly less effective than standard cognitive–behavioral treatment. In contrast, subjects initially treated with interpersonal therapy had continued to improve after termination, and by one year had caught up to the cognitive–behavioral condition on every index of outcome.

The finding that cognitive–behavioral treatment outperformed the behavioral intervention is consistent with the postulated mechanisms of change in the dominant cognitive–behavioral model; however, the unanticipated efficacy of interpersonal therapy at follow-up raises important questions for theoretical accounts of bulimia nervosa. Since interpersonal therapy did not address food or weight issues directly, through what mechanisms did it exert its beneficial effects on the focal symptoms of this disorder? In addition, how did a modality lacking any emphasis on relapse prevention prove so successful in maintaining, indeed, enhancing, treatment gains?

Fairburn and colleagues speculated that the decrease in bulimic behavior achieved through interpersonal therapy may have been mediated through effects on negative self-evaluation. They noted that "the patients who respond seem to develop an increased sense of self-worth and competence and, as a result, their tendency to evaluate themselves largely in terms of their weight lessens in intensity" (Fairburn, 1988, p. 641). Improvements in eating behavior were hypothesized to follow from these basic changes in self-concept. The temporal pattern of improvements in various domains of functioning across the cognitive–behavioral and interpersonal cells supported the assumption that these treatments operated through different mediating mechanisms, and was inconsistent with the alternative hypothesis that bulimia nervosa responds to any credible psychological intervention (Fairburn *et al.*, in press, b).

Two investigations have compared cognitive–behavioral treatment to the administration of antidepressant drugs. Mitchell (Mitchell *et al.*, 1990) implemented a 4-cell design in which all subjects received imipramine or pill placebo, and half additionally participated in an intensive group intervention that included cognitive–behavioral components. Attrition was highest in the drug-alone condition, moderate in the combined drug/group cell, and minimal amongst subjects receiving placebo with or without group psychotherapy. At the end of treatment, the group therapy intervention appeared markedly superior to drugs in suppressing bulimic symptoms; the combination of both modalities did not produce incremental benefit over psychotherapy alone in binging or purging, but contributed to greater reductions in depression and anxiety.

Agras (Agras *et al.*, 1992) assigned subjects to a 16- or 24-week course of desipramine with or without individual cognitive–behavioral treatment, or to cognitive–behavioral therapy alone. The complex pattern of results suggested superiority for cognitive–behavioral therapy alone or in combination with drugs at a 16-week assessment point. By follow-up assessment at 32 weeks, subjects who had received an extended course of desipramine in addition to cognitive–behavioral treatment were doing significantly better than those in drug-alone cells. It was also determined that subjects withdrawn from medication at 16 weeks were less likely to relapse if they had additionally participated in cognitive–behavioral therapy.

Several reviewers have suggested that antidepressant drugs and cognitive–behavioral therapy may exert their effects on bulimic behavior through directly opposite mechanisms (Craighead and Agras, 1991; Fairburn *et al.*, 1992, Wilson, 1993). Medication may facilitate dietary restraint by suppressing appetite, while cognitive techniques seek to decrease restraint by encouraging subjects to consume regular, ample meals and reintroduce avoided food into their diets. Studies have confirmed that imipramine-treated subjects continue to restrict their caloric intake after intervention, while those participating in cognitive–behavioral therapy increase the consumption of nonpurged calories significantly more (Rossiter *et al.*, 1988a,b). This difference may explain the better maintenance of treatment gains following cognitive–behavioral treatment, since restrained eating is often cited as an important causal variable in the development and maintenance of bulimic symptoms.

OBESITY

As noted at the beginning of this chapter, cognitive elements have not figured prominently in etiological theories of obesity. The lack of a comprehensive cognitive model reflects the assumption that no single set of causal or maintaining variables can account for the sole attribute, excess body weight, possessed in common by this heterogeneous population. Some attempts have been made to identify cognitive factors such as restraint and distorted body image that may contribute to the condition of obesity in subgroups of affected individuals. In recent years, increased attention has been paid to negative views of the self that represent consequences rather than causes of obesity.

The cognitive approach has also made minimal contributions to intervention. Cognitive techniques are typically employed as supportive elements intended to enhance the efficacy of behavioral treatment packages, which have dominated the field for the past 25 years. The results of the orthodox behavioral approach, with or without appended cognitive components, have been discouraging. Treatment typically sustains weight loss in only 5% of participants over a 4-year period (Kramer *et al.*, 1989; Brownell and Jeffrey, 1987). This extremely high rate of relapse, together with accumulating information about metabolic factors and the genetics of weight, contribute to a growing recognition that powerful biologic determinants are the principal forces against which the obese must contend. In the past several years a cognitive perspective has begun to inform the treatment of obesity in a radically different direction. Rather than simply using cognitive techniques to combat attitudes that interfere with adherence to weight control regimens, it is increasingly suggested that a cognitive–behavioral approach may be beneficial in restructuring obese clients' views of the nature of their problem. Cognitive tactics can be employed to teach obese individuals that what the world sees as a disorder often represents normal variation in body size, to persuade them that dieting is a contributor rather than a solution to their distress, and to help them develop coping strategies for responding to the social prejudice that may represent the greatest adverse consequence of their physical status.

The organization of this section of the chapter must reflect the general state of theory and research on cognitive variables in obesity: it will be a somewhat disjointed overview of disparate topics, with no discernible unifying themes. After a brief review of the characteristics of the obese population, we shall highlight the few cognitive themes that have generated research activity, examine the contribution of cognitive strategies to intervention, and finally consider, under a separate heading, the phenomenon of binge-eating in the obese.

Diagnosis of Obesity

Obesity is a condition in which bodily energy stores (usually in the form of fat) are excessively large (Garrow, 1986). The standard commonly applied in determining obesity is deviation from a height–weight actuarial data table (e.g., Metropolitan Life Insurance Company, 1983). Although total body weight is only a gross approximation of relative body fat, individuals 20–30% or more above "ideal" weight for height are generally designated obese.

While obesity may be accompanied by various forms of psychopathology, it is generally acknowledged that the obese as a group do not differ from normal-weight individuals on measures of psychological adjustment and personality (Striegel-Moore and Rodin, 1986; Wadden and Stunkard, 1987). Therefore, obesity cannot be regarded as a psychopathological entity, and has been excluded from psychiatric diagnostic systems such as the DSM. Regrettably, equivalence with the manifestly pathological conditions of anorexia nervosa and bulimia nervosa is suggested by the common heading of "eating disorders" under which all three are subsumed. In fact, it is not clear that the obese as a group eat any differently from the normal-weight as a group (Brownell and Wadden, 1991). In the minority who do (the obese binge-eaters), significant psychological symptomatology is often present (Marcus *et al.*, 1990); although it remains controversial whether this subgroup should qualify for a discrete psychiatric label, it is certainly inappropriate to characterize the whole population as in any sense "disordered."

Cognitive Themes in Obesity Research

Restraint

Restraint is the disposition to restrict food intake for the purpose of reducing or managing body weight. When dieting efforts are disrupted by cognitive cues (such as the perception of having eaten an impermissible quantity or type of food), emotional states (including depression, anxiety, and perhaps elation), or pharmacological factors (such as the consumption of alcohol), restrained eaters show a paradoxical tendency to overeat.

In the classic experimental paradigm, a subset of restrained and unrestrained eaters are directed to eat a fixed amount of food such as ice cream or a milkshake, typically presented in the context of a "taste perception" study. When participants are subsequently given the opportunity to consume another food or drink ad lib, unrestrained subjects who have received a preload tend to eat less, while preloaded restrained subjects often manifest counterregulation, consuming *more* than restrained subjects who have not yet eaten. The mechanism underlying counterregulation may be partly physiological: it is assumed that many restrained eaters are in a chronic state of deprivation brought about by restrictive dieting. Counterregulation is also a strongly cognitive phenomenon that seems to be driven by the belief that since dietary boundaries have been violated by ingesting a "forbidden" substance at preload, restraint is already broken and eating behavior disinhibited.

The construct of restraint was first proposed by Herman (Herman and Mack, 1975; Hibscher and Herman, 1977) to account for periodic overeating among obese dieters. According to Herman's account, it is the *dieting* in which obese individuals habitually engage that drives their eating behavior, rather than any inherent characteristics of such individuals such as overreliance on external cues (Schachter, 1971) or maintaining a sub-set-point weight (Nisbett, 1968). It follows that similar behavior should be manifested by normal-weight individuals who attempt to manage their weight through dieting; thus, not all restrained eaters who demonstrate the counterregulation effect will be overweight (and not all obese individuals will be restrained eaters, since some resist social pressure to diet).

The restraint hypothesis, subsequently refined by Herman and Polivy (1984), has generated an extraordinary volume of experimental research (for reviews, see Charnock, 1989; Heatherton *et al.*, 1988; Ruderman, 1986; Stunkard and Wadden, 1990). Studies have quite consistently affirmed the existence of counterregulation, at least in the normal-weight restrained subject with whom most of this research has been conducted. The construct has more recently been applied to the study of binge-eating in bulimia nervosa (Polivy and Herman, 1985; Rossiter *et al.*, 1989; Ruderman, 1985; Wardle and Beinart, 1981), and appears to hold considerable promise for our understanding of this form of eating disturbance (Ruderman, 1985).

Curiously, the highly generative restraint hypothesis has been most controversial when applied to the population that originally stimulated its formulation: the obese. Although the great majority of overweight individuals score high on measures of restraint, they do not consistently demonstrate counterregulation following consumption of a preload (Ruderman, 1986; Stunkard and Messick, 1985; Stunkard and Wadden, 1990). Ruderman and Wilson (1979) reported a particularly well-designed study in which obese and normal-weight subjects were exposed to two versions of the classic "taste test" manipulation. Although restraint predicted eating behavior better than weight status, the counterregulation effect was much stronger among normal-weight restrained subjects than among obese restrained subjects. The authors also reanalyzed data from two separate restraint studies (Hibscher and Herman, 1977; Spencer and Fremouw, 1979) in order to examine the relationship between weight status and counterregulation. They concluded that "taken as a whole, the data from these three experiments indicate that counterregulation is not a typical obese behavior" (Ruderman and Wilson, 1979, p. 589).

The failure to find expected effects even among obese subjects who score high on restraint scales has been attributed to a number of variables. Several authors have suggested that the measurement of restraint is responsible for observed anomalies. Heatherton *et al.* (1988) note that the most widely used inventory, the revised Restraint Scale, exhibits a different factor structure with obese subject pools, perhaps because of ceiling effects. Others identify problems with the Restraint Scale itself, which has been widely criticized for incorporating items on weight variability (which contribute to a Weight Fluctuation factor) along with items concerning deliberate restraint (loading on a Concern for Dieting factor). Observing that elevated scores in obese subjects are often a function of the endorsement of Weight Fluctuation items (Blanchard and Frost, 1983; Drewnowski *et al.*, 1982; Ruderman, 1985), some have suggested that the Restraint Scale possesses poor construct validity as a measure of dietary restraint for this population (Stunkard and Messick, 1985). Not all investigations confirm the relationship between high weight and the Weight Fluctuation factor, however (Lowe, 1984), and Heatherton *et al.* (1988) insist that weight variability is itself more closely related to dieting than to obesity.

Heatherton *et al.* (1988) favor an alternative explanation for the attenuated counterregulation of obese subjects. Noting that such individuals may establish a "diet boundary" that is different from that drawn by normal-weight restrained eaters, they maintain that identical preloads should not be expected to produce the same degree of counterregulation in both groups, since the effect is dependent on the judgment that acceptable limits for intake have been violated. They emphasize that personal quotas for the kind and quantity of food deemed acceptable must be assessed individually. Some indirect support for this proposal was provided in a study by Knight and Boland (1989), who found that disinhibition in normal-weight restrained eaters was governed by the "forbidden" quality of foods rather than the amount of calories consumed. Unfortunately, relatively few restraint experiments have included a determination of individual diet boundaries for subjects from either population of restrained eaters.

Another interpretation implicates sample characteristics of the overweight employed in restraint research. McCann *et al.*, (1992) recently reported that obese subjects attending a weight reduction clinic *did* manifest counterregulatory behavior. They suggested that disconfirmatory results in other studies may have been a function of testing overweight college students who may have a lower level of concern for restricting their intake.

The strong defense of the applicability of restraint to the obese population is in one sense surprising. The originators of restraint theory have elsewhere espoused the contemporary view that overweight individuals do not, as a group, eat differently from normal-weight individuals (Spitzer and Rodin, 1981; Thompson *et al.*, 1982). Stunkard and Wadden (1990) point out that, in retrospect, it is understandable that the restraint construct appears to have limited applicability to obesity. They observe:

> The Restraint Scale was developed when both externality theory and behavioral theories proposed that obese people ate in a distinctive manner, and the Restraint Scale was developed to measure aspects of this behavior. Since then it has become apparent that there is little or no support for the externality theory, and little evidence of a distinctive eating style among the obese." (p. 80)

Present data do suggest that the phenomena of restraint and disinhibition are likely to contribute to our knowledge of the cognitive and behavioral experience of some obese individuals (especially obese binge-eaters), as well as that of normal-weight bulimics. A great deal remains to be learned about these complex variables, notably, about the role of cognitive variables such as dichotomous thinking styles and schema-driven information processing (e.g., Jansen *et al.*, 1988; King *et al.*, 1991). Studies are also examining the relationship between restraint and more pervasive cognitive sets such as poor self-esteem (Polivy *et al.*, 1988) and general irrational beliefs, with conflicting findings reported by Ruderman (1985) and Jansen *et al.* (1988).

Progress in future research will depend in part on the resolution of persistent controversies in the measurement of restraint. In addition to the problems noted earlier, concerns have been expressed about a number of issues: the influence of social desirability, which is likely to be particularly pronounced in its effects on obese subjects (Stunkard and Messick, 1985); the tendency of restraint scale scores to reflect dieting history as well as current dieting behavior (Charnock, 1989; Lowe *et al.*, 1991); and the advisability of the routine practice of depending on an artificial median split to designate individuals as restrained or unrestrained eaters (Stein, 1988). Alternatives to the Restraint Scale have been developed in an attempt to overcome some of these difficulties (Stunkard and Messick, 1985; Van Strien *et al.*, 1986), and there is evidence that these scales measure somewhat different constructs (Laessle *et al.*, 1989b). One interesting proposal suggests that assessment of the separate dimensions of cognitive restraint and physiological deprivation might help to resolve some of the inconsistencies in the restraint literature and facilitate the construction of an eating disorder typology (Charnock, 1989).

While it seems certain that the construct of restraint will continue to be elaborated, qualified, and refined by ongoing research, it has already made a substantial contribution to the eating disorder field. After summarizing the cognitive factors that support disinhibition in restrained eaters, Wardle (1988) concludes that problems of intake regulation may result whenever eating "shifts from being a free behavior to a rule-governed behavior, in which intentions are at variance with other biologically and psychologically derived motivations" (p. 608). This central insight of restraint theory underscores the profound influence of cognition in eating disorders, and has significant implications for the understanding and remediation of each of the conditions discussed in this chapter.

Body Image

The construct of "body image" has been defined as the "evaluation of one's size, weight, or any other aspect of the body that determines physical appearance" (Thompson, 1990, p. 1). The phenomenon can be subdivided into a perceptual component (accuracy of body size estimation), a subjective component (satisfaction, evaluation, and anxiety regarding body size), and a behavioral component (avoidance of situations inducing negative evaluation and anxiety).

The concept of body image disturbance has been extensively (though often unsatisfactorily) researched in anorexia nervosa and bulimia nervosa, and carries diagnostic significance in the latter. Its theoretical role in obesity, however, remains unclear. It is difficult to avoid invoking the construct when faced with a 75-lb. anorexic who claims to "feel fat," or a 125-lb. bulimic who considers her average-sized body gargantuan and grotesque. But what conceptual relevance does the notion of a disturbance in body image hold for a 300-lb. individual who sees himself or herself as overweight, and has internalized the disparagement with which most of society regards such a body type? Empirical work in this area has addressed several issues: do the obese display deficits in the ability to estimate their body size accurately, is this deficit a causal and/or maintaining variable for excess body weight, and are such factors as distress, self-esteem, social avoidance, and dieting influenced by the perception and evaluation of body image in the obese?

The results of research concerning the first two of these questions are confusing and contradictory. In body size estimation tasks, the obese have sometimes been found less accurate (Cappon and Banks, 1968; Grinker,

1973) and sometimes equally or more accurate (Garner *et al.*, 1978; Leon *et al.*, 1978) than normal controls or clinical samples. The effect of weight loss on size estimation is also unclear. Some studies have reported that successful reducers continue to overestimate their size (Glucksman and Hirsch, 1969), while others suggest that they become more accurate (Chwast, 1978; Gardner *et al.*, 1989). It is probable that some of the marked inconsistency in these findings is attributable to method variance (Fisher, 1986), as is the case in the equally muddled literature on size estimation in anorexia nervosa and bulimia nervosa (Ben-Tovim, 1991; Cash and Brown, 1987; Garner *et al.*, 1987b; Hsu and Sobkiewicz, 1991; Slade, 1985). Another portion of the variance may be due to heterogeneity across samples of obese subjects.

Research has borne the common sense assumption that overweight individuals as a whole are unhappy with their appearance (Thompson, 1990). They possess a body type that is almost universally viewed as aesthetically and medically undesirable, and are often held personally accountable for their willful failure to conform to social norms for weight and shape. Wooley (1991) writes that:

> unlike other victims, the obese are regarded as wholly responsible for their condition, choosing it everyday by their deviant eating patterns. They are regarded, as countless studies have shown, as morally, intellectually, and emotionally inferior. . . . Obese are regularly subjected to the most condescending moralization and instruction. (p. 1)

A recent study verified the hypothesized linkage between attributions about the cause of obesity and condemnation of this body type. Allison *et al.*, (1991) administered two new measures, the Attitudes Toward Obese Persons scale and the Beliefs About Obese Persons scale, to samples of undergraduate and graduate students as well as members of a national obesity organization. The pattern of results suggested that subjects who believe that overweight individuals can (and presumably should) control their weight also hold more negative attitudes about the obese. Given the prevalence of stereotypes about the implications of excess weight, it is understandable that many obese persons also view their bodies with contempt, and seek relief through repeated attempts at weight control.

Weight Locus of Control

Interest in locus of control (LOC) in obesity research stems from its hypothesized relationship with dependency and self-regulation skills (Striegel-Moore and Rodin, 1986). Individuals with an internal LOC are believed to be more effective in the use of self-reinforcement, and are thought to exert more control over impulses. A derivative assumption is that such individuals should be able to restrain the inclination to eat and thus enjoy greater success in losing weight. Weight locus of control (WLOC) has been defined as the subset of cognitions that describe "the expectancy that one can affect or control, at least in part, one's own weight" (Stotland and Zuroff, 1990).

The postulated connection between general LOC and successful weight loss has not been supported consistently in empirical research. Both positive (Balch and Ross, 1975; Ross *et al.*, 1983; Saltzer, 1982) and negative results (Gormally *et al.*, 1980; Tobias and MacDonald, 1977; Wallston *et al.*, 1976) have been obtained. Conflicting findings have been attributed to the employment of general rather than weight-specific measures of LOC, and the use of inventories with unexamined psychometric properties (Stotland and Zuroff, 1990). Another possible explanation for these inconsistencies may be time sampling biases resulting from the premise that WLOC is a stable rather than fluctuating predisposition. The assessment of WLOC at single, rather than multiple points of time may obscure meaningful relationships between the expectancy of control and the successful maintenance of weight loss.

While the clinical utility of WLOC measures remains equivocal, it is possible that they might prove useful in tracing attributional changes over the course of short- and long-term weight loss attempts. Preliminary evidence suggests that individuals are more likely to attribute lack of success to themselves rather than to diet regimens (Jeffrey *et al.*, 1990; Goodrick *et al.*, 1992). Given the high probability of diet failure, research on the iatrogenic effects of such experiences seems especially warranted.

Self-Statements about Weight, Food, and Dieting

Several investigators have attempted to examine the relationship between "maladaptive private monologues" and the development and maintenance of obesity (Mahoney and Mahoney, 1976). Israel *et al.* (1985) asked subjects to rate the degree to which they were likely to have "positive" (weight-loss facilitating) or "negative" (weight-loss impeding) cognitions. In a college student sample, heavier subjects reported a greater incidence of both positive and negative food-related cognitions; however, no relationship between weight and cognitions was discerned in a sample of subjects enrolled in a weight-control program. O'Connor and Dowrick (1987) administered a cognitive questionnaire to samples of normal weight, overweight, and previously overweight subjects. Obese subjects were more likely to experience and to believe selected food- and weight-related cognitions, particularly extreme and self-defeating beliefs such as "I ate more than I should have — now my whole diet is blown." The degree and duration of obesity did not predict either the frequency or strength of belief in these self-statements. Hunt and Rosen (1981) collected self-monitored cognitions from normal-weight and nondieting obese college students through the use of a signaling device. No group differences were obtained in the proportion of thoughts categorized as food related, distorted, or negative. The low power of analyses imposed by small sample size (7 per cell) may be responsible for the failure to detect expected differences; however, the findings are also consistent with the hypothesis that distorted beliefs are more a function of dieting behavior than of weight status.

The few studies that have administered cognitive questionnaires designed for anorexics and bulimics to obese subjects have identified both similarities and differences among these groups. The partially cognitive Eating Disorder Inventory differentiates the obese and formerly obese from eating-disordered individuals (Garner *et al.*, 1983b); however, group means on this measure may obscure obese subtypes that closely resemble anorexic and bulimic samples (Thurstin *et al.*, 1988), and scores have been found to predict adherence to low-calorie treatment regimens (Abrams, 1991). Phelan (1987) found that obese subjects resembled bulimics on measures of self-perception and beliefs about their ability to diet, but did not endorse the same salient beliefs about the magical properties of food or the dependence of self-worth upon weight.

Inconsistencies across these studies may be attributable in part to differences in the obese samples assessed. As we will discuss in a subsequent section, cognitive distortions seem to be most closely associated with the binge-eating subgroup of the obese, whose proportion probably varied across the subject pools employed. Most importantly, the scanty data available suggest that negative cognitions about food and weight are correlated with dieting behavior rather than weight; thus, studies assessing obese subjects who are actively trying to restrict their food intake should be more likely to find evidence of distinctive cognitive content and styles.

Schematic Processing

Although the experimental investigation of weight and food schemata in obesity preceded the study of similar phenomena in anorexia nervosa and bulimia nervosa, the former area of inquiry has remained essentially dormant in recent years, while research proceeds at a lively pace in the latter. A seminal paper was published by Markus *et al.* (1987), outlining a theoretical model of weight self-schemata and information processing in the obese, and reporting a series of relevant studies. The investigators determined that individuals who are schematic for weight endorsed "fat" adjectives more frequently and rapidly than aschematic subjects, showed clearer and more consistent discriminations in responding to body silhouette stimuli, and recorded longer latencies in judging the types of foods they would like to eat. These differences did not correspond to the objective weight status of subjects as obese, overweight, or normal-weight, but rather to their disposition to perceive themselves as heavy and to characterize weight as a personally relevant domain. The authors concluded that "a significant component of *being fat* is *thinking fat*" (p. 70), and hypothesized that the tendency to evaluate a wide range of stimuli with reference to body weight may contribute to a variety of cognitive, behavioral, and affective differences between individuals who are schematic or aschematic for body weight.

Only a few other studies have examined aspects of cognitive processing in the obese population. Conforto and Gershman (1985) failed to detect differences between obese and normal-weight subjects in the incidental recall and semantic processing of food and nonfood words. King *et al.* (1991) found that obese as well as anorexic and restrained subjects tended to recall significantly more weight- and food-related items after reading a descriptive passage.

The same kinds of methodological and conceptual problems reviewed in our earlier section on the assessment of schemata in anorexia and bulimia will undoubtedly apply to the investigation of this neglected domain; in particular, it will be essential to tease apart the transitory effects of dieting from more stable differences in cognitive structures. One informative line of research may be an examination of the role of cognitive processing over the course of highly probable events in the life of an obese individual: as a precursor to the decision to diet, as a consequence of dieting and weight loss, and in the aftermath of weight regain.

Cognitive–Behavioral Treatments for Obesity

Cognitive components have been a recommended part of behavioral treatment packages for obesity for decades (e.g., Ferster *et al.*, 1962; Mahoney and Mahoney, 1976). As follow-up studies began to detect extremely high rates of weight regain after treatment termination, the position of cognitive techniques in the standard therapeutic regimen became increasingly secure. Behaviorists often attributed poor maintenance of weight loss to the influence of cognitive processes such as faltering motivation and disinhibition following dietary transgressions; therefore, it seemed logical to prevent such unwelcome cognitive interference by enhancing self-efficacy and emphasizing relapse prevention strategies. In addition, new experimental evidence that cognitive variables exert considerable influence over appetite and weight regulation strengthened the theoretical basis for cognitive techniques (Bennett, 1988). Unfortunately, since the specific contribution of adjunctive cognitive elements has rarely been examined in the vast behavioral literature, the validity of these assumptions remains unestablished. At present, it is possible to state only that the behavioral approach, now almost inevitably including cognitive bits and pieces, has yet to demonstrate long-term effectiveness in the control of obesity.

The few investigations that have been designed to test either the efficacy of "purely" cognitive treatments or the incremental benefit of cognitive elements in behavioral programs do not provide strong support for the modality. The two studies that have obtained favorable results were both marred by major methodological flaws (Block, 1980; Dunkel and Glaros, 1978). More adequate tests of the effectiveness of cognitive elements have consistently yielded negative findings. Collins *et al.* (1986) compared group-administered cognitive, behavioral, and combined treatments with a nutrition–exercise control condition. No significant benefits accrued from the addition of cognitive techniques to behavior therapy, while cognitive techniques alone were only marginally more effective than the control condition. DeLucia and Kalodner (1990) reported that the addition of self-statement modification to a basic behavioral regimen neither increased weight loss nor improved maintenance over a brief 3-month follow-up.

Bennett (1986a,b) reported a pair of studies in which self-instructional training was compared to several control conditions (1986a) or to a behavioral cue avoidance and a social pressure control condition (1986b). Self-instructional training proved no more powerful than any of the control conditions in either study, and was inferior to behavioral treatment in the stronger comparison. Follow-up at one year revealed a gradual upward trend toward pretreatment weight across cells.

Only two of these six studies examined the differential effects of alternative treatments on cognitive variables (Bennett, 1986b; DeLucia and Kalodner, 1990). With the exception of one inventory used by DeLucia and Kalodner (1990), the cognitive measures employed were study-specific instruments with unknown psychometric properties. In both studies, significant cognitive changes were evident after either cognitive or behavioral intervention, suggesting that it may not be necessary to target cognitive processes directly to obtain improvements in this domain. Moreover, cognitive shifts did not appear to be sufficient to produce desired behavioral changes. Subjects receiving the cognitive treatment alone in the Bennett (1986b) study reported increased self-efficacy expectations without an accompanying increase in weight loss. Bennett concluded that "cognitive restructuring had the limited effect of making subjects feel that dieting had become easier, but did not help them to diet more effectively" (p. 235).

In sum, existing research provides little support for the efficacy of cognitive techniques in the production and maintenance of weight loss. It should be emphasized that most of the studies examining the relative efficacy of cognitive elements constitute rather weak tests of their potential contribution. None included the sustained treatment course currently recommended for obesity; the results of behavioral trials support a minimum treatment duration of 16 weeks (Brownell and Jeffrey, 1987). None presented cognitive and behavioral strategies in an integrated fashion, analogous to that recommended for anorexia nervosa and bulimia nervosa (Fairburn, 1985; Garner and Bemis, 1982) and other psychiatric conditions (Hollon and Beck, 1986). Cognitive strategies typically consisted of attempts to modify superficial cognitive content, were often cursorily described, and were usually implemented by relatively inexperienced graduate student therapists. Most included brief follow-up periods that might be insufficient to detect the differential maintenance of treatment effects hypothesized to represent the principal benefit of cognitive intervention. Future studies must redress these shortcomings before the potential utility of cognitive strategies can be gauged.

Most importantly, the cognitive perspective should also guide future research to focus on the iatrogenic effects of diet failure and return to pretreatment weight status. Unsuccessful attempts to control obesity can instill a sense of hopelessness, despair, and self-derogation in novice and career dieters (Wooley and Garner, 1991). Recent evidence also suggests that weight cycling has adverse physiological sequelae (Lissner *et al.*, 1991) that may carry health implications equal or greater in magnitude to those associated with the steady persistence of obesity. As weight regain is the *typical* outcome of all contemporary interventions for this condition, the ethical implications of continuing to advocate ineffective and possibly harmful treatment programs seems inescapable (Lustig, 1991). Moreover, the minority of reducers who are successful in maintaining weight loss after intervention manifest a number of psychological changes that bear closer scrutiny. Successful dieters score high on measures of restraint (Bennett, 1986b; Bjorvell *et al.*, 1986), the same complex variable that has been linked to the *maintenance* of obesity and vulnerability to binge-eating in other research. Subjects who are able to sustain weight loss following treatment may do so at the expense of developing a "healthy narcissism about their appearance and physical condition that for many has the qualities of a minor obsession" (Colvin and Olson, 1983, p. 294). Just how "healthy" this preoccupation may prove in the long run awaits extended follow-up research capable of evaluating its broad-spectrum effects on other aspects of psychological and interpersonal functioning.

As we noted at the beginning of this section, some experts have begun to advocate a dramatically different approach to counseling obese clients. Wooley (1991) states:

> I personally believe that it is time to leave fat people alone. If we do involve ourselves in their lives, it should be to help them recover from dieting, improve their body image, develop weapons against social prejudice, and improve their health through all means except dieting. I don't really think many will be worse for it, and very many will be better. (p. 3)

Brownell (1991) recommends the implementation of educational programs to provide those seeking weight loss with more accurate information about the biological limits constraining body weight and shape, and guidelines for determining "reasonable" personal goals for body size. Garner and Wooley (in press) advise that the first responsibility of therapists and physicians should be candor about the ineffectiveness of treatment, supplemented when indicated and desired with cognitive–behavioral techniques to promote the normalization of food intake and to encourage moderate exercise. Although some descriptive accounts of similar approaches have been published (e.g., Ciliska, 1991), no comparative data are yet available on the effects of such interventions on the weight, health, beliefs, or general adjustment of obese subjects.

Binge-Eating in the Obese

Clinicians and researchers have shown increasing interest in a subgroup of the obese who report frequent binge-eating episodes but do not purge. These individuals seem to differ from the general obese population in many important respects; however, it is not clear whether or how they should be accommodated into the psychiatric classification scheme. Many, perhaps most, would qualify for the diagnosis of bulimia nervosa, since DSM-III-R criteria for bulimia do not specify weight level and allow the "compensatory behavior" criterion to be satisfied by strict dieting, fasting, or excessive exercise in lieu of purgation. Others would have to be consigned to the category of "eating disorder not otherwise specified," or would receive no psychiatric label.

This dispersal of binge-eating subjects seems unsatisfactory to many observers. Some experts believe that the application of a single label to bingers who do and do not purge obscures meaningful distinctions between these groups of subjects, and suggest subclassification of bulimia nervosa into purging and nonpurging types. Others express concern that the grouping of normal-weight and overweight bingers ignores the treatment implications of weight status, and prefer to identify "obese binge-eaters" as a separate category. Finally, some advocate subsuming all nonpurging binge-eaters under a common heading such as "compulsive overeating" or "binge-eating disorder" without reference to weight or compensatory behavior.

The latter proposal has won powerful proponents, who have nominated "binge-eating disorder" for entry into DSM-IV. Supporters contend that distinctive symptomatology and the presence of significant psychiatric comorbidity justify the inclusion of this syndrome in a manual of mental disorders, and maintain that the adoption of consistent diagnostic standards will facilitate data collection. Critics argue that it would be premature to form a separate diagnostic category on the basis of current evidence (Fairburn *et al.*, 1993). They recommend that individuals who do meet criteria for bulimia nervosa should continue to be assigned to this well-established category, and the remainder studied extensively before a new disorder is codified.

The following inclusionary features are specified for the proposed binge-eating disorder: (1) recurrent episodes of binge-eating; (2) indications of loss of control during most episodes; (3) marked distress about binge-eating; and (4) a minimum average frequency of 2 episodes per week across a 6-month period (Wilson and Walsh, 1991). An exclusionary criterion is fulfillment of all diagnostic requirements for bulimia nervosa, which, in addition to the first, second, and fourth criteria above, specify the use of one or more compensatory practices, and the presence of distorted attitudes about weight and shape.

It is not clear why the latter attitudinal criterion has been omitted from proposed criteria for binge-eating disorder. Preliminary data suggest that individuals likely to qualify for this diagnosis differ from nonbinging obese subjects in their greater dissatisfaction with weight and shape (Marcus *et al.*, 1988), greater emphasis on the body for self-appraisal (Wilson *et al.*, 1993), greater fear of gaining weight (Wilson *et al.*, 1993), greater preoccupation with eating (Marcus *et al.*, 1988, 1990), and greater tendency to express general cognitive distortions such as dichotomous thinking (Fremouw and Heyneman, 1983). These subjects also score higher than the nonbinging obese on measures of restraint (Marcus *et al.*, 1988), and exhibit the "feast or famine" consummatory patterns characteristic of purging bulimics (Rossiter *et al.*, 1992). Moreover, they consistently display higher levels of psychopathology (Kolotkin *et al.*, 1987; Marcus *et al.*, 1988), typically falling in between obese nonbinging and normal-weight bulimic comparison samples (Kirkley *et al.*, 1992; Prather and Williamson, 1988).

If these apparent differences from the general obese population and similarities to the bulimic population buttress the argument that binge-eating without purgation merits inclusion in DSM-IV, they do not demonstrate the need for a category separate from bulimia nervosa. Although it is not yet possible to determine what proportion of subjects meeting proposed binge-eating disorder criteria would also meet current bulimia nervosa criteria, available evidence suggests that most would qualify for both diagnoses. Thus, the question of whether a new category should be added to DSM-IV is linked to a decision about whether dieting should be retained as a possible compensatory behavior in bulimia nervosa. Tentatively, it appears that the behavior of binging carries the most significance as a predictor of attitudes, behavior, and psychological distress, while the additional presence of purgation places individuals father along the spectrum of psychiatric disturbance.

Whether bulimia nervosa or binge-eating disorder is the most appropriate category assignment for these individuals, it is clear that they constitute a substantial minority of the obese population, or at least of that subgroup seeking assistance with weight reduction. One survey using the proposed criteria for binge-eating disorder found an average frequency of 30% across 3 weight-control samples and a rate of 71.2% within a self-help program intended for "compulsive overeaters" (Spitzer *et al.*, 1992). The prevalence of binge-eating disorder among obese respondents across 3 community samples was a much more modest 4.4% (yielding an overall prevalence of 2% across community subjects in all weight categories). Both advocates and critics of the "new diagnosis" proposal concur that this subgroup of the obese is likely to have distinctive problems that are not adequately addressed by the conventional weight reduction programs in which most probably enroll. In fact, research confirms that obese binge-eaters do even more poorly in behavioral treatment regimens than overweight subjects as a group (Gormally *et al.*, 1980; Keefe *et al.*, 1984; Marcus *et al.*, 1988; Wilson, 1976).

Some observers reason that since obese bingers appear more similar to normal-weight binge–purgers than to obese nonbingers, they would be more appropriately treated by programs designed for the former, specifically, cognitive–behavioral regimens focused on the discouragement rather than the promotion of dietary restraint (Kirkley *et al.*, 1992). As in the established cognitive–behavioral model for bulimia nervosa, the primary therapeutic goals of such programs are the normalization of aberrant eating patterns and the modification of dysfunctional attitudes about food, weight, and shape. Importantly, weight reduction is not emphasized in this approach, and may be seen as contraindicated until binge episodes have been eliminated.

Two controlled trials suggest that this approach can produce some short-term reduction of binge-eating in the obese. Telch *et al.* (1990) found that a 10-week cognitive–behavioral group treatment reduced binge-eating by

94% and eliminated episodes in 79% of participants; in contrast, subjects in a waitlist condition reduced binge-eating by a mere 9%, and no subject was free of episodes at final assessment.

It was not clear that the cognitive–behavioral treatment worked through intended cognitive mechanisms, however, as it did not alter attitudes about eating and weight. Wilson, *et al.* (1993) notes that the apparent intransigence of distorted beliefs in the obese binge-eating population contrasts markedly with the consistent evidence of cognitive change following similar treatments for bulimia nervosa. He suggests that this difference may explain the disturbing rate of relapse already evident at a 10-week follow-up in the Telch *et al.* (1990) study. Although treatment gains are typically stable over long periods in bulimics who have received cognitive–behavioral therapy, they eroded rapidly and substantially among the obese binge-eaters, in whom the average binge reduction figure dropped to 69% and the abstinence rate to 49%. While it is possible that differences in the implementation of the cognitive–behavioral treatment accounted for the poorer maintenance of improvements, it seems plausible that these relapse rates reflect a basic distinction between normal and overweight binge-eaters. Even after achieving symptom control, the obese must contend with the objective fact that their appearance does not conform to social norms or preferences. In the absence of attitudinal change, these individuals may be unable to relinquish the goal of losing weight, and may be vulnerable to recurrence of the diet/binge cycle as they continue the struggle to reduce.

A second study conducted by the same group of investigators (Wilfley *et al.*, in press) examined the relative effectiveness of cognitive–behavioral treatment compared to interpersonal therapy, using the model adapted for bulimia by Fairburn *et al.* (1991b). Active treatments were administered in a group format for 16 weeks. Participants in the two therapy conditions improved more than waitlist subjects, with interpersonal therapy producing nonsignificantly higher rates of binge reduction and abstinence. At 1-year follow-up the therapy conditions appeared equally effective. Binge-eating rates had risen slightly from the end-of-treatment levels but remained significantly below pretreatment rates. Neither treatment effected weight loss. Echoing the conclusions of Fairburn *et al.* (in press, a) with reference to bulimia, the investigators speculated that the two modalities may work through distinctive mechanisms and may be differentially effective with different patient subgroups; however, the omission of attitudinal measures prevents the examination of mechanisms or the assessment of correlations between belief change and relapse.

It appears from these early results that cognitive–behavioral treatment may be modestly, though not uniquely, effective in the short-term modification of binge-eating in the obese. It remains to be established whether this approach — or any other form of intervention — can effect changes in core beliefs or sustain long-term reductions of symptomatic behavior. Clearly, a resolution of the controversies surrounding appropriate diagnostic criteria for this subgroup must be achieved before research can proceed in a maximally informative manner. The data reviewed here suggest that the presence and modifiability of cognitive variables such as distorted attitudes toward weight and shape may be important indicators of both fundamental similarities and differences between obese nonbinging, obese binging, and normal-weight binge–purging individuals.

CONCLUSION

In the decade since comprehensive cognitive–behavioral models of anorexia nervosa and bulimia nervosa were articulated, substantial progress has been made in examining their validity and utility for the understanding and treatment of these disabling conditions. A few elements of the conceptual framework are strongly supported by empirical evidence, while many of its most distinctive components, such as the role of schematic processing, have just begun to be subjected to experimental evaluation. Cognitive–behavioral therapy is solidly established as the current treatment of choice for bulimia nervosa; the most interesting questions for the next generation of research concern the identification of the therapeutic mechanisms through which this modality and other effective forms of psychotherapy may operate. Surprisingly little is known about the efficacy of cognitive–behavioral treatment for anorexia nervosa; the few available data suggest only that a narrow emphasis on beliefs about food and weight is insufficient to resolve its tenacious symptomatology. The role of cognition in the maintenance and modification of obesity is even less clear. Although there is suggestive evidence that cognitive factors contribute to many of the secondary complications of this condition, it has yet to be established that interventions targeting these variables will prove any more successful than existing techniques.

If progress has been uneven across the different areas reviewed in this chapter, cumulative knowledge about the eating disorders has advanced rapidly, and insights obtained from the study of each condition continue to inform our understanding of the others. Perhaps the most significant contribution of the cognitive–behavioral approach applies equally to all: an increased recognition of the havoc that can result when socially sanctioned beliefs about the value of thinness impel individuals to attempt to exert control over normal biological states through the exercise of willpower.

REFERENCES

Abrams, M. (1991). The Eating Disorders Inventory as a predictor of compliance in a behavioral weight-loss program. *International Journal of Eating Disorders, 10*, 355–360.

Agras, W. S., Rossiter, E. M., Arnow, B., Schneider, J. A., Telch, C. F., Raeburn, S. D., Bruce, B., Perl, M., and Koran, L. M. (1992). Pharmacologic and cognitive–behavioral treatment for bulimia. *American Journal of Psychiatry, 149*, 82–87.

Allison, D. B., Basile, V. C., and Yuker, H. E. (1991). The measurement of attitudes toward and beliefs about obese persons. *International Journal of Eating Disorders, 10*, 599–607.

Balch, P., and Ross, A. W. (1975). Predicting success in weight reduction as a function of locus of control: A unidimensional and multidimensional approach. *Journal of Consulting and Clinical Psychology, 43*, 119.

Bemis, K. M. (1983). A comparison of functional relationships in anorexia nervosa and phobia, In P. L. Darby, P. E. Garfinkel, D. M., Garner, and D. V. Coscina (Eds.), *Anorexia nervosa: Recent developments in research* (pp. 403–415). New York: Alan R. Liss.

Bemis, K. M. (1986). *A comparison of the subjective experience of individuals with eating disorders and phobic disorders.* Unpublished doctoral dissertation, University of Minnesota, Minneapolis, MN.

Bennett, G. A. (1986a). An evaluation of self-instructional training in the treatment of obesity. *Addictive Behaviors, 11*, 125–134.

Bennett, G. A. (1986b) Cognitive rehearsal in the treatment of obesity: A comparison against cue avoidance and social pressure. *Addictive Behaviors, 11*, 225–237.

Bennett, G. A. (1988). Cognitive–behavioral treatments for obesity. *Journal of Psychosomatic Research, 32*, 661–665.

Bennett, W., and Gurin, J. (1982). *The dieter's dilemma.* New York: Basic Books.

Ben-Tovim, D. I. (1991). Women's body attitudes: A review of measurement techniques. *International Journal of Eating Disorders, 10*, 155–167.

Ben-Tovim, D. I., and Walker, M. K. (1991). Further evidence for the Stroop Test as a quantitative measure of psychopathology in eating disorders. *International Journal of Eating Disorders, 10*, 609–613.

Ben-Tovim, D. I., Walker, M. K., Fok, D., and Yap, E. (1989). An adaptation of the Stroop test for measuring shape and food concerns in eating disorders: A quantitative measure of psychopathology? *International Journal of Eating Disorders, 6*, 681–687.

Bjorvell, H., Rossner, S., and Stunkard, A. (1986). Obesity, weight loss, and dietary restraint. *International Journal of Eating Disorders, 5*, 727–734.

Blanchard, F., and Frost, R. O. (1983). Two factors of restraint: Concern for dieting and weight fluctuation. *Behaviour Research and Therapy, 21*, 259–267.

Block, J. (1980). Effects of rational emotive therapy on overweight adults. *Psychotherapy: Theory, Research and Practice, 17*, 277–280.

Brownell, K. D. (1991). Dieting and the search for the perfect body: Where physiology and culture collide. *Behavior Therapy, 22*, 1–12.

Brownell, K. D., and Jeffrey, R. W. (1987). Improving long-term weight loss: Pushing the limits of treatment. *Behavior Therapy, 18*, 353–374.

Brownell, K. D., and Wadden, T. A. (1991). The heterogeneity of obesity: Fitting treatments to individuals. *Behavior Therapy, 22*, 153–177.

Bruch, H. (1978). *The golden cage: The enigma of anorexia nervosa*. Cambridge, MA: Harvard University Press.

Cappon, D., and Banks, R. (1968). Distorted body perception in obesity. *Journal of Nervous and Mental Disease, 146*, 465–467.

Cash, T. F., and Brown, T. A. (1987). Body image in anorexia nervosa and bulimia nervosa. *Behavior Modification, 11*, 487–521.

Casper, R. C., and Davis, J. M. (1977). On the course of anorexia nervosa. *American Journal of Psychiatry, 134*, 974–977.

Casper, R. C., Offer, D., and Ostrov, E. (1981). The self-image of adolescents with acute anorexia nervosa. *Journal of Pediatrics, 98*, 656–661.

Channon, S., de Silva, P., Hemsley, D., and Perkins, R. (1989). A controlled trial of cognitive–behavioral and behavioral treatment of anorexia nervosa. *Behaviour Research and Therapy, 27*, 529–535.

Channon, S., and Hayward, A. (1990). The effect of short-term fasting on processing of food cues in normal subjects. *International Journal of Eating Disorders, 9*, 447–452.

Channon, S., Hemsley, D., and de Silva, P. (1988). Selective processing of food words in anorexia nervosa. *British Journal of Clinical Psychology, 22*, 137–138.

Charnock, D. J. K. (1989). A comment on the role of dietary restraint in the development of bulimia nervosa. *British Journal of Clinical Psychology, 28*, 329–340.

Chwast, R. (1978). The interrelationship among accuracy of body size perception, body satisfaction and the body image in obese and non-obese women. Unpublished doctoral dissertation, Case Western Reserve University, Cleveland, OH.

Ciliska, D. (1991). *Beyond dieting: Psychoeducational interventions for chronically obese women: A non-dieting approach*. New York: Brunner/Mazel.

Clark, D. M. (1986). A cognitive approach to panic. *Behaviour Research and Therapy, 24*, 461–470.

Clark, D. A., Feldman, J., and Channon, S. (1989). Dysfunctional thinking in anorexia and bulimia nervosa. *Cognitive Therapy and Research, 13*, 377–387.

Collins, R. L., Rothblum, E. D., and Wilson, G. T. (1986). The comparative efficacy of cognitive and behavioral approaches to the treatment of obesity. *Cognitive Therapy and Research, 10*, 299–318.

Colvin, R. H., and Olson, S. B. (1983). A descriptive analysis of men and women who have lost significant weight and are highly successful at maintaining the loss. *Addictive Behaviors, 8*, 287–295.

Conforto, R. M., and Gershman, L. (1985). Cognitive processing differences between obese and nonobese subjects. *Addictive Behaviors, 10*, 83–85.

Connors, M. E., Johnson, C. L., and Stuckey, M. K. (1984). Treatment of bulimia with brief psychoeducational group therapy. *American Journal of Psychiatry, 141*, 1512–1516.

Cook, J. A. M., Jones, N., and Johnston, D. W., (1989). The effects of imminent minor surgery on the cognitive processing of health and interpersonal threat words. *British Journal of Clinical Psychology, 28*, 282–282.

Cooper, J. P., Morrison, T. L., Bigman, O. L., Abramowitz, S. I., Levin, S., and Krener, P. (1988). Mood changes and affective disorder in the bulimic binge–purge cycle. *International Journal of Eating Disorders, 7*, 469–474.

Cooper, M. J., Anastasiades, P., and Fairburn, C. G. (1992). Selective processing of eating-, shape-, and weight-related words in persons with bulimia nervosa. *Journal of Abnormal Psychology, 101*, 352–355.

Cooper, P. J., and Bowskill, R. (1986). Dysphoric mood and overeating. *British Journal of Clinical Psychology, 25*, 155–156.

Cooper, P. J., and Fairburn, C. G. (1984). Cognitive behaviour therapy for anorexia nervosa; Some preliminary findings. *Journal of Psychosomatic Research, 28,* 493–499.

Cooper, Z., and Fairburn, C. G. (1987). The eating disorder examination: A semi-structured interview for the assessment of the specific psychopathology of eating disorders. *International Journal of Eating Disorders, 6,* 1–8.

Cox, G. L., and Merkel, W. T. (1989). A qualitative review of psychosocial treatments for bulimia. *Journal of Nervous and Mental Disease, 177,* 77–84.

Craighead, L. W., and Agras, W. S. (1991). Mechanisms of action in cognitive-behavioral and pharmacological interventions for obesity and bulimia nervosa. *Journal of Consulting and Clinical Psychology, 59,* 115–125.

Crisp, A. H. (1980). *Anorexia nervosa: Let me be.* London: Academic Press.

Dalgleish, T., and Watts, F. N. (1990). Biases of attention and memory in disorders of anxiety and depression. *Clinical Psychology Review, 10,* 589–604.

Davis, R., Freeman, R., and Solyom, L. (1985). Mood and food: An analysis of bulimic episodes. *Journal of Psychiatric Research, 19,* 331–335.

Davis, R., Freeman, R. J., and Garner, D. M. (1988). A naturalistic investigation of eating behavior in bulimia nervosa. *Journal of Consulting and Clinical Psychology, 56,* 273–279.

DeLucia, J. L., and Kalodner, C. R. (1990). An individualized cognitive intervention: Does it increase the efficacy of behavioral interventions for obesity? *Addictive Behaviors, 15,* 473–479.

Demitrack, M. A., Lesem, M. D., Listwak, S. J., Brandt, H. A., Jimerson, D. C., and Gold, P. W. (1990). CSF oxytocin in anorexia nervosa and bulimia nervosa: Clinical and pathophysiologic considerations. *American Journal of Psychiatry, 147,* 882–886.

Drewnowski, A., Riskey, D., and Desor, J. A. (1982). Feeling fat yet unconcerned: Self-reported overweight and the restraint scale. *Appetite. Journal for Intake Research, 3,* 273–279.

Dunkel, L. D., and Glaros, A. G. (1978). Comparison of self-instructional and stimulus control treatments for obesity. *Cognitive Therapy and Research, 2,* 75–78.

Elmore, D. K., and de Castro, J. M. (1990). Self-rated moods and hunger in relation to spontaneous eating behavior bulimics, recovered bulimics, and normals. *International Journal of Eating Disorders, 9,* 179–190.

Fairburn, C. G. (1983). Bulimia: Its epidemiology and management. *Psychiatric Annals, 13,* 953–961.

Fairburn, C. G. (1985). Cognitive–behavioral treatment for bulimia. In D. M. Garner and P. E. Garfinkel (Eds.), *Handbook for psychotherapy for anorexia nervosa and bulimia* (pp. 160–192). New York: Guilford Press.

Fairburn, C. G. (1988). The current status of psychological treatments for bulimia nervosa. *Journal of Psychosomatic Research, 32,* 635–645.

Fairburn, C. G., and Garner, D. M. (1988). Diagnostic criteria for anorexia nervosa and bulimia nervosa: The importance of attitudes to shape and weight. In D. M. Garner and P. E. Garfinkel (Eds.), *Diagnostic issues in anorexia nervosa and bulimia nervosa* (pp. 36–55). New York: Brunner/Mazel.

Fairburn, C. G., Cooper, P. J., Cooper, M. J., McKenna, F. P., and Anastasiades, P. (1991a). Selective information processing in bulimia nervosa. *International Journal of Eating Disorders, 10,* 415–422.

Fairburn, C. G. Jones, R., Peveler, R. C., Carr, S. J., Solomon, R. A., O'Connor, M. E., Burton, J., and Hope, R. A. (1991b). Three psychological treatments for bulimia nervosa. *Archives of General Psychiatry, 48,* 463–469.

Fairburn, C. G., Agras, W. S., and Wilson, G. T. (1992). The research on the treatment of bulimia nervosa: Practical and theoretical implications. In G. H. Anderson and S. H.

Kennedy (Eds.), *The biology of feast and famine: Relevance to eating disorders.* New York: Academic Press.

Fairburn, C. G., Jones, R., Peveler, R. C., Hope, R. A., and O'Connor, M. (in pressb). Psychotherapy and bulimia nervosa: The longer-term effects of interpersonal therapy, behaviour therapy, and cognitive behaviour therapy. *Archives of General Psychiatry.*

Fairburn, C. G., Welch, S. L., and Hay, P. J. (1993c). The classification of recurrent overeating: The "binge eating disorder" proposal. *International Journal of Eating Disorders, 13,* 155–159.

Ferster, C. B., Nurnberger, J. I., and Levitt, E. E. (1962). The control of eating. *Journal of Mathetics, 1,* 87–109.

Fisher, S. (1986). *Development and structure of the body image, Vol 1.* Hillsdale, NJ: Erlbaum.

Foa, E. B., Feske, U., Murdock, T. B., Kozak, M. J., and McCarthy, P. R. (1991). Processing of threat-related information in rape victims. *Journal of Abnormal Psychology, 100,* 156–162.

Frankenberg, F., Garfinkel, P. E., and Garner, D. M. (1982). Anorexia nervosa: Issues in prevention. *Journal of Preventive Psychiatry, 1,* 469–483.

Franko, D. L., Zuroff, D. C., and Bendiksen, I. (1988). *Further validation of the Bulimic Thoughts Questionnaire.* Paper presented at the Third International Conference on Eating Disorders, New York.

Freeman, C. P. L., and Munro, J. K. M. (1988). Drug and group treatments for bulimia/bulimia nervosa. *Journal of Psychosomatic Research, 32,* 647–660.

Fremouw, W. J., and Heyneman, N. E. (1983). Cognitive styles and bulimia. *The Behavior Therapist, 6,* 143–144.

Gardner, R. M., Morrell, J., Urrutia, R., and Espinoza, T. (1989). Judgments of body size following significant weight loss. *Journal of Social Behavior and Personality, 4,* 603–613.

Garner, D. M. (1986a). Cognitive therapy for anorexia nervosa. In K. D. Brownell and J. P. Foreyt (Eds.), *Handbook of eating disorders: Physiology, psychology, and treatment of obesity, anorexia, and bulimia* (pp. 301–327). New York: Basic Books.

Garner, D. M. (1986b). Cognitive therapy for bulimia nervosa. *Adolescent Psychiatry, 13,* 358–390.

Garner, D. M. (1987). Psychotherapy outcome research with bulimia nervosa. *Psychotherapy and Psychosomatics, 48,* 129–140.

Garner, D. M. (1988). Anorexia nervosa. In M. Hersen and C. G. Last (Eds.), *Child behavior therapy casebook,* (pp. 263–276). New York: Plenum.

Garner, D. M., and Bemis, K. M. (1982). A cognitive–behavioral approach to anorexia nervosa. *Cognitive Therapy and Research, 6,* 123–150.

Garner, D. M., and Bemis, K. M. (1985). Cognitive therapy for anorexia nervosa. In D. M. Garner and P. E. Garfinkel (Eds.), *Handbook of psychotherapy for anorexia nervosa and bulimia* (pp. 107–146). New York: Guilford Press.

Garner, D. M., and Wooley, S. (in press). Confronting the failure of behavioral and dietary treatments for obesity. *Clinical Psychology Review.*

Garner, D. M., Garfinkel, P. E., and Moldofsky, H. (1978). Perceptual experiences in anorexia nervosa and obesity. *Canadian Psychiatric Association Journal, 23,* 249–260.

Garner, D. M., Garfinkel, P. E., and Olmsted, M. P. (1983a). An overview of the socio-cultural factors in the development of anorexia nervosa. In P. L. Darby, P. E. Garfinkel, D. M. Garner, and D. V. Coscina (Eds.), *Anorexia nervosa: Recent developments in research* (pp. 65–82). New York: Alan R. Liss.

Garner, D. M., Olmsted, M. P., and Polivy, J. (1983b). Development and validation of a multidimensional eating disorder inventory for anorexia nervosa and bulimia. *International Journal of Eating Disorders, 2,* 15–34.

Garner, D. M., Garfinkel, P. E., and O'Shaughnessy, M. (1985a). The validity of the distinction between bulimia with and without anorexia nervosa. *American Journal of Psychiatry, 142*, 581–587.

Garner, D. M., Rockert, W., Olmsted, M. P., Johnson, C., and Coscina, D. V. (1985b). Psychoeducational principles in the treatment of bulimia and anorexia nervosa. In D. M. Garner and P. E. Garfinkel (Eds.), *Handbook of psychotherapy for anorexia nervosa and bulimia* (pp. 513–572). New York: Guilford Press.

Garner, D. M., Fairburn, C. G., and Davis, R. (1987a). Cognitive–behavioral treatment of bulimia nervosa. *Behavior Modification, 11*, 398–431.

Garner, D. M., Garfinkel, P. E., and Bonato, D. P., (1987b). Body image measurement in eating disorders. *Advances in Psychosomatic Medicine, 17*, 119–133.

Garrow, J. S. (1986). Physiological aspects of obesity. In K. D. Brownell and J. P. Foreyt (Eds.), *Handbook of eating disorders: Physiology, psychology, and treatment of obesity, anorexia, and bulimia* (pp. 45–62). New York: Basic Books.

Glucksman, M. L., and Hirsch, J. (1969). The response of obese patients to weigh reduction. III. The perception of body size. *Psychosomatic Medicine, 31*, 1–17.

Goldberg, S. C., Halmi, K. A., Eckert, E. D., Casper, R. C., Davis, D. M., and Roper, M. (1980). Attitudinal dimensions in anorexia nervosa. *Journal of Psychiatric Research, 15*, 239–151.

Goodrick, G. K., Raynaud, A. S., Pace, P. W., and Foreyt, J. P. (1992). Outcome attributions in a very low calorie diet program. *International Journal of Eating Disorders, 12*, 117–120.

Gormally, J., Rardin, D., and Black, S. (1980). Correlates of successful response to a behavioral weight control clinic. *Journal of Counseling Psychology, 27*, 179–191.

Grinker, J. (1973). Behavioral and metabolic consequences of weight reduction. *Journal of the American Dietetic Association, 62*, 30–34.

Heatherton, T. F., and Baumeister, R. F. (1991). Binge eating as escape from self-awareness. *Psychological Bulletin, 110*, 86–108.

Heatherton, T. F., Herman. C. P., Polivy, J., King, G. A., and McGree, S. T. (1988). The (mis)measurement of restraint: An analysis of conceptual and psychometric issues. *Journal of Abnormal Psychology, 97*, 19–28.

Herman, C. P., and Mack, D. (1975). Restrained and unrestrained eating. *Journal of Personality, 43*, 647–660.

Herman, C. P., and Polivy, J. (1984). A boundary model for the regulation of eating. In A. B. Stunkard and E. Stellar (Eds.), *Eating and its disorders* (pp. 141–156). New York: Raven Press.

Hibscher, J. A., and Herman, C. P. (1977). Obesity, dieting and the expression of "obese" characteristics. *Journal of Comparative and Physiological Psychology, 91*, 374–380.

Hollon, S. D., and Beck, A. T. (1986). Cognitive and cognitive–behavioral therapies. In S. L. Garfield and A. E. Bergin (Eds.), *Handbook of psychotherapy and behavior change* (3rd ed.) (pp. 443–482). New York: Wiley.

Hope, D. A., Rapee, R. M., Heimberg, R. G., and Dombeck, M. J. (1990). Representations of the self in social phobia: Vulnerability to social threat. *Cognitive Therapy and Research, 14*, 177–189.

Hsu, L. K. G. (1990). Experiential aspects of bulimia nervosa: Implications for cognitive behavioral therapy. *Behavior Modification, 14*, 50–65.

Hsu, L. K. G., and Sobkiewicz, T. A. (1991). Body image disturbance: Time to abandon the concept for eating disorders? *International Journal of Eating Disorders, 10*, 15–30.

Hunt, D. A., and Rosen, J. C. (1981). Thoughts about food by obese and nonobese individuals. *Cognitive Therapy and Research, 5*, 317–322.

Israel, A. C., Stolmaker, L., and Andrian, C. A. G. (1985). Thoughts about food and their relationship to obesity and weight control. *International Journal of Eating Disorders, 4,* 549–558.

Jansen, A., Merckelbach, H., Oosterlaan, J., Tuiten, A., and van den Hout, M. (1988). Cognitions and self-talk during food intake of restrained and unrestrained eaters. *Behaviour Research and Therapy, 26,* 393–398.

Jeffery, R. W., French, A. S., and Schmid, T. L. (1990). Attributions for dietary failures: Problems reported by participants in the hypertension prevention trial. *Health Psychology, 9,* 315–329.

Johnson, C., and Larson, R. (1982). Bulimia: An analysis of moods and behavior. *Psychosomatic Medicine, 44,* 341–351.

Johnson, C., Lewis, C., and Hagman, J. (1984). The syndrome of bulimia: Review and synthesis. *Psychiatric Clinics of North America, 7,* 247–273.

Kaye, W. H., Gwirtsman, H. E., George, D. T., Weiss, S. R., and Jimerson, D. C. (1986). Relationship of mood alterations to bingeing behavior in bulimia. *British Journal of Psychiatry, 149,* 479–485.

Keefe, P. H., Wyshogrod, D., Winberger, E., and Agras, W. S. (1984). Binge eating and outcome of behavioral treatment of obesity: A preliminary report. *Behaviour Research and Therapy, 22,* 319–321.

Keys, A., Brozek, J., Henschel, A., Mickelson, O., and Taylor, H. I. (1950). *The biology of human starvation* (Vol 2). Minneapolis: University of Minnesota Press.

King, G. A., Polivy, J., and Herman, C. P. (1991). Cognitive aspects of dietary restraints: Effects on person memory. *International Journal of Eating Disorders, 10,* 313–321.

Kirkley, B. G., Kolotkin, R. L., Hernandez, J. T., and Gallagher, P. N. (1992). Binge eaters, and obese nonbinge eaters on the MMPI. *International Journal of Eating Disorders, 12,* 221–228.

Knight, L. J., and Boland, F. J. (1989). Restrained eating: An experimental disentanglement of the disinhibiting variables of perceived calories and food type. *Journal of Abnormal Psychology, 98,* 412–420.

Kolotkin, R. L., Revis, E. S., Kirkley, B. G., and Janick, L. (1987). Binge eating in obesity: Associated MMPI characteristics. *Journal of Consulting and Clinical Psychology, 55,* 872–876.

Kramer, F. M., Jeffery, R. W., Forster, J. L., and Snell, M. K. (1989). Long-term follow-up of behavioral treatment for obesity: Patterns of weight regain among men and women. *International Journal of Obesity, 13,* 123–136.

Laberg, J. C., Wilson, G. T., Eldredge, K., and Nordby, H. (1991). Effects of mood on heart rate reactivity in bulimia nervosa. *International Journal of Eating Disorders, 10,* 169–178.

Laessle, R. G., Zoettl, C., and Pirke, K. M. (1987). Metaanalysis of treatment studies for bulimia. *International Journal of Eating Disorders, 6,* 647–653.

Laessle, R. G., Bossert, S., Hank, G., Hahlweg, H., and Pirke, K. M. (1989a). Cognitive processing in bulimia nervosa: Preliminary observations. *Annals of New York Academy of Sciences, 575,* 543–544.

Laessle, R. G., Tuschl, R. J., Kotthaus, B. C., and Pirke, K. M. (1989b). A comparison of the validity of three scales for the assessment of dietary restraint. *Journal of Abnormal Psychology, 98,* 504–507.

Leon, G. R., Bemis, K. M., Meland, M., and Nussbaum, D. (1978). Aspects of body image perception in obese and normal weight youngsters. *Journal of Abnormal Child Psychology, 6,* 361–371.

Levine, M. P., and Smolak, L. (1989). *Toward a developmental psychopathology of eating disorders: The example of the middle school transition.* Paper presented at the 8th National Converence of the National Anorexic Aid Society, Columbus, OH.

Lingswiler, V. M., Crowther, J. H., and Stevens, M. A. P. (1987). Emotional reactivity and eating in binge eating and obesity. *Journal of Behavioral Medicine, 10,* 287–299.

Lingswiler, V. M., Crowther, J. H., and Stevens, M. A. P. (1989). Affective and cognitive antecedents to eating episodes in bulimia and binge eating. *International Journal of Eating Disorders, 8,* 533–539.

Lissner, L., Odell, P. M., D'Agostino, R. B., Stokes, J., Kreger, B. E., Belanger, A. J., and Brownell, K. D. (1991). Variability in body weight and health outcomes in the Farmingham population. *New England Journal of Medicine, 324,* 1839–1844.

Lowe, M. R. (1984). Dietary concerns, weight fluctuation and weight status: Further explorations of the restraint scale. *Behaviour Research and Therapy, 22,* 243–248.

Lowe, M. R., Whitlow, J. W., and Bellwoar, V. (1991). Eating regulation: The role of restraint, dieting, and weight. *International Journal of Eating Disorders, 10,* 461–471.

Lustig, A. (1991). Weight loss programs: Failing to meet ethical standards? *Journal of the American Dietetic Associations, 91,* 1252–1254.

MacLeod, C. M. (1991). Half a century of research on the Stroop effect: An integrative review. *Psychological Bulletin, 109,* 163–203.

MacLeod, C. M., Mathews, A., and Tata, P. (1986). Attentional bias in emotional disorders. *Journal of Abnormal Psychology, 95,* 15–20.

Mahoney J., and Mahoney, (1976). *Permanent Weight Control.* New York: Norton.

Marcus, M. D., Wing, R. R., and Hopkins, J. (1988). Obese binge eaters: Affect, cognitions, and response to behavioral weight control. *Journal of Consulting and Clinical Psychology, 56,* 433–439.

Marcus, M. D., Wing, R. R., Ewing, L., Kern, E., Gooding, W., and McDermott, M. (1990). Psychiatric disorders among obese binge eaters. *International Journal of Eating Disorders, 9,* 69–77.

Markus, H. (1990). Unresolved issues of self-representation. *Cognitive Therapy and Research, 14,* 241–253.

Markus, H., Hamil, R., and Sentis, K. P. (1987). Thinking fat: Self-schemas for body weight and the processing of weight relevant information. *Journal of Applied Social Psychology, 17,* 50–71.

Mathews, A., and MacLeod, C. (1987). An information-processing approach to anxiety. *Journal of Cognitive Psychotherapy, 1,* 105–115.

McCann, K. L., Perri, M. G., Nezu, A. M., and Lowe, M. R. (1992). An investigation of counterregulatory eating in obese clinic attenders. *International Journal of Eating Disorders, 12,* 161–169.

McNally, R. J., Kaspie, S. P., Riemann, B. C., and Zeitlin, S. B. (1990). Selective processing of threat cues in posttraumatic stress disorder. *Journal of Abnormal Psychology, 99,* 398–402.

Metropolitan Life Insurance Company (1983). 1983 Height and weight tables. *Statistical Bulletin, 64,* 3–9.

Mitchell, J. E., Pyle, R. L., Eckert, E. D., Hatsukami, D., Pomeroy, C., and Zimmerman, R. (1990). A comparison study of antidepressants and structured intensive group psychotherapy in the treatment of bulimia nervosa. *Archives of General Psychiatry, 47,* 149–157.

Mizes, J. S. (1990). Criterion-related validity of the Anorectic Cognitions Questionnaire. *Addictive Behaviors, 15,* 153–163.

Mizes, J. S., and Klesges, R. C. (1989). Validity, reliability, and factor structure of the Anorectic Cognitions Questionnaire. *Addictive Behaviors, 14,* 589–594.

Nisbett, R. E. (1968). Taste, deprivation, and weight determinants of eating behavior. *Journal of Personality and Social Psychology, 10,* 107–116.

O'Connor, J., and Dowrick, P. W. (1987). Cognitions in normal weight, overweight, and previously overweight adults. *Cognitive Therapy and Research, 11,* 315–326.

Peveler, R. C., and Fairburn, C. G. (1989). Anorexia nervosa in association with diabetes mellitus: A cognitive-behavioral approach to treatment. *Behaviour Research and Therapy*, 27, 95–99.

Phelan, P. W. (1987). Cognitive correlates of bulimia: The Bulimic Thoughts Questionnaire. *International Journal of Eating Disorders*, 6, 593–607.

Polivy, J., and Herman, C. P. (1985). Dieting and binging: A causal analysis. *American Psychologist*, 40, 193–201.

Polivy, J., Heatherton, T. F., and Herman, C. P. (1988). Self-esteem, restraint and eating behavior. *Journal of Abnormal Psychology*, 97, 354–356.

Prather, R. C., and Williamson, D. A. (1988). Psychopathology associated with bulimia, binge eating, and obesity. *International Journal of Eating Disorders*, 7, 177–184.

Rosen, J. C. (1987). A review of behavioral treatments for bulimia nervosa. *Behavior Modification*, 11, 464–486.

Ross, M. W., Kalucy, R. S., and Morton, J. E. (1983). Locus of control in obesity: Predictors of success in a jaw-wiring programme. *British Journal of Medical Psychology*, 53, 49–56.

Rossiter, E. M., Agras, W. S., and Losch, M. (1988a). Changes in self-reported food intake in bulimics as a consequence of antidepressant treatment. *International Journal of Eating Disorders*, 7, 779–783.

Rossiter, E. M., Agras, W. S., Losch, M., and Telch, C. F. (1988b). Dietary restraint of bulimic subjects following cognitive–behavioral or pharmacological treatment. *Behaviour Research and Therapy*, 26, 495–498.

Rossiter, E. M., Wilson, G. T., and Goldstein (1989). Bulimia and dietary restraint. *Behaviour Research and Therapy*, 4, 465–468.

Rossiter, E. M., Agras, W. S., Telch, C. F., and Bruce, B. (1992). The eating patterns of nonpurging bulimic subjects. *International Journal of Eating Disorders*, 11, 111–120.

Ruderman, A. J. (1985). Restraint, obesity and obesity. *Behaviour Research and Therapy*, 23, 151–156.

Ruderman, A. J. (1986). Dietary restraint: A theoretical and empirical review. *Psychological Bulletin*, 99, 247–262.

Ruderman, A. J., and Wilson, G. T. (1979). Weight, restraint, cognitions, and counterregulation. *Behaviour Research and Therapy*, 17, 581–590.

Russell, G. F. M., Campbell, P. G., and Slade, P. D. (1975). Experimental studies on the nature of the psychological disorder in anorexia nervosa. *Psychoneuroendocrinology*, 1, 45–56.

Safran, J. D., Segal, Z. V., Hill, C., and Whiffen, V. (1990). Refining strategies for research on self-representations in emotional disorders. *Cognitive Therapy and Research*, 14, 143–160.

Saltzer, E. B. (1982). The weight locus of control (WLOC) scale: A specific measure for obesity research. *Journal of Personality Assessment*, 46, 620–628.

Scanlon, E., Ollendick, T. H., and Bayer, K. (1986). *The role of cognitions in bulimia: An empirical test of basic assumptions*. Paper presented at the annual meeting of the Association for the Advancement of Behavior Therapy, Chicago.

Schachter, S. (1971). Some extraordinary facts about obese humans and rats. *American Psychologist*, 26, 129–144.

Schlundt, D. G., Johnson, W. G., and Jarrell, M. P. (1985). A naturalistic functional analysis of eating behavior in bulimia and obesity. *Advances in Behaviour Research and Therapy*, 7, 149–162.

Schmidt, N. B., and Telch, M. J. (1991). *Selective processing of body shape and food cues in high and low restraint subjects*. Poster presented at the annual meeting of the Association for the Advancement of Behavior Therapy, New York.

Schotte, D. E., McNally, R. J., and Turner, M. L. (1990). A dichotic listening analysis of body weight concern in bulimia nervosa. *International Journal of Eating Disorders*, 9, 109–113.

Schulman, R. G., Kinder, B. N., Gleghorn, A., Powers, P. S., and Prange, M. (1986). The development of a scale to measure cognitive distortions in bulimia. *Journal of Personality Assessment, 50*, 630–639.

Segal, Z. V. (1988). Appraisal of the self-schema construct in cognitive models of depression. *Psychological Bulletin, 103*, 147–162.

Slade, P. (1982). Towards a functional analysis of anorexia nervosa and bulimia nervosa. *British Journal of Clinical Psychology, 21*, 167–179.

Slade, P. (1985). A review of body image in anorexia nervosa and bulimia nervosa. *Journal of Psychiatric Research, 19*, 255–265.

Spencer, J. A., and Fremouw, W. J. (1979). Binge eating as a function of restraint and weight classification. *Journal of Abnormal Psychology, 88*, 262–267.

Spitzer, R. L., and Rodin, J. (1981). Human eating behavior: A critical review of studies in normal weight and overweight individuals. *Appetite. Journal for Intake Research, 2*, 293–299.

Spitzer, R. L., Devlin, M., Walsh, B. T., Hasin, D., Wing, R., Marcus, M., Stunkard, A., Wadden, T., Yanovski, S., Agras, S., Mitchell, J., and Nonas, C. (1992). Binge eating disorder: A multisite field trial of the diagnostic criteria. *International Journal of Eating Disorder, 11*, 191–203.

Stein, D. M. (1988). The scaling of restraint and the prediction of eating. *International Journal of Eating Disorders, 7*, 713–717.

Steinberg, S., Tobin, D., and Johnson, C. (1990). The role of bulimic behaviors in affect regulation: Different functions for different patient subgroups? *International Journal of Eating Disorders, 9*, 51–55.

Stotland, S., and Zuroff, D. C. (1990). A new measure of weight locus of control: the dieting beliefs scale. *Journal of Personality Assessment, 54*, 191–203.

Striegel-Moore, R., and Rodin, J. (1986). The influence of psychological variables in obesity. In K. D. Brownell and J. P. Foreyet (Eds.). *Handbook of Eating Disorders*. New York: Basic Books.

Striegel-Moore, R., McAvay, G., and Rodin, J. (1986). Psychological and behavioral correlates of feeling fat in women. *International Journal of Eating Disorders, 5*, 935–947.

Stroop, J. R. (1935). Studies of interference in serial verbal reactions. *Journal of Experimental Psychology, 18*, 643–662.

Stunkard, A. J., and Messick, S. (1985). The three-factor eating questionnaire to measure dietary restraint, disinhibition, and hunger. *Journal of Psychosomatic Research, 29*, 71–83.

Stunkard, A. J., and Wadden, T. A. (1990). Restrained eating and human obesity. *Nutritional Reviews, 48*, 78–86.

Telch, C. F., Agras, W. S., Rossiter, E. M., Wilfley, D., and Kenardy, J. (1990). Group cognitive–behavioral treatment for the nonpurging bulimic: An initial evaluation. *Journal of Consulting and Clinical Psychology, 58*, 629–635.

Thompson, D. A., Berg, K. M., and Shatford, L. A. (1987). The heterogeneity of bulimic symptomatology: Cognitive and behavioral dimensions. *International Journal of Eating Disorders, 6*, 215–234.

Thompson, J. K. (1990). *Body image disturbance*. New York: Pergamon.

Thompson, J. K., Jarvie, G. J., Lahey, B. B., and Cureton, K. J. (1982). Exercise and obesity: Etiology, physiology, and intervention. *Psychological Bulletin, 91*, 55–79.

Thurstin, A. H., Weinsier, R. L., Linton, P. H., and Crist, D. A. (1988). An eating disorder inventory-based typology of outpatient obese individuals. *Journal of Substance Abuse, 1*, 45–53.

Tobias, L. L., and MacDonald, M. L. (1977). Internal locus of control and weight loss: An insufficient condition. *Journal of Consulting and Clinical Psychology, 45*, 647–653.

Turnbull, J., Freeman, C. P. L., Barry, F., and Henderson, A. (1989). The clinical characteristics of bulimic women. *International Journal of Eating Disorders, 8,* 399–409.

Van Strien, T., Frijters, J. E. R., Bergers, G. P. A., and Defares, P. B. (1986). The Dutch Eating Behavior Questionnaire (DEBQ) for assessment of restrained, emotional and external eating behavior. *International Journal of Eating Disorders, 5,* 295–315.

Vitousek, K. B. (1990). Cognitive–behavioral treatment of weight preoccupation. Workshop presented at the annual meeting of the Association for the Advancement of Behavior Therapy, San Francisco, CA, November, 1990.

Vitousek, K. B., and Ewald, L. (1992). Self-representation in the eating disorders: The cognitive perspective. In Z. Segal and S. Blatt (Eds.), *Self-representation in emotional disorders: Cognitive and psychodynamic perspectives* (pp. 221–257). New York: Guilford Press.

Vitousek, K. B., and Hollon, S. (1990). The investigation of schematic content and processing in eating disorders. *Cognitive Therapy and Research, 14,* 191–214.

Vitousek, K. B., Daly, J., and Heiser, C. (1991a). Reconstructing the internal world of the eating-disordered individual: Overcoming denial and distortion in self-report. *International Journal of Eating Disorders, 10,* 647–666.

Vitousek, K. B., Garner, D. M., and Hollon, S. D. (1991b). *The assessment of cognitive processes in eating disorders.* Unpublished manuscript, University of Hawaii.

Vitousek, K., Ewald, L., Mew, L., and Manke, F. (1992). *Interpretation of ambiguous stimuli in the eating disorders: The influence of contextual cues.* Manuscript submitted for publication.

Wadden, T. A., and Stunkard, A. J. (1987). Psychopathology and obesity. *Annals of the New York Academy of Science, 499,* 55–65.

Walker, M. K., Ben-Tovim, D. I., Jones, S., and Bachok, N. (1992). Repeated administration of the Adapted Stroop test: Feasibility for longitudinal study of psychopathology in eating disorders. *International Journal of Eating Disorders, 12,* 103–105.

Wallston, B. S., Wallston, K. A., Kaplan, G. D., and Maides, S. A. (1976). Development and validation of the health locus of control (HLC) scale. *Journal of Consulting and Clinical Psychology, 44,* 580–585.

Wardle, J. (1988). Cognitive control of eating. *Journal of Psychosomatic Research, 32,* 607–612.

Wardle, J., and Beinart, H. (1981). Binge eating: A theoretical review. *British Journal of Clinical Psychology, 20,* 97–109.

Wilfley, D. E., Agras, W. S., Telch, C. F., Rossiter, E. M., Schneider, J. A., Cole, A. G., Sifford, L., and Raeburn, S. D. (in press). Group cognitive–behavioral therapy and group interpersonal psychotherapy for the nonpurging bulimic: A controlled comparison. *Journal of Consulting and Clinical Psychology.*

Williamson, D. A., Kelley, M. L., Davis, C. J., Ruggiero, L., and Veitia, M. C. (1985). The psychophysiology of bulimia. *Advances in Behaviour Research and Therapy, 7,* 163–172.

Wilson, G. T. (1976). Obesity, binge eating, and behavior therapy: Some clinical observations. *Behavior Therapy, 7,* 700–701.

Wilson, G. T., (1989). Bulimia nervosa: Models, assessment, and treatment. *Current Opinion in Psychiatry, 2,* 790–794.

Wilson, G. T. (1993). Psychological and pharmacological treatment of bulimia nervosa: A research update. *Applied and Preventive Psychology: Current Scientific Perspectives, 2,* 35–42.

Wilson, G. T., and Smith, D. (1989). Assessment of bulimia nervosa: An evaluation of the eating disorder examination. *International Journal of Eating Disorders, 8,* 173–179.

Wilson, G. T., and Walsh, B. T. (1991). Eating disorders in the DSM-IV. *Journal of Abnormal Psychology, 100,* 362–365.

Wilson, G. T., Nonas, C. A., and Rosenblum, G. D. (1993). Assessment of binge-eating in obese patients. *International Journal of Eating Disorders, 13,* 25–33.

Wolchik, S. A., Weiss, L., and Katzman, M. A. (1986). An empirically validated, short-term psychoeducational group treatment program for bulimia. *International Journal of Eating Disorders, 5*, 21–34.

Wooley, S. (1991). Obesity: Winners and losers in the marketing of false hope. *NAAS Newsletter, 14*, 1–5.

Wooley, S. C., and Garner, D. M. (1991). Obesity treatment: The high cost of false hope. *The Journal of the American Dietetic Association, 91*, 1248–1251.

Zotter, D. L., and Crowther, J. H. (1991). The role of cognition in bulimia nervosa. *Cognitive Therapy and Research, 15*, 413–426.

Substance Use Disorders: Cognitive Models and Architecture

Mark S. Goldman and Bruce C. Rather

University of South Florida

The scientific investigation of alcohol and substance abuse forces a head-on confrontation with the mind–body problem. Drugs are chemical agents but have effects on emotions and behaviors; the use of a drug is essentially a behavioral event but physiological systems are inevitably involved. Hence, the phenomenon of alcohol and drug abuse provides an ideal locus for the scientific pursuit of these interrelationships. Ultimately, our ability to prevent and treat these conditions can only be enhanced by a better understanding of the manner in which the behavioral and pharmacological spheres interconnect.

Improved understanding of the biological end of this continuum has come about using laboratory techniques that continue to advance in sophistication. On the behavioral side, precision rarely achieved in psychology in measuring observable activity has come through the use of operant methodology. A number of psychopharmacological phenomena are, however, not fully or easily addressed at either the strictly biological (reductionist) or the purely behavioral (molar) level. These phenomena readily lend themselves to the use of methods and theories of cognitive science. The introduction of cognitive concepts has, in turn, opened new areas of

PSYCHOPATHOLOGY AND COGNITION

inquiry that would not have been explored using conventional psycho-pharmacological or behavioral approaches.

In most instances, approaches based on cognitive science do not replace existing formulations, but instead augment or provide a different level of explanation. As one example, the phenomenon of behavioral tolerance could be addressed using traditional concepts in classical and operant conditioning. Recent formulations, however, have usefully employed models derived from cognitive science to expand understanding of inter-vening mechanisms. In this chapter, we will explore cognitive models guided by the belief that theoretical approaches that integrate well with explanations at other levels of analysis (e.g., behavioral, biological) are more promising for the development of psychological science than the free-standing "mini-theory" approach, which pays little attention to scientific integration.

This chapter will emphasize recent work in the alcohol realm, partly because this is the area with which we are most familiar, and because much of the research and theorizing we will discuss have been used first for explaining alcohol use and abuse. We will begin by presenting infor-mation that led to the need for mediational mechanisms of the kind that cognitive science can provide. Discussion of some early evidence that shows the utility of cognitive models for explaining these phenomena will follow, along with a general presentation of a variety of models from cog-nitive science that may prove helpful in guiding future research.[1]

ANTECEDENTS OF SUBSTANCE USE

A body of research over the past two decades has confirmed that alco-holism and drug abuse do not spring full-blown into existence at the mo-ment of first contact with the substance. These behavioral patterns develop over time (albeit faster in some than in others), and are linked to a wide range of antecedent ("risk") variables, many of which appear prior to the onset of any use, and certainly prior to abuse. Some of the variables may merely cooccur with some regularity with other variables that are related to the actual processes by which consumption is influenced (i.e., "mark-ers"). Other variables may more directly influence the development of use

[1]For psychopharmacologists and others uncomfortable with the term "cognitive": dictionary definitions of cognitive generally refer to the action of "knowing," which implies a "knower." Since "cognitive" explana-tions for mediational processes can imply, therefore, that the substrate for behavioral control is a "knower" (or homunculus) in the head, the term cognitive justifiably may be regarded as tautological. If, however, the term is limited to the postulation of systems for processing information that is initially received by the senses, and ultimately influences behavior, the term loses much of its circularity, and becomes little different from any mechanistic intervening variable (see Bolles, 1972; Goldman et al., 1987).

or abuse. The range of these variables is quite extensive and full coverage is beyond the scope of the current paper. The reader is recommended to a number of recent sources that thoroughly review identified antecedent variables in the alcoholism field (Burk and Sher, 1988; Hawkins *et al.*, 1992; MacDonald and Blume, 1986; Russell *et al.*, 1985; Sher, 1991; Windle and Searles, 1990). A similar group of variables have also been identified for drug risk (see Glantz and Pickens, 1992; Hawkins *et al.*, 1992). Controversy exists over whether variables that represent early childhood and adolescent environment or those emanating from genetically influenced biological characteristics are the predominant influences on the eventual development of alcohol problems (Murray *et al.*, 1983; Peele, 1986; Searles, 1988). The consensus in the field tends, however, toward a multicomponent position that includes both sets of variables, possibly arranged in different combinations, which may result in different pathways to alcoholism and drug abuse (Cloninger, 1987; Zucker, 1987).

Although the identification of these variables represents a significant research advance, it is important to appreciate that most are only *descriptive* characteristics of an individual's physical and social environment, behavioral patterns, or neurophysiology. The mechanisms by which these variables actually manifest their influence over consumption remain, in most cases, either completely unspecified or only vaguely implied. Advances in this field clearly depend on better understanding of the processes and mechanisms that bridge the temporal and logical gap between antecedents and eventual drinking outcomes. Bridging processes must be offered of a relatively long-term nature, such as those that carry forward the influence of genetically inherited physical characteristics or early family environment, as well as processes that operate over a much shorter term. Short-term processes must explain how a single drinking or drug use experience influences the probability of engaging in a subsequent experience, or even how consumption of a single drink within one drinking episode might affect the probability of taking the next drink. The most theoretically attractive processes (due to parsimony) would be those that help explain control over both time frames.

To demonstrate how the identification of risk variables often fails to specify actual mechanisms by which substance use may be controlled, it will be helpful to review some of the most highly supported antecedent variables in terms of their explanatory power. In the sociocultural realm, gender (Harfond and Mills, 1978; Margulies *et al.*, 1977; Smart and Gray, 1979), socioeconomic status (Cahalan and Cisin, 1968), race (Donovan *et al.*, 1983; Harfond and Mills, 1978; Harfond and Spiegler, 1983), ethnic and religious affiliations (Burkett, 1980; Cahalan and Cisin, 1968; Knupfer and Room, 1967; Wilsnack and Wilsnack, 1980), family environment (Benson and Heller, 1987; Harfond and Spiegler, 1983; Margulies *et al.*, 1977; West and Prinz, 1987), and peer influences (Jessor and Jessor, 1975) have been identified as predictive of drinking (and substance use) behavior. In each case, these are categorical and descriptive variables and not mechanisms by which later use may be influenced. Instead, we must ask what it is about gender, or socioeconomic status (SES), or ethnic affiliation that plays a role in eventual drinking/drug use patterns. It is evident that children of different gender, SES, and ethnic affiliation are exposed to different models and messages that impart some learning that affects later consumption and behavior.[2] Family process variables (e.g., cohesion, disruption), which clearly play an influential role (Barnes, 1977; Zucker, 1976; Zucker and Gomberg, 1986), are also inadequate as a causal explanation. Exactly *how* does a child's experience within a distressed family affect drinking or drug use decisions later in life? Implicit in current literature is that such children may carry a residual of emotional distress *but also* learn to anticipate that alcohol or other drugs can relieve such distress.

Even reductionistic approaches that emphasize the underlying biological substrate do not automatically reveal processes by which consumption is actually influenced. For example, Schuckit (1987, p. 304) remarks in connection with genetic transmission that "the actual mechanism for the expression of vulnerability (still) needs to be studied." A brief review of some of the most well known biological markers of alcoholism risk makes this problem more evident. Why, for example, should differing isoenzymes of aldehyde dehydrogenase (Harada *et al.*, 1982; Newlin, 1989) place individuals at different levels of risk for the development of alcoholism? Aldehyde dehydrogenase is an enzyme involved in the metabolism of alcohol. There is no suggestion that such an enzyme directly controls neurophysiological pathways that influence complex behavioral decision making. Instead, it is supposed that individuals react differently to alcohol because of these differing isoenzymes, and thus experience (and remember) alcohol to have differing degrees of pleasure/aversiveness. Similar analyses can apply to neuropharmacological substrates often connected with alcoholism, such as the GABA and NMDA receptor complex (Allan and Harris, 1987; Celentano *et al.*, 1988; Glowa *et al.*, 1989; Greenberg *et al.*, 1984;

---

[2]An alternative explanation is, of course, that such variables may serve as markers of later social behavior patterns. That is, being male in childhood is an indication that one is likely to be male as an adult and spend time with other males. If males drink more than females, then the risk associated with this variable may be merely that it is an indicator of later social pressure. The same may be true for SES, or ethnic affiliation. However, individuals from risk groups often continue to demonstrate greater risk even after disconnecting to some extent from the earlier risk group (for example, individuals of certain ethnic religious affiliation who continue to demonstrate drinking patterns similar to those of their original group despite no longer interacting with such individuals as an adult).

Hoffman *et al.*, 1989; Morrow *et al.*, 1988), differing dopamine receptor alleles (Blum *et al.*, 1990; Cloninger, 1991; Noble *et al.*, 1991), or variations in neurotransmitter activity (Alexopoulos *et al.*, 1983; Tabakoff *et al.*, 1988). In fact, these concepts are even applicable to the control of substances with known sites of activity such as particular receptors (e.g., benzodiazepines; morphine). Prior to physical addiction, use of these substances reflects a behavioral choice, which must depend, in part, on memories of pleasurable or pain-reducing effects. It is, of course, arguable that even addictive behavior is, in part, dependent on information about drug effects (in order for the user even to identify what is "craved").

Individuals at high risk for alcoholism have also been suggested to have variations in the P_3, or other components of the event-related potential (Begleiter and Porjesz, 1988; Porjesz and Begleiter, 1985) and perhaps low levels of EEG slow-wave activity (Gabrielli *et al.*, 1982; Pollock *et al.*, 1983). Once again, workers in these areas suggest that somehow these abnormal electrical outputs of the brain reflect aversive states, and that alcohol serves as a reinforcer by regularizing (diminishing) these aversive states. No direct control is inferred, but rather the influence on alcohol consumption is presumed to be indirect, that is, individuals learn to use alcohol as a means of controlling aversive states.

Other important risk factors are those temperament/personality variables that have been linked to eventual development of alcoholism and other drug use. Antisocial personality, sensation-seeking, and reward-seeking characteristics have all been suggested as indicators of high risk (Sher *et al.*, 1991; Zucker and Gomberg, 1986). In regard to drug-abuse vulnerability, recently identified dimensions of affectivity, for example, positive and negative, and arousal (Ford, 1987; Watson and Clark, 1984; Watson and Tellegen, 1985) have also been regarded as risk factors (Pandina *et al.*, 1992). In none of these cases, however, is the effect presumed to be specific for alcoholism or drug use; rather, it is presumed that these individuals' needs for excitement and reward, or their lessened response to punitive consequences, may make the reward value of alcohol (or drugs) relatively greater. Once again, the process by which altered reinforcement value actually influences drug-use behavior remains unspecified.

Even the most specific mechanism proposed, that of individual differences in innate or acquired reactivity (the reciprocal of tolerance), may require some further conceptual elaboration. Even if we presume that alcohol/drug use is somehow more reinforcing for some individuals (e.g., see Newlin and Thomson, 1990, for a review of alcohol reward effects), one is left with the need to explain how an individual instance of a rewarding experience then influences a future episode of alcohol or drug use. Of course, traditional behavioral and psychopharmacological explanations eschew the use of intervening variables to explain these type of phenomena, but even such researchers have become more accepting of possible cognitive mediation of both alcohol and drug use. For example, psychobiological researchers such as Jaffe (cited in Barnes, 1988, p. 417) have noted that "memory may be the real biological basis of drug dependence" and Wise (1988, pp. 124–125) indicates that "significant craving results from the memory of past positive reinforcement." In making these observations, both researchers reflect the understanding that no researcher in any area of investigation has yet demonstrated that any particular biological factor "commandeers" consumption activity in the absence of some form of cognitive mediation.

COGNITIVE MEDIATION OF SUBSTANCE ABUSE

Although psychology has since its inception debated the utility of intervening variables and hypothetical constructs for explaining behavior, a number of reasons for examining cognitive mediational processes in the alcohol and drug realm go beyond the traditional arguments about the utility of these concepts. The most pragmatic reason is perhaps that cognitive psychology and, more generally, cognitive science, has been making great strides in recent years, and the application of some of these concepts to the alcohol and drug field may prove useful as a source of productive new approaches. As we shall see, cognitive approaches have become quite sophisticated, and in some applications rival the sophistication found in more biologically oriented approaches. Furthermore, the search for cognitive mediators is important because many of the antecedents identified as risk variables in this field happen at an early point in a person's life, may not be obvious or distinguishable when they occur, or are not easily changed (e.g., ethnicity). Hence, investigation of cognitive mediational processes that offer some attendant ability for restructuring cognitive influences may present a new opportunity for understanding, preventing, and treating these problem behaviors. Finally, and perhaps most importantly, most current models of risk are highly multivariate, and include a large number of complex variables that interact in complicated ways. If a limited number of mediational "final common pathways," such as memory function, could be identified, the possibility of controlling these behaviors becomes greatly simplified.

Alcohol Expectancies

Although a number of concepts from cognitive psychology have by now found their way into the literature on alcohol and drug abuse, the most frequently invoked (and perhaps oldest) cognitive concept is that of expectancy. The concept of expectancy began to be used in the alcohol field when classical placebo effects, which had always been regarded as trivial and an experimental nuisance, began to be seen as an important factor in determining psychopharmacological effects. Expectancy, or the anticipation of a systematic if/then relationship between events and objects, has always been a central concept in cognitive approaches to psychology, and has been expanded and increased in sophistication with recent developments in cognitive psychology. It may be suggested, in fact, that the term expectancy itself may be somewhat outdated when applied to modern cognitive formulations (Goldman, 1989).

Some aspects of the modern-day expectancy concept can undoubtedly be traced to notions of basic associational processes dating back to William James (1890/1983), as well as to concepts emanating from other early schools of psychology (e.g., Gestalt). Tolman (1932) introduced the modern conception of expectancy as an intervening variable that comes between a stimulus and response and is stored in memory, that is, it is stored for utilization in future situations. These ideas obviously can be used to account for vicarious or observational learning, and thereby provide the basis for work by such individuals as Bandura (1977). MacCorquodale and Meehl (1954) further systematized Tolman's theory to account for any learning that is acquired by the organism in the absence of performance, and Rotter (1954) highlighted the probabalistic nature of expectancy. In 1972, Bolles explicitly suggested that the pure associative concept of reinforcement be replaced with the concept of expectancy, and Mischel (1973) was influential in employing these same concepts for explaining human learning. Since that time, sophisticated expectancy formulations have been offered to explain operant and classical conditioning (Anderson, 1983; Rescorla, 1988), and have been usefully employed to produce computer programs that mimic human behavior (Newell, cited in Waldrop, 1988). In addition, psychopathology (Alloy and Tabachnik, 1984), hypnosis (Kirsch, 1985), psychotherapy (Kirsch, 1990), interpersonal processes (Jones, 1986; Miller and Turnbull, 1986), and affect (Carver and Scheier, 1990), have been productively approached using expectancy formulations.

Placebo Studies

The expectancy concept was first brought into the alcohol field in a variety of studies in which expectancy was operationally defined in terms of whether the subject was led to believe they would be receiving an active drug (independently of whether they actually did). Using a completely crossed variant of a simple placebo design called the "balanced" placebo design (Marlatt and Rohsenow, 1980), a succession of studies showed that alcoholics' craving and loss of control might be attributed to expectancy effects, as might a variety of social and emotional effects in nonalcoholics, including sexuality, aggression, and anxiety or tension reduction (see Goldman *et al.*, 1987; Hull and Bond, 1986). Psychomotor and performance measures have appeared less attributable to expectancy effects (see Hull and Bond, 1986), but anticipation of alcohol consumption can minimize the deterioration in performance normally seen after alcohol consumption (i.e., the compensation for alcohol effect; George *et al.*, 1990; Ross and Pihl, 1988; Williams *et al.*, 1981). Although some have argued that findings from balanced placebo studies may have been artifacts of experimenter demands (Knight *et al.*, 1986), it is difficult to dismiss all placebo effects as purely the result of experimental artifact. Such expectancy effects have also been found for other psychoactive drugs (e.g., Fillmore and Vogel-Sprott, 1992).

Psychometric Approaches to Expectancies

To permit quantification and exploration of expectancies in relation to different subject populations, a variety of assessment instruments have been psychometrically derived to measure expectancylike characteristics. Items on these scales have included "reasons for drinking," "attitudes about alcohol," and "effects of alcohol use." It is sometimes difficult to compare findings across scales because some scales include items that tap value judgments about goodness or badness of drinking or other specific characteristics of drinking situations. Regardless of these differences, however, some common findings directly bear upon the etiology of alcohol and drug use. First, expectancies have been identified in all age and drinker groups, ranging from elementary-aged children (Gaines *et al.*, 1988; Miller *et al.*, 1990; Noll *et al.*, 1990) to adolescents prior to and following drinking onset (Chrisitiansen and Goldman, 1983; Christiansen *et al.*, 1982; Christiansen *et al.*, 1989) to college age (Brown, 1985a) and adult abstainers, social drinkers, and even alcoholics (Brown *et al.*, 1985). Similar expectancies have been identified for nicotine (Brandon and Baker, 1992), marijuana and cocaine (Jaffe, 1992; Jaffe *et al.*, 1989; Schafer and Brown, 1991), and mixed drugs (Wong *et al.*, 1991). If we include cognitive structures with other labels (e.g., schema) in this set, cognitions relating to alcohol use and its effects have even been identified in pre-school-aged children (Noll *et al.*, 1990). With regard to alcohol expectancies, some questions have been raised about precise factor structure (Leigh, 1989), but as we shall see, such uncertainties are likely inherent to the manner in which expectancies are stored in memory (Goldman *et al.*, 1991).

Identification of expectancies in drinker and drug-using groups, using a variety of different questioning techniques, has been important, but by itself would have sparked only limited interest. What is most striking is that the level of expectancies found in these different age and drinking groups is related to a number of important criterion variables connected to drinking, including drinking levels themselves. The relationship has also been shown to be relatively independent of other experiences that drinkers encounter, such as the effects of being in an alcohol treatment program (Brown *et al.*, 1985). Furthermore, when the expectancy-measuring instrument is constructed so as to be sensitive to situational variations in alcohol use, expectancy affirmation also can predict the amount that an individual drinks on a single occasion (Levine and Goldman, 1989). To be sensitive to situational variation, however, the instrument must be constructed so that scales are relatively invariant across a number of prototypic drinking situations (Levine and Goldman, 1989). Such a criterion is not easy to achieve, however, due to natural fluctuations in the structure of expectancies (see later modeling results).

In addition to drinking itself, some laboratory studies have shown that the behaviors individuals expect in themselves after drinking are consistent with the behaviors they actually demonstrate upon alcohol administration (George *et al.*, 1989; Roehling and Goldman, 1987; Rohsenow and Bachorowski, 1984; Sher, 1985). This finding has been somewhat inconsistent, however, suggesting the need for further adjustments in theory, or methodological refinements to reduce variability. One primary source of the discrepant findings from such research may be the variable success of investigators in producing a laboratory context that sufficiently mimics prior drinking experiences so as to permit confidence that expectancies have actually been activated.

A number of studies have also successfully related alcohol expectancies to risk status (family history positive or negative for alcoholism) (Brown *et al.*, 1987; Sher *et al.*, 1991; and others), although these findings also have not been uniform (Sher *et al.*, 1991). It is difficult to know if inconsistencies among these studies are due to variations in the instruments used, or to the limited theoretical relationship between alcohol expectancies and family history of alcoholism. After all, it is only those alcoholic families that convey higher expectancies about alcohol effects that should produce such expectancies in their children. Similarly, only family history positive individuals who experience differential reactivity to alcohol should maintain such expectations after alcohol exposure (not all children of alcoholics necessarily carry genetic risk). Since these relationships are not perfect, it is likely that some inconsistencies *should* be found when examining expectancies in the context of family history for alcoholism. Measured alcohol expectancies have also been shown to predict treatment outcome in alcoholics (Brown, 1985b); those alcoholics with higher expectancies generally were less successful during follow-up, and treated alcoholics and members of Alcoholics Anonymous who had not been drinking for some time showed lowered expectancies for alcohol effects (Connors *et al.*, 1990; Rather and Sherman, 1989).

Expectancies as Mediators

In 1955, in connection with their position on construct validation, Cronbach and Meehl averred that the utility of an unobservable construct was supported when that construct, as measured by specific operations, proved to be well integrated within a network of theoretically consistent criterion variables. The findings reviewed above constitute the beginnings of an interlocking system of relationships, which Cronbach and Meehl (1955) called a nomological network. The theoretical utility of alcohol expectancies can only be demonstrated to a point by empirical relationships with criterion variables, however. What is necessary is research that simultaneously shows the relationship of expectancies to antecedent risk variables and criterion variables such as drinking. Other recent studies have successfully filled this gap in the literature using a correlational design suggested by Baron and Kenny (1986), or variants of this design using covariance structure modeling techniques. In these designs, a variable is indicated to be a mediator if it can be shown to explain a significant portion of the variance in the relationship between an antecedent and a consequent (or a predictor and a criterion). In the Baron and Kenny (1986) approach, these relationships are demonstrated using multiple regression techniques, while in covariance structure modeling the relationships are demonstrated using simultaneous structural equations. Using these designs, a number of studies have now shown that expectancies mediate a significant portion of the influence on antecedents such as family history of alcoholism, sensation-seeking, and/or antisocial personality, family cohesiveness, and other significant risk indicators in adults (Henderson and Goldman, 1987; Sher *et al.*, 1991; Stacy *et al.*, 1991), and in adolescents (Smith and Goldman, 1990, 1992).

Origin of Expectancies

Given that expectancies have been identified in all age and drinker groups, including those with and without drinking experience, it appears safe to argue that expectancies can be acquired both from observational learning in the absence of alcohol (Bandura, 1985), and from direct experience with alcohol use (see Goldman *et al.*, 1987). Since placebo studies have, however, shown the affective and behavioral effects of alcohol to be somewhat discontinuous from actual pharmacological effects, it is necessary to inquire as to why expectancies of such effects were even acquired by humans. That is, if alcohol does *not* consistently (or perhaps even through direct pharmacological actions) render one relaxed, social, sexually aroused, for example, how did such expectancies arise? It is insufficient to say that such effects were observed in parents or significant others. From what source were their expectancies acquired? Although other drugs of abuse seem to have much more direct pharmacological effects through neuropharmacological pathways and reward systems, there may also be placebo (expectancy) effects of these drugs as well (for example, marijuana and nicotine undoubtedly have such characteristics). The ethical/legal difficulties of performing drug placebo studies with major drugs of abuse constrains such research, however.

To explain how alcohol may come to produce some affective and behavioral outcomes (and associated expectancies) in the absence of direct pharmacological induction, it appears necessary to postulate a means for alcohol to render behavior more "plastic," or shapable by circumstances. Although a number of models have been suggested (e.g., see Weintraub and Goldman, 1983), a cognitively oriented model has recently been the subject of much interest. This attention-allocation model (Josephs and Steele, 1990) notes two alcohol effects that are central to its operation: (1) alcohol has been shown to consistently impair the capacity to engage in controlled, effortful processing, that is, processing that requires attention (e.g., Birnbaum *et al.*, 1980; Schneider *et al.*, 1984); and (2) Alcohol narrows attention to the most immediate internal and external cues (e.g., Moskowitz and DePry, 1968; Rosen and Lee, 1976). Thus, the variable effects of alcohol are explained, in a given situation, by which cues are currently most salient and how much of one's attentional resources are currently occupied. For example, Josephs and Steele (1990) found that as attentional demands of a distracting activity increased, so did alcohol's reduction of anxiety concerning a future stressful situation. However, when attentional resources were not occupied, anxiety increased. Alcohol is hypothesized to cause what has been called "alcohol myopia, a state of shortsightedness in which superficially understood, immediate aspects of experience have disproportionate influence on behavior and emotion" (Steele and Josephs, 1990, p. 923). These theorists then go on to explain why commonly expected alcohol effects are most likely those induced by this "myopic" condition.

Recent Cognitive Concepts as Mediational Mechanisms

To provide cognitive explanations for the full range of important phenomena in the alcohol and drug use field, including urges, craving, and tolerance, it is necessary to review more recent cognitive concepts. Note, however, that some of these concepts are more heuristic than scientifically precise, and most are not mutually exclusive. In fact, many of these concepts work best together to provide a comprehensive picture. Rather than attempting to review all the issues and controversies pertaining to each of these concepts, only general descriptions are provided to assist with subsequent discussions. The reader is encouraged to consult the recent, more comprehensive, references cited in the text.

Episodic and Semantic Memory

Although episodic and semantic memory have been distinguished by some theorists as separate memory systems (Squire, 1992; Tulving, 1972, 1985) the same underlying system may provide the substrate for both. Episodic memory is autobiographical in character and includes events as they were experienced (albeit sometimes in distorted form). In contrast, semantic memory is thought to be a lexicon of abstract knowledge and rules that are stored without reference to the events during which they were acquired (Chang, 1986). Sometimes episodic and semantic memory are collectively referred to as declarative memory (Squire, 1992). Alcohol and drug expectancies can readily be conceived as stored in a semantic system after acquisition in a real-life context, which also provides for episodic storage.

Procedural Memory

A second general information storage system frequently distinguished from declarative memory is the procedural memory system, which includes motor skills acquired through practice, and rules and strategies that are not retrievable to conscious awareness. While information in declarative memory is often assumed to be stored in lists or networks, information in procedural memory is theorized to be stored in sequences. Hence, a motor skill sequence tends to run its typical course once the sequence is initiated (consider the similarity of this concept to some aspects of "loss-of-control" drinking). A number of recent theorists (e.g., Squire, 1992) have referred to this type of memory as *non*declarative to recognize that it includes more than motor skill learning.

Attention and Consciousness

Although many definitions of the term attention are possible, appreciation of the theories to be presented subsequently requires the understanding of attention as selective control over information utilized by the system.

Another way of understanding attention is in terms of top–down versus bottom–up processing. Top–down processing refers to control by some form of central executive, whereas bottom–up processing refers to control that emanates from the natural selectivity of the peripheral sensory system or systems further along in the processing sequence that back up the sensory systems. Top–down selection of information into awareness is thought to be possible within a limited number of channels, although arguments have also been made for multiple resource systems (Wickens, 1984; see Logan, 1988) (multiple activities may, however, require "switching" of attention). Hence, attending to more than one source of information at the same time is highly demanding. Outside of active awareness, however, the information-processing capacity of the brain is thought to be virtually unlimited.

Automatic versus Controlled Processing

Closely related to the description of attention are recent distinctions between automatic versus controlled processing (Hasher and Zacks, 1979; Schneider and Shiffrin, 1977; Shiffrin and Schneider, 1977; see Logan, 1988). As an example, early in the acquisition of a complex habit, such as learning to drive a car, considerable effort and attention must be given to all the details of driving. Such processing is considered to be controlled, or conceptually driven. After practice, however, these procedures become virtually automatic so that little effort and attention are necessary. This shift is adaptive in that it permits a variety of behaviors to be carried out simultaneously without overloading the limited-capacity attention system. However, such processing can also be problematic in cases such as alcohol and drug use in which automatic processes that control consumption may appear to both the consumer and the observer to be beyond the individual's control.

Priming: Implicit and Explicit

Other aspects of attention are highlighted in another cognitive concept, that of priming. Priming refers to the presentation of a stimulus that influences a subsequent behavior. A priming stimulus may or may not be presented in a manner that allows for conscious awareness. Hence, the terms explicit (within awareness), and implicit (outside awareness) are applied (Graf and Mandler, 1984; Meyer and Schvaneveldt, 1971; see Schacter, 1992). Primes help activate aspects of memory pertaining to a particular stimulus category and thereby facilitate retrieval of elements from that category (Caramazza et al., 1976; Rips et al., 1973). This concept can be applied to alcohol and drug use and abuse when stimuli such as the sights, sounds, or smells that relate to alcohol or drugs precipitate an unplanned instance of use.

Prototypes and Exemplars

In early theories of conditioning, a response was understood to be associationally related to a specific stimulus; in fact, it was even inferred by some theorists that each unique stimulus was connected to a unique response. In modern cognitive conceptions, a response need not be related to a highly specific and unique stimulus but, instead, repeated presentation of stimuli may result in the storage of some limited and generalized stimulus representation of a particular stimulus category (Smith and Medin, 1981). A generalized stimulus that represents the most important key features of an object or event, or, in connectionist models, the averaging of a number of stimulus presentations over time, is referred to as a *prototype*. If, instead, a particular stimulus from the array of all possible stimuli of that type becomes representative of the category, this stimulus is referred to as an *exemplar*. For example, an alcoholic need not necessarily learn to experience urges and craving in relation to every single bar he or she encounters, but rather distill out of his/her experience with bars a "barlike" stimulus complex that represents the category. In some instances this representation may be a particular bar, such as the bar on the television show "Cheers." Such a representation would be an exemplar.

Encoding Specificity

It has been theorized that memories are most strongly activated in connection with the specific stimulus contexts and encoding processes that were originally present during acquisition, and empirical support for this position has been obtained. This principle has been referred to in the cognitive literature as encoding specificity (Tulving, 1985). Encoding specificity has much in common, of course, with the older psychopharmacology term "state-dependent" learning, and even with classical concepts of stimulus generalization and discrimination. A unique feature of the encoding concept is, however, that the prior history of the organism (previously stored memories) and the manner of encoding (e.g., stimulus features vs. semantic meaning) are emphasized as influencing the storage process.

Fuzzy Categories

Real-world categories are not discrete, but at their boundaries tend to blend with each other, and often have overlapping features. For example, as categories, trucks and cars might be readily distinguishable, but for certain vehicles such as station wagons or off-road vehicles, the decision about appropriate placement may not be easy. Hence, when dealing with information systems such as expectancies, the typical psychometric requirement that scales (categories) be totally discrete and independent may be neither reasonable nor possible (see Goldman *et al.*, 1991). In fact, such characteristics of categories have been actually built into modern computer decision making in the form of "fuzzy" logic (Gupta and Yamakawa, 1988; Zimmerman, 1987).

Application of Cognitive Processes as Mediators of Alcohol and Drug Phenomena

Expectancy Operation

To tie expectancy concepts to recent theory in cognitive psychology, it is helpful to recall that Tolman (1932) originally posited expectancies to be specific memory content. It has been proposed (Goldman, 1989; Goldman *et al.*, 1991; Rather *et al.*, 1992) that alcohol (and drug) expectancies are essentially information about substance use and its consequences, acquired initially in an episodic format via modeling of parents and peer groups, and exposure to media. Expectancies are also acquired in episodic memory based upon one's own early experience with alcohol consumption. Though recent work suggests that all individuals may hold much the same range of expectancy content, the probability that such content may influence behavior is a function of differential experiences, due either to differences in family and peer usage of alcohol and drugs, or to differential personal reactivity to alcohol. Rather than completely remaining in episodic (autobiographical) format, an abstract representation of this information is stored in semantic format as pure information about alcohol and drug effects, which can be activated in connection with any alcohol- or drug-related situation.

To understand *how* these stored bits of information may influence ongoing behavior, it is helpful to borrow from the work of Newell (1973), Lang (1985), and Bower and Cohen (1982). The conceptualizations of these theorists would suggest that, in addition to expectancies of alcohol effects, memories of stimulus configurations (prototypes or exemplars) previously associated with alcohol use are also stored, as are memories of past emotions and motor patterns (essentially the "programs" for these behaviors). Such representations of emotional and motor patterns are also understood to be directly linked to actual physiological/emotional control mechanisms in the brain, which are, in turn, connected to peripheral autonomic mechanisms and skeletal muscle patterns. When the individual encounters an

external stimulus configuration that sufficiently matches a stored prototype or exemplar, the system is activated to produce drinking (or drug use)
behavior and associated emotional and motor activities. In other terms,
sufficient activation of alcohol and/or drug expectancies is presumed to
provide a "go" signal for actual substance use and its associated emotional/
motor behaviors. As we shall see subsequently, it is also possible that
activation of expectancies of sedation can actually give a "no-go" signal,
which influences the system to shut down. Such theorizing integrates well
with recent biopsychological theories that suggest that drug reinforcement
is associated with activation of brain neurochemical systems that normally mediate appetitive (approach) behavior (Gray, 1982; Panksepp, 1982;
Stewart *et al.*, 1984; Wise, 1988; Wise and Bozarth, 1987). Understood this
way, the expectancy memory system may operate largely in an automatic
fashion, without much conscious attention and decision making. Such
automatic operation does not, however, preclude top–down or (conceptual)
control that breaks in on automatic patterns to direct drinking episodes or
to curtail drinking.

With increasing drinking experience, it may be assumed that the behavioral repertoire associated with drinking becomes increasingly automatic
and a stereotyped cognitive (e.g., typical patterns of expectancy activation)
and motor sequence develops. Motor systems are involved in the move-
ments necessary for alcohol consumption, as is skeletal muscle activity,
which is both agonistic and antagonistic (e.g., behavioral tolerance) to
actual alcohol effects. At this point, the expectancy and motor sequences
can be regarded as automatic and residing in part in the procedural memory store. As a consequence, alterations of the drinking behavior become
more problematic and require considerable effort.

It is important to note that the presence of the chemical substance is not
required for activation of the above processes. All that is required is that a
stimulus be encountered that can activate this system. Such a stimulus
need not be the substrate itself. Hence, this type of theory can easily
explain placebo effects, as well as phenomena such as cue reactivity (which
is a kind of placebo effect in which the presence of the substance serves as
the stimulus cue) as well as substance abusers' subjective report of craving
and urges.

Cravings, Urges, and Tolerance

Also building upon Lang's (1985) conception of a propositional information network, Baker *et al.* (1987) offered a similar theory to model the
cognitive structure of urges. Baker *et al.* (1987) posited that urges are affective states and that two urge systems derive from the two components of

affect, positive-affect urges and negative-affect urges. The positive-affect urge system corresponds to the activation of the appetitive-motivational system (e.g., Gray, 1982; Panksepp, 1982; Wise, 1988) previously described. When stimulus conditions provide a sufficient match to the encoded information regarding previous drug use, the urge network will be activated and the person will report increased urges and positive affect leading to seeking out and self-administering drugs. In addition to drug availability, stimuli associated with prior drug use, a priming dose of the drug, and/or positive affect can "turn on" this system.

The negative-affect urge system is strongly associated with drug withdrawal. Conditioning processes in drug tolerance and drug dependence have been formulated in cognitive terms (Poulos and Cappell, 1991; Siegel, 1983; Siegel et al., 1988; Tiffany and Baker, 1986; Vogel-Sprott, 1992), and it has been suggested that such conditioned drug effects form the substrate of drug urges and cravings (Poulos et al., 1981). Siegel's (1975) theory of drug tolerance states that stimuli reliably paired with administration of a drug become conditioned stimuli that elicit behavioral responses opposite in direction to the direct effects of the drug. These "compensatory" responses dampen the direct drug effects, thereby resulting in reduction of the overall drug response (i.e., tolerance). Hence, presentation of the drug-related stimulus is theorized to cause activation of the information system relating to previous experience with the drug, which in turn triggers compensatory behavioral responses. It is presumed that activation of the compensatory response, in the absence of the drug, will be experienced as withdrawal and craving and increase the probability of drug use. The negative-affect urge system (Baker et al., 1987) then may trigger urges whenever any sort of negative affect is experienced, due to its subjective similarity to withdrawal effects. Baker and Tiffany (1985) argue that compensatory responses need not be posited as part of the mechanics of tolerance, but that habituation processes, based upon the decreased salience of cues that have already been stored in memory, can account for these effects. Poulos and Cappell (1991) suggest, however, that a comprehensive explanation of all drug tolerance effects does, in fact, require the postulation of compensatory responding, but in the more general context of activation of biological mechanisms of homeostasis.

Regardless of the precise substrate for tolerance, however, Tiffany (1990) carried cognition-dependent theorizing even further, noting that the correlations between physiological responses, self-reported urges, and observed drug use behavior are not strong. Building upon this disconnection between self-reported urges and drug consumption, Tiffany (1990) suggests that much of the urge system is essentially automatic (nonconscious). Therefore, activation of this system can *independently* trigger drug use behavior and/or self-reported urges. He goes on to indicate, based on theories of automaticity, that such automaticity in connection with urges develops through practice (in this case repeated use of a drug), that different processes are responsible in experienced and unexperienced subjects, that urges require consistent and unique stimulus conditions, and that some level of nonautomatic processing is always involved.

Cue Reactivity

Cue reactivity, which refers to measurable, behavioral effects that occur immediately after the presentation of a drug or alcohol stimulus cue, can also be brought within the explanatory net of a cognitive regulation system. Researchers have found that presentation of alcohol cues (e.g., smelling a preferred beverage) results in increased salivation in alcoholic but not in nonalcoholic subjects (Monti *et al.*, 1987; Pomerleau *et al.*, 1983). Both alcoholic and nonalcoholic subjects report greater urges to drink (Cooney *et al.*, 1987; Monti *et al.*, 1987) and increased expectations of pleasant alcohol effects (Cooney *et al.*, 1987) upon presentation of relevant alcohol cues. These events have been explained using Pavlovian conditioning models. But since Pavlovian conditioning has itself been explained using expectancy formulations (see Rescorla, 1988), an expectancy (cognitive) system is an obvious candidate for the development of theories of cue reactivity. From this perspective, alcohol cues would be thought to induce these behavioral effects by first activating a cognitive system. The particular pattern of behavioral effects for any given person would depend on the strength of activation and the nature of previously stored information.

Contributions from Cognitive Science to the Understanding of Cognitive Architecture

The above selected concepts from cognitive psychology serve to fill in gaps in our understanding of alcohol and substance abuse, and, as shall be seen later, generate new studies on these phenomena. Another line of thinking, more appropriately referred to as cognitive or information *science*, subsumes cognitive psychology, but also includes work from a variety of other fields such as computer science and linguistics (Simon and Kaplan, 1990). Some concepts emanating from cognitive science go beyond those from cognitive psychology in that models are tested on a computer for their capability to mimic behavioral functions. Proposed memory structures that store information and then utilize such information for the ongoing control of behavior have been referred to as cognitive architectures. After a brief review of historical and conceptual developments in this area that help explain the importance of this work, we shall present some possible models of the cognitive architecture for alcohol expectancies.

The Universal Machine

Prior to the years immediately before World War II, all machines were designed specifically for the unique task they were to perform. That is, their components were designed to perform specific functions, which might or might not be useful in any other machine. During World War II, Alan Turing began work on what would later be called the "universal machine," and which clearly had application to the development of computers. For the present purposes, however, it is important to appreciate that the concept of the universal machine had applicability far beyond the development of computers. This concept had direct bearing on models of human brain function. The essence of the universal machine was that it was a model for a mechanistic substructure that could be *programmed* and thereby configured to perform virtually any task. That is, the same fundamental machine could accomplish many different tasks, depending upon the instructions provided for it and the information available to it. Hence, the core of such a machine was flexibility of purpose; a model was provided that could handle many different kinds of problems presented to it, and could possibly even adapt (i.e., "learn") and develop in the face of changing environmental demands (Turing, 1950). Ideas about such architectures provide a fertile ground for developing initial models of the structures that control alcohol and drug use.

It remains possible, of course, that human brain function is totally unrelated to the manner in which a computer functions, but recent findings in cognitive and neural science suggest that some functional characteristics may be shared. For example, for any machine to have flexible output, it appears requisite that the machine process small units, or bits, of information. Storage and recombination of small units permit flexible assembly into larger, operational structures that can accomplish different functions (Pylyshyn, 1990). It may be instructive to contrast this emphasis on elementary units with the practice in some areas of psychology such as personality theory and psychopathology, to postulate complex constructs that are opaque as to operative mechanism (e.g., antisocial personality). In such cases, comprehensive understanding requires further specification of functional mechanisms. Intrinsic to the concept of the universal machine is the fact that the final productions of such a machine (e.g., behavioral analogues) derive from computations of some kind performed upon elemental units. The modeling of neural operation as a universal machine changes earlier conceptions of behavior as the product of reflex arcs to behavior as combinations of bits of information. It must, however, be recognized that even the concept of a simple reflex arc is inherently a computational model in which the computations are performed by physiological events that occur in successive neurons and across successive synapses. Hence, in a general sense, computational modeling should not be viewed as a radically new approach, but one that is quite readily integrated with other conceptions of human brain functioning and behavioral processing.

Basic Architectures

Although many variations in basic architecture have been proposed and actually used in computers and computer models, the present explication of cognitive processes in alcohol and drug abuse can be assisted by reducing these models to three highly simplified types. The vast majority of computers currently in operation employ Von Neumann architecture (named after the physicist who originally specified their design) (see Simon and Kaplan, 1990). Such architecture includes an addressable memory capable of storing both a program and data, input and output devices, and the capability of processing stored information. Computers based upon this design are fast because of high speed electronics, but always require serial (sequential) step-through of all operations. A greatly simplified version of the Von Neumann architecture is presented in Fig. 8.1.

To avoid the speed limitations intrinsic to serial processing, computer scientists and psychologists have also explored models in which information can be processed in a parallel fashion, so that many "pieces" of information can be handled simultaneously, with decisions arising from the overall pattern of information that results. Such a scheme can also be configured so that a central "director" (program and central processing unit) is not required, and control emanates from the relationship that develops among elementary units. As noted below, such configurations (which can be referred to as "networks") have appeal for the modeling of neural systems (or at least portions of such systems).

A number of aspects of human functioning have suggested models that have a network structure, which, depending on content, may be referred to as either connectionist or symbolic. One major characteristic of neural operation that has stimulated and constrained the development of such models is processing time. Since neurons operate in the time scale of milliseconds, human processes (the simplest of which take on the order of one hundred milliseconds) can only involve one hundred or so steps. Feldman (1985) has called this the "100-step program" constraint. Hence, all activities between simple neural events and overt behaviors must not require more than one hundred or so sequential processes. For instance,

Information Bits

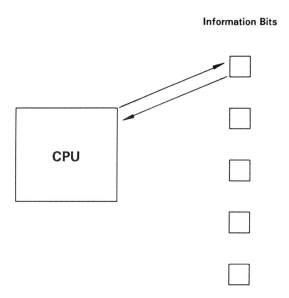

Figure 8.1.   Simplified version of a serial processing system.

although the act of recognition may appear simple from the vantage point of human behavior, the process requires the identification of a stimulus as a particular stimulus despite all its possible permutations (consider the various ways in which the letter *a* might be written); it is at present simply impossible to build a full recognition system in a serial format that takes only one hundred steps. This constraint requires that human neural functioning must involve considerable parallel processing through network structures: processing that can sample information from a large number of information storage points all in the first step and gradually assemble the information relevant to the particular stimulus configuration by narrowing down the combination of these elements over successive steps that could fit within the 100-step program constraint. A parallel or network system is depicted in Fig. 8.2.

Connectionist networks may be distinguished from symbolic systems by the information that is stored in each. Connectionist systems are essentially highly simplified and schematized neurons that are interconnected by a network. These "neurons," or elements in the network, simply have a capacity to either activate or not activate upon receipt of a prespecified pattern of stimulation. No "representation" of any "real-world" object or

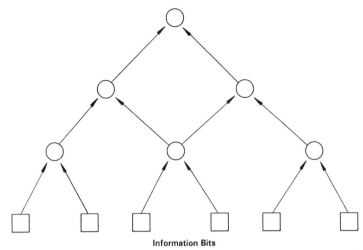

Information Bits

Figure 8.2.   Simplified version of a network or parallel processing system.

event is stored. The network adapts to carry out a particular function ("learns") by adjustments in the strengths of connections among the elements (see Gluck and Bower, 1988). In symbolic systems, the elements are symbols or representations of meanings. Once again, however, higher decision making depends on assemblies of these more molecular symbols stored at various locations in the network.

Another important distinction between these fundamental architectures is that the Von Neumann structure is essentially a "top–down" model in which a program must be provided to direct the operations that assemble larger structures. In both network approaches, assembly of more elementary bits of information into larger order structures can occur in a "bottom–up" fashion, that is, no higher order external direction is necessary, but rather the pattern of activation of elements determines the ultimate product. Consequently, an additional reason for favoring the network architecture for models of human functioning (apart from their speed of operation) is that these models preclude the need for higher order directors or "homunculi." Of course, it is quite possible that the functioning human system actually employs all variations on these architectures, possibly at different levels of functioning. For example, there may be a basic neural (biological hardware) level, a highly parallel connectionist level that translates neural functioning into computations, and a higher order symbolic level (Simon and Kaplan, 1990). The symbolic level may also be viewed as assembling even further into a higher order semantic or knowledge level (Pylyshyn, 1990). Hence, organized symbol structures or schemata may emerge at the top of this hierarchy from operations at levels more basic, which, in turn, feed back on (control) lower systems. Alternatively, top–down control of a system may be exercised by another system that has already assembled a "program" to direct the operations of the original system. The reader is recommended to read Simon and Kaplan (1990), Pylyshyn (1990), Newell *et al.* (1990), and Rumelhart (1990) for more detailed explication of these concepts.

Deciphering the Cognitive Architecture of Alcohol and Drug Use

To initiate inquiry into a possible architecture that is most useful for understanding the governance of alcohol and drug use and abuse, it is helpful to select a working model. For a variety of reasons, a network model would appear to be a good candidate for this initial model. As pointed out by Rather *et al.* (1992): (1) network models are parsimonious and do not require postulation of multiple independently measured constructs; (2) Network models are process oriented in that they go beyond prediction based upon linear combinations and variables and instead emphasize the process by which behavioral outcomes are controlled. Specifically, network models offer a mechanism for learning and flexibility based upon activation and strength of connections (Simon and Kaplan, 1990). Also, Newell (1973) notes that the huge variety that any organism encounters in the external world requires a system that can constantly be readjusted by integrating new elements. A network model is readily adaptable to such "combinatorial" memory structure and does not require a complete reconfiguration whenever new variations on stimulus configurations are encountered; and (3) network models are readily integrated with certain basic operations of the nervous system (Barinaga, 1990) and can provide a rather direct model for parallel processes that must operate in the eye, ear, and other parts of the brain (Simon and Kaplan, 1990). In fact, Chang (1986) recommends network theory as a useful general theory of cognitive representation from which more specific theories can be developed, including those that permit integration of processes that control emotional reactivity and motor programs (Lang, 1985). In his recent discussion of cognitive architecture, Estes (1991) averred that memory "traces can be viewed as vectors or lists, as nodes in network or as points in multidimensional space" (p. 12).

The point of entry into investigation of the cognitive architecture of alcohol and drug abuse, in keeping with Estes (1991), is to assume that information relevant to such use is stored in a multidimensional space or network. A further assumption is that elements to be entered into the network or multidimensional space have some measurable psychological distance from each other. That is, it is assumed that elements reside within a true Euclidean space and are therefore separated from each other by a Euclidean distance metric. Simply put, some elements are psychologically closer together than others, and are therefore more likely to be activated together. If such an assumption is made, techniques such as multidimensional scaling (MDS) and cluster analysis can be applied to determine their configuration. With MDS (Kruskal and Wish, 1978; Schiffman *et al.*, 1981) and cluster analysis (Johnson, 1967; Sneath and Sokal, 1973) elements can be located or "mapped" relative to each other in multidimensional space. Cluster analysis assumes no underlying dimensions, but instead determines what elements are located most closely to others, relative to all other elements being examined. This process shall be elaborated subsequently, but a quick review of MDS and clustering may assist understanding. As an example of MDS, if we were to take a group of major United States cities and provide a matrix of distances between them, MDS could be used to actually plot a map that would closely resemble a map of the United States. Specifically, a monotonic function is found using MDS algorithms, which locates each entry (city) in multidimensional space (which can be graphed) in relation to each other point. This "mapping" is then compared for "goodness of fit" to the relations among the entries as determined by the Euclidean distance inputs. Hierarchical cluster analysis, which also shall be used in some examples, does not assume a dimensional space, but instead groups elements in a hierarchical fashion based on their Euclidean distance. At the primary level, elements are grouped with other elements to which they are closest (according to a prespecified decision rule) and then, in turn, groups of elements are grouped with other groups of elements, and so on, until all elements constitute one overall hierarchical tree, which, as we shall see, looks much like a cognitive network.

The assumption of Euclidean distance as the metric among elements allows for a primary function of both MDS and clustering, that is, the graphic or pictorial representation of psychological elements. Such visual displays often provide an understanding of the processes that may govern the relationships among the elements that go beyond that which can be determined using traditional correlational techniques. Another advantage of these techniques is that their output can be used as a core element in a validational network that includes a divergent set of methods. Even true experiments can be built on findings from MDS and clustering and then carried out to test the consistency of such findings with the graphic representations. In relation to memory research, for example, distances between category elements determined by MDS have been used to successfully predict reaction times to judgments about whether items belong in a category (Rips *et al.*, 1973; Shoben, 1976), and to predict the order of recall of items in a free-recall situation (Caramazza *et al.*, 1976). Even more striking is that lists of items to be learned in free-recall paradigms can be organized to permit easier acquisition if the items are arranged in accord with distances determined by MDS solutions (Cooke *et al.*, 1986). Hence, there is good reason to believe that the "maps" generated using these methods actually reflect some unobservable psychological (associative) distance between elements (Nosofsky, 1992).

One other assumption is necessary before actual data sets can be examined. To provide content for entry into the MDS and cluster analytic procedures, it is assumed that the elements stored in the network are bits of information about emotional and behavioral consequences of alcohol use (if other drugs were the target, the outcomes of other drug use would be entered). These elements are essentially what have been called expectancies in earlier research on this topic. It must be understood, however, that unlike expectancies, which are defined as information about "if–then" relationships, the only information contained in these networks pertains to outcomes (the "then" portion of the expectancy). Alcohol use (the "if") is connected to these outcomes by a higher order architectural scheme. That is, it is assumed that when a stimulus associated with alcohol use sufficiently matches a stored representation of a signal for alcohol consumption (e.g., setting), the network of information relating to these outcomes becomes activated in some fashion. For the present purposes, we will assume a simple notion of spreading activation (Collins and Loftus, 1975), although a variety of types of activation could be specified.

In recent work (Rather *et al.*, 1992), expectancy elements were specified using a group of English words (usually adjectives) that were established by judges and statistical methods (coefficient alphas) to encompass or "bracket" the essential meaning of a particular expectancy. Expectancy elements (referred to as nodes in an information network) were defined in this manner because adjectives taken from the general English language lexicon have many different meanings that go well beyond their connection to alcohol or drug use. To preclude these extraneous meanings from obscuring their special meaning when connected to alcohol use, *multiple* items were included to define a *single* alcohol expectancy "meaning" (or in psychometric terms, to reduce measurement error).

Initial Empirical Modeling

At this point, mathematical procedures such as MDS and cluster analysis for modeling an alcohol expectancy network can be applied to these "isomeaning" expectancy elements. We explain the rationale for using these approaches instead of more traditional factor analytic techniques thus: flexibility of a machine to handle a wide variety of situations and to be adaptable to changing circumstances requires that information be stored in small units. The possibility of combining and recombining such units into higher order aggregations that are specifically organized in response to particular stimulus inputs allows for this ongoing adaptability. The basic assumption of factor analysis (excluding principal components) is just the opposite, namely, that operation of higher order unobserved (theoretical) variables is responsible for observed variation in lower order variables (responses to measured variables or "indicators"). Hence, factor analysis, or the search for common variance in a correlation matrix, may not be the most applicable approach to determining operational (molecular) elements. The problem is identical to that encountered by researchers attempting to understand intelligence. Consider Sternberg (1985), "First, the model of [mental] maps and the factor-analytic methods used to instantiate it had little, if anything, to say about mental processes. Yet, two individuals could receive the same score on a mental-ability test through very different processes, and indeed, by getting completely different items correct. . . ." (p. 1114).

It may be argued, of course, that each item on an alcohol expectancy instrument actually does reflect ("indicate") the central operation of some limited number of processes that manifest themselves in a variety of ways, and in differing situations. For example, if alcohol does have some fundamental capacity to influence anxiety mechanisms in a downward direction, then a variety of consequences such as relaxation, increased social assertiveness, or improved sexuality might emanate from this single, central process. While it is critical that we understand such central mechanisms (and factor analysis of expectancy lists might offer some insight into such mechanisms), the *operation* of expectancies may still be best understood as based on accumulated bits of information, stored in memory. These bits may be collected over time by each individual as a consequence of both vicarious and direct experience with the effects of alcohol. The reason for postulating this sort of operational mechanism is that the information-processing system that actually influences drinking is not likely to have direct access to basic physiological processes that produce (in part) subjective or observable alcohol effects; only *information about the specific manifestations of these processes* can be stored to influence future decision making. Complicating the picture still further, however, is the possibility that each individual organizes these separate pieces of information about consequences into higher order structures, that is, schemata, which are reflected in factor structure. Whether the best level of analysis for deciphering operational processes is ultimately at the molecular or molar level remains to be determined. However, the molecular approach is new to this field and offers as yet unexamined avenues for research.

Connected with this issue are the related topics of expectancy items as information elements versus "indicators," and item-response theory. While these topics are too extensive to elaborate in this context, it is sufficient to say that the above arguments are not meant to suggest that individual responses to expectancy items are error free and/or reflect precisely what is stored in memory. It is important to appreciate, however, that correlational and factor analytic techniques, while addressing the question of response error, have generally been of less utility for constructing operational models of cognitive functioning than computational models, which are based upon more basic elements or "bits" of information.

The construction of an observable, measurable, proxy for such "software elements" is, therefore, a fundamental step when undertaking empirical modeling of networks. As indicated by Simon and Kaplan (1990), the most basic elements may be simple pattern recognition elements coupled by weighted connections between these elements [as hypothesized in connectionist or parallel distributing processing (PDP) models]. Since expectancies have been researched to date at the semantic (or meaning) level, however, the most appropriate place to begin empirical modeling is at the symbolic (semantic) network level. (Such a network is *not* identical to traditional conceptions of semantic memory. Episodic information may also be stored in a network format.)

Our approach to the initial construction of elementary semantic units used category generation techniques (Battig and Montegue, 1969) that called for samples of relevant subjects to generate as many single words as possible that represented the emotional, social, and behavioral (motor) consequences of alcohol use. It is, of course, theorized that these words are connected to stored representations of prior direct or observed experiences with these effects. As noted above, item groups that would "bracket" a single common meaning most related to particular alcohol consequences were used. Individual items (four for each group) were presented in a Likert-style format, and the total score for all four items was used as an index of the strength of the expectation for that particular expectancy outcome. For psychometric reasons, each word used was allowed to appear in only one word group. (It must be recognized, however, that exclusive grouping is somewhat artificial because in normal operation, a network combines and recombines elements in such a way that some overlap may occur in the meaning of word groupings. Unique and completely distinctive meaning is also limited because word groupings would rarely, if ever, be activated alone in the absence of activation of other word groupings.) Since the meaning of each word grouping represents the intersection of the meanings of its elements, the distinctive meaning represented by each word group is referred to as a "node."

Once these hypothetical "nodes" have been constructed, a number of mathematical techniques can be applied to help decipher how they are likely stored in relation to each other. The subject set to which application is made can be humans in general, or various subsets of humans, such as individuals of different drinking level, gender, or age. As discussed earlier, these techniques, which include MDS and cluster analysis, assume a Euclidean metric. In some models (e.g., spreading activation), the coactivation of nodes as a function of distance is built into the fabric of the theory: nodes are presumably stimulated by a hypothetical "wave" of activation that spreads across the network in which they are located and diminishes over distance (Collins and Loftus, 1975). It is not necessary, however, to assume actual spread of activation across an actual physical space, but only that the Euclidean distance between nodes is reflective of the probability of their coactivation. It is also important to understand that these techniques are not necessarily mutually exclusive (or even mutually exclusive with factor analytic techniques, despite some different mathematical assumptions), but can be used together on the same data set to reveal and highlight different aspects of the corelationships.

In our recent paper using college students (Rather *et al.*, 1992), MDS procedures were used to locate expectancy nodes in multidimensional space according to their location on particular dimensions that represent some set of psychological characteristics that they possess. As seen in Fig. 8.3, the multidimensional scaling solution was quite revealing about the relational architecture of these expectancy nodes at the semantic level. A two-dimensional solution appeared to be best, with one dimension representing positive/prosocial to negative/antisocial characteristics, and the second dimension representing arousal to sedation. Most important, however, was the relationship (location) of the nodes to each other. Nodes representing partying and fun appeared close together (funny, energetic, sociable, jolly, verbal), with nodes representing sedation (mellow, sleepy) located farther away, and nodes representing negative effects (dangerous, unhappy, nervous, mean) located at the greatest distance. Ancillary procedures, which will not be elaborated here (PREFMAP; a multiple regression procedure), showed that all levels of drinkers associated first to the partying and prosocial effects, whereas aversive effects were quite remote associates (Rather *et al.*, 1992). Hence this MDS "mapping" showed that individuals seek positive effects from alcohol use, while being relatively undeterred by possible aversive outcomes. However, heavy drinkers also were less likely to see sedating effects as part of the outcome matrix,

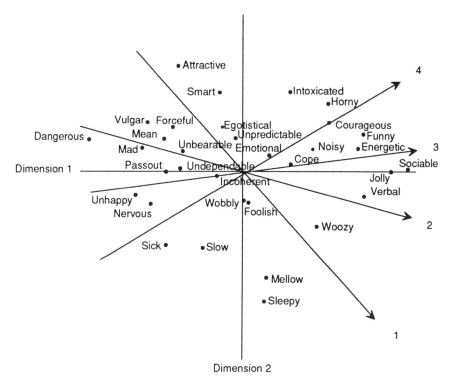

Figure 8.3 Multidimensional scaling of alcohol expectancy word groups (nodes) with PREFMAP preference vectors of four drinking groups. 1, Light drinkers; 2, light/moderate drinkers; 3, moderate/heavy drinkers; 4, heavy drinkers. (From Rather et al., 1992, p. 180. © 1992 by the American Psychological Association.)

whereas light drinkers had a relatively high association level to such sedating effects.

Cluster Analysis

Although MDS permits the visualization of the relationship among expectancy nodes, it assumes an underlying set of dimensions in order to locate nodes in multidimensional space. While each of these dimensions represents a psychological scale that characterizes aspects of these nodes, it is not necessary to assume that psychological dimensions are actually present in a hypothetical cognitive architecture that controls their activa-

Arbitrary Distance Units

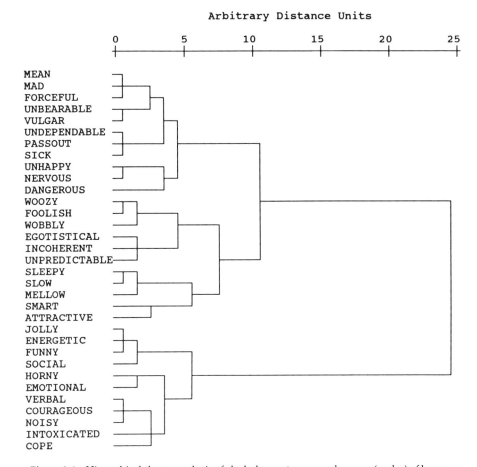

Figure 8.4 Hierarchical cluster analysis of alcohol expectancy word groups (nodes) of heavy drinkers.

tion. Furthermore, network structures are assumed to be hierarchical, with nodes assembling in ever larger groupings to determine overall meaning, as well as critical thresholds that will energize further effects. MDS, by itself, does not map the hierarchical structure of the hypothesized network. Other methods, falling under the heading of cluster analysis, also assume a Euclidean distance metric, but do not require the assumption of dimensionality and can permit hierarchical grouping of nodes. To demonstrate how cluster analytic methods can reveal a hierarchical network of expec-

Arbitrary Distance Units

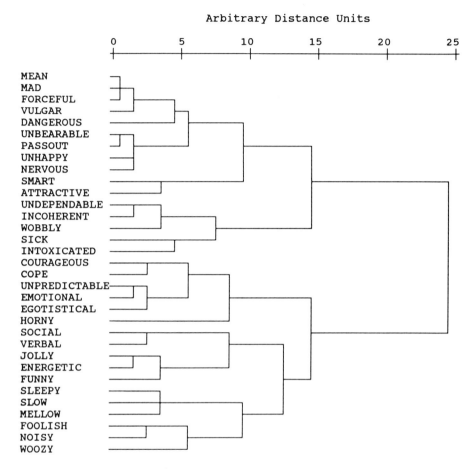

Figure 8.5 Hierarchical cluster analysis of alcohol expectancy word groups (nodes) of light drinkers.

tancies, Fig. 8.4 and Fig. 8.5 show separate cluster analyses for heavy and light drinkers (using a complete linkage method) performed on the same alcohol expectancy nodes as those that appeared in the above MDS solution (Rather *et al.*, 1992).

The most immediate impression upon examination of (the left side of) either figure is that nodes begin by joining other nodes in small groups (of two or three) and then these groups are, in turn, grouped together in ever enlarging clusters. At the final clustering, all elements are joined together.

The points at which clumpings of nodes join together are, of course, higher order nodes, which represent meanings that derive from the combined meanings of lower order nodes. The "dendrogram" or "hierarchical tree" shown in these clustering diagrams also depicts the psychological distance between nodes in the form of the length of the horizontal lines (in arbitrary units), which must be traversed before nodes are joined (either directly or after joining with other nodes). It may be hypothesized that the farther apart two nodes are, the less likely they are to be coactivated.

Simultaneous inspection of Fig. 8.4 and Fig. 8.5 reveals interesting contrasts between the hypothetical networks of heavy and light drinkers. It can be seen that the light drinkers require many more steps in distance before higher order joining occurs. In addition, even at the lowest order of assembly, a number of nodes of the heavy drinkers are joined after merely one step, whereas the lighter drinkers join few nodes after only one step, or even after a few steps. Even more striking is the overall configuration of the two dendrograms. The heavy drinkers (see the bottom of the figure) quickly group together a set of nodes reflecting sociability, fun, and arousal. Further, this grouping stands by itself, unconnected to all remaining expectancies of sedation and aversive effects until the last level of grouping in the hierarchy. Such an arrangement suggests that heavy drinkers quickly activate expectations of prosocial, "partying" like outcomes, and do not readily cross-connect such expectancies with either sedation or aversive effects. Contrast this structure with the light drinkers, who are not only less likely (note the longer distances) to coactivate the network, but immediately include expectations of sedation and silly behavior along with expectations of social and energizing outcomes at the first level of the network. Such structure suggests that light drinkers' network structure may serve to damp activation by incorporating expectations of sedation and unwanted outcomes into the configuration immediately upon any activation of the network. To extend this empirically based theorizing one step further, it may be judged from this structure that light drinkers' dampened expectancy networks are less likely to reach threshold levels of activation that would, in turn, trigger extensive further drinking and/or behavioral outcomes that would reinforce the use of alcohol.

Systematic Cross-Validation

Although highly informative about hypothetical network structure, the data used for the aforementioned MDS and clustering models were based upon subjects' responses to unipolar scaling of each expectancy word. That is, each word was presented to each subject separately. Subjects then rated their subjective probability of occurrence for each of these effects.

Scaling was then accomplished by comparing the subjective cumulative probability of each word group with the subjective cumulative probability of other word groups. [In simple terms, the total length of the line representing all four words in one group (node) was compared with the analogous line for each other group (node).] Although a quite legitimate means of assessing distance, this method is nevertheless indirect. A more direct method requires subjects to directly rate the similarities between each set of word pairs until all pairings have been exhausted. Such a procedure was, in fact, undertaken for the expectancy words noted above, and essentially replicated the structure described above (Rather and Goldman, 1991). Note that in the case of direct comparisons, it is not possible to use word groups because the matrix of comparisons of a large number of words with each other would require an unwieldy number of judgments for each subject. Hence, this systematic replication not only used direct comparisons but used only the single words most representative of the original word groups (nodes). Even with single word representation, the expectancy structure remained stable and comparable with the original structure. Comparability was not based on visual judgment, but also included regression analyses of MDS dimensions. (We will subsequently discuss how these hypothetical networks may suggest prevention and intervention strategies.)

Addition of Empirically Derived Networks to Cognitive Models

The visualization of expectancy networks allows us to amplify the cognitive models discussed earlier by using MDS and clustering. For example, these empirically derived models support the theory that the drinking and other behaviors demonstrated by heavy drinkers is in part related to differential cognitive structure. That is, heavy drinkers have both different and tighter (decreased distance) organization among expectancy nodes. Hence, it may be assumed that heavier drinkers have a variety of energizing and euphoric outcomes immediately accessible upon exposure to an alcohol-related stimulus complex. The activation of positive, social, and arousing expectancies without interference from aversive and sedating expectancies may, in turn, activate motor and affective systems that encourage further drinking and social and affectively arousing experiences. Hence, in heavier drinkers it appears that the pattern recognition elements that detect the presence of a drinking situation further trigger activation of expectancy elements that are related to more drinking, as well as to socially and affectively positive experiences. These, in turn, activate cognitive representations of the same affective and motor patterns, which, finally, are linked to peripheral autonomic and skeletal motor systems that actually produce the same behavioral patterns. Heavier drinkers' consumption appears to be little tempered by sedating and aversive effects, which are tightly grouped to each other, but organized quite separately from the activating effects. In contrast, light drinkers have expectations that can dampen drinking built into the structure of their empirically derived networks from the first level, so that ongoing drinking is modulated by competition among elements that are inconsistent regarding the affective and behavioral patterns that are triggered.

These differing structures are often reflected in the spontaneous remarks of alcoholic persons seen in treatment. A quite typical comment was made by a medical professional in his mid-thirties, who was being seen for after-work drinking that was excessive (approximately 6–8 shots of vodka each evening) to the point that his in-hospital performance the subsequent day was threatened. He said that his daily workload was intensely demanding, and he felt entitled to some fun at the end of each workday. Alcohol had long been involved with "partying" for him; his biggest difficulty in giving up drinking was his inability to create a sense of fun and excitement in the absence of alcohol. Note that he did not "party" in the conventional sense each evening. The sense of "partying" was due almost entirely to his use of alcohol. Without alcohol, each day was experienced solely as filled with the demand for his output, without any "payoff" that followed his efforts. Contrast this experience with individuals we all encounter who deliberately limit their alcohol consumption in a social gathering for fear that too much drinking will make them sleepy.

Theorizing derived from empirically derived models also permits linkage between the long- and short-term effects of expectancy operation. Long-term antecedents, such as childhood experiences, affect the storage of expectancy nodes. The resulting expectancy network is, in turn, available for activation proximate to a drinking occasion. The particular nodes that are most accessible then determine behavioral outcomes.

Structured in such a manner, ongoing regulation of drinking can be viewed as highly automatic, consistent with Tiffany's (1990) view of the operation of urges. (In this sense, urges may be merely a more subjectively extreme version of the processes that regulate all drinking.) Such a system does not require conscious attention and deliberation, particularly for heavy drinkers. The activation of relatively consistent positive, social, and energizing effects in heavy drinkers does not produce competition among nodes for final control of behavioral outcomes. Hence, no need arises in the system of the heavy drinker to reconcile divergent commands for top–down intervention. In contrast, competition and inconsistency among expectancy nodes in lighter drinkers may force more conscious attention to drinking decisions.

This type of theorizing leads to the possibility that one way of preventing and/or treating excessive alcohol use is to produce more competition and inconsistency among operational expectancy nodes. Our beginning efforts to produce such effects will be reviewed shortly. Although beyond the scope of this chapter, as well as the current level of progress in this area, it is important to note that these empirical methods for modeling expectancy networks may eventually permit the development of mathematical algorithms that can be tested in a computer for their ability to mimic drinking behavior and its attendant effects. The use of such computational algorithms is one basis for developing precise scientific theories about behavioral control. As shown by Nosofsky (1986, 1992) and others, scaling procedures based on Euclidean distances are readily adaptable to the development of computational models for category formation, and such models have already been proposed (e.g., ALCOVE; Kruschke, 1992).

Evidence for Automaticity

In a sense, the most compelling evidence for automatic operation of the aforementioned processes is the profound experience of "loss of control" that is a fundamental part of most concepts of addiction. In part, this term refers to the observation of drinking or drug use that persists in a self-destructive manner until some external force stops it (e.g., unconsciousness), but an essential ingredient in this concept is the sense of the user that he or she did not intend to drink or use substances to the degree that he/she in fact eventually did. Behavior displayed in the presence of only limited awareness and intention is the essence of automatic processing. Although the layperson's perception of behavior in the absence of awareness has always been with us (most of us can recall arriving home from work coupled with the memory that we had not the slightest realization of how we drove the route), cognitive psychology has offered some research designs that allow the testing of such automatic processing. The basic paradigm for demonstrating implicit memory is to present some stimulus that is not explicitly indicated to priming of the subject, or a stimulus that may even be totally unrecognized by the subject, and then to show that performance on a separate task is influenced. Although research demonstrating such implicit priming of alcohol or drug use is limited at this point, two recent studies in our laboratory serve to demonstrate the effect. The first study (Chenier and Goldman, 1992) used a fragment-completion task, which called for subjects to fill in missing letters in a list of word fragments. The word lists included fragments of both expectancy words and neutral words. Subjects completed these lists in what they thought was a location of convenience (a laboratory room). For some subjects this location included a considerable display of wall-mounted alcohol advertising, while for other subjects the room was kept visually sterile. Debriefing sessions showed that subjects remained unaware that these differences had any meaning for the study at hand. Nevertheless, subjects in the room with alcohol advertising successfully completed significantly more fragments of expectancy words than subjects in the neutral conditions. Although a variety of research designs have been developed to demonstrate automaticity, one key feature of automaticity is performance in the absence of attention and directed effort. This aspect of automaticity can be tested using implicit memory tasks such as the above fragment-completion task (Schacter, 1992).

Even more to the point, Roehrich and Goldman (1992) showed that implicit priming of alcohol expectancy stimuli could result in greater drinking. Subjects volunteered for what they thought was a study of learning and memory, in which they were called on to name the colors in which words were printed (i.e., the Stroop paradigm). Without any cuing of the subjects regarding this fact, the words used were either expectancy or neutral words. Subjects also were shown segments of the television shows "Cheers" or "Newhart" and were told they would be later asked to recall specific events in these shows. The presentation of expectancy versus neutral words and the "Cheers" (bar environment) versus "Newhart" (neutral environment) videos, were completely crossed in a 2 × 2 experimental design. Subjects were told they would be called on to complete the second phase of this study after a 30-minute wait. Each subject was then asked if, rather than just waiting for the 30 minutes, they would be interested in participating in an unrelated consumer survey to help pass the time. Almost all subjects agreed to such participation and moved down the hall to a room in which they were told their task was to taste-rate beverages that might be coffee, sparkling water, or beer. In actuality, all subjects were asked to taste beer in a standard taste-rating format (Marlatt and Rohsenow, 1980), which required them to provide their reactions to the taste of the beers (the beers were actually nonalcoholic).

In summary, the results of this study showed that subjects that had received expectancy words in the Stroop paradigm drank more beer than those receiving neutral words; those viewing the segment of "Cheers" drank even more; and those receiving both expectancy words and the "Cheers" segment drank the most. These effects were additive and independent, with each added alcohol stimulus producing a significant increment in drinking. Debriefing showed that subjects had no idea that the two experiments were connected (some subjects were even concerned that their consumption of beer in the consumer survey might somehow damage their ability to participate in the follow-up of the memory study).

These results support automatic processing of alcohol information. However, the demonstration of automatic control of drinking, even in social drinkers, does not rule out top–down or conceptual control. In fact, on an ongoing basis there is likely a dynamic, shifting balance between top–down and more automatic levels of control. Subjects may deliberately decide to go out and get "drunk" on a particular night, or may, conversely, decide that drinking is inappropriate for religious or other reasons and consequently avoid drinking. Nevertheless, this evidence does suggest that not all drinking is deliberately controlled in "social" drinkers. Since automatic control derives from experience (practice), it may also be that the more experience one has with drinking or even the more drinking-enhancing messages one receives (even in childhood prior to one's own drinking via observational learning), the more likely that drinking is not under volitional control. In effect, "loss-of-control" drinking may not be the purview of solely the "addict."

Expectancy Challenge

Since the above results indicate that a cognitive network can be activated to produce increased drinking, an obvious question is whether the same network can be manipulated to decrease drinking. Although it might be theoretically possible to manipulate the cognitive structure to produce deactivation (that is, place it closer to a resting state and further away from the threshold of further activation), one would not expect this temporary fluctuation in activation state to be a lasting effect. The more interesting possibility, and one having more obvious application to intervention and treatment, would be to challenge expectancies in order to alter the network in a way that would result in reduced drinking. Three recent studies directly address the possibility of challenging expectancies to alter drinking patterns, and four additional studies bear upon applying such challenge to intervention and prevention work. The first two of the three studies designed to lower drinking by challenging expectancies used female subjects and assisted with the development of challenge methods. The first of these studies (Henderson and Goldman, 1987) used a limited expectancy challenge procedure that consisted primarily of administration of a placebo alcohol beverage and subsequent disclosure of the placebo nature of this beverage after subjects had engaged in intoxicatedlike behavior. The context was a rating session of the attractiveness of males (appearing on slides taken from advertising copy), with the ostensible purpose of showing that alcohol use changes judgments of attractiveness. After subjects had not actually consumed alcohol, the women engaged in behaviors that they themselves were quite shocked to discover were the result of a placebo manipulation. The next study (Massey and Goldman, 1988; see Goldman *et al.*, 1991, p. 142) piloted a more extensive challenge, in which subjects were encouraged to attend to everyday cues that stimulate the formation of alcohol expectancies (such as alcohol advertising), and asked to undergo a challenge procedure in which subjects were told that they might or might not be receiving alcohol, but their job was to identify whom among them had received the alcohol. One hundred percent of subjects showed inaccuracies in their ability to identify subjects that actually received alcohol. Both studies found short-term decreases in drinking relative to control groups.

In the third and most extensive study to date (Darkes and Goldman, in press), the subjects were light- to heavy-drinking males, repeated challenge sessions were incorporated, and an instrument designed to measure short-term changes in expectancy was employed to see if changes in drinking paralleled changes in measured expectancies. As in the study by Massey and Goldman (1988), subjects were challenged to identify whom among them had actually received alcohol. Some males below legal drinking age were also included. These underage subjects were not administered beverages, but were also challenged to identify subjects who had actually received alcoholic beverages. As in earlier studies, the purpose of the challenge procedure was to undermine (lower the probability) of association between drinking and expectancy nodes. An additional purpose of this manipulation was to reinforce the competing interpretation that alcohol's social and sexual consequences may be, in part, placebo effects. Once again, the subjects receiving an expectancy challenge lowered their drinking in the two weeks subsequent to the manipulation, compared to control groups. Equally important, measured expectancies decreased to parallel decreases in drinking; those subjects that lowered their drinking decreased their expectancies, whereas subjects who did not lower drinking showed no change in expectancies.

Although these findings have obvious implications for prevention and intervention strategies, the absence of extensive, long-term follow-up precludes statements about their ultimate impact in this arena. These results are, however, consistent with the few prior reports of prevention and/or treatment using expectancy theory. Goldman and Klisz (1982) described the use of expectancy concepts in a single-case methodology. Brown *et al.* (1988), showed that VA patients with higher social and physical expectancies benefited more from social-skills training than patients with lower social expectancy scores (as measured by clinical ratings). Baer *et al.* (in 1991) have been incorporating with some success an expectancy challenge that is part of a multicomponent prevention program on a college campus, although no independent assessment of the effects of expectancy challenge was possible. Kraus *et al.* (1990) have recently suggested that the development of alcohol expectancies in elementary-aged school children can be slowed using films that attempt to undermine expectancies. It is important to point out that a critical aspect of expectancy challenge as a preventative or therapeutic modality is that it attempts to undermine incentive mechanisms. That is, it is presumed that altering the cognitive structure of individuals will directly alter the mechanisms that control drinking. Contrast this approach with most existing prevention and intervention strategies that attempt to suppress incentive-driven behavior ("Just Say No," "Alcohol is Destroying Your Life"). This difference is best characterized by the comment of a recent subject who returned for follow-up evaluation after participating in an expectancy challenge program (Darkes and Goldman, in press): "You guys sure took all the fun out of my drinking. Every time I took a drink I felt as though I was kidding myself if I let go and partied."

CONCLUSION

This chapter attempts to demonstrate the increasing convergence between theories originally articulated to account for different aspects of alcohol and drug use and abuse (e.g., risk carry-over, tolerance, craving), but which have begun to blend with each other as gaps in our knowledge base are filled. The use of expectancy formulations to explain both animal and human research on behavioral tolerance is particularly noteworthy in this regard. A number of other theories could be considered cognitive in nature, but were not included in this chapter because they do not easily fit within this theoretical fabric and/or are variants of covered approaches. Such theories, for example, coping theory, some aspects of personality theory, self-awareness theory, and self-handicapping theory should be examined for a complete understanding of this research area (see Blane and Leonard, 1987). It should be obvious that the latter portions of this chapter represent new approaches in this field, which are as yet insufficiently supported by research to allow for much confidence in their eventual utility. Nevertheless, they do follow significant advances in other areas of cognitive science, and will hopefully offer as much direction for substance abuse research as they have in their original areas of application.

It would be of obvious benefit to the field if the wide array of risk factors recently identified in the alcohol and substance abuse arena could be reduced to a few pathways of actual influence over consumption and addiction so that our capacity to understand these processes can be improved. It is also of obvious advantage if these pathways can be accessed for prevention and intervention efforts. Approaches based on cognitive science offer just this sort of possibility.

ACKNOWLEDGMENTS

Portions of this research were supported by National Institute on Alcohol Abuse and Alcoholism Grants RO1AA05946, RO1AA06123, and R37AA08333 to Mark S. Goldman. Appreciation is expressed to Jack Darkes, who reviewed the manuscript, and Yvette Myers, who did the typing.

REFERENCES

Alexopoulus, G. S., Lieberman, K. W., and Frances, R. J. (1983). Platelet MAO activity in alcoholic patients and their first degree relatives. *American Journal of Psychiatry, 140*, 1501–1504.

Allan, A. M., and Harris, R. A. (1987). Acute and chronic ethanol treatments alter GABA receptor-operated chloride channels. *Pharmacology Biochemistry Behavior, 27* 665–670.

Alloy, L. B., and Tabachnik, N. (1984). Assessment of covariation by humans and animals: The joint influence of prior expectations and current situational information. *Psychological Review, 91*, 112–149.

Anderson, J. R. (1983). A spreading activation theory of memory. *Journal of Verbal Learning and Verbal Behavior, 22*, 261–295.

Baer, J. S., Kivlahan, D. R., Fromme, K., and Marlatt, G. A. (in press). Secondary prevention of alcohol abuse with college student populations: A skills training approach. In *Self-control and the addictive behaviors* N. Heather, W. R. Miller, and L. Greeley (eds.), (pp. 339–356). New York: MacMillan.

Baker, T. B., and Tiffany, S. T. (1985). Morphine tolerance as habituation. *Psychological Review, 92*, 78–108.

Baker, T. B., Morse, E., and Sherman, J. E. (1987). The motivation to use drugs: A psychobiological analysis of urges. In P. Clayton Rivers (Ed.), *Alcohol and addictive behavior: Nebraska symposium on motivation 1986* (pp. 257–323). Lincoln, NE: University of Nebraska Press.

Bandura, A. (1977). *Social learning theory.* Englewood Cliffs, NJ: Prentice-Hall.

Bandura, A. (1985). *Social foundations of thought and action.* Englewood Cliffs, NJ: Prentice-Hall.

Barinaga, M. (1990). The mind revealed? *Science, 249*, 856–858.

Barnes, D. M. (1988). The biological tangle of drug addiction. *Science, 241*, 415–417.

Barnes, G. M. (1977). The development of adolescent drinking behavior: An evaluative review of the impact of the socialization process within the family. *Adolescence, 12*, 572–589.

Baron, R. M., and Kenny, D. A. (1986). The moderator-mediator variable distinction in social psychological research: Conceptual, strategic and statistical considerations. *Journal of Personality and Social Psychology, 51*, 1173–1182.

Battig, W. F., and Montague, W. E. (1969). Category norms for verbal items in 56 categories: A replication and extension of the Connecticut category norms. *Journal of Experimental Psychology Monograph, 80*, Part 2, 1–46.

Begleiter, H., and Porjesz, B. (1988). Potential biological markers in individuals at high risk for alcoholism. *Alocholism, 12*, 488–493.

Benson, C. S., and Heller, K. (1987). Factors in the current adjustment of young adult daughters of alcoholic and problem drinking fathers. *Journal of Abnormal Psychology, 90*, 305–312.

Birnbaum, I. M., Johnson, M. K., Hartley, J. T., and Taylor, T. H. (1980). Alcohol and elaborative schemas for sentences. *Journal of Experimental Psychology: Human Learning and Memory, 6*, 293–300.

Blane, H. T., and Leonard, K. E. (Eds.). (1987). *Psychological theories of drinking and alcoholism*. New York: Guildford.

Blum, K., Noble, E. P., Sheridan, P. J., Montgomery, A., Ritchie, T., Jagadeeswaran, P., Nogami, H., Briggs, A. H., and Cohn, J. B. (1990). Allelic association of human dopamine D_2 receptor gene in alcoholism. *Journal of the American Medical Association, 263*, 2055–2060.

Bolles, R. C. (1972). Reinforcement, expectancy, and learning. *Psychological Review, 79*, 394–409.

Bower, G. H., and Cohen, P. R. (1982). Emotional influences in memory and thinking: Data and theory. In M. Clark and S. Fiske (Eds.), *Affect and cognition* (pp. 291–331). Hillsdale, NJ: Erlbaum.

Brandon, T. H., and Baker, T. B. (1992). The smoking consequences questionnaire: The subjective utility of smoking in college students. *Psychological Assessment: A Journal of Consulting and Clinical Psychology, 3*, 484–491.

Brown, S. A. (1985a). Expectancies versus background in the prediction of college drinking patterns. *Journal of Consulting and Clinical Psychology, 53*, 123–130.

Brown, S. A. (1985b). Reinforcement expectancies and alcoholism treatment outcome after a one-year follow-up. *Journal of Studies on Alcohol, 46*, 304–308.

Brown, S. A., Goldman, M. S., and Christiansen, B. A. (1985). Do alcohol expectancies mediate drinking patterns of adults? *Journal of Consulting and Clinical Psychology, 53*, 512–519.

Brown, S. A., Creamer, V. A., and Stetson, B. A. (1987). Adolescent alcohol expectancies in relation to personal and parental drinkig patterns. *Journal of Abnormal Psychology, 96*, 117–121.

Brown, S. A., Millar, A., and Passman, L. (1988). Utilizing expectancies in alcohol treatment. *Psychology of Addictive Behavior, 2*, 59–65.

Burk, J. P., and Sher, K. J. (1988). The "forgotten children" revisited: Neglected areas of COA research. *Clinical Psychology Review, 8*, 285–302.

Burkett, S. R. (1980). Religiosity, beliefs, normative standards and adolescent drinking. *Journal of Studies on Alcohol, 41*, 662–671.

Cahalan, D., and Cisin, I. H. (1968). American drinking practice: A summary of findings from a national probability sample. I. Extent of drinking by population subgroups. *Quarterly Journal of Studies on Alcohol, 29*, 130–151.

Caramazza, A., Hersh, H., and Torgerson, W. S. (1976). Subjective structures and operations in semantic memory. *Journal of Verbal Learning and Verbal Behavior, 15*, 103–117.

Carver, C. S., and Scheier, M. F. (1990). Origins and functions of positive and negative affect: A control process view. *Psychological Review, 97*, 19–35.

Celentano, J. J., Gibbs, T. T., and Farb, D. H. (1988). Ethanol potentiates GABA- and glycine-induced chloride currents in chick spinal cord neurons. *Brain Research, 455*, 377–380.

Chang, T. M. (1986). Semantic memory: Facts and models. *Psychological Bulletin, 99*, 199–220.

Chenier, G., and Goldman, M. S. (1992). *Implicit priming of an alcohol expectancy network*. Paper presented at the 100th Annual Meeting of the American Psychological Association, Washington, D.C.

Christiansen, B. A., and Goldman, M. S. (1983). Alcohol-related expectancies versus demographic/background variables in the prediction of adolescent drinking. *Journal of Consulting and Clinical Psychology, 51*, 249–257.

Christiansen, B. A., Goldman, M. S., and Inn, A. (1982). Development of alcohol-related expectancies in adolescents: Separating pharmacological from social-learning influences. *Journal of Consulting and Clinical Psychology, 50*, 336–344.

Christiansen, B. A., Smith, G. T., Roehling, P. V., and Goldman, M. S. (1989). Using alcohol expectancies to predict adolescent drinking behavior at one year. *Journal of Consulting and Clinical Psychology, 57,* 93–99.

Cloninger, C. R. (1987). Neurogenetic adaptive mechanisms in alcoholism. *Science, 236,* 410–416.

Cloninger, C. R. (1991). D_2 dopamine receptor gene is associated but not linked with alcoholism. *Journal of the American Medical Association, 266,* 1833–1834.

Collins, A. M., and Loftus, E. F. (1975). A spreading-activation theory of semantic processing. *Psychological Review, 82,* 407–428.

Cooke, N. M., Durso, F. T., and Schvaneveldt, R. W. (1986). Recall and measures of memory organization. *Journal of Experimental Psychology: Learning, Memory, and Cognition, 12,* 538–549.

Connors, G. J., Tarbox, A. R., Faillace, L. A. (1990). *Changes in alcohol expectancies and drinking behavior among treated problem drinkers.* Paper presented at the Annual Meeting of the American Psychological Association, Boston, Massachusetts.

Cooney, N. L., Gillespie, R. A., Baker, L. H., and Kaplan, R. F. (1987). Cognitive changes after alcohol cue exposure. *Journal of Consulting and Clinical Psychology, 55,* 150–155.

Cronbach, L. J., and Meehl, P. E. (1955). Construct validity in psychological tests. *Psychological Bulletin, 52,* 281–302.

Darkes, J., and Goldman, M. S. (in press). Expectancy challenge and drinking reduction: Experimental evidence for a mediational process. *Journal of Consulting and Clinical Psychology.*

Donovan, J. E., Jessor, R., and Jessor, L. (1983). Problem drinking in adolescence and young adulthood. A follow-up study. *Journal of Studies on Alcohol, 44,* 109–137.

Estes, W. K. (1991). Cognitive architectures from the standpoint of an experimental psychologist. *Annual Review of Psychology, 42,* 1–28.

Feldman, J. A. (1985). Connectionist models and their applications: Introduction. *Cognitive Science, 9,* 1–2.

Fillmore, M., and Vogel-Sprott, M. (1992). Expected effect of caffeine on motor performance predicts the type of response to placebo. *Psychopharmacology, 106,* 209–214.

Ford, M. E. (1987). *Humans as self-constructing living systems: A developmental perspective on behavior and personality.* Hillsdale, NJ: Erlbaum.

Gabrielli, W. F., Mednick, S. A., Volavka, J., Pollock, V. E., Schulsinger, F., and Itil, T. M. (1982). Electroencephalograms in children of alcoholic fathers. *Psychophysiology, 19,* 404–407.

Gaines, L. S., Brooks, P. H., Maisto, S., Dietrich, M., and Shagena, M. (1988). The development of children's knowledge of alcohol and the role of drinking. *Journal of Applied Developmental Psychology, 9,* 441–457.

George, W. H., Derman, K. H., and Nochajski, T. H. (1989). Expectancy set, self-reported expectancies, and predispositional traits: Predicting interest in violence and erotica. *Journal of Studies on Alcohol, 50,* 541–551.

George, W. H., Raynor, J. O., and Nochajski, T. H. (1990). Resistance to alcohol impairment of visual–motor performance: II. Effects of attentional set and self-reported concentration. *Pharmacology, Biochemistry, and Behavior, 36,* 261–266.

Glantz, M., and Pickens, R. (Eds.). (1992). *Vulnerability to drug abuse.* Washington, D.C.: American Psychological Association.

Glowa, J. R., Crawley, J., Suzdak, P. D., and Paul, S. M. (1989). Ethanol and the GABA receptor complex: Studies with the partial inverse benzodiazepine receptor agonist Ro 15-4513. *Pharmacology, Biochemistry, & Behavior, 31,* 767–772.

Gluck, M. A., and Bower G. H. (1988). Evaluating and adaptive network model of human learning. *Journal of Memory and Language, 27,* 166–195.

Goldman, M. S. (1989). Alcohol expectancies as cognitive-behavioral psychology: Theory and practice. In T. Loberg, W. R. Miller, P. E. Nathan, and G. A. Marlatt (Eds.), *Addictive behaviors: Prevention and early intervention* (pp. 11–30). Amsterdam: Swets & Zeitlinger.

Goldman, M. S., and Klisz, D. K. (1982). Behavioral treatment of an alcoholic: The unvarnished story. In W. M. Hay and P. E. Nathan (Eds.), *Clinical case studies in the behavioral treatment of alcoholism* (pp. 23–48). New York: Plenum.

Goldman, M. S., Brown, S. A., and Christiansen, B. A. (1987). Expectancy theory: thinking about drinking. In H. T. Blane and K. E. Leonard (Eds.), *Psychological theories of drinking and alcoholism* (pp. 181–226). New York: Guilford Press.

Goldman, M. S., Brown, S. A., Christiansen, B. A., and Smith, G. T. (1991). Alcoholism etiology and memory: Broadening the scope of alcohol expectancy research. *Psychological Bulletin, 110*, 137–146.

Graf, P., and Mandler, G. (1984). Activation makes words more accessible, but not necessarily more retrievable. *Journal of Verbal Learning and Verbal Behavior, 23*, 553–568.

Gray, J. A. (1982). *The neuropsychology of anxiety: An inquiry into the functions of the septohippocampal system*. New York: Oxford University Press.

Greenberg, D. A., Cooper, E. C., Gordon, A., and Diamond, I. (1984). Ethanol and the gammaaminobutyric acid-benzodiazepine receptor complex. *Journal of Neurochemistry, 42*, 1062–1968.

Gupta, M. M., and Yamakawa, T. (Eds.). (1988). *Fuzzy logic in knowledge-based systems, decision, and control*. Amsterdam: Elsevier.

Harada, S., Agarwahl, D. P., Goedde, H. W., Tagaki, S., and Ishikawa, B. (1982). Possible protective role against alcoholism for aldehyde dehydrogenase isoenzyme deficiency in Japan. *Lancet, 2*, 827.

Harfond, T. C., and Mills, G. S. (1978). Age-related trends in alcohol consumption. *Journal of Studies on Alcohol, 39*, 207–210.

Harfond, T. C., and Spiegler, D. L. (1983). Developmental trends of adolescent drinking. *Journal of Studies on Alcohol, 44*, 181–188.

Hasher, L., and Zacks, R. T. (1979). Automatic and effortful process in memory. *Journal of Experimental Psychology: General, 108*, 356–388.

Hawkins, J. D., Catalano, R. F., and Miller, J. Y. (1992). Risk and protective factors for alcohol and other drug problems in adolescence and early adulthood: Implications for substance abuse prevention. *Psychological Bulletin, 112*, 64–105.

Henderson, M. A., and Goldman, M. S. (1987). *Effect of a social manipulation on expectancies and subsequent drinking*. Paper presented at the annual meeting of the Association for Advancement of Behavior Therapy Convention, Boston, MA.

Hoffman, P. L., Rabe, C. S., Moses, F., and Tabakoff, B. (1989). N-Methyl-D-Aspartate receptors and ethanol: Inhibition of calcium flux and cyclic GMP production. *Journal of Neurochemistry, 52*, 1937–1940.

Hull, J. G., and Bond, C. F. (1986). Social and behavioral consequences of alcohol consumption and expectancy: A meta-analysis. *Psychological Bulletin, 99*, 347–360.

Jaffe, A. (1992). Cognitive factors associated with cocaine abuse and its treatment: An analysis of expectancies of use. In T. Kosten and H. Kieber (Eds.), *Clinicians guide to cocaine addiction* (pp. 128–150). New York: Guilford Press.

Jaffe, A. J., Kilbey, M. M., and Rosenbaum, G. R. (1989). Cocaine related expectancies: Their domain and implications for treatment. *Pharmacology, Biochemistry, & Behavior, 32*, 1094.

James, W. (1983). *The principles of psychology*. Cambridge, MA: Harvard University Press. (Original work published).

Jessor, R., and Jessor, S. L. (1975). Adolescent development and the onset of drinking: A longitudinal study. *Journal of Studies on Alcohol, 36*, 27–51.

Johnson, S. C. (1967). Hierarchical clustering schemes. *Psychometrika, 32,* 241–254.

Jones, E. E. (1986). Interpreting interpersonal behavior: The effects of expectancies. *Science, 234,* 41–46.

Josephs, R. A., and Steele, C. M. (1990). The two faces of alcohol myopia: Attentional mediation of psychological stress. *Journal of Abnormal Psychology, 99,* 115–126.

Kirsch, I. (1985). Response expectancy as a determinant of experience and behavior. *American Psychologist, 40,* 1189–1202.

Kirsch, I. (1990). *Changing expectations: A key to effective psychotherapy.* Pacific Grove, CA: Brooks/Cole.

Knight, L. J., Barbaree, H. E., and Boland, F. J. (1986). Alcohol and the balanced-placebo design: The role of experimenter demands in expectancy. *Journal of Abnormal Psychology, 95,* 335–340.

Knupfer, G., and Room, R. (1967). Drinking patterns and attitudes of Irish, Jewish and White Protestant American men. *Quarterly Journal of Studies on Alcohol, 28,* 676–699.

Kraus, D., Smith, G. T., and Ratner, H. H. (1990). *Modifying alcohol-related expectancies in school-aged children.* Paper presented at the annual meeting of the American Psychological Association, Boston, MA.

Kruschke, J. K. (1992). ALCOVE: An exemplar-based connectionist model of category learning. *Psychological Review, 99,* 22–44.

Kruskal, J. B., and Wish, M. (1978). *Multidimensional scaling.* (Sage University Paper series on Quantitative Applications in the Social Sciences, #07-011). London: Sage Publications.

Lang, P. J. (1985). The cognitive psychophysiology of emotion: Fear and anxiety. In A. H. Tuma and J. D. Maser (Eds.), *Anxiety and anxiety disorders.* Hillsdale, NJ: Erlbaum.

Leigh, B. C. (1989). In search of the seven dwarves: Issues of measurement and meaning in alcohol expectancy research. *Psychological Bulletin, 105,* 361–373.

Levine, B., and Goldman, M. S. (1989). *Situational variations in expectancies.* Paper presented at the 97th Annual Meeting of the American Psychological Association, New Orleans, LA.

Logan, G. D. (1988). Toward an instance theory of automatization. *Psychological Review, 95,* 492–527.

MacCorquodale, K. M., and Meehl, P. E. (1954). Preliminary suggestions as to a formalization of expectancy theory. *Psychological Review, 60,* 53–60, 125–129.

MacDonald, D. I., and Blume, S. B. (1986). Children of alcoholics. *American Journal of Diseases of Children, 140,* 750–754.

Margulies, R. Z., Kessler, R. C., and Kandel, D. B. (1977). A longitudinal study of onset of drinking among high school students. *Quarterly Journal of Studies on Alcohol, 38,* 879–912.

Marlatt, G. A., and Rohsenow, D. J. (1980). Cognitive processes in alcohol use: Expectancy and the balanced placebo design. In N. K. Mello (Ed.), *Advances in substance abuse: Behavioral and biological research* (pp. 159–199). Greenwich, CT: JAI Press.

Massey, R., and Goldman, M. S. (1988). *Manipulating expectancies as a means of altering alcohol consumption.* Paper presented at the 96th annual convention of the American Psychological Association, Atlanta, GA.

Meyer, D. E., and Schvaneveldt, R. W. (1971). Facilitation in recognizing pairs of words: Evidence of a dependence between retrieval operations. *Journal of Experimental Psychology, 90,* 227–234.

Miller, D. T., and Turnbull, W. (1986). Expectancies and interpersonal process. *Annual Review of Psychology, 37,* 233–256.

Miller, P. M., Smith, G. T., and Goldman, M. S. (1990). Emergence of alcohol expectancies in childhood: A possible critical period. *Journal of Studies on Alcohol, 51,* 343–349.

Mischel, W. (1973). Toward a cognitive social learning reconceptualization of personality. *Psychological Review, 80*, 252–283.

Monti, P. M., Binkoff, J. A., Abrams, D. B., Zwick, W. R., Nirenberg, T. D., and Liepman, M. R. (1987). Reactivity of alcoholics and nonalcoholics to drinking cues. *Journal of Abnormal Psychology, 96*, 122–126.

Morrow, A. L., Suzdak, P. D., Karanian, J. W., and Paul, S. M. (1988). Chronic ethanol administration alters gamma-aminobutyric acid, pentobarbital and ethanol-mediated 36Cl-uptake in cerebral cortical synaptoneurosomes. *Journal of Pharmacology and Experimental Therapy, 246*, 158–164.

Moskowitz, H., and DePry, D. (1968). Differential effect of alcohol on auditory vigilance and divided attention. *Quarterly Journal of Studies on Alcohol, 29*, 54–63.

Murray, R. M., Clifford, C. A., and Gurling, H. M. D. (1983). Twin adoption studies: How good is the evidence for a genetic role. In M. Galanter (Ed.), *Recent developments in alcoholism* (pp. 25–48). New York: Plenum.

Newell, A. (1973). Production systems: Models of control structures. In W. G. Chase (Ed.), *Visual information processing* (pp. 463–526). New York: Academic Press.

Newell, A., Rosenbloom, P. S., and Laird, J. E. (1990). Symbolic architectures of cognition. In M. I. Posner (Ed.), *Foundations of cognitive science* (pp. 93–131). Cambridge, MA: MIT Press.

Newlin, D. B. (1989). The skin-flushing response: Autonomic, self-report, and conditioned responses to repeated administrations of alcohol in Asian men. *Journal of Abnormal Psychology, 98*, 421–425.

Newlin, D. B., and Thomson, J. B. (1990). Alcohol challenge with sons of alcoholics: A critical review and analysis. *Psychological Bulletin, 108*, 383–402.

Noble, E. P., Blum, K., Ritchie, T., Montgomery, A., and Sheridan, P. J. (1991). Allelic association of the D_2 dopamine receptor gene with receptor-binding characteristics in alcoholism. *Archives of General Psychiatry, 48*, 648–654.

Noll, R. B., Zucker, R. A., and Greenberg, G. S. (1990). Identification of alcohol by smell among preschoolers: Evidence for early socialization about drugs occurring in the home. *Child Development, 61*, 1520–1527.

Nosofsky, R. M. (1986). Attention, similarity, and identification-categorization relationship. *Journal of Experimental Psychology: General, 115*, 39–57.

Nosofsky, R. M. (1992). Similarity scaling and cognitive process models. *Annual Review of Psychology, 43*, 25–53.

Pandina, R. J., Johnson, V., and Labouvie, E. W. (1992). Affectivity: A central mechanism in the development of drug dependence. In M. Glantz and R. Pickens (Eds.), *Vulnerability to drug abuse* (pp, 179–209). Washington, D.C.: American Psychological Association.

Panksepp, J. (1982). Toward a general psychobiological theory of emotions. *Behavior Brain Science, 5*, 407–467.

Peele, S. (1986). The implications and limitations of genetic models of alcoholism and other addictions. *Journal of Studies on Alcohol, 47*, 63–73.

Pollock, V. E., Volavka, J., and Goodwin, D. W. (1983). The EEG after alcohol administration in men at risk for alcoholism. *Archives of General Psychiatry, 40*, 857–861.

Pomerleau, O. F., Fertig, J., Baker, L., and Cooney, N. L. (1983). Reactivity to alcohol cues in alcoholics and nonalcoholics: Implications for a stimulus control analysis of drinking. *Addictive Behaviors, 8*, 1–10.

Projesz, B., and Begleiter, H. (1985). Human brain electrophysiology and alcoholism. In R. E. Tarter and D. H. van Thiel (Eds.), *Alcohol and the brain* (pp. 139–182). New York: Plenum.

Poulos, C. W., and Cappell, H. (1991). Homeostatic theory of drug tolerance: A general model of physiological adaptation. *Psychological Review, 98*, 390–408.

Poulos, C. W., Hinson, R. and Siegel, S. (1981). The role of Pavlovian processes in drug tolerance and dependence: Implications for treatment. *Addictive Behaviors, 6*, 205–211.

Pylyshyn, Z. W. (1990). Computing in cognitive science. In M. I. Posner (Ed.), *Foundations of cognitive science* (pp. 49–91). Cambridge, MA: MIT Press.

Rather, B. C., and Goldman, M. S. (1991). *Differences in the memory organization and structure of alcohol expectancies*. Paper presented at the 99th Annual Meeting of the American Psychological Association, San Francisco, CA.

Rather, B. C., and Sherman, M. F. (1989). Relationship between alcohol expectancies and length of abstinence among Alcoholics Anonymous members. *Addictive Behaviors, 14*, 531–536.

Rather, B. C., Goldman, M. S., Roehrich, L., and Brannick, M. (1992). Empirical modeling of an alcohol expectancy memory network using multidimensional scaling. *Journal of Abnormal Psychology, 101*, 174–183.

Rescoria, R. A. (1988). Pavlovian conditioning. *American Psychologist, 43*, 151–160.

Rips, L. J., Shoben, E. J., and Smith, E. E. (1973). Semantic distance and the verification of semantic relations. *Journal of Verbal Learning and Verbal Behavior, 12*, 1–20.

Roehling, P. V., and Goldman, M. S. (1987). Alcohol expectancies and their relationship to actual drinking experiences. *Psychology of Addictive Behaviors, 1*, 108–113.

Roehrich, L., and Goldman, M. S. (1992). *Priming the pump: Alcohol expectancy activation increases drinking behavior*. Paper presented at the 100th Annual Meeting of the American Psychological Association, Washington, D.C.

Rohsenow, D. J., and Bachorowski, J. A. (1984). Effects of alcohol and expectancies on verbal aggression in men and women. *Journal of Abnormal Psychology, 93*, 418–432.

Rosen, L. J., and Lee, C. L. (1976). Acute and chronic effects of alcohol use on organizational processes in memory. *Journal of Abnormal Psychology, 85*, 309–317.

Ross, D. F., and Pihl, R. O. (1988). Alcohol, self-focus and complex reaction-time performance. *Journal of Studies on Alcohol, 49*, 115–125.

Rotter, J. B. (1954). *Social learning and clinical psychology*. New York: Prentice-Hall.

Rumelhart, D. E. (1990). The architecture of mind: A connectionist approach. In M. I. Posner (Ed.), *Foundations of cognitive science* (pp. 49–91). Cambridge, MA: MIT Press.

Russell, M., Henderson, C., and Blume, S. (1985). *Children of alcoholics: A review of the literature*. New York: Children of Alcoholics Foundation.

Schacter, D. L. (1992). Understanding implicit memory: A cognitive neuroscience approach. *American Psychologist, 47*, 559–569.

Schafer, J., and Brown, S. A. (1991). Marijuana and cocaine effect expectancies and drug use patterns. *Journal of Consulting and Clinical Psychology, 59*, 558–565.

Schiffman, S. S., Reynolds, M. L., and Young, F. W. (1981). *Introduction to multidimensional scaling*. New York: Academic Press.

Schneider, W., and Shiffrin, R. M. (1977). Controlled and automatic human information processing: I. Detection, search, and attention. *Psychological Review, 84*, 1–66.

Schneider, W., Dumais, S. T., and Shiffrin, R. M. (1984). Automatic and controlled processing and attention. In R. Parasuraman and D. R. Davies (Eds.), *Varieties of attention* (pp. 1–27). New York: Academic Press.

Schuckit, M. A. (1987). Biological vulnerability to alcoholism. *Journal Consulting and Clinical Psychology, 55*, 301–309.

Searles, J. S. (1988). The role of genetics in the pathogenesis of alcoholism. *Journal of Abnormal Psychology, 97*, 153–167.

Sher, K. J. (1985). Subjective effects of alcohol: The influence of setting and individual differences in alcohol expectancies. *Journal of Studies on Alcohol, 46*, 137–146.

Sher, K. J. (1991). *Children of alcoholics: A critical appraisal of theory and research*. Chicago: University of Chicago Press.

Sher, K. J., Walitzer, K. S., Wood, P. A., and Brent, E. E. (1991). Characteristics of children of alcoholics: Putative risk factors, substance use and abuse, and psychopathology. *Journal of Abnormal Psychology, 100*, 427–448.

Shiffrin, R. M., and Schneider, W. (1977). Controlled and automatic human information processing: II. Perceptual learning, automatic attending, a general theory. *Psychological Review, 84*, 127–190.

Shoben, E. J. (1976). The verification of semantic relations in a same-different paradigm: An asymmetry in semantic memory. *Journal of Verbal Learning and Verbal Behavior, 15*, 365–379.

Siegal, S. (1975). Evidence from rats that morphine tolerance is a learned response. *Journal of Comparative and Physiological Psychology, 89*, 498–506.

Siegal, S. (1983). Classical conditioning, drug tolerance and drug dependence. In Y. Israel, F. B. Glaser, H. Kalant, R. E. Popham, W. Schmidt, and R. G. Smart (Eds.), *Research advances in alcohol and drug problems* (Vol. 7, pp. 207–246). New York: Plenum.

Siegal, S., Krank, M. D., and Hinson, R. E. (1988). Anticipation of pharmacological and nonpharmacological events: Classical conditioning and addictive behavior. *Journal of Drug Issues, 17*, 83–110.

Simon, H. A., and Kaplan, C. A. (1990). Foundations of cognitive science. In M. I. Posner (Ed.), *Foundations of cognitive science* (pp. 1–47). Cambridge, MA: MIT Press.

Skinner, B. F. (1938). *The behavior of organisms: An experimental analysis*. New York: Appleton-Century-Crofts.

Smart, R. G., and Gray, G. (1979). Parental and peer influences as correlates of problem drinking among high school students. *International Journal of the Addictions, 10*, 869–882.

Smith, G. T., and Goldman, M. S. (1990). *Toward a mediational model of alcohol expectancies*. Paper presented at the 98th Annual Meeting of the American Psychological Association, Boston, MA.

Smith, G. T., and Goldman, M. S. (1992). *Children's alcohol expectancies and their implication for prevention of alcoholism*. Paper presented at the Society for Research in Child Development Convention, Seattle, WA.

Smith, E. E., and Medin, D. L. (1981). *Categories and concepts*. Cambridge, MA: Harvard University Press.

Sneath, P. H. A., and Sokal, R. R. (1973). *Numerical taxonomy*. San Francisco: Freeman.

Squire, L. R. (1992). Memory and the hippocampus: A synthesis from findings with rats, monkeys, and humans. *Psychological Review, 99*, 195–231.

Stacy, A. W., Newcomb, M. D., and Bentler, P. M. (1991). Cognitive motivation and drug use: A 9-year longitudinal study. *Journal of Abnormal Psychology, 100*, 502–515.

Steele, C. M., and Josephs, R. A. (1990). Alcohol myopia: It's prized and dangerous effects. *American Psychologist, 45*, 921–933.

Sternberg, R. J. (1985). Human intelligence: The model is the message. *Science, 230*, 1111–1118.

Stewart, J., de Wit, H., and Eikelboom, R. (1984). Role of unconditioned and conditioned effects in the self-administration of opiates and stimulants. *Psychological Review, 91*, 251–268.

Tabakoff, B., Hoffman, P. L., Lee, J. M., Saito, T., Willard, B., and De Leon-Jones, F. (1988). Differences in platelet enzyme activity between alcoholics and nonalcoholics. *New England Journal of Medicine, 318*, 134–139.

Tiffany, S. T. (1990). A cognitive model of drug urges and drug-use behavior: Role of automatic and nonautomatic processes. *Psychological Review, 97*, 147–168.

Tiffany, S. T., and Baker, T. B. (1986). Tolerance to alcohol: Psychological models and their application to alcoholism. *Annals of Behavioral Medicine, 8*, 2–3, 7–12.

Tolman, E. G. (1932). *Purposive behavior in animals and man*. New York: Appelton-Century-Crofts.

Tulving, E. (1972). Episodic and semantic memory. In E. Tulving and W. Donaldson (Eds.), *Organization of memory* (pp. 381–403). New York: Academic Press.

Tulving, E. (1985). How many memory systems are there? *American Psychologist, 40*, 385–398.

Turing, M. A. (1950). Computing machinery and intelligence. *Mind, 59*, 433–460.

Vogel-Sprott, M. (1992). *Alcohol tolerance and social drinking: Learning the consequences*. New York: Guilford Press.

Waldrop, M. M. (1988). Soar: A unified theory of cognition? *Science, 241*, 296–298.

Watson, D., and Clark, L. (1984). Negative affectivity: The disposition to experience aversive emotional states. *Psychological Bulletin, 96*, 465–490.

Watson, D., and Tellegen, A. (1985). Toward a consensual structure moood. *Psychological Bulletin, 98*, 219–235.

Weintraub, A. L., and Goldman, M. S. (1983). Alcohol and proactive interference: A test of response eccentricity theory of alcohol's psychological effects. *Addictive Behaviors, 8*, 151–166.

West, M. O., and Prinz, R. J. (1987). Parental alcoholism and childhood psychopathology. *Psychological Bulletin, 102*, 204–218.

Wickens, C. D. (1984). Processing resources in attention. In R. Parasuraman and R. Davies (Eds.), *Varieties of attention* (pp. 63–102). New York: Academic Press.

Windle, M., and Searles, J. S. (Eds.). (1990). *Children of alcoholics: Critical perspectives*. New York: Guilford Press.

Williams, R. M., Goldman, M. S., and Williams, D. L. (1981). Expectancy and pharmacological effects of alcohol on human cognitive and motor performance: The compensation for alcohol effect. *Journal of Abnormal Psychology, 90*, 267–270.

Wilsnack, R. W., and Wilsnack, S. C. (1980). Drinking and denial of social obligations among adolescent boys. *Journal of Studies on Alcohol, 41*, 1118–1133.

Wise, R. A. (1988). The neurobiology of craving: Implications for the understanding and treatment of addiction. *Journal of Abnormal Psychology, 97*, 118–132.

Wise, R. A., and Bozarth, M. A. (1987). A psychomotor stimulant theory of addiction. *Psychological Review, 94*, 469–492.

Wong, C. J., Newlin, D. B., Better, W. E., and Pretorius, M. B. (1991). *The ARC drug expectancy questionnaire: An instrument for assessing expectancies concerning use of cocaine, heroin, marijuana, alcohol, and nicotine*. Paper presented at the annual meeting of the Association for Advancement of Behavior Therapy Convention, New York, NY.

Zimmerman, H. J. (1987). *Fuzzy sets, decision-making, and expert systems*. Norwell, MA: Klower Academic.

Zucker, R. A. (1976). Parental influences on the drinking patterns of their children. In M. Greenblatt and M. A. Schuckit (Eds.), *Alcoholism problems in women and children*. New York: Grune & Stratton.

Zucker, R. A. (1987). The four alcoholisms: A developmental account of the etiologic process. In P. Clayton Rivers (Ed.), *Alcohol and addictive behavior, Nebraska symposium on motivation*. Lincoln and London: University of Nebraska Press.

Zucker, R. A., and Gomberg, E. S. L. (1986). Etiology of alcoholism reconsidered: The case for a biopsychosocial process. *American Psychologist, 41*, 783–793.

9

Psychopathy and Cognition

Joseph P. Newman and John F. Wallace

University of Wisconsin

> It is not easy to convey this concept, that of a biologic organism outwardly intact, showing excellent peripheral function, but centrally deficient or disabled in such a way that abilities, excellent at the only levels where we can formally test them, cannot be utilized for sane purposes or prevented from regularly working toward self-destructive and other seriously pathologic results. (p. vii)

This description of psychopathy, taken from Cleckley's (1976) preface to his book *The Mask of Sanity*, leaves little doubt concerning the formidable challenges that face investigators seeking to characterize cognitive processing anomalies in psychopathy.

Because there are no immediate indications of psychopathology, one cannot easily identify a psychopath, let alone characterize his or her deficits. To the contrary, the psychopath's "superficial charm and good intelligence; absence of delusions and other signs of irrational thinking; and absence of nervousness or psychoneurotic manifestations" convey a convincing representation of mental health (Cleckley, 1976, p. 337). Despite their apparent assets, other characteristics of the psychopath present a less flattering image. They include: unreliability, untruthfulness and insincerity, lack of remorse or shame, inadequately motivated antisocial behavior, poor judgment and failure to learn from experience, pathologic egocentricity and incapacity to love, general poverty in major affective reactions, unresponsiveness in general interpersonal relations, and failure to follow any life plan (Cleckley, 1976). A moment's reflection reveals that these attributes are difficult or impossible to discern from casual interactions with the psychopath; they must be deduced by observing his or her behavior over an extended period of time or through the use of case history materials.

The purpose of this chapter is to review the current status of cognitive research and theorizing in psychopathy. Before proceeding, however, it is important to discuss our use of the psychopathy construct and to differentiate it from related constructs. In the course of its long and perplexing history, this construct has assumed diverse meanings and has been known by a variety of terms (e.g., moral insanity, constitutional psychopathic inferiority, sociopathy, antisocial personality disorder). Nevertheless, historical reviews of the topic (e.g., Millon, 1981; Pichot, 1978) underscore two major themes, which, as will be apparent shortly, correspond to the current distinction between psychopathy and antisocial personality disorder.

DEFINING THE PSYCHOPATH

Beginning with Pinel (1809), who used the term *manie sans delire* to signify a disorder that, unlike other forms of mental illness, did not involve a disorder of the mind (i.e., reasoning), the hallmark of the disorder has been poorly regulated behavior that is both self-defeating and socially unacceptable. The confusion surrounding the disorder derives from two competing strategies that have been used to elaborate the diagnosis. One tradition emphasizes the biopsychological aspect of Pinel's description. Typically, such accounts posit some innate dysfunction (e.g., in physiological systems mediating affect) as the explanation for the psychopath's defect in self-governance. Although persistent social deviance and antisocial behavior may be more likely in such cases, they are not regarded as the defining features of the disorder. The second approach places greater weight on the person's social maladjustment. According to Millon (1981), for instance, Benjamin Rush and J. C. Prichard took "Pinel's morally neutral clinical observation of defects in 'passion and affect' and turned it into a social condemnation" (p. 186). This emphasis on chronic, irresponsible behavior prompted these early writers to focus on moral depravity and defective moral faculties as potential explanations for the disorder. Although the relatively recent concept of *sociopathy* places greater responsibility for the disorder on social, as opposed to psychological, factors, the emphasis on moral depravity is no less apparent.

In the extreme, both definitions have proven problematic. The first definition, emphasizing innate personality processes that contribute to maladaptive behavior, led to the formation of a wastebasket category that included virtually all personality disorders. On the other hand, defining the concept based on social deviance criteria has resulted in repeated calls to abandon the diagnosis, which, it is argued, is more accurately regarded as a sociological as opposed to a psychiatric phenomenon (e.g., Blackburn, 1988).

Though the concepts have evolved considerably, these two traditions (i.e., defective self-governance; antisocial character) appear to underlie the current distinction between psychopathy and the DSM-III-R diagnosis of Antisocial Personality Disorder (APD). Most recent references to the term "psychopathy" refer to the definition provided by Cleckley (1976). Though many of his illustrative cases involve criminal behavior, Cleckley took great care to dissociate the disorder from common criminality (see also Karpman, 1948). Consistent with the first tradition, Cleckley places the source of the problem within the individual. His own explanation was to propose a type of semantic dementia that could be seen in psychopaths' tendency to say one thing and do another. However, his most important contribution was to provide a poignant description of the psychopath, which, in capturing the essential features of the disorder, appears to identify a specific problem that sets it apart from other expressions of psychopathology and criminal behavior (Hart and Hare, 1989).

In contrast to Cleckley's emphasis on the psychological characteristics of the individual, the DSM-III-R APD diagnosis (American Psychiatric Association, 1987) has more in common with the second historical tradition. According to the manual,

> the essential feature of this disorder is a pattern of irresponsible and antisocial behavior beginning in childhood and early adolescence and continuing into adulthood. . . . Lying, stealing, truancy, vandalism, initiating fights, running away from home, and physical cruelty are typical childhood signs. In adulthood the antisocial pattern continues, and may include failure to honor financial obligations, to function as a responsible parent or to plan ahead, and an inability to sustain consistent work behavior. (p. 342)

Although this stable pattern of antisocial behavior may, in fact, indicate the existence of a personality disorder, the emphasis on antisocial conduct to the relative exclusion of personality processes is reminiscent of the value-laden concept of "moral insanity."

While there is, as yet, a paucity of hard evidence to document the importance of distinguishing between psychopathy and antisocial personality disorder (cf. Hare 1990), the APD diagnosis identifies a larger subset of criminal offenders (Hare, 1985) and is more likely to include individuals whose conduct problems reflect primarily the consequences of an underprivileged upbringing, substance abuse, and inadequate intellectual/social skills. The APD diagnosis, with its emphasis on chronic antisocial behavior per se, may also fail to identify psychopathic individuals whose higher socioeconomic status, above average intelligence, and excellent social skills enable them to avoid detection or to display their personality disorder in a less stereotypic fashion (see Widom, 1977). Finally, using antisocial behavior as the *sine qua non* of psychopathy may interfere with our ability to identify the precursors of this disorder in children before a pattern of chronic antisocial behavior has developed.

In this chapter, we use the term psychopathy to designate the syndrome described by Cleckley (1976). In practice, however, it is not possible to separate a construct from the method used to assess it. During the past decade, Hare's (1980, 1990) Psychopathy Checklist (PCL) has become the standard for operationalizing the psychopathy construct (cf. Thomas-Peter, 1992). Hare and his colleagues have amassed a sizable body of evidence demonstrating the high reliability, internal and external validity, and discriminant validity of the PCL (Hare *et al.*, 1990; Hart and Hare, 1989). Recent reports by Harpur and others (Harpur *et al.*, 1989; Kosson *et al.*, 1990) indicate that the checklist, though sufficiently homogeneous to be regarded as unifactorial, has two correlated subfactors: one corresponding to the egocentric, manipulative, and callous personality characteristics of the psychopath and the other to their impulsive, antisocial traits and lifestyle. Importantly, to score in the psychopathic range on the PCL, it is necessary to have both components of psychopathy to a significant degree. Though this definition may still fail to identify many noncriminal psychopaths, it provides a relatively conservative definition. At this point in time, we believe that a relatively narrow definition will be most productive in identifying meaningful psychological correlates of the disorder. For this reason, our review of the research literature on psychopathy will not be exhaustive. Instead, we will focus on relatively recent studies employing Cleckley's (1976) conceptualization of psychopathy.

PSYCHOPATHIC BEHAVIOR: A COGNITIVE VIEWPOINT

As might be expected from a disorder that has its origins in a condition referred to as manie sans delire, cognitive factors have not been prominent in theoretical accounts of psychopathy and, predictably, research on the topic has been sparse. Nevertheless, in spite of the absence of intellectual impairment and signs of irrational thinking in psychopaths, there is little evidence that their powers of reasoning are effective in guiding their day-to-day activities. From a psychological perspective, it is the discrepancy between psychopaths' apparent *capacity for* good judgment and their *exer-*

cise of good judgment that represents the most important and intriguing aspect of the syndrome.

To illustrate this discrepancy, Grant (1977) relates the self-observation of a twenty-two-year-old psychopath "whose intelligence was beyond question to anyone who knew him" (p. 60).

> "I always know damn well I shouldn't do these things, that they're the same as what brought me to grief before. I haven't forgotten anything. It's just that when the time comes I don't think of anything else. I don't think of anything but what I want now. I don't think about what happened last time, or if I do it just doesn't matter. It would never stop me." (p. 60)

What is the explanation for this failure of self-regulation? By definition, we have already ruled out inadequate intelligence and irrational thinking. Most influential theories of psychopathy regard the problem as a breakdown in the socialization process that results from some underlying, biologically based, motivational and/or emotional disturbance (e.g., Eysenck, 1964; Hare, 1965; Lykken, 1957; Quay, 1965). Lykken (1982), for example, has argued that most salient features of the disorder may be explained by a relative incapacity for fear. In contrast to nonpsychopaths, whose fear of punishment, social rebuke, and the unknown causes them to weigh their actions carefully, the psychopath is relatively unmotivated by such considerations. Given their lack of concern for future consequences, psychopaths are free to act on their impulses and to indulge their immediate desires. Moreover, this tendency to pursue their own needs without regard for others causes them to appear callous, egocentric, and remorseless. Although freedom from fear does not directly explain their lack of attachment to others, their egocentric and immature behavior is likely to stress relationships and interfere with the development of mutual affections. For example, during childhood the psychopath's carefree demeanor may elicit rejection and/or attempts at control by parents, setting the stage for an oppositional approach to interactions with authority. In addition, Lykken notes that without fear, children may have little need for reassurance and, consequently, may not come to view others as a source of comfort or tender affections. In sum, the lack of fear of negative consequences combined with the lack of tender, prosocial feelings for others leads the psychopath to be relatively unmotivated to adjust his or her behavior to the expectations and dictates of society.

Returning to the clinical observation just noted, Lykken's (1982) conceptualization of the psychopath underscores the person's low subjective weighing of potential negative consequences. Specifically, the amount of anxiety generated by potential punishment is not sufficient to outweigh his inclination to act on immediate urges. In light of his stated concern about the consequences, however, an alternative conceptualization is that the man's behavior reflects some cognitive processing deficit.

Though the possibility of a cognitive deficit in psychopathy has for the most part been viewed as secondary or incidental to an affective/motivational disturbance, a model for considering this possibility has been provided by Shapiro (1965) in his brilliant essays, *Neurotic Styles*. Moreover, Shapiro's characterization of the psychopath's cognitive style goes well beyond their failure to anticipate punishment. Although this aspect of psychopathy is noted, it is regarded as only one of many consequences of a more pervasive breakdown in the cognitive processing that underlies deliberate action.

The distinction between urges and deliberate action is fundamental to Shapiro's concept of the *impulsive style*. "In the normal person, the whim or the half-formed inclination to do something is the beginning of a complex process, although, if all is well, it is a smooth and automatic one" (1965, p. 140). The essence of his argument is that the active mental processes that normally translate incipient motives into deliberate actions are "short-circuited" in the psychopath. What is the nature of this "complex process"? According to Shapiro, it involves a type of elaboration whereby a passing thought or whim accrues interest and emotional support owing to its association with preexisting aims and interests. As discussed below, this integrative process is fundamental to the development of sustained goals, affective depth, lasting affections, self-restraint, sound judgment, and what is often referred to as "conscience."

The process of integrating current experience or whims with preexisting values enables a person to develop a perspective on behavior that goes beyond his or her immediate concerns. Such perspective, in turn, makes possible sustained commitments to ideas, ideals, and courses of action. Without this perspective, it is difficult to develop long-term goals and to resist impulses, and a person's thoughts and goals tend to shift erratically. Shapiro (1965) views this process as a prerequisite for contemplating behavior in terms that transcend one's own immediate interests. Moreover, in providing a context for the person's commitment to a course of action, the process of integrating current motivations with more stable interests and goals enhances their ability to tolerate frustration, endure boredom, take pride in their behavior, and acknowledge responsibility for their behavioral choices.

In addition to *stabilizing behavior* by uniting immediate considerations with long-standing values, Shapiro (1965) argues convincingly that the process of integrating present and past experience is necessary for the development of *affective depth* and meaningful interpersonal relationships. As an example, Shapiro discusses the difference between experiencing a sexual impulse and a sustained, whole-hearted reaction that derives from associating a potential partner with established attitudes of affection, readiness for intimacy, and other life anticipations (p. 144). Though not discussed in any detail, it is safe to assume that other affective expressions become enriched to a similar extent as they are elaborated on by preexisting, personally meaningful, associations.

Shapiro (1965) states that "the *cognition* of impulsive people is characterized by an insufficiency of active integrative processes that is comparable to the insufficiency of integrative processes on the affective side. . . ." The psychopath remains "oblivious to the drawbacks or complications that would give another person pause and might otherwise give him pause as well" (pp. 147–149). His cognition is not active, searching, and directed by stable interests. It lacks the planning, concentration, reflectiveness, objectivity, and judgment that come from a more analytic and integrative perspective. Relating a clinical example similar to Grant's (1977), Shapiro remarked that it is "not pertinent information that was lacking or unavailable to this man but rather the active, searching attention and organizing process that normally puts such information to use" (p. 149).

Beyond its implications for long-range, goal-directed behavior, affective depth, and reflective cognitive processing, Shapiro's (1965) conceptualization of psychopathy is informative with regard to *morality and the development of conscience*. According to Shapiro, "conscience and moral values are not elemental psychological faculties, but involve and depend on a number of cognitive and affective functions" (p. 163). For Shapiro, differences between psychopaths and nonpsychopaths with respect to moral conduct "are not primarily matters of moral scruple on the part of the normal person or the lack of them on the part of the psychopathic character; they are matters of interest and automatic cognitive tendency" (p. 166).

Thus, Shapiro's (1965) characterization of the psychopath suggests that their callous, antisocial behavior reflects, to a significant degree, *a deficit in automatic processes*, which preclude meaningful analysis and modulation of behavior. In comparison to theories that focus on inadequate fear (e.g., Lykken, 1982), Shapiro's perspective is at once more specific and more far reaching. Rather than regarding psychopathic behavior as deliberate behavior, reflecting an inappropriate balance of approach and avoidance considerations, Shapiro focuses on the process that enables such decisions to be made. The psychopath's impulsive style entails much more than a weak avoidance motive and/or a strong motive to approach (cf. Fowles, 1980). Specifically, appropriate response modulation and self-control are considered to reflect the outcome of a dynamic process involving the person's ability *to realize* and *be guided by* the "meaning" of their actions. In suggesting that inhibitory cues accrue less readily to previously punished responses in psychopaths, thereby reducing their ability to anticipate and avoid punishment, Shapiro easily explains the psychopath's failure to utilize such information. However, psychopaths' difficulty using cues for punishment is, by no means, the only example of their constrained perspective.

Finally, in addressing psychopaths' cognitive style, Shapiro (1965) recognized the difficulty and perhaps futility in trying to distinguish between cognitive and affective modes of functioning. "Both areas of functioning and the modes that respectively characterize them exist together, each is hardly imaginable without the other, and, in all likelihood, they develop together." (pp. 154–155). Psychopaths' difficulty integrating current whims with past experience apparently interferes with their ability to appreciate the emotional and moral significance of events as well as their ability to adopt a critical perspective on their own behavior. Conveniently, and correctly we think, this perspective indicates that the goal of developing a cognitive perspective on psychopathy will be facilitated by incorporating past research and theory regarding the psychopath's deficient "affective response."

THEORIES OF PSYCHOPATHY: A COGNITIVE PERSPECTIVE

As noted above, traditional theories of psychopathy have emphasized biologically based differences in arousal, emotional reactivity, and fear conditioning. Increasingly, however, these theories are being reformulated and/or elaborated to accommodate recent advances in cognitive psychology. In this section, we briefly review the traditional theories while highlighting the emerging, cognitive perspective. To date, with minor exceptions (e.g., Millon, 1981; Widom, 1976), consideration of cognitive factors in psychopathy has been limited to "cognitive deficits" as opposed to "cognitive distortions" (see Ch. 1, this volume).

One of the earliest and most important perspectives on psychopathy was provided by Eysenck (1964) within the framework of his theory of introversion–extraversion. Eysenck has proposed that socialized, altruistic behavior is learned via Pavlovian conditioning.

> The newborn and the young child have . . . to acquire a "conscience" through a process of conditioning; in other words, on thousands of occasions, when they behave in an antisocial manner, parents, teachers, peers, and others punish them in a variety of ways, thus associating through Pavlovian conditioning antisocial thoughts and actions with disagreeable consequences. As a result of this conditioned "conscience," such individuals will refrain from contemplating or carrying out antisocial activities because the contemplation or carrying out is

accompanied by conditioned feelings of fear/anxiety, anticipation of punishment, and guilt. (Eysenck and Gudjonsson, 1989, p. 111)

Psychopathy, like criminality, is regarded by Eysenck as a biologically based predisposition to "low arousability/arousal" that causes such individuals to condition more slowly and, therefore, socialize less readily than noncriminal, nonpsychopathic individuals. In addition to retarding the development of fearful and guilty responses, psychopaths' low level of arousal is hypothesized to motivate sensation-seeking and risk-taking behavior (see also Quay, 1965, 1977), increasing the likelihood that psychopaths will come into conflict with society.

Building on Eysenck's (1964, 1977) theory, Trasler (1978) has proposed a social learning perspective on psychopathy that places greater emphasis on cognitive factors. Like Eysenck, Trasler acknowledges the importance of physiological factors and early conditioning for the development of appropriate self-restraint later in life. However, he argues that such restraints can "not be explained in terms of the immediate contingencies, or even in terms of the reinforcement history of the individual" (p. 277) because, in most cases, they develop in the absence of any direct experience with punishment. According to Trasler, human beings employ cognitive abilities to organize related experiences and verbal instruction into "structures" such as rules, reasons, motives, and intentions that mediate the evaluation and inhibition of socially undesirable behaviors. With regard to psychopaths, he suggests that their "idiosyncratic inability to make use of perceptions which would normally result in changes in behavioral disposition" (p. 286) precludes the development of internalized responses that make exploitative acquisition, physical aggression, and sexual misconduct "unthinkable" for others. Thus, internalization of societal rules and principles via conditioning and social instruction promotes socialization by altering a person's perception of social situations and the range of acceptable responses. Trasler (1978) concludes that psychopaths are "not automata, driven to commit infractions of the law by factors beyond their control, but people whose decisions and choices, and whose immediate options and alternatives, are different from those which confront non-criminals" (p. 287).

Another important perspective on psychopathy has developed from Hare's careful and extensive investigations regarding the psychopath's psychophysiological reaction to the threat of punishment. Although his theory continues to evolve as research evidence accumulates, the central tenet of Hare's theoretical perspective has remained relatively constant: cues for punishment elicit less fear arousal in psychopaths than in nonpsychopaths. For instance, using skin conductance as an index of fear arousal,

Hare (1965) found that psychopaths displayed a steeper temporal gradient of fear than did nonpsychopaths as they watched a numerical "countdown" to administration of an electric shock. Relative to nonpsychopaths, then, it appears that psychopaths experience less anticipatory anxiety in response to the cues preceding the occurrence of an aversive event.

Hare (1970) elucidated the significance of this finding using Mowrer's two-factor theory of avoidance learning. According to Mowrer (1947), a person's (internal) fear response acts as a stimulus for operant behavior aimed at reducing the associated, unpleasant drive state. Moreover, to the extent that the behavior is successful in reducing fear, it is experienced as reinforcing and is emitted more readily on subsequent occasions. Thus, the experience of fear is fundamental to avoidance learning (i.e., behaving so as to reduce the risk of punishment) and may also promote the development of prosocial behavior as illustrated by the following example. A young child contemplating some socially proscribed behavior, such as lying or stealing, is likely to experience fear as a result of past punishments for this behavior. This conditioned emotional response may, in turn, cause the child to *inhibit* the behavior (i.e., display *passive* avoidance). To the extent that this "prosocial behavior" (i.e., deciding not to lie/steal) is followed by fear reduction, it will be strengthened and increase the probability that the child will emit prosocial behaviors in the future. Mednick and his colleagues (e.g., Mednick and Hutchings, 1978), in particular, have emphasized the role of fear reduction in motivating the development of socialization. Based on evidence that psychopaths display slower electrodermal recovery, he has proposed that psychopaths experience less immediate and, therefore, less powerful reinforcement following the inhibition of socially proscribed behavior (cf. Hare, 1978).

In more recent summaries of his research, Hare (1978, 1986) has deemphasized fear conditioning and adopted a cognitive interpretation of psychopaths' reaction to punishment. Specifically, he has suggested that psychopaths are especially adept at "gating out" or attenuating stimuli associated with punishment. Although this response appears to be effective in reducing fear, ignoring such cues may contribute to the psychopath's difficulty avoiding punishment. In a related vein, Hare and his colleagues (Jutai and Hare, 1983) have proposed that psychopaths are more adept at screening out irrelevant stimuli. Thus, Hare's more recent theorizing holds that psychopaths possess a relatively unique attentional style that enables them to screen out distracting and/or threatening cues but that, unfortunately, contributes to the psychopath's failures of avoidance learning.

The concept of arousal has played a major role in these and other important theories of psychopathy (e.g., Quay, 1965). However, unidimensional theories of arousal are no longer regarded as tenable and their application to psychopathy has been criticized (see Mawson and Mawson, 1977). Unidimensional theories of arousal were based on the activity of the ascending reticular activation system (ARAS; e.g., Malmo, 1959), but more recent considerations of arousal recognize multiple physiological substrates that involve limbic structures as well as the ARAS (e.g., Routtenberg, 1968). Not surprisingly, these changes have resulted in a fresh perspective on the role of arousal in psychopathy.

Based primarily on this shift in emphasis from the ARAS to the septohippocampal system (SHS), Gray (1970) proposed a major modification of Eysenck's (1964) theory of introversion–extraversion and, by extension, psychopathy. Whereas Eysenck's model emphasizes general arousal and conditionability, Gray's use of the SHS caused him to propose that the introversion–extraversion dimension reflects sensitivity to signals for punishment (i.e., fear conditionability). More recently, Gray (1982, 1987) has characterized SHS functioning as a type of behavioral inhibition or anxiety system that mediates a person's reaction to threatening stimuli.

The implications of Gray's model for psychopathy have been addressed in detail by Fowles (1980). Elaborating on the three interacting brain systems described by Gray (1987), he proposed a "three-arousal model" comprised of a behavioral activation system (BAS), behavioral inhibition system (BIS), and a general arousal system that we shall refer to as the nonspecific arousal system (NAS). The BAS reacts to stimuli associated with reward and active avoidance by increasing activity in the NAS and initiating active, goal-directed behavior (i.e., approach or active avoidance). The BIS reacts to signals for punishment and nonreward (i.e., omission of expected rewards) by increasing NAS activity, inhibiting ongoing behavior, and redirecting attention to significant stimuli. The NAS not only responds to increases in BAS and BIS activity, but also functions to intensify the behavioral outputs of these two systems (i.e., by increasing the speed and intensity of *approach behavior* or by facilitating response inhibition and *inspection of environmental cues*). Psychopathy, according to Fowles (1980), may be explained by the single assumption of a weak BIS.

It should be noted, however, that the BIS comprises several physiological subsystems, subserving numerous interrelated psychological processes. For example, in order to detect potential threats, the BIS must monitor environmental stimuli and anticipated responses. After a threat is detected, other connections act to increase "arousal" and facilitate rapid cognitive processing and/or evasive action (see Wallace *et al.*, 1991; Wallace and Newman, 1992). In addition to detecting potential threats, the BIS also plays a crucial role in the inhibition of behavior and must, therefore, be coordinated with the motor response system. This coordination involves evaluation of potential responses, interruption of ongoing or anticipated motor behavior, and decision making concerning the relative merits of approach and avoidance (see Gray, 1987). Thus, citing a weak or dysfunctional BIS implicates a complex array of physiological and psychological processes and leaves unspecified which component of the BIS is dysfunctional.

Strictly speaking, postulating a globally weak BIS implies that cues for punishment are less readily detected and that, once detected, they elicit less arousal, less inhibition, and less stimulus processing. In support of this contention, Fowles (1980, 1988) notes that psychopaths display low levels of fear arousal (i.e., fewer skin conductance responses); are more sensitive to reward cues than to punishment cues; and are less likely than nonpsychopaths to inhibit ongoing behavior in response to cues for punishment.

The implications of the Gray/Fowles model for cognitive processing in psychopaths have not been addressed by these authors. However, it follows from the function of the BIS that psychopaths would tend to allocate attention preferentially to reward cues as opposed to punishment cues and that they would less readily reallocate attention to environmental stimuli in response to cues for punishment.

The relevance of SHS functioning for psychopathy was also the focus of another paper published in 1980. Expanding on earlier suggestions by Hare (1970) and Gray (1970), Gorenstein and Newman (1980) proposed a model for psychopathy and other "syndromes of disinhibition" based on an analogy to the behavioral consequences of septal lesions in animals. Whereas other authors had noted the potential etiological significance of the SHS based on similarities between the laboratory deficits shown by psychopaths and those associated with SHS dysfunction, we argued that, regardless of its etiological significance, the functional analogy could be exploited by using the more extensive and precise literature on SHS dysfunction to generate novel hypotheses concerning the "perceptual, motivational, cognitive and other psychological peculiarities" (p. 308) displayed by psychopaths and other disinhibited individuals.

As in psychopathy, the poor *passive avoidance* learning of animals with septal lesions was often attributed to poor fear conditioning and insensitivity to punishment. However, animals with septal lesions display adequate, and sometimes superior, *active avoidance* learning. Passive avoidance refers to *withholding specific behaviors* to reduce the risk of punishment whereas active avoidance refers to *emitting specific behaviors* to reduce the risk of punishment. Moreover, animals with septal lesions often have difficulty withholding inappropriate (i.e., premature) responses in tasks involving rewards only. Combined, such evidence suggests that septal lesions interfere with an animal's ability to inhibit goal-directed behavior based on feedback from the environment. Finally, it has been noted that cues for punishment, omission of expected rewards, and the delivery of punishment itself, often increase the intensity of goal-directed behavior in septal animals rather than leaving them unaffected. This paradoxical facilitation of behavior is not consistent with "insensitivity to punishment," but it is precisely what would be expected if aversive stimuli produce increases in "nonspecific arousal" without interrupting the dominant (i.e., ongoing) response set (see Dickinson, 1974).

Thus, one hypothesis derived from the "septal model" is that psychopaths' apparent insensitivity to punishment reflects a more fundamental deficit in *response modulation*. Response modulation involves suspending a dominant response set in order to accommodate feedback from the environment. According to this hypothesis, once focused on some goal-directed behavior, psychopaths would be relatively unable to interrupt their response set in order to accommodate less immediate, and other less salient, considerations such as the prospect of punishment and future rewards (Newman *et al.*, 1983; Newman *et al.*, 1985). Consequently, psychopaths are prone to emit and perseverate maladaptive responses despite the availability of cues indicating the need to revise their response strategy. In contrast to earlier theories, which emphasize deficient fear conditioning and sensitivity to punishment per se, response modulation highlights the importance of integrating competing (e.g., approach and avoidance) motivations. Although a failure to inhibit punished responses may reflect weak avoidance motivation, it could also reflect difficulty interrupting approach behavior.

In cognitive terms, "response modulation entails a brief shift of attention from the organizing and implementation of goal-directed action to its evaluation" (Newman, 1991, p. 174). To the extent that psychopaths fail to interrupt an ongoing response set in reaction to unexpected punishments and the omission of expected rewards, they are not only less likely to accommodate this feedback, but they will also spend less time reflecting on (i.e., process less deeply) the particular stimulus context and response that preceded the aversive event. Thus, in addition to impairing self-regulation in the immediate present, the psychopath's failure to pause following negative feedback also interferes with his or her ability to profit from experience because they are less likely to recognize similar problem situations and/or defective responses in the future (Newman, 1987). Finally, in contrast to reflective individuals, whose cognitive style inclines them to develop coping strategies that enhance *predictive control* over the environment (learning to anticipate problems), psychopaths' difficulty learning from punishment predisposes them to develop coping strategies involving *instrumental control* (learning to handle problems; Patterson and Newman, in press).

An alternative perspective on the cognitive implications of our physiological animal model of psychopathy has recently been proposed by Gorenstein (1991). According to Gorenstein, psychopathy reflects a central deficit in the ability to "develop or maintain the abstract mental representations that are required to initiate and sustain any higher form of behavioral activity" (p. 116). As a result of this problem, the psychopath is relatively unable "to remove himself psychologically from a situation and evaluate performance by measuring it against some internal standard or code" (p. 116). Thus, according to Gorenstein (1991), the psychopath's "behavior is largely dependent on external cues, inveterate habit, biological drives, or other determinants of 'stereotypical' or 'dominant' responding" (p. 127).

Three other theories of psychopathy deserving comment include Schachter and Latane's (1964) discussion of the cognitive consequences of autonomic hyperreactivity in psychopathy, Gough's (1948) "sociological" or role-taking theory of psychopathy, and Millon's (1981) interpersonal formulation.

Based on their observation that psychopaths display greater heart-rate elevations following exogenously administered adrenalin and other "more or less stressful stimuli" (p. 264), Schachter and Latane (1964) proposed that psychopaths are "more responsive to virtually every titillating event, whether only mildly provoking or dangerously threatening . . ." and that because "almost every event provokes strong autonomic discharge then, in terms of internal autonomic cues, the subject feels no differently during times of danger than during relatively tranquil times" (pp. 266–267). According to Schachter, the autonomic hyperreactivity of psychopaths disrupts their ability to apply appropriate emotional labels to their experiences, causing them to interpret both socially defined "emotional situations" and socially defined "unemotional situations" inappropriately. Although the empirical support for this theory has been questioned (e.g., Hare, 1972), other investigators continue to comment on the potential significance of this formulation (e.g., Goldman *et al.*, 1971; Finn *et al.*, 1990; Mawson and Mawson, 1977; Tarter, 1979).

Gough (1948) has described psychopaths as deficient in role taking, which, according to Gough, includes the ability to perceive and evaluate one's own behavior from the perspective of another. Lacking this objectification of the self, psychopaths have difficulty relating to others in a manner that is conducive to forming lasting attachments, as well as in progressing beyond an egocentric and uninsightful perspective on their behavior.

Moreover, difficulty anticipating other people's reactions to their behavior may impede the psychopath's ability to display appropriate self-control.

In contrast to other theorists considered, Millon's (1981) characterization of psychopaths highlights their *cognitive distortions*. According to Millon, psychopaths regard the world as a hostile, "dog-eat-dog" place and consequently are hypervigilant and hypersensitive to insults and challenges. They "magnify minor slights into major insults and slanders" meriting retaliation. Their hostile expectations, suspiciousness, and confrontational style, in turn, elicit hostile behavior from others and so justify their perceptions, creating a "vicious cycle." This characterization of the psychopath has much in common with the hostile attributional style displayed by aggressive children (see Dodge and Crick, 1990). In light of the potential relation between psychopathy and childhood aggression, this similarity in social cognition may be worthy of note.

Summary

This brief review of theoretical perspectives on psychopathy reveals considerable agreement. From an information-processing perspective, the central issue concerns psychopaths' failure to accommodate cues for punishment and other potentially significant stimuli by switching attention from the implementation of behavior to the inspection of environmental stimuli. The overlap appears to result from the relative unanimity concerning psychopaths' primary characteristic: their failure to employ available cues for the purpose of inhibiting punished, or otherwise inappropriate, behavior (i.e., deficient passive avoidance learning). Remarkably, there is also convergence concerning a potential physiological substrate for psychopathy. The relevance of septo-hippocampal functioning for psychopathy has been implicated in one form or another by Gorenstein and Newman (1980), Gray (1970), Hare (1970), Mawson and Mawson (1977), Trasler (1978) and, indirectly, by Fowles (1980).

Which psychological processes are responsible for the breakdown in self-regulation displayed by psychopaths? It is here that the theoretical perspectives on psychopathy diverge. One group of theories focuses on the role of arousal in precluding adequate fear conditioning. Whereas some have proposed that low arousal interferes with the development of conditioned responses to punishment cues (e.g., Eysenck, 1964; Hare, 1965), others have argued that excessive autonomic (cardiovascular) reactivity precludes meaningful differentiation between emotionally relevant and emotionally irrelevant cues, rendering most, if not all, cues essentially useless (e.g., Schachter and Latane, 1964). Hare's revised theory (e.g., 1978) appears to integrate these disparate perspectives; hyperreactivity within the cardiovascular system is held to "gate out" aversive stimuli, thus reducing the emotional impact of such cues as well as the psychopath's ability to learn their significance.

In contrast to explanations emphasizing insensitivity to punishment, several theorists have suggested that hypersensitivity to reward may underlie psychopaths' inhibitory deficits (e.g., Gorenstein and Newman, 1980; Quay, 1988; Scerbo et al., 1990; Shapiro et al., 1988). According to these theorists, psychopaths' failure to inhibit punished responses reflects a bias to focus attention on reward cues to the extent that it interferes with processing cues for punishment (Newman et al., 1983, 1985).

Rather than focusing on sensitivity to rewards or punishments, other theories attribute psychopaths' inhibitory failures to difficulty switching attentional (Harpur and Hare, 1990) or response (Newman, 1987, 1991a) sets. According to these theories, once psychopaths adopt a dominant attentional or response set, they are relatively unable to alter that set to accommodate other information from the environment.

Having set out these related but competing theories concerning the factors responsible for the psychopath's failures of self-regulation, we turn now to our review of the empirical evidence.

LABORATORY EVIDENCE

Rather than reviewing the laboratory evidence on psychopathy in relation to the particular theories, our review is organized according to the type of research, that is, according to the methods used and questions asked. This category-based strategy is at once more efficient and more conducive to the development of a cognitive reformulation of the evidence.

Autonomic Conditioning Data

In light of their apparent insensitivity to punishment, it is not surprising that one of the earliest and most often investigated questions in psychopathy concerns autonomic conditioning to cues for punishment (e.g., Lykken, 1957; Hare, 1965). As this literature has already been the subject of numerous reviews (e.g., Hare, 1978; Mawson and Mawson, 1977; Siddle and Trasler, 1981), we will simply summarize the principal findings.

One of the earliest and most important studies in this area was reported by Hare in 1965. Hare monitored skin conductance (SC) as incarcerated psychopaths and nonpsychopaths were shown the numbers 1 to 12 in sequence. Subjects were informed in advance that an intense electric shock would be delivered when the number 8 appeared. In comparison to nonpsychopaths, who showed a pronounced increase in SC as the number 8 approached, the rise in SC displayed by psychopaths was smaller, less rapid, and began later. Similar findings have been observed in several other studies (e.g., Hare and Craigen, 1974; Lippert and Senter, 1966; Ogloff and Wong, 1990). In fact, psychopaths' attenuated SC responses in anticipation of aversive stimuli is among the best replicated findings in the field.

There is also a substantial amount of agreement concerning the interpretation of this observation. According to Hare (1970, 1978), the SC data provide an index of the extent to which subjects experience fear in anticipation of aversive events. In addition, as noted by Hare (1978) and others (e.g., Fowles, 1980), research by Szpiler and Epstein (1976) provides useful perspective on this measure. Szpiler and Epstein (1976) reported that subjects who believed that they could reduce punishment by emitting an avoidance response displayed fewer nonspecific SC responses than subjects who believed that shocks were uncontrollable. While supporting the association between SC responses and fear/anxiety, these data demonstrate that response uncertainty, or "helplessness" as this term was used by Mandler (1972), may also play an important role in determining "fear arousal."

In contrast to findings for SC, psychopaths anticipating aversive events display increases in heart rate (HR) that are equal to or greater than those shown by nonpsychopaths (Hare and Quinn, 1971; Hare and Craigen, 1974). Although group differences in HR during anticipation of punishment have been reported less consistently than differences in SC responding, this finding has been the subject of much theoretical speculation.

Drawing upon theoretical developments in psychophysiology that link HR acceleration with stimulus reducing (e.g., Graham and Clifton, 1966; Lacey, 1967) and "active coping" (Obrist, 1976), Hare (1978) has proposed that "the particular pattern of electrodermal and cardiovascular reactivity to threat found in psychopathic subjects is related to the operation of efficient coping mechanisms which reduce the salience (and hence the guiding and arousing functions) of premonitory cues, and which make the anticipated stimulus less aversive" (p. 124). However, this interpretation is not uniformly accepted. Siddle and Trasler (1981), for example, find it implausible that "a stimulus which elicits a cardiac acceleration can be attenuated by some process which is thought to be controlled by that same cardiac acceleration" (p. 293). In addition, because other investigators employing similar paradigms have reported HR acceleration in nonincarcerated subjects resembling that displayed by psychopaths, these authors regard the absence of HR acceleration in Hare's nonpsychopaths as more noteworthy. Moreover, the fact that psychopaths sometimes display smaller SC responses than nonpsychopaths despite the absence of any signal that might facilitate active coping raises additional questions concerning the mechanism responsible for psychopaths' attenuated SC. Nevertheless, though disputing the particular mechanism (i.e., Hare's interpretation of the HR data), Siddle and Trasler (1981) arrive at a similar conclusion based on an analysis of electrodermal recovery in psychopaths.

Ogloff and Wong (1990) recently reported the results of a study designed to shed further light on this issue. HR and SC were recorded while psychopaths and controls participated in a countdown procedure similar to the one employed by Hare (1965). In one condition, subjects were told that they could avoid the unpleasantly loud tones by pressing a button just before the tone was scheduled to be delivered. In the second condition, the tones could not be avoided. Across conditions, psychopaths displayed significantly lower resting SC than nonpsychopaths. Moreover, in contrast to controls who displayed significant increases in SC level as the tone approached, psychopaths showed smaller increases. Significant group differences were also apparent in the HR data. Overall, psychopaths displayed a significantly greater increase in HR during the countdown than nonpsychopaths. However, this main effect was qualified by a Group × Condition × Countdown interaction: whereas HR acceleration was generally greater in the condition involving the unavoidable tone than in the condition allowing avoidance, the increase in HR preceding the unavoidable tone was significant for the psychopaths only.

Overall, the Ogloff and Wong (1990) data provide additional evidence that psychopaths display lower SC and higher HR in anticipation of aversive events. In addition, the data are consistent with Hare's proposal that psychopaths employ an effective coping response in anticipation of aversive stimuli. In the condition providing an external means of coping (i.e., an active avoidance response), psychopaths displayed remarkably little HR acceleration. However, when the tone was unavoidable, their HR acceleration was pronounced. Unlike nonpsychopaths, who tended to have lower SC levels in the active avoidance condition than in the condition with the unavoidable tone, the SC curves for psychopaths in the two conditions were nearly identical. Although apparently supporting Hare's (1978) formulation, these results do not necessarily settle the issue. First, Ogloff and Wong (1990) note that "somewhat surprisingly, no differences were found between psychopaths' and nonpsychopaths' ratings of tone intensity" (p. 243). Consequently, aside from the SC data, there is no evidence that psychopaths were, in fact, more effective in coping with or reducing the aversiveness of the stimuli. Moreover, because psychopaths' SC data were indistinguishable in the two conditions despite differences in HR acceleration, it is not entirely clear that the HR acceleration in the unavoidable tone condition was responsible for psychopaths' low SC level.

An alternative interpretation of these data is that the relatively low SC levels exhibited by psychopaths in the two conditions reflect their lower level of response uncertainty and/or evaluation. In contrast to controls who may experience increases in arousal due to the anticipation of possible instrumental and/or emotional reactions to the aversive stimuli, which, in turn, may be regarded as unacceptable (see Mandler, 1972), the lack of SC responding seen in psychopaths may indicate their disinclination to anticipate and/or evaluate such responses (Schalling, 1978). Psychopaths' HR acceleration, on the other hand, might simply provide a meaningful indication of their reaction to the stressful situation. In other words, psychopaths may not be more successful than controls in dealing with stress, they may simply manifest their stress differently. Equating HR with motor readiness and SC with response uncertainty (cf. Fowles, 1980), psychopaths' autonomic reaction to stressful situations might be viewed as reflecting a bias toward *instrumental* (i.e., motoric) as opposed to *predictive* (i.e., cognitive) control (see Mineka and Kihlstrom, 1978; Patterson and Newman, in press). From this perspective, the directional fractionation (high HR and low SC) displayed by psychopaths may reflect a greater dissociation between their motor- and stimulus-processing faculties.

Although this formulation has much in common with the interpretation proposed by Fowles (1980), he regards psychopaths as relatively insensitive to punishment and interprets their HR acceleration in response to punishment cues as stemming from the reduced inhibitory influence of their behavioral inhibition system. In contrast, we are suggesting that psychopaths' and nonpsychopaths' divergent reactions to stressful situations reflect differences in the nature, rather than differences in the magnitude, of their responses. Whereas nonpsychopaths react to punishment with a combination of behavior activation and inhibition, the inhibitory component of psychopaths' reaction to stressful events, which relies on the association between stimulus information and motor planning, is noticeably absent. Nevertheless, the arousal component of their reaction to punishment appears to be intact, resulting in a paradoxical facilitation of ongoing behavior (see Newman, 1987; Nichols and Newman, 1986; Patterson and Newman, in press).

This interpretation of the data is offered as a tentative hypothesis intended to facilitate the integration of psychophysiological and behavioral research domains. We hasten to assert that the "correct" interpretation of these autonomic data is far from clear. As noted by the psychophysiologists contributing the research (e.g., Hare, 1978; Siddle and Trasler, 1981), the data are open to a variety of interpretations. In order to resolve these ambiguities, it is essential that psychophysiologists begin to conduct their investigations in the context of meaningful behavioral paradigms (Arnett *et al.*, 1993; Siddle and Trasler, 1981).

Behavioral Findings on Reaction to Punishment and Passive Avoidance Learning

As was the case for the autonomic conditioning data, the literature on avoidance learning in psychopaths has been reviewed on several occasions (e.g., Blackburn, 1983; Brantley and Sutker, 1984; Fowles, 1980; Hare, 1986). Thus, our review of this literature will also be abbreviated.

Avoidance of Electric Shocks

The seminal study on avoidance learning in psychopaths was published by Lykken in 1957. Subjects were instructed to learn a complex sequence of lever presses that would take them through the 20 steps or choice points of a "mental maze" task. There were four response alternatives at each choice point. Pressing the correct lever turned on a green light and moved subjects to the next step in the maze, whereas pressing two of the other levers turned on a red light and signaled subjects that they would have to continue their search for the correct response. Of particular importance, a fourth lever at each choice point was associated with administration of an electric shock. Subjects were not instructed to avoid the electric shocks — they were not even told that shocks were avoidable. Instead, Lykken deliberately misled subjects into thinking that shocks were noncontingent in order to determine whether anxiety reduction would motivate learning of this *latent*, passive avoidance contingency. As predicted, "primary sociopaths" (i.e., low-anxious psychopaths) displayed the poorest passive avoidance learning, although both primary and "neurotic sociopaths" performed significantly more poorly than the nonincarcerated, normal control group. The importance of this finding is enhanced by several reported replications (e.g., Schachter and Latané, 1964; Schmauk, 1970).

A study by Chesno and Kilmann (1975) provides additional evidence for deficient avoidance learning in psychopaths. In this experiment, 90 male prisoners were subdivided into six groups formed by crossing two levels of psychopathy (based on Cleckley ratings) with three levels of anxiety (assessed via self-report). Subjects viewed a series of 10 2-digit numbers displayed on a white screen for 2 seconds followed by a 2-second intertrial interval. Their task was to learn by trial and error which numbers signaled that they should press a button to avoid a brief electric shock and which numbers indicated that they should withhold responding to avoid the shock. To assess the effect of background stimulation on avoidance learning, one-third of the subjects performed the task while continuous, 35-db white noise was played through their headphones; one-third received randomly interrupted 65-db white noise; and one-third received intermittent, 95-db white noise. Shocks were administered by an experimenter who sat next to the subject during the task.

In the minimal stimulation condition (35 db), low-anxious psychopaths committed significantly more avoidance errors than low-anxious nonpsychopaths, whereas anxious psychopaths committed significantly *fewer* avoidance errors than anxious nonpsychopaths. Both low-anxious psychopaths and high-anxious controls displayed significantly poorer avoidance learning in this condition than did the same groups under conditions providing greater stimulation. Although these results are sometimes cited as evidence for deficient passive avoidance learning in psychopaths (e.g., Siddle and Trasler, 1981), the results do not support this contention. Overall, the psychopaths committed significantly more active than passive avoidance errors. In other words, they underresponded. Moreover, high-anxious controls actually committed nonsignificantly more passive avoidance errors than low-anxious psychopaths in the minimal stimulation condition. Although inspection of the means suggests that low-anxious psychopaths in the minimal stimulation condition may have committed more passive avoidance as well as more active avoidance errors than low-anxious controls, the specific comparisons were not reported.

Chesno and Kilmann's (1975) interpretation of these data focuses on the importance of stimulation level. Whereas low-anxious psychopaths performed more poorly than the various control groups when stimulation was low, they performed at least as well as controls when stimulation was high. Based on the assumption that level of arousal in low-anxious psychopaths is suboptimal, the authors proposed that these subjects had no need to commit shocked errors in the high-stimulation conditions but that "primary sociopaths were most likely to commit and *benefit* by these errors when other stimulation was minimal" (p. 148). As noted by the authors, their results are also consistent with theories invoking Mowrer's two-factor theory (Eysenck, 1964; Hare, 1965). That is, fear conditioning appeared to be insufficient to sustain avoidance learning without the boost in arousal derived from the higher levels of external stimulation.

Chesno and Kilmann's (1975) findings are somewhat difficult to reconcile with Hare's (1978) gating out theory because active avoidance responses were available to subjects as in the Ogloff and Wong (1990) study. Thus, there would be little reason to screen out the stimuli. Perhaps, it could be argued, low-anxious psychopaths chose to gate out the stimuli under the minimal stimulation condition, but that the intermittent white noise used in the high-stimulation conditions disrupted their active coping responses. These data are also problematic for the Gray/Fowles model because in their view active avoidance is not mediated by the behavioral inhibition system, yet psychopaths' active avoidance was as impaired as their passive avoidance. Moreover, these data are not readily explained by theoretical explanations associated with our laboratory.

In light of the difficulty that recent theoretical formulations have in accommodating these data, it is worth noting several unusual aspects of the study. First, although the exact cell sizes are not reported, it appears that means were based on only five subjects per cell. Second, data from the first seven blocks of trials were discarded and only the last five blocks of acquisition trials were analyzed. As this strategy probably eliminated those trials during which subjects acquired the discrimination, the task has little or no significance for avoidance *learning*. Finally, of the 50 trials analyzed, low-anxious psychopaths did not respond on more than half (13/25) of the trials presenting an opportunity to avoid shocks by pressing the button. Such findings suggest that psychopaths were simply unconcerned about the punishments.

Avoidance of Monetary Punishments

The preceding studies on avoidance of electric shocks raise concerns about psychopaths' motivation to perform the task requirements. As noted by Lykken (1957), the level of anxiety engendered by the latent shock contingency may have been insufficient to motivate passive avoidance learning in psychopaths. Similarly, Chesno and Kilmann (1975) concluded that electric shocks may "benefit" psychopaths by increasing arousal to a more comfortable level. Thus, it is unclear whether psychopaths have difficulty *learning* punishment contingencies or are simply less willing to *perform* them.

A study by Schmauk (1970) examined passive avoidance learning in psychopaths and controls using three types of punishment: saying "wrong" (i.e., social punishment), electric shocks, and subtracting $.25 from an $8.00 cash stake. Using a slightly modified version of the Lykken (1957) task, he found that low-anxious psychopaths performed more poorly than nonpsychopaths in the electric shock and social punishment conditions. Of particular significance, however, these groups did not differ when passive avoidance errors resulted in loss of money. In light of their adequate performance when monetary punishment was used, Schmauk's findings reinforce concerns about the motivation of low-anxious psychopaths to avoid electric shocks. Unfortunately, the psychopathic and nonpsychopathic subjects used in this study were recruited from two different populations (county prison vs. noninstitutionalized farm workers and hospital attendants). Thus, it is also possible that the monetary punishments had greater motivational significance for the incarcerated psychopaths than for nonincarcerated controls, as the latter have access to more diverse sources of income (Gorenstein, 1991).

Although Schmauk's (1970) findings suggest that psychopaths and controls do not differ in avoidance learning when monetary punishments are employed, a study by Siegel (1978) provides evidence to the contrary. Siegel (1978) developed a card-playing task involving 11 specially arranged decks of standard playing cards and standard poker chips. Each deck was comprised of 40 cards and was constructed to include a predetermined percentage of punishments ranging from 0 to 100% in 10% increments. Subjects were told that, for each deck of cards, they could play as many cards as they wished by turning them over one at a time. Alternatively, they could stop playing at any time and go on to the next deck. Subjects won a chip worth $.01 each time that they turned over a number card and they lost $.01 each time that a face card was turned over. Analyses employed a measure of response suppression, defined as the percentage of cards not played within the base line time limit (i.e., the time taken to play all 40 cards of the 0% deck, which was also the first deck played by all subjects).

As predicted, psychopaths displayed significantly less suppression and earned significantly less money than the nonpsychopathic offenders and nonoffender controls. More detailed analysis of the data revealed that the group differences in suppression were significant for the 40% through 80% decks only (see Fig. 9.1). Siegel (1978) interpreted these results as support for his hypothesis that response suppression in psychopaths would be weakest when the probability of punishment was most uncertain. However, in light of the fact that psychopaths displayed less suppression than controls on every deck of cards, it is possible that the absence of group differences at the extreme probabilities derives from lack of variability (i.e., floor and ceiling effects) rather than from differences in the "certainty" of punishment.

Of particular relevance for this presentation are the recall and expectancy data reported by Siegel (1978). Immediately after playing the 30% and 70% decks, Siegel asked subjects (1) to recall "the percentage of punishment cards played" and (2) to estimate "the chances that the next card from that deck would be a punishment card" (p. 517). All three groups demonstrated excellent *recall*: the figures were 31.2% and 72.4% for psychopaths, 32.77% and 70.62% for nonpsychopathic controls, and 30.26% and 73.51% for nonoffender controls. Psychopaths and controls also gave similar *estimates* concerning the next card for the 30% deck. However, psychopaths' estimate for the 70% deck (55.2%) was significantly lower

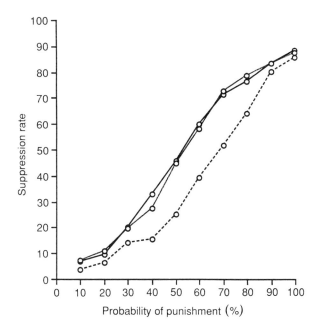

Figure 9.1. Number of cards played as a function of percent punishment and psychopathy. ---○---, psychopathic offenders; —○—, nonpsychopathic offenders; ···●···, nonoffenders. (From Siegel, 1978. ©1978 by the American Psychological Association. Adapted by permission.)

than that of the nonpsychopath (69.1%) and nonoffender (71.2%) control groups. Despite demonstrating knowledge of the payoffs, as evidenced by their recall, psychopaths appear less able or less inclined to integrate such information with expectations about the future.

In 1987, Newman *et al.* proposed an alternative interpretation of these findings derived from the septal model (Gorenstein and Newman, 1980). Specifically, we suggested that availability of reward serves to establish a dominant response set, which, in psychopaths, is relatively resistant to interruption by punishment or other forms of feedback from the environment. In contrast to Siegel's procedure, we employed a single deck of 100 playing cards presented via a computer monitor and $.05 rewards and punishments. The probability of reward was high initially to establish a dominant response set for reward (i.e., 90% reward, 10% punishment) but then decreased by 10% with each block of 10 cards until the probability of reward decreased to 0%. (Recall that Siegel (1978) required subjects to play

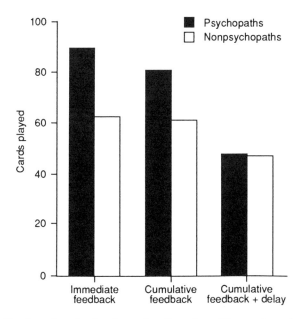

Figure 9.2. Number of cards played as a function of condition and psychopathy. (From Newman et al., 1987.)

a deck with 100% reward prior to allowing them to choose among the remaining decks.) We employed three conditions: one involving immediate feedback only; a second provided subjects with immediate feedback plus a cumulative display of all cards played; and a third condition involved an enforced, 5-second delay after each response, during which the immediate and cumulative feedback remained on the display. As predicted, psychopaths played more cards and lost more money than nonpsychopathic offenders in the condition involving immediate feedback only. Moreover, psychopaths tended to play more cards than controls even when they were provided with a cumulative display illustrating the declining probability of reward and increasing probability of punishment. In marked contrast to the other conditions, psychopaths and controls terminated the game at an equally appropriate time when subjects were prevented from responding immediately after receiving feedback (see Fig. 9.2).

Both card-playing studies provide evidence that psychopaths perseverate responding for reward despite the availability of information contraindicating that response. Importantly, Siegel's (1978) assessment of recall demonstrates that psychopaths had indeed encoded the relevant information successfully. The crucial question then, is why didn't they use it? According to Siegel, psychopaths have a "magical" belief in their immunity to uncertain punishments and that superstitious logic is "a major pathognomonic characteristic of psychopathy" (p. 514). Alternatively, the results of these studies suggest that once psychopaths set their sights on some goal such as winning money, they are less likely than nonpsychopaths to interrupt their reward-seeking behavior or accommodate information that is inconsistent with their goal. Despite the fact that psychopaths demonstrated awareness of the payoffs in the Siegel study and were given a graphic display of the payoffs in our study, psychopaths' behavior suggests that they were either unable or uninclined to make use of this information.

The discrepancy between a psychopath's understanding or verbal report on the one hand and their behavior on the other has been noted frequently in the psychopathy literature (Cleckley, 1976; Hare, 1986; Gorenstein and Newman, 1980). One possibility suggested by Shapiro's (1965) characterization of psychopathy is that this discrepancy reflects a deficit in the automatic accrual of meaningful associations to anticipated actions *while* psychopaths are engaged in goal-directed behavior. However, if psychopaths are asked to recall the probability of punishment in the interval between playing cards, they are capable of producing the information readily and accurately. Even while performing a task, if their reward-seeking behavior is interrupted and feedback is presented, psychopaths are apparently capable of using this information to exercise good judgment and alter a maladaptive response set. The fact that psychopaths did not perseverate responding in our enforced delay condition suggests that their poor suppression in the other conditions reflects a failure to accommodate information rather than superstitious logic or lack of motivation to avoid loss of money.

In contrast to the ambiguity concerning psychopaths' motivation to avoid electric shocks, it is generally agreed that psychopaths are adequately motivated to avoid loss of money (e.g., Schmauk, 1970). Nevertheless, based on the previous data, it is impossible to determine conclusively whether psychopaths' poor performance on the card-playing tasks reflects perseveration of reward seeking or a lack of responsiveness to monetary punishments. To address this issue, Newman and Kosson (1986) modified the go/no-go discrimination task developed by Chesno and Kilmann (1975). Rather than punishing errors with electric shocks, subjects lost $.10 from their cash stake whenever they committed a passive avoidance (commission) or active avoidance (omission) error. Under these conditions, psychopaths appeared no less responsive to monetary punishments than controls and they performed both passive and active avoidance contingencies as well as the nonpsychopathic prison controls.

Despite their proficient passive avoidance in the punishment-only condition, psychopaths committed significantly more passive avoidance errors than controls on the same task when it involved competing reward and punishment contingencies, that is, when correct responses were followed by $.10 rewards and incorrect responses (i.e., passive avoidance errors) were punished by taking away $.10. In light of their adequate performance in the punishment-only condition, it is difficult to argue that psychopaths' poor avoidance in the reward–punishment condition reflected lack of motivation, insensitivity to punishment, or a general inability to inhibit inappropriate responses. Rather, we interpreted the data as evidence that once psychopaths adopt a dominant response set for reward, they are less likely than controls to shift attention to process the cues associated with delivery of punishment (see also Newman *et al.*, 1985).

Although our interpretation of the results is reasonable in light of the response perseveration displayed by psychopaths in the card-playing tasks described above, the task employed by Newman and Kosson (1986) provided no direct assessment of response perseveration or allocation of attention. Thus, we (Newman *et al.*, 1990) conducted a follow-up study using a modified version of the passive avoidance task to examine the extent to which subjects suspended approach behavior following monetary punishments. Following each response, subjects viewed a feedback display that included the stimulus to which they had responded and a statement indicating either that they had been correct and won $.10 or that they had been incorrect and lost $.10. Of particular relevance, this display remained on the monitor for a maximum of 5 seconds or until subjects pressed a button to end the display and initiate the next trial. The computer measured this response latency without the subject's knowledge. The amount of time that subjects paused after reward was subtracted from the amount of time that they paused after punishment to arrive at an estimate of the amount of time that subjects suspended approach behavior to process negative feedback (i.e., reflectivity).

Because preliminary analyses revealed significant psychopathy by anxiety interactions for both passive avoidance learning and reflectivity, hypotheses were tested using low-anxious psychopaths and low-anxious controls only. Consistent with predictions, low-anxious psychopaths showed significantly less inclination to pause after negative feedback and committed significantly more passive avoidance errors than low-anxious controls. Moreover, regression analysis was used to examine the association between pausing after punishment and learning from punished errors (i.e., passive avoidance errors) after controlling for the amount of time that subjects paused following rewards. The longer that subjects paused following punishment, the fewer passive avoidance errors they made. These findings clarify the potential contribution of reward contingencies and response perseveration to the psychopath's failure to profit from punishment. To the extent that psychopaths persist in a dominant response set for reward, they are less likely to pause and process negative feedback and, therefore, less likely to develop an association between a particular response and an aversive outcome. This mechanism has both short-term and long-term consequences for passive avoidance: regarding the former, perseverating a maladaptive response set may result in the immediate administration of punishments as it did in the card-playing task (e.g., Newman *et al.*, 1987). With regard to the latter, failure to pause and process cues for punishment may hamper a person's ability to anticipate and therefore avoid inappropriate responses in the future as it did in the passive avoidance task.

Therefore, in contrast to results reported by Schmauk (1970), several recent studies suggest that psychopaths perform more poorly than controls on avoidance learning tasks involving monetary punishments. As noted by Newman *et al.* (1990), a salient difference between avoidance learning tasks revealing group differences and those that do not concerns the use of competing reward and punishment contingencies. In the experiments reported by Siegel (1978) and Newman *et al.* (1987), subjects began responding for reward and were then required to alter the established response set to avoid losing money. Similarly, subjects in the reward–punishment conditions reported by Newman and Kosson (1986) and Newman *et al.* (1990) typically master the discrimination by responding to both good and bad stimuli before learning to inhibit responses that are followed by punishment. In contrast to these studies, the punishment contingency employed by Schmauk (1970) was salient from the outset of the task and there was no competing reward contingency. In the punishment-only condition employed by Newman and Kosson (1986), the punishment contingencies were also salient from the outset and there was no competing reward contingency. In these later examples, we suggest that psychopaths performed as well as controls because there was no requirement to revise an established response set.

Obviously, the requirement to alter a dominant response set is not the only difference between these two sets of tasks. Whereas those revealing differences involved monetary rewards as well as punishments, no group differences were observed in the tasks involving punishments only. Thus, it is possible that availability of reward is sufficient to disrupt avoidance learning independent of the requirement to alter a dominant response set.

To address this hypothesis, Newman *et al.* (1990) modified their avoidance learning task to establish independent reward and punishment contingencies that would cause subjects to allocate attention to both contingencies from the outset of the task. This strategy was intended to create a task that involved monetary rewards and punishments, but that obviated the requirement to alter a dominant response set in a manner analogous to our punishment-only condition. Under these conditions, we found absolutely no evidence that psychopaths were less likely to pause following punishment or more likely to commit passive avoidance errors in comparison to controls.

Though the experiment just described is in need of replication because the subjects had participated in previous studies, the results suggest an interesting interpretation. Psychopaths do not appear to be less able or less motivated than controls to perform avoidance contingencies when doing so is the focus of their attention. However, when avoidance contingencies are "latent" or introduced after subjects have established their goals, controls appear to shift their attention and process the association between their responses and the occurrence of punishment automatically, whereas psychopaths experience difficulty with this type of information processing. Without a "time out" (e.g., the enforced delay employed by Newman *et al.*, 1987) or some other method for facilitating integration of new information, psychopaths tend to perseverate their ongoing response set.

In contrast to explanations emphasizing hyposensitivity to punishment or hypersensitivity to reward, this analysis of psychopaths' deficient self-regulation attributes their problem to difficulty altering a dominant response set based on the accrual of additional, inhibitory associations to the prepared response. An important consequence of this response modulation deficit concerns the complex nature of motivationally relevant stimuli such as punishment and frustration. As noted by Gray (1987) and others (e.g., Caplan, 1970; Dickinson, 1974, 1975), punishment typically increases nonspecific arousal as well as behavioral inhibition. If, as proposed, nonspecific arousal increases the intensity of behavior (and psychopaths' reaction to aversive stimuli often involves increased nonspecific arousal without a counterbalancing increase in behavioral inhibition, as noted above), then aversive stimuli may paradoxically increase rather than decrease the intensity of their ongoing behavior.

To examine the effects of punishment stimuli on the responding of psychopathic and nonpsychopathic subjects, we recently conducted a study in which we (1) trained subjects to inhibit responses when a particular stimulus was present in order to avoid punishment, and then (2) presented this cue for punishment while subjects performed a visual search reaction time test. Even though the conditioned stimulus was unrelated to performance in the second phase, subjects were expected to respond more slowly when the cue was present than when it was absent, because of its inhibitory associations. As expected, there were no group differences in Phase 1, but a significant Psychopathy × Trial type interaction in Phase 2 revealed that, unlike controls, who responded more slowly when the punishment cue was present, psychopaths responded more quickly on the cue-present trials (Newman, 1991b).

The implications of this discussion for psychopathy are several. First, assessing sensitivity to punishment using measures of response suppression may be inadequate because difficulty altering a dominant response set may limit response suppression even though a person experiences a strong punishment-induced increase in arousal. Second, the psychopath's *reaction* to punishment appears to involve an increase in nonspecific arousal without a concomitant increase in response inhibition. Third, to the extent that it does, this aspect of the syndrome would make it especially difficult for psychopaths to display self-control in situations involving frustration, punishment, or other affects involving arousal as well as inhibitory components. Thus, in addition to its lack of inhibitory influence over behavior, the arousal component of punishment may actually disrupt self-control in psychopaths.

The results of a recent experiment assessing delay of gratification are consistent with the possibility that punishment has an "activating" effect on psychopaths (Newman *et al.*, 1992). On each of 50 trials, subjects were given a choice between two responses. In Condition REW, subjects could either respond immediately and be rewarded (win $.05) on 40% of the trials or they could wait 10 seconds and respond to a second button that was rewarded on 80% of the trials. A second condition (REW + PUN) provided monetary punishments as well as rewards. Whenever subjects did not win $.05, $.05 were taken away. In this condition, the probabilities were set to 70% reward (30% punishment) for the immediate button and 90% reward (10% punishment) for the delayed response in order to match the expected earnings used in Condition REW. In a third condition (EQ), subjects had to wait 10 seconds before responding to either button, and the payoffs were identical to those in Condition REW.

The principal finding in this study was a Psychopathy × Anxiety × Condition interaction. Although we had expected a more general deficit in delay of gratification among low-anxious psychopaths, their delay behavior depended on Condition. Whereas low-anxious psychopaths performed at least as well as controls in Conditions REW and EQ, they displayed the *poorest* delay of gratification in Condition REW + PUN. Thus, the addition of a punishment contingency to the delay task had a significant, adverse effect on the performance of low-anxious psychopaths.

Investigations of Attention

Psychophysiological Studies

In reviewing the theoretical perspectives on psychopathy, we noted that psychopaths' failures to accommodate cues for punishment have been attributed increasingly to attentional factors. For instance, several authors have suggested that psychopaths overallocate attention to events of immediate motivational significance to the neglect of less salient or less immediate considerations (Jutai and Hare, 1983; Newman *et al.*, 1983; Kosson and Newman, 1986). A related hypothesis is that psychopaths "gate out" aversive stimuli and/or are less open to environmental stimuli (Hare, 1978; Siddle and Trasler, 1981).

One of the first studies of this type was reported by Jutai and Hare (1983). Event-related potentials (ERPs) to irrelevant tone pips were recorded while subjects either sat quietly or played an engaging video game. N100 was used as an index of subjects' attentional response to the tones. Although the groups did not differ when they simply listened passively to the tones, psychopaths displayed smaller N100 responses than controls during the early trials of the video game condition.

The fact that group differences were specific to the condition involving an engaging primary task appears to support the *"overfocusing hypothesis."* According to the overfocusing hypothesis, however, poor secondary task performance results from overallocation of attention to the primary task. Thus, clear support for this hypothesis requires evidence of increased attention to the primary task (e.g., the video game) in addition to decreased attention to a secondary task (e.g., attentional responses to tones; see Kosson and Newman, 1989). However, psychopaths performed no better than controls on the video game. Without evidence for an attentional trade-off of this type, the smaller ERPs displayed by psychopaths are equally consistent with alternative interpretations. For example, psychopaths may be superior at screening out irrelevant stimuli (Hare, 1978); they may have less overall attentional capacity (Harpur and Hare, 1990); the perceptual-motor requirements of the video game may have demanded more attentional capacity from psychopaths than from controls, resulting in less "spare capacity"; or, perhaps associated with anomalous feedback circuits in the brain, the effortful organization of goal-directed behavior associated with playing the video game may have directly suppressed stimulus intake in psychopaths, while leaving this function unaffected in controls (see Smith *et al.*, 1992).

A related study reported by Jutai *et al.* (1987) recorded ERPs while subjects performed an "oddball" paradigm requiring them to press a button whenever the less frequent of two phonemes occurred. Again, the task was performed under single-task (oddball task only) and dual-task conditions (i.e., oddball task plus video game). Data were reported for N100, P300 (a response usually elicited by unpredictable stimulus events requiring a response), and slow positive wave (SW). The SW is a response that "begins 200–300 msec after stimulus presentation and peaks at approximately 500–700 msec. It is elicited by the same sorts of events as P300, and may reflect an attempt to reduce uncertainty about the outcome of stimulus evaluation" (Jutai *et al.*, 1987, p. 176).

Both groups performed equally well on the oddball task, the video game, and the dual task involving the simultaneous performance of the oddball and video-game tasks. In addition, there were no group differences in N100 or P300 when the oddball task was performed alone and, according to the authors, there was no evidence of SW activity in either group when the oddball task was performed alone. Although no group differences were found in the N100 or P300 components of the ERP during the dual task, Jutai *et al.* (1987) reported that P300 latencies to the target tended to be longer for psychopaths than for controls ($p < .10$). Moreover, they noted that the significant increase in P300 latency associated with performance of the oddball task under dual-task versus single-task conditions was due primarily to psychopaths, although this interaction also fell short of conventional statistical significance ($p < .10$). According to the authors, their principal finding was that psychopaths displayed significantly larger SW amplitudes than controls in the dual-task condition.

In discussing this finding, Jutai *et al.* (1987) noted that because two target phonemes never occurred sequentially, it should have been easy for subjects to learn that detecting a target stimulus on a trial following presentation of a target was highly improbable. Thus, they proposed that the relatively large SW seen in psychopaths indicates that they "failed to learn as much as Group NP about the likelihood that a target would appear on a subsequent trial, and, consequently, equivocated about stimulus probability" (p. 182). Thus, similar to our conclusion regarding the performance of psychopaths on the card-playing tasks reported by Siegel (1978) and Newman *et al.* (1987), these results suggest that psychopaths have difficulty accommodating information such as conditional probabilities while engaged in perceptual-motor processing.

Results from two other studies (Forth and Hare, 1989; Raine and Venables, 1988) have been interpreted as evidence for *enhanced processing of relevant information* by psychopaths. Using an oddball paradigm under single-task conditions, Raine and Venables reported larger P300 amplitudes at their parietal recording site for psychopaths than for nonpsychopaths in response to the rare *visual target*. Although this finding was interpreted as evidence of enhanced information processing, it should be noted that psychopaths' performance on the continuous performance task was no better than that of controls. In fact, inspection of the means revealed that controls performed nonsignificantly better than psychopaths on three of the four measures reported. Moreover, the authors noted evidence of slower P300 recovery in psychopaths, a finding reminiscent of the SW data reported by Jutai *et al.* (1987). In light of the performance data, one may question whether the ERPs reflect enhanced information processing or simply greater cognitive effort, perhaps to compensate for some processing defect.

Forth and Hare (1989) assessed contingent negative variation (CNV) during a reaction-time task involving monetary payoffs. Although no group differences in CNV were observed in the interval immediately preceding the signal to respond (i.e., the imperative stimulus), the authors reported that psychopaths displayed larger CNVs than controls during the second immediately following the "warning stimulus." In addition to indicating that an imperative stimulus was imminent, the warning stimulus signaled whether subjects would win or lose money on that trial. Together with results reported by Raine and Venables (1988), these findings provide additional evidence that psychopaths are not simply unmotivated or unresponsive to the requirements of experimental tasks. To the contrary, they suggest that, in comparison to controls, psychopaths may actually engage in more effortful allocation of attention to relevant task demands.

Behavioral Studies

Several authors have noted that investigations of attention employing ERPs are necessarily limited because they do not provide behavioral evidence of overfocusing (Harpur and Hare, 1990; Jutai, 1989; Kosson and Newman, 1986). In order to remedy this problem, Kosson and Newman (1986) employed a visual-search task and an auditory probe reaction-time task under single- and dual-task conditions. One group of subjects was instructed to perform as well as possible on the visual task and to allocate attention to the auditory task only to the extent that it would not interfere with performance on the visual task (Focused-Attention Condition). A second group of subjects was instructed to divide their attention equally between the two tasks. Based on the overfocusing hypothesis, we predicted that psychopaths would display superior performance on the visual task and relatively poor performance on the auditory task relative to controls in the focused-attention condition. No differences were expected in the divided-attention condition, because the requirement to distribute attention was apparent from the outset of the task.

The findings provided little support for our hypotheses. Although psychopaths performed as well as controls on the visual task in the focused-attention condition, they were not significantly better. In addition, reaction times to auditory probes were significantly slower in psychopaths than in controls regardless of condition. Finally, psychopaths committed significantly more errors than controls on the visual-search task in the divided-attention condition. Thus, even though psychopaths appeared to have less attentional capacity available for the auditory task than controls, we found no evidence of superior performance on the visual task as required by the overfocusing interpretation. Moreover, our instruction to divide attention between the two tasks caused psychopaths to perform more poorly than controls on both tasks, perhaps indicating that it took more cognitive capacity for psychopaths to comply with this request to manage their attentional resources (see Kosson and Newman, 1986).

More recently, we examined the overfocusing hypothesis by assessing the ability of psychopaths and nonpsychopaths to alter a dominant response set in the context of a cued reaction-time task (Howland *et al.*, in press). On each trial, a warning stimulus and an imperative stimulus were presented. Subjects' task was to press a button with their left hand or right hand depending upon whether the imperative stimulus occurred on the left or right side of the computer display. Warning stimuli were predictive of imperative stimulus location on 80% of the trials and were therefore presumed to establish a dominant response set. In addition, monetary payoffs were determined by response speed. We predicted that psychopaths would overfocus on the expected location and have more difficulty than controls altering their response set on trials involving invalid cues (i.e., when the warning stimuli signaled the location of the imperative stimulus incorrectly).

The results provided partial support for our hypotheses. Psychopaths committed more errors than controls when subjects were led to expect a right-handed response (warning stimulus on the right) but the imperative stimulus required a left-handed response. No significant differences were obtained for the switch trials involving preparation of a left-handed response or in analyses of reaction time. However, despite the fact that psychopaths appeared to have greater difficulty than controls in altering a set to respond with their right hand, we found no evidence that they responded more quickly or more accurately when the imperative stimulus was correctly predicted by a right-handed warning stimulus. Thus, as in the Kosson and Newman (1986) study, these results provide some evidence that psychopaths are less efficient than controls in processing unexpected information, but contrary to the overfocusing hypothesis, this lack of efficiency is not associated with superior performance on facets of the task upon which attention is focused. Moreover, these observations appear to parallel the ERP findings reported by Jutai and his colleagues (1987).

Harpur and Hare (1990) have recently described a study in which they examined the overfocusing hypothesis using a visual, cued reaction time task. Visual cues, predicting the location of the imperative stimuli 67% of the time, were presented to the left or right of a fixation point at stimulus onset asynchronies (SOAs) of 50, 150, 650, and 1000 msecs. Differences in reaction time between valid and invalid cuing trials enabled the authors to assess "exogenous facilitation, occurring at early SOAs (50–150 msecs) as a result of a cue drawing attention rapidly to the cued location; endogenous facilitation developing from 200 msecs on, as a result of the predictive validity of the cue; (and) inhibition of return, apparent at SOAs of 650 and 1000 msecs, and acting to inhibit responding to a target at a previously cued location" (p. 17).

Psychopaths and controls did not differ in exogenous orienting of attention or on the inhibition of return measures. However, psychopaths displayed significantly greater orienting than controls to the cued side at SOAs of 650 and 1000 msecs. The authors interpreted this evidence of stronger endogenous orienting in psychopaths as support for the overfocusing hypothesis.

Like the psychophysiological evidence presented by Forth and Hare (1989) and Raine and Venables (1988), these data appear to indicate that active, effortful allocation of attention to salient events is exaggerated in psychopaths relative to controls. As noted previously, however, in the absence of behavioral evidence demonstrating superior primary-task performance coupled with compromised secondary-task performance, we hesitate to interpret such evidence as support for the overfocusing hypothesis. Alternatively, the management of attentional resources in psychopaths may be more dependent on effortful/controlled information processing than it is in control subjects, perhaps owing to some situation-specific defect in the automatic allocation of attention to relevant stimuli. By this account, psychopaths' greater reliance on cuing stimuli may reflect an active coping strategy employed to compensate for a more fundamental problem in the flexible allocation of attention to relevant cues.

We recently completed two studies that raise additional doubts regarding the standard overfocusing hypothesis. In one case, we employed a verbal memory task commonly used to evaluate overfocusing engendered by background noise and monetary incentives (e.g., Hockey and Hamilton, 1970; Davies and Jones, 1975). Eight stimulus words were presented, one at a time, and arranged so that each word appeared in one of the four corners of the computer monitor. Prior to the presentation, subjects were told that they would be asked to recall the words in order and that they would be paid according to how many words they recalled. Following the presentation, subjects were asked to recall the words as instructed, but they were also asked to indicate the corner in which the word was displayed. In this task, word recall is the primary task and recall of word *location* is the secondary task, presumably reflecting spare capacity. Contrary to predictions based on the overfocusing hypothesis, no significant group differences were observed in primary or secondary task.

The second study involved a follow-up to the cuing-task study reported by Howland *et al.* (in press). Because the cues employed by Howland *et al.* signaled both the likely location of the imperative stimulus and the likely response (left or right), the dominant response set established was both attentional and motor. To disentangle these processes, we developed a task to assess difficulty switching an attentional set independent of motor preparation. On each trial, two rectangles appeared, one on either side of the monitor. On 80% of the trials, an *X* appeared in the right hand rectangle in one of three locations, indicating that subjects should press the left, middle, or right button on their response panel. The response requirements of the task were minimized because correct responses were rewarded regardless of response speed and because subjects could not anticipate which button they would have to press. On the other hand, attentional demands were maximized by presenting the *X* briefly and following it with a masking stimulus. On 20% of the trials, the *X* appeared in the left rectangle and thus required subjects to switch attention from the right to the left side of the monitor in order to perceive the location of *X*. Although the task was sensitive enough to reveal significant group differences between high- and low-anxious subjects, there was no evidence that psychopaths had more difficulty switching attention than controls (Howland and Newman, 1991).

The tasks used to assess overfocusing in these last two studies did not involve difficult response requirements: In both cases, subjects made their responses after the timed portion of the trial had ended. These experiments provided no evidence of differential attentional effects. On the other hand, attentional anomalies were reported by Jutai *et al.* (1987) who used a demanding perceptual-motor task (video game), and by Howland *et al.* (in press) who used a speeded reaction-time task. Overall, we might speculate that the use of a demanding perceptual-motor task is an important factor determining whether psychopaths appear less responsive than controls to the presentation of unexpected stimuli. Moreover, it appears that observing deficient secondary-task performance in psychopaths may depend upon the use of more cognitively demanding tasks such as processing conditional probabilities (Jutai *et al.*, 1987).

Investigations of Neuropsychological Performance

An alternative method for analyzing cognitive performance in psychopaths involves the use of traditional neuropsychological tests. Although neuropsychological tests are frequently used to make inferences about potential brain damage, they may also be used to assess functional strengths and weaknesses regardless of their implications for structural brain abnormalities.

As noted by Hart *et al.* (1990), hypotheses concerning neuropsychological performance in psychopaths are often based on similarities between the behavior of psychopaths and brain-damaged patients (e.g., Elliott, 1978; Flor-Henry, 1976; Gorenstein, 1982). To date, however, there is no convincing evidence that psychopaths display clinically significant levels of neuropsychological impairment.

The most active area of neuropsychological assessment in psychopaths involves measures of frontal functioning because, like patients with frontal damage, psychopaths appear to be deficient in "executive functions" (see Elliot, 1978; Gorenstein, 1991; Kandel and Freed, 1989). As noted by Schalling (1978), the "similarities between psychopathic behavior and the effects of frontal lesions are noteworthy in view of current neuropsychological models which emphasize the importance of these parts of the brain for persistence and consistency of behaviour, for the regulation of attention and activation processes, and for affective responsiveness (Luria, 1973; Nauta, 1971)" (pp. 94–95). Schalling and Rosen (1968) conducted one of the first studies in this area using the Porteus Maze test, which assesses planning and foresight and is therefore considered relevant to frontal functioning (Lezak, 1983). Criminal psychopaths, diagnosed using Cleckley criteria, were found to exhibit more rule-breaking and carelessness relative to nonpsychopathic offenders. Though Sutker *et al.* (1972) reported a failure to replicate this finding, their subjects were assigned to groups using MMPI criteria.

More recently, Gorenstein (1982) reported that psychopaths performed more poorly than controls on other measures with presumed relevance to frontal functioning [i.e., the Wisconsin Card Sorting Test (WCST); the sequential matching memory test; and the Necker Cube task]. Our discussion will focus on the WCST. In this task, subjects are shown a series of display cards containing one of four different *shapes* (e.g., squares, circles), printed in one of four different *colors*, and varying in *number* (i.e., from one to four). Subjects are instructed to sort the cards into piles under the four sample cards laid out in front of them. The task involves sorting according to different rules: subjects must first sort cards according to color, then, after a criterion is met, according to shape, and finally according to number. Each time that the rule changes, subjects are forced to alter an established set and sort according to a new rule. The task yields several different performance measures, including perseverative and nonperseverative errors. Perseverative errors occur when a subject incorrectly sorts a card according to the previous rule. The remaining errors are considered nonperseverative.

Gorenstein (1982) predicted that, like frontal patients, psychopaths would find it relatively difficult to alter a dominant set and would, therefore, commit more perseverative errors than controls. As predicted, psychopaths committed more perseverative, and no more nonperseverative, errors than controls. However, unsuccessful attempts to replicate this finding have cast doubt on the findings (Devonshire et al., 1988; Hare, 1984; Hoffman et al., 1987; Sutker and Allain, 1987).

Using a computerized version of the WCST, Howland and Newman (1987) examined the performance of psychopathic and nonpsychopathic offenders under different experimental conditions. In one condition, subjects were provided with monetary rewards and punishments after each response, whereas subjects in the other condition merely received feedback (i.e., "correct" or "wrong") via the computer monitor. No significant differences were obtained in the condition involving feedback only. However, when an experimenter delivered monetary rewards and punishments after each response, psychopaths committed significantly more perseverative errors and achieved fewer categories than controls. Moreover, in contrast to controls who paused to reflect (i.e., slowed down) when monetary punishment signaled a change in the sorting rule, psychopaths either responded more quickly (following the first rule change) or displayed no change in response speed at all. Despite random assignment of subjects to groups and a lack of group differences in intelligence overall, group differences in intelligence occurred within conditions. Thus, our findings should be regarded as tentative and in need of replication.

As noted above, certain WCST results appear to contradict other evidence, indicating that psychopaths perseverate dominant response sets (e.g., Siegel, 1978; Newman et al., 1987). There are, however, two salient differences between procedures demonstrating groups differences and those that do not. First, the tasks revealing group differences employed monetary rewards and punishments. The importance of this factor has been discussed previously. Second, there are important differences between the *measures of perseveration*. Similar to measures of response perseveration used to assess septal dysfunction, the card-playing tasks establish a particular response in the presence of particular cues. In marked contrast, the WCST involves rule learning and flexibility in the application of these rules. The rules for responding in the WCST are not represented in the external environment and they are not associated with a specific response because the correct response can only be determined after examining the next card to be sorted. The factors responsible for the perseveration of *abstract, sorting rules* may well be different from those accounting for the psychopaths' difficulty altering a *specific prepared response* (i.e., dominant response set).

With regard to more general assessments of neuropsychological performance in psychopaths, Hart et al. (1990) recently reported the results of a large-scale neuropsychological "screening" that employed two samples of psychopathic and nonpsychopathic offenders. The battery of tests administered to the first sample ($N = 90$) included the Trail-Making Test, Visual Retention Test, Auditory-Verbal Learning Test, and Visual Organization Test. The battery administered to the second sample ($N = 167$) included the Trail Making Test, Controlled Word Association Test, Vocabulary and Block Design subtests of the WAIS-R, and a measure of reading ability. Multivariate analysis of variance conducted on each sample revealed no significant differences ($F < 1.00$ in both cases). However, the authors note that psychopaths tended ($p < .06$) to perform more poorly than controls on the Trail-Making Test in one sample.

Smith *et al.* (1992) recently completed a detailed investigation of neuropsychological performance in psychopaths. Only right-handed subjects with estimated IQ scores of 75 or greater, and whose records (plus interview data) revealed no evidence of serious head injuries were included. Moreover, we employed a thorough assessment of drug and alcohol symptoms to control for this potentially confounding variable. Finally, based on numerous studies indicating that the performance of psychopaths may be moderated by level of anxiety, psychopaths and controls were subdivided into high- and low-anxious groups using the Welsh anxiety scale. The test battery included Block Design, the Controlled Oral Word Association Test, Digit Span, Finger Tapping, Paired Associates, the Short Category Test, the Stroop Color-Word Test, and the Trail Making Test.

Although group differences were predicted for six of the twelve dependent measures (the other six measures were included to control for general performance), only two of the tasks [Block Design and the Trail Making Test (B form)] revealed significantly poorer performance in low-anxious psychopaths than in low-anxious controls. Nevertheless, the fact that these differences were obtained despite the use of well-matched subject groups and that the differences remained significant even after partialling out intelligence, substance abuse, and performance on the six control measures, increases our confidence that this is not a spurious finding.

We consider it noteworthy that Block Design and Trails were the only two tasks in the entire battery that involve perceptual–motor integration. That is, both tasks required subjects to shift frequently between planning motor behavior (e.g., tracing and assembling the blocks) and analyzing stimulus materials. Given that both tasks are widely used, it is somewhat surprising that this finding has not been reported previously (cf. Hart *et al.*, 1990). Though the results are in need of replication, it seems likely that our decision to examine performance within level of anxiety was an important factor. When the data were reanalyzed, collapsing across anxiety, the differences between psychopaths and controls disappeared.

Investigations of Language and Verbal Functioning

Nearly all of the research in this area of cognitive functioning has been conducted by Hare and his colleagues. Moreover, Hare *et al.* (1988) have provided an excellent summary of the work. Thus, our discussion of their findings will be brief and limited to those studies with direct relevance to the topic of this chapter.

As noted previously, Cleckley (1976) used the term "semantic dementia" to connote his belief that psychopaths are characterized by a type of neuropsychological defect that interferes with their ability to experience the affect or meaning associated with their words. Hare and his colleagues have pursued this lead using a variety of behavioral and psychophysiological methods.

Hare and McPherson (1984) used a dichotic listening task in which 22 sets of 3 words were delivered via stereophonic headphones to one ear or the other. Recall was assessed following each trial (i.e., simultaneous presentation of one set to each ear) and the total number of words recalled from each ear was analyzed. A significant Group × Ear interaction indicated that psychopaths showed a smaller right ear advantage than nonpsychopaths. The results were interpreted as evidence that language functions are less strongly lateralized in psychopaths than in controls.

Lateralization of language functions has also been assessed using divided visual-field studies. Using a relatively simple task, Hare (1979) found superior recognition of words presented to the right (RVF; left hemisphere), as opposed to left visual field (LVF; right hemisphere) in both psychopathic and nonpsychopathic subjects. However, in a similar study that employed word categorization tasks of varying complexity, Hare and Jutai (1988) reported a Group × Visual Field interaction associated with performance in the relatively difficult, abstract categorization task. In contrast to nonpsychopathic and noncriminal controls, who displayed the expected RVF advantage (i.e., more LVF than RVF errors), psychopaths

displayed a LVF advantage (i.e., more RVF than LVF errors). Like the dichotic listening data, these findings were taken as evidence that psychopaths are characterized by atypical cerebral organization of language.

In an effort to assess whether the affective and semantic components of
language are integrated as well in psychopaths as in controls, Williamson
et al. (1991) presented subjects with a lexical decision task involving emotional and neutral words. Stimuli were presented briefly in the LVF or RVF
and subjects had to indicate, as quickly as possible, whether or not the
letter string was a word. Overall, there were no group differences in accuracy and the accuracy of both groups was greater for emotional than for
neutral words. However, analysis of the reaction time data revealed a significant Group × Word Type interaction indicating that controls, but not
psychopaths, responded more quickly to emotional than to neutral words.
Although not statistically significant, ERP data were consistent with this
finding. The authors concluded that words convey less information to psychopaths than they do to other individuals. Once again, we note that
psychopaths' processing of cues from the environment is less complete or
less efficient than controls' while they are preparing to make a particular
response.

Summary and Integration

As already noted, the majority of experimental studies on psychopathy
has been concerned with understanding psychopaths' failure to utilize
information to regulate approach behavior. However, with the exception of
their poorer passive avoidance learning (e.g., Lykken, 1957; Newman and
Kosson, 1986; Newman *et al.*, 1987; Siegel, 1978), the observed group differences appear to reflect processing anomalies as opposed to performance
deficits. Nevertheless, given the relevance of passive avoidance learning to
the uninhibited, antisocial behavior that characterizes psychopaths, it
could be argued that the critical performance deficit has been discovered
and that the goal of current research is primarily to explain the factors
mediating its expression.

The idiosyncratic processing of punishment cues, attentional probes,
and language described in our review provides significant insight in this
regard. Psychopaths display less electrodermal activity in anticipation of
punishment, but they are no less responsive on cardiovascular measures.
While there can be little doubt that psychopaths are anticipating the aversive events in the countdown procedures, their autonomic psychophysiology reveals that they anticipate or experience stressful events differently
than controls. Group differences in allocation of attention are also informative even though evidence of processing deficiencies has been relatively

rare. Kosson and Newman (1986) found that psychopaths displayed slower reaction times on an auditory discrimination task performed in a dual-task context, and Howland *et al.* (in press) reported that psychopaths had more difficulty inhibiting a dominant response set on trials involving an unexpected shift in the location of the imperative stimulus. Other studies suggest that psychopaths display enhanced allocation of attention to stimuli with immediate motivational significance. Overall, research employing traditional neuropsychological tests suggest that these reliable performance measures are unable to detect meaningful differences between psychopaths and controls (Hart *et al.*, 1990). Nevertheless, such studies raise the possibility that low-anxious psychopaths may be less adept than controls at speeded, perceptual-motor integration (Schalling, 1978; Smith *et al.*, 1992). Finally, research on language processing in psychopaths provides intriguing evidence for processing anomalies. The data appear to indicate that the association of words with meaning and affect occurs less readily or less automatically in psychopaths than in controls. Although psychopaths are able to use words appropriately and perform well on measures of verbal intelligence, the semantic and affective components of their response appear to be elicited less automatically.

Overall, we have observed no hint of a cognitive deficit among psychopaths on measures of abstract reasoning, short- or long-term memory, rule learning, motor speed, verbal skills, or attentional concentration. In addition, they appear to have no difficulty learning and performing complex contingencies as long as the requirements of the task are clear from the outset. However, consistent with Shapiro's (1965) portrayal of the psychopath as deficient in the capacity to integrate current urges and relevant associations automatically, our review highlights differences between psychopaths and controls regarding their ability to use incidental information to enhance, elaborate upon, or otherwise achieve perspective on a dominant or ongoing response set. Whereas this process occurs in a relatively automatic manner for most people, it may necessitate the use of a higher proportion of controlled processing resources in psychopaths.

Throughout this chapter, we have employed the terms "automatic" and "controlled" processing without elaborating on or qualifying our use of these terms. Following Schneider *et al.* (1984), we regard automatic processing as "a fast, parallel, fairly effortless process that is not limited by short-term memory capacity, is not under direct subject control, and is responsible for the performance of well-developed skilled behaviors" (p. 1). Controlled processing has been used to designate a "slow, generally serial, effortful, capacity-limited, subject-regulated processing mode that must be used to deal with novel or inconsistent information" (p. 2). Though impulsive individuals are often described as responding automatically in the absence of controlled deliberation, the switch to controlled processing itself is, in part, mediated by automatic processes. This aspect of attention was brought to light using the analogy of the "cocktail party phenomenon" (see Neisser, 1966). Even when our attention is devoted to an engaging conversation, we automatically notice and direct our attention to significant stimuli in the environment such as the mention of our name. Presumably, we can disregard distracting stimuli while remaining sufficiently attuned to the environment so that we may detect significant stimuli and shift our attention in the event that controlled analysis of stimuli appears warranted. A defect in the automatic processing that underlies this ability to screen, detect, and redirect attention in response to significant stimuli would provide a cogent mechanism for the motivational, affective, and cognitive idiosyncracies described by Shapiro (1965).

In addition, a deficit in this type of automatic processing provides a satisfying explanation for the experimental results that we have reviewed. Consider the data on passive avoidance learning. The poor passive avoidance learning of psychopaths is most readily observed in tasks involving a "latent" punishment contingency (e.g., Lykken, 1957; Schmauk, 1970), a changing probability of punishment (Newman et al., 1987; Siegel, 1978) and, to a lesser extent, in tasks involving competing reward/punishment contingencies (e.g., Newman and Kosson, 1986; Newman et al., 1990). Particularly in the first two paradigms, subjects first become engaged in goal-directed behavior and subsequently are required to notice the latent contingency or changing probabilities in order to avoid excessive punishments. Thus, recognizing the necessity of altering one's dominant response set in reaction to these "unattended" contingencies may rely largely on the strength of automatic processing. On the other hand, psychopaths perform at least as well as controls on equally demanding tasks when the various components of the task are manifest from the outset (e.g., Newman and Kosson, 1986, Punishment-Only Condition; Newman et al., 1990, Study 2).

A deficiency in automatic information processing when a dominant response set has been established is also consistent with psychopaths' performance in divided attention paradigms. Although psychopaths registered the presentation of tone pips while they are sitting passively, the N100 component of their ERPs indicate that the tones were registered less well under conditions involving a complex perceptual-motor task (Jutai and Hare, 1983). Similarly, their perception of speech phonemes appeared to be less certain while performing the same perceptual-motor task even though their response to the phonemes was indistinguishable from controls' under base-line conditions (Jutai et al., 1987). Psychopaths' reaction times to auditory probes were slower than those of controls under dual-task conditions while they attempted to focus or divide (i.e., intentionally allocate) their attention, although no group differences were apparent in the base-line, single-task assessments (Kosson and Newman, 1986). As noted in our review, the evidence for enhanced attention shown by psychopaths in response to salient, primary-task stimuli is likely to reflect the utilization of controlled information-processing resources.

Though we find the data from avoidance learning and divided-attention paradigms most compelling, we believe that the autonomic conditioning data, neuropsychological findings, and the results of investigations of language functions in psychopaths are also compatible with our hypothesis. Because the performance requirements of most traditional neuropsychological tests are manifest, adequate performance relies primarily on controlled processing. In spite of this fact, a lack of efficiency in the automatic encoding of perceptual information while simultaneously organizing motor responses would place subjects at a disadvantage on measures such as the Trail Making Test and Block Design and may explain the fact that low-anxious psychopaths performed more poorly than controls on these measures. The relatively poor performance of psychopaths on the Porteus Mazes is also consistent with this formulation.

Incorporating the important data on language functioning requires only the eminently reasonable assumption that the priming of semantic and affective associations by words relies upon automatic information processing. Whereas word definitions may be generated using controlled processing, the rapid priming of associated meanings by words probably reflects automatic processing primarily. Importantly, conceptualizing the language anomalies in terms of priming suggests a connection to the priming of personal constructs by internally generated as well as by environmentally mediated stimuli. Recent investigations of the role of primes in activating "self-guides" (e.g., Higgins *et al.*, 1986) may be especially important for understanding psychopaths' failure to place their current motivations in a larger perspective. Although we do not wish to add to the confusion surrounding the psychological interpretation of SC responding, it is not unreasonable to suggest that it would be influenced by the priming of particular associations and, therefore, partially dependent upon automatic processing.

Finally, our proposal provides a novel and potentially important perspective on the tendency of psychopaths to display disinhibited behavior following punishment and frustrative nonreward. Whereas the evidence for response facilitation (i.e., increases in response speed) following punishment is less powerful for psychopaths than for impulsive college students (e.g., Nichols and Newman, 1986; Patterson *et al.*, 1987), the reaction of low-anxious psychopaths does appear to involve a breakdown in cognitive reflectivity (e.g., Newman *et al.*, 1990) and self-control as measured by delay of gratification (Newman *et al.*, 1992). Our explanation for the observed group differences under such circumstances does not involve differences in affective responding per se — we assume that monetary punishments engender emotional responding in psychopaths and non-psychopaths alike. Rather, we propose that psychopaths' performance is more disrupted by punishments than controls' because it is more heavily dependent upon controlled information processing. Thus, in spite of the fact that psychopaths are sometimes capable of displaying self-restraint, especially when immediate incentives are provided (e.g., delay of gratification; reward-only condition), the use of control processing to maintain self-control becomes increasingly difficult when negative feedback elicits emotional responding and reduces the ability to engage in control processing.

IMPLICATIONS FOR THE STUDY AND TREATMENT OF PSYCHOPATHY

Before discussing some of the implications of this cognitive hypothesis, several points are in need of clarification. First, to our knowledge there has been no direct assessment of automatic processing efficiency in psychopaths. Though their performance on a variety of tasks suggests a problem of this type, our proposal is in need of direct investigation to determine whether psychopaths do, in fact, display a deficit in automatic processing while they are engaged in the effortful organization (i.e., deliberate planning and/or implementation) of goal-directed behavior.

Second, we are *not* proposing that psychopaths have a general deficit in automatic processing. Psychopaths' deficit appears to be limited to circumstances in which they are actively engaged in the formulation and implementation of goal-directed behavior. Nevertheless, these are precisely the conditions under which automatic processing is needed to monitor feedback from the environment and assess the suitability of one's response strategy.

Third, we do not mean to imply that psychopaths are completely unable to make use of automatic processing while organizing goal-directed behavior. Although we again note the need for experimental investigation, we suspect that psychopaths simply have a higher threshold for processing information that is peripheral to the organization of goal-directed behavior.

Fourth, our proposal is not intended to supplant the theoretical perspectives on psychopathy outlined earlier in this chapter. We recognize that an apparent defect in automatic information processing might result from poor conditioning, a weaker emotional/arousal response to motivationally significant cues, weaker internal representations, or difficulty modulating dominant response sets. The significance of our proposal derives largely from its attempt to link existing theories of psychopathy with advances in human information processing.

Finally, in proposing this cognitive interpretation of psychopathic behavior, we do not wish to downplay the contribution of biological factors. Indeed, as noted earlier, there is considerable consensus regarding the potential importance of septo-hippocampal system (SHS) functioning for understanding psychopathy. Moreover, as illustrated by the following description, Gray's characterization of the SHS (e.g., Gray, 1982, 1987) is quite compatible with our hypothesis.

> The septo-hippocampal system (together with a number of other closely related structures . . .) has the central task of comparing, quite generally, actual with expected stimuli. The system functions in two modes. If actual stimuli are successfully matched with expected ones ('match'), it functions in 'checking mode' and behavioural control rests with other (unspecified) brain mechanisms. If there is discordance between actual and expected stimuli . . . or if the predicted stimulus is aversive . . . — conditions that are jointly termed 'mismatch' — the septo-hippocampal system takes direct control over behaviour and now functions in 'control mode' (1987, p. 293).

In order to accomplish this "comparator" function, the SHS must have access to several types of information:

> "the present state of the world, stored past environmental regularities (learned by way of Pavlovian conditioning), the next intended step in the motor program, and stored past relationships between such steps and changes in the environment (learned by way of instrumental conditioning). (1987, p. 294)

Our proposal regarding a situation-specific deficit in automatic processing corresponds to Gray's characterization of the comparator function of the SHS. The checking of actual and expected stimuli is regarded as an automatic process that is necessary for self-regulation because it mediates the switch to controlled processing. Although Gray uses the term "mismatch" to describe cues for punishment, it seems clear that such stimuli must also "match" specific templates that determine a person's expectations. Moreover, we expect that people develop a wide variety of templates of this type with preestablished implications for behavior (i.e., a punishment cue may carry inhibitory associations). Following Shapiro (1965), we believe that people have internal representations for personal goals, interests, and a variety of other considerations besides threat stimuli. Such cognitive structures probably play an active role in the top–down screening of, and sensitivity to, meaningful associations. To the extent that we are attuned to particular stimuli because of their acquired significance, they will more readily reach threshold and trigger an automatic attentional response. Whether psychopaths' higher threshold for processing peripheral stimuli reflects a deficit in top–down processing of this type or a problem in the bottom–up registration of such cues while organizing goal-directed behavior requires further study. It is possible that both processes are operating, with a situation-specific deficit in bottom–up processing interfering with the encoding of significant stimuli and development of cognitive structures that are necessary for top–down processing (see Patterson and Newman, in press).

Implications for Research

With the preceding qualifications in mind, we will briefly consider some implications of our proposal for research on psychopathy. Perhaps most importantly, our proposal provides a framework for generating hypotheses and advancing knowledge about psychopathy using recent advances in cognitive psychology. For example, our proposal establishes a context for using priming procedures and other cognitive methods to evaluate the difficulty that psychopaths experience in making use of environmental feedback and stored representations of response–outcome associations to guide behavior. In contrast to motivational/emotional theories, which focus on psychopaths' inadequate response to punishment, a defect in automatic processing of the type outlined above appears capable of explaining the more general inability of psychopaths to achieve a meaningful perspective on their behavior.

The current perspective may also help to resolve confusion concerning the situation-specific evidence of reduced cognitive capacity in psychopaths relative to controls. As noted, the performance of psychopaths in attentional paradigms has occasionally been interpreted as evidence that they have less available cognitive capacity (Harpur and Hare, 1990; Kosson and Newman, 1986). Yet, their performance on standard measures of intelligence and neuropsychological performance suggests that, in general, they have as much cognitive capacity as controls. However, psychopaths will appear to have less cognitive capacity than controls when circumstances require them to devote controlled processing resources to accomplish aspects of a task that controls accomplish automatically (e.g., attending to changing probabilities).

Our proposal may also explain the difficulty that researchers have had in demonstrating performance deficits in psychopaths and clarify the necessary conditions for observing such deficits. Specifically, we suspect that psychopaths use controlled processing resources *to compensate* for their situation-specific weakness in automatic processing. Such reliance on controlled, as opposed to automatic, information processing may explain why psychopaths typically show no performance deficit when task requirements are explicit from the outset but perform poorly on tasks with latent or changing contingencies. Importantly, this formulation suggests that observing performance deficits in psychopaths will depend on situational factors that occupy or disrupt controlled processing. Thus, we would consider psychopaths to be at high risk for behaving maladaptively whenever affective responses, alcohol, fatigue, demanding primary tasks, or attention-eliciting stimuli (e.g., female experimenters; Kosson and Newman, 1986) significantly reduce their cognitive processing capacity and their ability to use controlled processing resources to regulate behavior.

Implications for Treatment

Our cognitive interpretation of psychopaths' self-regulatory deficit serves to bridge the gap between laboratory findings and clinical observations. Clinical descriptions of psychopathy emphasize a profound, but situation-specific, lack of insight regarding the meaning of their own behavior — a deficit that is most apparent while they are pursuing immediate goals or intoxicated with alcohol. Such characterizations are consistent with a defect in automatic processing of the type described. In contrast to nonpsychopaths, for whom urges act automatically to prime past associations, such perspective is achieved less readily in the psychopath. Their difficulty processing important cues, while engaged in goal-directed behavior, constrains their ability to consider the consequences of their behavior and to exercise good judgment.

If psychopaths' failure to accommodate incidental cues related to their behavior reflects a situation-specific deficit in *automatic processing* as proposed, attempts to remedy their problem are likely to require the use of *controlled processing*. Psychopaths do not automatically orient to important cues while performing other activities and they are less inclined to pause and reflect on response feedback while engaged in goal-directed behavior. For psychopaths, then, it is essential that they learn to pause and effortfully evaluate their plans before initiating behavior. In light of the fact that psychopaths are often regarded as impulsive, it is noteworthy that interviewers on our project report that psychopaths appear to be highly circumspect, at least initially. In contrast to controls, psychopaths are perceived initially as distant, hostile, and reserved. However, they tend suddenly to become confident, "smooth," and gregarious after sizing up the nature of the situation. Our laboratory assessments of response speed and errors seem to reveal a similar pattern — psychopaths begin cautiously and react more spontaneously after achieving some initial success on our tasks.

To the extent that psychopaths must rely on controlled processing resources to achieve self-regulation, it is essential that they learn to recognize *high-risk situations*. As noted previously, we would regard psychopaths as "at risk" for displaying disinhibited behavior whenever they (1) commit a large proportion of their attentional capacity to achieving an immediate goal or (2) experience a reduction in available cognitive capacity associated with significant affective responses, fatigue, or the use of alcohol. The experience of affect is considered to be especially problematic because it energizes behavior while disrupting behavioral controls. One might even contemplate the possibility that psychopaths have learned to avoid affective responses because they disrupt controlled processing and interfere with behavioral controls.

To this point, our discussion of *cognition* in psychopathy has focused almost exclusively on cognitive processing deficits. However, before concluding, it is essential to acknowledge that psychopaths and nonpsychopaths may also differ with regard to *cognition distortions* (i.e., particular attitudes and beliefs that shape their behavioral goals and reactions to situations independent of group differences in cognitive processing; see Ch. 1, this volume). In particular, psychopaths and nonpsychopaths differ in the extent to which they are committed to societal norms. As noted by Millon (1981), psychopaths tend to perceive the world as an unpredictable, hostile place and this perception is used to rationalize their tendency to fend for themselves without regard for the feelings, rights, or needs of others. Such beliefs may have developed as a result of an unfortunate upbringing, because of others' reactions to the psychopath's selfish, aggressive style, or because psychopaths have more difficulty than others anticipating and avoiding the negative reactions of others. However, regardless of their etiology, such beliefs assume greater importance for psychopaths than for controls because psychopaths' inherent biases with regard to interpreting and responding to the environment are more likely to go unchecked and be translated into action.

It is our belief that the processing deficit implicated in this review is not specific to psychopaths. Rather, we assume that the essential defect in automatic processing while organizing goal-directed behavior may be found in other groups or individuals whose absence of hostile expectations and whose disinclination to respond aggressively makes the diagnosis of psychopathy inappropriate. Documenting this possibility and determining the factors that eventuate in adaptive, prosocial manifestations of the diathesis might be an important step in developing early intervention strategies aimed at preventing psychopathy. In this regard, it is instructive to consider Yochelson and Samenow's (1977) recommendations concerning the cognitive "re-socializing" of psychopaths. By addressing the manner in which psychopaths think about the world and the rights of others, it may be possible to alter their response inclinations and limit the social consequences of their difficulty in self-regulation.

Finally, we wish to reconsider the concept of moral insanity discussed in the introduction. The preceding discussion should serve to clarify the distinction between inadequate self-regulation and the display of immoral conduct. Whereas a defect in self-control stemming from less efficient automatic processing may explain a person's failure to consider the consequences (or deeper meaning) of their actions, it does not, in itself, foster antisocial behavior. Although their self-control is hampered under certain conditions, psychopaths are capable of evaluating the moral implications of their behavior. As noted above, antisocial attitudes and beliefs are likely to be potent moderators of immoral behavior. The behavioral expression of psychopathy appears to reflect an unfortunate combination of a cognitive processing deficit and a lack of commitment to social mores.

FUTURE DIRECTIONS

First, the cognitive hypothesis put forth in this chapter is in need of direct investigation to verify the hypothesized defect in automatic processing and its presumed relation to the effortful organization of goal-directed behavior. If our hypothesis can be substantiated, its implications for treatment would, as suggested, involve teaching psychopaths about the peculiar limitations of their processing and about the types of situations in which their cognitive style is likely to get them into trouble. Unfortunately, if, as we expect, the hypothesized defect in cognitive processing is present at birth, it is likely to be associated with relatively important and stable effects on socioemotional development. Such factors make change difficult and point to the importance of prevention efforts. If there is merit to our proposal, it should be possible to develop screening measures for identifying the hypothesized cognitive deficit. Importantly, there would be no reason to identify individuals displaying the defect as psychopathic or even at high risk for this disorder. To the contrary, we suggest that the hypothesized defect might best be understood as a *learning disability*. Moreover, consistent with the learning disability analogy, successful interventions are likely to depend on *identifying* the problem in a timely fashion, *characterizing* the processing limitations clearly and specifically, *devising* appropriate methods for circumventing the problem, and *training* the individual in their use. Finally, as noted above, it would be essential for prevention efforts to address the social as well as the cognitive aspects of development. Paralleling the recent advances pertaining to the comorbidity of attention deficit disorder and conduct disorder, the long-term adjustment of individuals at risk for psychopathy will likely depend on their acceptance or rejection of social mores (see Mannuzza *et al.*, 1989).

ACKNOWLEDGMENTS

We thank Peter Arnett for his helpful comments, contributions to data collection, and assistance in preparing the figures. Preparation of this chapter was supported, in part, by Grant MH37711 from the National Institute of Mental Health. We express our appreciation to the Wisconsin Division of Corrections and the staff at Oakhill Correctional Institution for making our research on psychopathy possible.

REFERENCES

American Psychiatric Association. (1987). Diagnostic and Statistical Manual of Mental Disorders (3rd ed., revised). Washington, D.C.: American Psychiatric Association.

Arnett, P. A., Howland, E. W., Smith, S. S., and Newman, J. P. (1993). Autonomic responsivity during passive avoidance in incarcerated psychopaths. *Personality and Individual Differences, 14*, 173–185.

Blackburn, R. (1983). Psychopathy, delinquency and crime. In A. Gale and J. A. Edwards (Eds.), *Physiological correlates of human behavior* (pp. 187–203). New York: Academic Press.

Blackburn, R. (1988). On moral judgments and personality disorders: The myth of psychopathic personality revisited. *British Journal of Psychiatry, 153*, 505–512.

Brantley, P. J., and Sutker, P. B. (1984). Antisocial behavior disorders. In H. E. Adams and P. B. Sutker (Eds.), (pp. 439–478). *Comprehensive handbook of psychopathology*. New York: Plenum.

Caplan, M. (1970). Effects of withheld reinforcement on timing behavior of rats with limbic lesions. *Journal of Comparative Physiological Psychology, 71*, 119–135.

Chesno, F. A., and Kilmann, P. R. (1975). Effects of stimulation intensity on sociopathic avoidance learning. *Journal of Abnormal Psychology, 84*, 144–150.

Cleckley, H. (1976). *The mask of sanity* (5th ed.). St. Louis, MO: Mosby.

Davies, D. R., and Jones, D. M. (1975). The effects of noise and incentives upon attention in short-term memory. *British Journal of Psychology, 66*, 61–68.

Devonshire, P. A., Howard, R. C., and Sellars, C. (1988). Frontal lobe functions and personality in mentally abnormal offenders. *Personality and Individual Differences, 9*, 339–344.

Dickinson, A. J. (1974). Response suppression and facilitation by aversive stimuli following septal lesions in rats: A review and model. *Physiological Psychology, 2*, 444–456.

Dickinson, A. (1975). Suppressive and enhancing effects of footshock on food-reinforced operant responding following septal lesions in rats. *Journal of Comparative and Physiological Psychology, 88*, 851–861.

Dodge, K. A., and Crick, N. R. (1990). Social information-processing bases of aggressive behavior in children. *Personality and Social Psychology Bulletin, 16*, 8–22.

Elliott, F. (1978). Neurological aspects of antisocial behavior. In W. H. Reid (Ed.), *The psychopath: A comprehensive study of antisocial disorders and behaviors* (pp. 146–189). New York: Brunner/Mazel.

Eysenck, H. J. (1964). *Crime and personality*. London: Routledge & Kegan Paul.

Eysenck, H. J. (1977). *Crime and personality (3rd ed.)*. London: Routledge & Kegan Paul.

Eysenck, H. J., and Gudjonsson, G. H. (1989). *The causes and cures of criminality*. New York: Plenum.

Finn, P. R., Zeitouni, N. C., and Pihl, R. O. (1990). Effects of alcohol on psychophysiological hyperreactivity to nonaversive and aversive stimuli in men at high risk for alcoholism. *Journal of Abnormal Psychology, 99*, 79–85.

Flor-Henry, P. (1976). Lateralized temporal limbic dysfunction and psychopathology. *Annals of the New York Academy of Sciences, 280*, 777–797.

Forth, A. E., and Hare, R. D. (1989). The contingent negative variation in psychopaths. *Psychophysiology, 26*, 676–682.

Fowles, D. C. (1980). The three-arousal model: Implications of Gray's two factor learning theory for heart rate, electrodermal activity, and psychopathy. *Psychophysiology, 17*, 87–104.

Fowles, D. C. (1988). Psychophysiology and psychopathology: A motivational approach. *Psychophysiology, 25*, 373–391.

Goldman, H., Lindner, L., Dinitz, S., and Allen, H. (1971). The simple psychopath: Physiologic and sociologic characteristics. *Biological Psychiatry, 3*, 77–83.

Gorenstein, E. E. (1982). Frontal lobe functions in psychopaths. *Journal of Abnormal Psychology, 91*, 368–379.

Gorenstein, E. E. (1991). A cognitive perspective on antisocial personality. In P. A. Magaro (Ed.), *Annual review of psychopathology: Cognitive bases of mental disorders* (Vol. 1, pp. 100–133). Newbury Park, California: Sage Publications.

Gorenstein, E. E., and Newman, J. P. (1980). Disinhibitory psychopathology: A new perspective and a model for research. *Psychological Review, 87*, 301–315.

Gough, H. G. (1948). A sociological theory of psychopathy. *American Journal of Sociology, 53*, 359–366.

Graham, F. K., and Clifton, R. K. (1966). Heart rate change as a component of the orienting response. *Psychological Bulletin, 65*, 305–320.

Grant, V. W. (1977). *The menacing stranger: A primer on the psychopath*. Oceanside, NY: Dabor Science Publications.

Gray, J. A. (1970). The psychophysiological basis of introversion-extraversion. *Behavior, Research and Therapy, 8*, 249–266.

Gray, J. A. (1982). *The neuropsychology of anxiety*. New York: Oxford University Press.

Gray, J. A. (1987). *The psychology of fear and stress*. New York: Cambridge University Press.

Hare, R. D. (1965). A conflict and learning theory analysis of psychopathic behavior. *Journal of Research in Crime and Delinquency, 6*, 397–401.

Hare, R. D. (1970). *Psychopathy: Theory and research*. New York: Wiley.

Hare, R. D. (1972). Psychopathy and physiological responses to adrenalin. *Journal of Abnormal Psychology, 75*, 138–147.

Hare, R. D. (1978). Electrodermal and cardiovascular correlates of psychopathy. In R. D. Hare and D. Schalling (Eds.), *Psychopathic behavior: Approaches to research* (pp. 107–144). New York: Wiley.

Hare, R. D. (1979). Psychopathy and laterality of cerebral function. *Journal of Abnormal Psychology, 88*, 605–610.

Hare, R. D. (1980). A research scale for the assessment of psychopathy in criminal populations. *Personality and Individual Differences, 1*, 111–119.

Hare, R. D. (1982). Psychopathy and physiological activity during anticipation of an aversive stimulus in a distraction paradigm. *Psychophysiology, 19*, 266–271.

Hare, R. D. (1984). Performance of psychopaths on cognitive tasks related to frontal lobe function. *Journal of Abnormal Psychology, 93,* 133–140.

Hare, R. D. (1985). Comparison of procedures for the assessment of psychopathy. *Journal of Consulting and Clinical Psychology, 53,* 7–16.

Hare, R. D. (1986). Twenty years of experience with the Cleckley psychopath. In W. H. Reid, D. Dorr, J. I. Walker, and J. W. Bonner, III (Eds.), *Unmasking the psychopath: Antisocial personality and related syndromes.* New York: Norton.

Hare, R. D. (1990). *Manual for the revised psychopathy checklist.* Unpublished manuscript, Department of Psychology, University of British Columbia, Vancouver, Canada.

Hare, R. D., and Craigen, D. (1974). Psychopathy and physiological activity in a mixed-motive game situation. *Psychophysiology, 11,* 197–206.

Hare, R. D., and Jutai, J. W. (1983). Criminal history of the male psychopath: Some preliminary data. In K. T. Van Dusen and S. A. Mednick (Eds.), *Prospective studies of crime and delinquency* (pp. 225–236). Boston: Kluwer-Nijhoff.

Hare, R. D., and Jutai, J. W. (1988). Psychopathy and cerebral asymmetry in semantic processing. *Personality and Individual Differences, 9,* 329–337.

Hare, R. D., and McPherson, L. M. (1984). Psychopathy and perceptual asymmetry during verbal dichotic listening. *Journal of Abnormal Psychology, 93,* 141–149.

Hare, R. D., and Quinn, M. J. (1971). Psychopathy and autonomic conditioning. *Journal of Abnormal Psychology, 77,* 223–235.

Hare, R. D., Williamson, S. E., and Harpur, T. J. (1988). Psychopathy and Language. In T. E. Moffitt and S. A. Mednick (Eds.), *Biological contributions to crime causation.* Dordrecht, Netherlands: Nijhoff Martinus.

Hare, R. D., Harpur, T. J., Hakstian, A. R., Forth, A. E., Hart, S. D., and Newman, J. P. (1990). The revised psychopathy checklist: Descriptive statistics, reliability, and factor structure. *Journal of Consulting and Clinical Psychology: Psychological Assessment, 2,* 338–341.

Harpur, T. J., and Hare, R. D. (1990). Psychopathy and Attention. In J. Enns (Ed.), *The development of attention: Research and theory.* Amsterdam: North-Holland.

Harpur, T. J., Hare, R. D., and Hakstian, A. R. (1989). Two-factor conceptualization of psychopathy: Construct validity and assessment implications. *Psychological Assessment: A Journal of Consulting and Clinical Psychology, 1,* 6–17.

Hart, S. D., and Hare, R. D. (1989). Discriminant validity of the Psychopathy Checklist in a forensic psychiatric population. *Psychological Assessment: A Journal of Consulting and Clinical Psychology, 1,* 211–218.

Hart, S. D., Forth, A. H., and Hare, R. D. (1990). Performance of criminal psychopaths on selected neuropsychological tests. *Journal of Abnormal Psychology, 99,* 374–379.

Higgins, E. T., Bond, R., Klein, R., and Strauman, T. J. (1986). Self-discrepancies and emotional vulnerability: How magnitude, type and accessibility of discrepancy influence affect. *Journal of Personality and Social Psychology, 53,* 1004–1014.

Hockey, G. R. J., and Hamilton, P. (1970). Arousal and information selection in short-term memory. *Nature (London), 226,* 866–867.

Hoffman, J. J., Hall, R. W., and Bartsch, T. W. (1987). On the relative importance of "psychopathic" personality and alcoholism on neuropsychological measures of frontal lobe dysfunction. *Journal of Abnormal Psychology, 96,* 158–160.

Howland, E. W., and Newman, J. P. (1987). *The effect of incentives on Wisconsin Card Sorting Task performance in psychopaths.* Unpublished manuscript.

Howland, E. W., and Newman, J. P. (1991). *Differentiating the motor and attentional components underlying psychopaths' difficulty altering a dominant response set.* Unpublished data set.

Howland, E. W., Kosson, D. S., Patterson, C. M., and Newman, J. P. (in press). Altering a dominant response: Performance of psychopaths and low socialization college students on a cued reaction time task. *Journal of Abnormal Psychology*.

Jutai, J. W. (1989). Psychopathy and P3 amplitude: A commentary on Raine. *International Journal of Psychophysiology, 8*, 17–22.

Jutai, J. W., and Hare, R. D. (1983). Psychopathy and selective attention during performance of a complex perceptual-motor task. *Psychophysiology, 20*, 146–151.

Jutai, J. W., Hare, R. D., and Connolly, J. F. (1987). Psychopathy and event-related brain potentials (ERPs) associated with attention to speech stimuli. *Personality and Individual Differences, 8*, 175–184.

Kandel, E., and Freed, D. (1989). Frontal-lobe dysfunction and antisocial behavior: A review. *Journal of Clinical Psychology, 45*, 404–413.

Karpman, B. (1948). The myth of psychopathic personality. *American Journal of Psychiatry, 104*, 523–534.

Kosson, D. S., and Newman, J. P. (1986). Psychopathy and the allocation of attention in a divided attention situation. *Journal of Abnormal Psychology, 95*, 252–256.

Kosson, D. S., and Newman, J. P. (1989). Socialization and attentional deficits under focusing and divided attention conditions. *Journal of Personality and Social Psychology, 57*, 87–99.

Kosson, D. S., Smith, S. S., and Newman, J. P. (1990). Evaluating the construct validity of psychopathy in Black and White male inmates: Three preliminary studies. *Journal of Abnormal Psychology, 99*, 250–000.

Lacey, J. I. (1967). Somatic response patterning and stress: Some revisions of activation theory. In N. H. Appley and R. Trumbell (Eds.), *Psychological stress: Issues in Research* (pp. 14–44). New York: Appleton-Century-Crofts.

Lezak, M. D. (1983). *Neuropsychological assessment*. New York: Oxford University Press.

Lippert, W. W., and Senter, R. J. (1966). Electrodermal responses in the sociopath. *Psychonomic Science, 4*, 25–26.

Luria, A. R. (1973). *The working brain*. New York: Basic Books.

Lykken, D. T. (1957). A study of anxiety in the sociopathic personality. *Journal of Abnormal and Social Psychology, 55*, 6–10.

Lykken, D. T. (1982). Fearlessness: Its carefree charm and deadly risks. *Psychology Today* (September, 20–28).

Malmo, R. B. (1959). Activation: A neuropsychological dimension. *Psychological Review, 66*, 367–386.

Mandler, G. (1972). Helplessness: Theory and research in anxiety. In C. D. Spielberger (Ed.), *Anxiety: Current trends in theory and research* (Vol II, pp. 363–374). New York: Academic Press.

Mannuzza, S., Klein, R. G., Konig, P. H., and Giampino, T. L. (1989). Hyperactive boys almost grown up: IV. Criminality and its relationship to psychiatric status. *Archives of General Psychiatry, 46*, 1073–1079.

Mawson, A. R., and Mawson, C. D. (1977). Psychopathy and arousal: A new interpretation of the psychophysiological literature. *Biological Psychiatry, 12*, 49–74.

Mednick, S. A., and Hutchings, B. (1978). Genetic and psychophysiological factors in asocial behavior. In R. D. Hare and D. Schalling (Eds.), *Psychopathic behavior: Approaches to research* (pp. 239–254). New York: Wiley.

Millon, T. (1981). *Disorders of personality: DMS-III Axis II* (pp. 181–215). New York: Wiley.

Mineka, S., and Kihlstrom, J. F. (1978). Unpredictable and uncontrollable events: A new perspective on experimental neurosis. *Journal of Abnormal Psychology, 87*, 256–271.

Mowrer, O. H. (1947). On the dual nature of learning—a reinterpretation of "conditioning" and "problem-solving." *Harvard Educational Review, 17*, 102–148.

Nauta, W. J. H. (1971). The problem of the frontal lobe: A reinterpretation. *Journal of Psychiatric Research, 8*, 167–187.

Neisser, U. (1966). *Cognitive psychology*. New York: Appleton-Century-Crofts.

Newman, J. P. (1987). Reaction to punishment in extraverts and psychopaths: Implications for the impulsive behavior of disinhibited individuals. *Journal of Research in Personality*, 464–485.

Newman, J. P. (1991a). Self-regulatory failures in criminal psychopaths. *Published proceedings of the Third Symposium on Violence and Aggression*. University of Saskatoon Press.

Newman, J. P. (November, 1991b). *Response Modulation Deficits in Psychopaths*. Paper presented as part of a symposium on *Neuropsychological Approaches to Antisocial Behavior* at the annual meeting of the American Society of Criminology.

Newman, J. P., and Kosson, D. S. (1986). Passive avoidance learning in psychopathic and nonpsychopathic offenders. *Journal of Abnormal Psychology, 95*, 257–263.

Newman, J. P., Gorenstein, E. E., and Kelsey, J. E. (1983). Failure to delay gratification following septal lesions in rats: Implications for an animal model of disinhibitory psychopathology. *Personality and Individual Differences, 4*, 147–156.

Newman, J. P., Widom, C. S., and Nathan, S. (1985). Passive-avoidance in syndromes of disinhibition: Psychopathy and extraversion. *Journal of Personality and Social Psychology, 48*, 1316–1327.

Newman, J. P., Patterson, C. M., and Kosson, D. S. (1987). Response perseveration in psychopaths. *Journal of Abnormal Psychology, 96*, 145–148.

Newman, J. P., Patterson, C. M., Howland, E. W., and Nichols, S. L. (1990). Passive avoidance in psychopaths: The effects of reward. *Personality and Individual Differences*.

Newman, J. P., Kosson, D. S., and Patterson, C. M. (1992). Delay of gratification in psychopathic and nonpsychopathic offenders. *Journal of Abnormal Psychology, 101*, 630–636.

Nichols, S. L., and Newman, J. P. (1986). Effects of punishment on response latency in extraverts. *Journal of Personality and Social Psychology, 50*, 624–630.

Obrist, P. (1976). The cardiovascular–behavioral interaction — as it appears today. *Psychophysiology, 13*, 95–107.

Ogloff, J. P. R., and Wong, S. (1990). Electrodermal and cardiovascular evidence of a coping response in psychopaths. *Criminal Justice and Behavior, 17*, 231–245.

Patterson, C. M., and Newman, J. P. (in press). Reflectivity and learning from aversive events: Toward a psychological mechanism for the syndromes of disinhibition. *Psychological Review*.

Patterson, C. M., Kosson, D. S., and Newman, J. P. (1987). Reaction to punishment, reflectivity, and passive-avoidance learning in extraverts. *Journal of Personality and Social Psychology, 52*, 565–575.

Pichot, P. (1978). Psychopathic behaviour: A historical overview. In R. D. Hare and D. Schalling (Eds.), *Psychopathic behavior: Approaches to research* (pp. 55–70). New York: Wiley.

Pinel, P. (1809). *Traite medico-phiosophique sur l'alienation mentale* (2nd ed.). Paris: J. Ant. Brosson.

Quay, H. C. (1965). Psychopathic personality as pathological stimulation seeking. *American Journal of Psychiatry, 122*, 180–183.

Quay, H. C. (1977). Psychopathic Behavior: Reflections on its nature, origins, and treatment. In I. C. Uzgiris and F. Weizmann (Eds.), *The Structuring of experience* (pp. 371–382). New York: Plenum.

Quay, H. C. (1988). The behavioral reward and inhibition systems in childhood behavior disorder. In L. M. Bloomingdale (Ed.), *Attention deficit disorder* (Vol 3, pp. 176–186). Oxford: Pergamon.

Raine, A., and Venables, P. H. (1988). Enhanced P3 evoked potentials and longer recovery times in psychopaths. *Psychophysiology, 25*, 30–38.

Routtenberg, A. (1968). The two-arousal hypothesis: Reticular formation and limbic system. *Psychological Review, 75*, 51–80.

Schachter, S., and Latane, B. (1964). Crime, cognition and the autonomic nervous system. In H. R. Jones (Ed.), *Nebraska symposium on motivation* pp. 221–275. Lincoln: The University of Nebraska Press.

Schalling, D. (1978). Psychopathy-related personality variables and the psychophysiology of socialization. In R. D. Hare and D. Schalling (Eds.), *Psychopathic behavior: Approach to research* (pp. 85–106). New York: Wiley.

Schalling, D., and Rosen, A. (1968). Porteus Maze differences between psychopathic and non-psychopathic criminals. *British Journal of Social and Clinical Psychology, 7*, 224–228.

Schmauk, F. J. (1970). Punishment, arousal, and avoidance learning in sociopaths. *Journal of Abnormal Psychology, 76*, 325–335.

Schneider, W., Dumais, S. T., and Shiffrin, R. M. (1984). Automatic and control processing and attention. In R. Parasuraman and D. R. Davies (Eds.), *Varieties of attention* (pp. 1–27). New York: Academic Press.

Shapiro, D. (1965). *Neurotic styles*. New York: Basic Books.

Shapiro, S. K., Quay, H. C., Hogan, A. E., and Schwartz, K. P. (1988). Response perseveration and delayed responding in undersocialized aggressive conduct disorder. *Journal of Abnormal Psychology, 97*, 371–373.

Siddle, D. A. T., and Trasler, G. B. (1981). The psychophysiology of psychopathic behavior. In M. J. Christie and P. G. Mellett (Eds.), *Foundations of psychosomatics* (pp. 283–303). Chichester: Wiley.

Siegel, R. A. (1978). Probability of punishment and suppression of behavior in psychopathic and nonpsychopathic offenders. *Journal of Abnormal Psychology, 87*, 514–522.

Smith, S. S., Arnett, P. A., and Newman, J. P. (1992). Neuropsychological differentiation of psychopathic and nonpsychopathic criminal offenders. *Personality and Individual Differences, 13*, 1283–1245.

Sutker, P. B., and Allain, A. N. (1987). Cognitive abstraction, shifting, and control: Clinical sample comparisons of psychopaths and nonpsychopaths. *Journal of Abnormal Psychology, 96*, 73–75.

Sutker, P. B., Moan, C. E., and Swanson, W. C. (1972). Porteus Maze Test qualitative performance in pure sociopaths, prison normals and antisocial psychotics. *Journal of Clinical Psychology, 28*, 349–353.

Szpiler, J. A., and Epstein, S. (1976). Availability of an avoidance response as related to autonomic arousal. *Journal of Abnormal Psychology, 85*, 73–82.

Tarter, R. E. (1979). Etiology of alcoholism: Interdisciplinary integration. In P. E. Nathan, G. A. Marlatt, and T. Loberg (Eds.), *Alcoholism: New directions in behavioral research and treatment* (pp. 41–70). New York: Plenum.

Thomas-Peter, B. A. (1992). The classification of psychopathy: A review of the Hare vs Blackburn debate. *Personality and Individual Differences, 13*, 337–342.

Trasler, G. (1978). Relations between psychopathy and persistent criminality — Methodological and theoretical issues. In R. D. Hare and D. Schalling (Eds.), *Psychopathic behavior: Approach to research* (pp. 273–298). New York: Wiley.

Wallace, J. F., and Newman, J. P. (1990). Differential effects of reward and punishment cues on response speed in anxious and impulsive individuals. *Personality and Individual Differences, 11*, 999–1009.

Wallace, J. F., and Newman, J. P. (1992). Attentional processes mediating the breakdown of self regulation: Effects of neuroticism and stimulus significance. Submitted.

Wallace, J. F., Bachorowski, J., and Newman, J. P. (1991). Failures of response modulation: Impulsive behavior in anxious and impulsive individuals. *Journal of Research in Personality, 25,* 23–44.

Widom, C. S. (1976). Interpersonal and personal construct systems in psychopaths. *Journal of Consulting and Clinical Psychology, 44,* 614–623.

Widom, C. S. (1977). A methodology for studying noninstitutionalized psychopaths. *Journal of Consulting and Clinical Psychology, 45,* 674–683.

Williamson, S., Harpur, T. J., and Hare, R. D. (1991). Abnormal processing of affective words by psychopaths. *Psychophysiology, 28,* 260–273.

Yochelson, S., and Samenow, S. E. (1977). *The criminal personality, Volume 2: The change process.* New York: Jason Aronson.

Cognitive Factors in Marital Disturbance

Norman Epstein

University of Maryland, College Park

Donald H. Baucom

University of North Carolina at Chapel Hill

The current chapter differs from the others in this volume because the identified patient or client is not an individual; instead, it is a couple. From a cognitive–behavioral perspective, primary attention in marital discord is focused on the quality of the relationship, and the individual is important in how he or she contributes to that relationship. Consequently, the study of cognitions in marital distress can become quite complex because interest lies not only in the relationships among each individual's own cognitions, behavior, and emotions, but also in the interplay between the two partners' cognitions, behaviors, and emotions. Only through studying these interactive processes within each spouse and between spouses can we come to a clear understanding of marital discord from a cognitive–behavioral perspective. Even though cognitive–behavioral marital and family therapists (e.g., Epstein *et al.*, 1988) have acknowledged the importance of applying systems concepts such as circular causality to the study of distressed relationships, at the current time such a model of marital functioning remains a desired goal. Our present understanding of the role of cognition in marriage is rudimentary. This chapter will describe current knowledge about types of cognitive variables that may play roles in the quality of marital interaction, and will examine the initial theoretical models that have been offered to account for links between marital cognitions and problematic emotional and behavioral responses between spouses. In addition, we will present a more comprehensive model that integrates cognitive, behavioral, and affective components of marital interaction.

COGNITIVE VARIABLES PERTINENT TO
MARITAL FUNCTIONING

In order to study the role of cognitive variables in marriage, the various types of cognitions relevant to marital functioning must first be identified. Baucom *et al.* (1989a) proposed that there are at least five cognitive variables that need to be considered in understanding marital functioning: selective perception, attributions, expectancies, assumptions, and standards (see also Ch. 1, this volume).[1] Selective perception involves what aspects of one's own behavior, one's partner's behavior, and the couple's dyadic interaction the individual notices. This perceptual process is fundamental to the other cognitive processes and outcomes, because what is noticed provides the material for subsequent cognitive evaluations. When studying marital discord, researchers and clinicians are particularly interested in cognitive biases by which the individual or couple tends to notice particular aspects of the marital situation and ignores other aspects. Beck and his associates (Beck and Emery, 1985; Beck *et al.*, 1979) refer to this process as *selective abstraction.* For example, a husband's comment to his wife, "You always try to get your way" may reflect his attending to any instances in which she expresses her preferences assertively and his failing to notice the times when she asks him what he wants or when she acquiesces to his requests.

Second, once various events have been noted, at times partners are motivated to provide explanations or *attributions* for the behaviors that have

---

[1]Fincham *et al.* (1990a) have argued that this typology focuses on the content of "deliberate, effortful" conscious cognitions, rather than the largely unconscious "automatic" *processes* and underlying cognitive *structures* that mediate much of the rapid interaction between partners. Although we agree with Fincham *et al.* that much of the cognitive activity affecting partners' emotional and behavioral responses to each other occurs spontaneously and beyond awareness, we believe that the typology we previously outlined (selective abstraction, attributions, expectancies, assumptions, standards) includes both conscious, reflective identification of cognitive content *and* unconscious cognitions. It is important to differentiate between unconscious cognitive processes (e.g., by which incoming data about a partner's current behavior are evaluated in terms of the observing spouse's preexisting personal constructs about ways in which people express caring) and the resulting conscious cognitive products that researchers and clinicians typically assess by means of interviews and questionnaires. As Fincham *et al.* note, existing research on marital cognition has involved measurement of conscious cognitions, and new methodologies will be needed to assess cognitive processes and structures that are not immediately accessible to the respondent.

occurred. Although partners do not attempt to provide attributions for every small, routine behavior that transpires, they seem to be particularly motivated to provide explanations for unexpected or novel events, negative experiences, and behaviors that are personally relevant (cf. Baucom, 1987; Bradbury and Fincham, 1990; Holtzworth-Munroe and Jacobson, 1985). At least two major classes of attributions appear worthy of distinction. First, spouses make *causal attributions*, or attempts to explain *why* some marital event or behavior occurred. Second, spouses at times make *responsibility/ blame attributions*, in which they determine whether an individual who has been seen as a cause of an event should be blamed or held as culpable for the event. For example, a husband might conclude that his wife caused them to miss a social engagement because she arrived home late from work. He might not blame, however, if he viewed her lateness as being due to her admirable sense of duty in attending to an emergency that had arisen at her work at the last moment. Therefore, he would be less upset with her than he would have been if he attributed her lateness to her caring less about their relationship than about her career.

Third, spouses not only attempt to make attributions for events that have occurred, but they also attempt to make predictions about future marital events and the course that their relationship is likely to take. These *expectancies* for the future are important because they impact the individual's behavior and emotional responses. Thus, if a wife makes a broad prediction that her husband is not going to change and will continue to be uninterested in improving their relationship, she might feel depressed and lack motivation to engage in therapeutic tasks to alter the relationship. A spouse's expectancies also may involve more specific predictions about events, such as a husband's expectancy, "If I buy my wife a present, she'll find something wrong with it and exchange it for something else."

These expectancies are likely to be influenced by and are likely to influence the fourth class of cognitive variables, spouses' *assumptions* or beliefs about the characteristics and operations of people and relationships. Assumptions involve the individual's views about how things really *are*. Thus, based upon an individual's past experiences, the person comes to believe that certain objects and persons in the world have certain qualities and are related to one another in certain ways. For example, in the marital domain, a husband might believe that women are incapable of accomplishing tasks that require mechanical aptitude and that men are deficient in dealing with emotionally laden topics; these assumptions could exert a pervasive influence on his views as to how marital roles should be structured.

Whereas assumptions focus on the individual's beliefs of how things actually are, the fifth class of cognitions, *standards*, deals with what the individual believes partners and relationships *should* be like. Standards provide a template against which various marital behaviors and events are evaluated. If one's own behaviors do not meet one's standards for appropriate spousal behavior, then a sense of guilt, shame, failure, and/or depression might ensue. Similarly, if one's partner fails to measure up to one's standards for partner behavior, then disappointment and/or anger, among other emotions are likely to follow. (The particular emotional and behavioral responses to the violation of standards are likely mediated by other cognitive factors, such as the attributions provided for the partner's unacceptable behavior.) For example, if a wife holds a standard that partners should give top priority to spending time together but her husband often schedules leisure activities with his friends, she may be quite distressed. Her distress may take the form of depression if she makes an attribution that his violation of her standard is due to a loss of love for her, whereas she may be more likely to experience anger if she attributes his behavior to selfishness.

It is important to note that the assumptions and standards that an individual reports during a clinical interview or through responses to structured inventories may not be the ones determining his or her emotional and behavioral reactions to a partner. For example, an individual may consciously endorse a standard that power should be shared equally between two partners, but his or her consistent upset in situations when the other person attempts to negotiate decisions may reflect an unstated standard (perhaps beyond awareness) that is far less egalitarian. It is unlikely that the latter standard could be assessed by means of self-report inventories, whereas it might be identified deductively through a review of daily logs of upsetting interactions with the partner.

RESEARCH ON COGNITIVE VARIABLES IN MARRIAGE

Selective Abstraction

At least two types of investigations have been conducted that bear on the extent to which spouses selectively attend to marital events. First, several studies have examined the degree to which spouses agree about what has occurred in their marriage. To maximize the likelihood that differential reporting is a function of selective attention and not memory, investigators have asked spouses to report on what events have occurred during the past 24 hours. The results of these investigations indicate that spouses have relatively different perceptions of what events have occurred in a 24-hour period (Christensen and Nies, 1980; Christensen et al., 1983; Jacobson and Moore, 1981). Kappas calculated between husbands' and wives' reports of marital behavior average approximately .50. Calculating agreement rates differently, Jacobson and Moore (1981) concluded that husbands and wives typically agree less than 50% of the time on whether a given event has occurred during the past day. Even their rate of agreement about the occurrence of sex was as low as 60%. As might be expected, the agreement rate varies among couples, and the rate of agreement seems to be related to level of marital adjustment. Happy couples demonstrate a higher rate of agreement than do distressed couples.

Low rates of interspousal agreement are consistent with selective abstraction, but high rates of interspousal agreement do not necessarily indicate that the spouses are attending appropriately to the various stimuli in their environment. For example, in order to maintain their view of a highly satisfactory relationship, a husband and wife might both selectively attend to the same positive relationship events while ignoring negative behaviors. In order to address this issue, it is necessary to compare spouses' perceptions of relationship events with the ratings of outsiders who are not emotionally involved in the relationship and who can provide a more "detached" reporting of relationship events. Robinson and Price (1980) have conducted just such a study, in which trained raters coded the presence and absence of specific behaviors among distressed and nondistressed couples in the couples' homes. The couples also provided ratings of what behaviors had occurred during the same time period. Overall, the findings indicated rather poor correspondence between the spouses' and the raters' perceptions of what events had occurred, with correlations between the two averaging approximately .50. The correlations between raters and distressed spouses were lower than the correlations between the raters and nondistressed spouses. The distressed spouses tended to report 50% fewer pleasurable events than those identified by the outside raters. On the one hand, the possibility cannot be ruled out that the distressed spouses noticed the events coded as pleasurable by the raters but experienced those events as negative due to idiosyncratic factors (e.g., memories of past times when the same behaviors were parts of negative marital interaction patterns). On the other hand, the findings also are consistent with clinical reports of "negative tracking," in which members of distressed couples selectively notice negative marital events and overlook positive ones (Jacobson and Margolin, 1979).

Thus, differences in attending to what events have occurred appear to be a way of life for most couples, but these differences are accentuated among distressed couples. In particular, distressed couples might not note many of the positive behaviors that occur in their marriages. These findings coincide with the complaints of distressed spouses that "You always notice what I do wrong, but you never seem to notice when I do something right."

Attributions

Influenced by the seminal work of Heider (1958), Jones and Davis (1965), and Kelley (1973), researchers have invested a great deal of effort in attempting to understand how individuals explain events that occur in their lives. Whereas much of the early work on attributions in social psychology focused on interactions in which the individuals did not know each other, in recent years marital researchers have studied attributions within the context of intimate relationships such as marriage. There are a number of questions about attributions in marriage that might be posed, such as (1) whether attributions predict subsequent behaviors and emotional responses or (2) whether attributions are meaningfully related to other maritally related cognitions. The primary focus to date, however, has been on establishing whether there is a relation between the type of attributions that spouses make for marital events and their level of marital adjustment.

The relation between marital attributions and marital adjustment has been studied in a number of different ways. For example, spouses have been presented with either hypothetical situations or events from their own relationships. Attributions have been assessed from self-report measures and videotaped interactions. These various strategies raise numerous methodological and conceptual issues (see Baucom *et al.*, 1989a, for a recent discussion of these methodological issues). However, in spite of these diverse research strategies, there is some consistency in the findings. Overall, the results indicate that distressed couples tend to make attributions that might be labeled as "distress-maintaining," whereas nondistressed couples provide "relationship-enhancing" attributions (Holtzworth-Munroe and Jacobson, 1985). That is, in providing causal explanations for a marital event, unhappy couples tend to provide explanations that focus on negative aspects of the partner and/or the relationship. For example, members of distressed couples frequently explain negative marital events by viewing the partner as the cause of the problem and seeing the cause of the problem as exerting a global influence on the marriage; similarly, they see the cause of the problem as stable or unlikely to change in the future. Conversely, nondistressed couples explain the causes of positive events as likely to influence many aspects of the marriage and likely to continue into the future (see Baucom and Epstein, 1990, or Bradbury and Fincham, 1990, for a review).

In addition to asking couples to provide explanations for why an event has occurred, some investigators have asked couples to offer responsibility attributions for marital events. That is, when a positive event has occurred, are the causal agents worthy of praise; similarly, when a negative event occurs, should the causal agents be blamed. Although based on a smaller body of research than the findings regarding causal attributions, the over-all pattern of findings indicates that "an association exists between marital dissatisfaction and the tendency to view positive partner behaviors as less intentional, less positive in intent, motivated by selfish concerns, and less worthy of praise" (Bradbury and Fincham, 1990, p. 5). When considering a partner's negative behavior, distressed spouses view the partner as (1) hav-ing a negative intent; (2) demonstrating a negative attitude toward the respondent; (3) selfishly motivated; and (4) worthy of blame (Bradbury and Fincham, 1990). Thus, within distressed marriages, each spouse is likely to blame the other for negative events and view the partner as worthy of little praise for positive events.

This pattern of causal and responsibility attributions is extremely im-portant in understanding how marital distress can be maintained, even when a partner is attempting to improve the relationship. If one spouse does not view that the partner caused the positive changes or does not believe that the partner's behavior is worthy of praise, then positive changes from the partner are unlikely to have their intended effect (and be reinforced). Likewise, if any remaining negative relationship events are attributed to the partner, are seen as stable and pervasive, and viewed as worthy of blame to the partner, then the impacts of these negative behav-iors are likely to be maximized.

Expectancies

Individuals attend to stimuli in their environment and attempt to ex-plain why various events have occurred so that they may respond adap-tively, produce desired outcomes, and avoid aversive outcomes. In order to accomplish these goals, individuals need to be able to make predictions or form expectancies about future events and the consequences of certain actions. Thus, the accurate development and application of expectancies or predictions about the future is a highly adaptive process that allows effi-cient and effective interaction in human relationships. However, the for-mation of distorted expectancies is possible as a result of multiple factors. For example, due to selective abstraction, one spouse might note only certain aspects of the partner's behavior. Making predictions based on only a portion of the relevant behavior is fraught with risks, such as underesti-mating the likelihood that one's partner will be upset if one behaves in a particular way. Furthermore, even if the spouse notices the relevant infor-mation available, this information must be processed appropriately in or-der to make accurate predictions. For example, if a spouse makes distorted attributions for a partner's behavior, then this attribution is likely to influ-ence expectancies about future behavior. Thus, if a husband accurately perceives his wife's negative behavior and makes an inference that his wife behaved negatively because of a desire to hurt him, he might then develop an expectancy that she will attempt to hurt him in the future in similar situations.

Similarly, predictions about future behavior made from observations of a partner's past or current behavior can be distorted by the assumptions that an individual holds about covariation among people's characteristics (see the discussion of assumptions, below). For example, one man heard his wife say that she was staying at work late because of her dedication to completing a major project, and he then became upset as he formed an expectancy that she would not put much time and effort into childrearing if they had children in the future. Exploration of the husband's cognitions revealed that he held a basic assumption that a woman's investment in work and her investment in family were negatively correlated.

Bandura (1977) has distinguished between outcome expectancies and efficacy expectancies (he uses the terms *expectancy* and *expectation* inter-changeably). An outcome expectancy involves an individual's belief that a certain action will result in a certain outcome. Thus, a husband might believe that if he shares more of his feelings and thoughts with his wife, then they will feel closer to each other. An efficacy expectancy, on the other hand, involves an individual's belief concerning whether he or she is able to carry out the action in question. In the above example, the husband might have a negative efficacy expectancy that he will not be *able* to share more of his thoughts and feelings with his wife, even though he held a positive outcome expectancy that successfully doing so would lead to the desired closeness between them. Doherty (1981a,b) proposed that spouses' efficacy expectancies are important determinants of marital conflict resolution. If a spouse believes that either of the partners is unable to engage in behaviors needed to bring about some important change in the relationship, then he or she is unlikely to attempt to bring about such changes, thus exhibiting symptoms of learned helplessness (Seligman, 1975).

Pretzer *et al.* (1991) employed a self-report questionnaire to assess spouses' expectancies about their marriages, along with their attributions for partners' behaviors. They found that the more an individual attributed marital problems to his or her own behavior, the more that person believed that the couple would be able to improve their marital relationship in the future, thus demonstrating a linkage between attributions and expectancies. Also, individuals evidencing a higher expectancy of improvement in the relationship demonstrated lower levels of depression, and less attribution of causality for relationship problems to the partner's behavior, personality traits, lack of love, and malicious intent.

Understanding spouses' expectancies is important because their expectancies are likely to exert a major influence on spouses' moods and willingness to attempt to make relationship changes. Rotter (1954) has distinguished between *specific expectancies*, which concern predictions for a certain situation (e.g., "If I forget my wife's birthday, she will be furious"), and *generalized expectancies*, which are more global and stable ("No matter what I do, my partner will not want to spend time alone with me"). This distinction is useful because specific expectancies are likely to be more easily disconfirmed and amenable to change than generalized expectancies. Several disconfirming experiences concerning a specific expectancy might lead the individual to question that expectancy. However, several disconfirmations of a generalized expectancy might lead the person to conclude that these examples are merely exceptions to the rule and that the expectancy still holds.

Assumptions

Assumptions and standards are two types of cognitions that theorists typically refer to as "schemata," "knowledge structures," and "cognitive structures" (Nisbett and Ross, 1980; Seiler, 1984; Turk and Speers, 1983). Seiler (1984) notes that cognitive structures are the fairly stable internalized representations that an individual has regarding rules for categorizing things and events, for solving problems, and for taking action toward particular goals. In regard to marriage, cognitive structures serve as templates for processing ongoing marital events.

Marital assumptions involve an individual's beliefs about, for example, the characteristics of males and females, what a particular spouse is like, and how events occur in an intimate relationship. It is likely that some of an individual's assumptions about marriage and the partners involved develop from personal experiences *outside* the current marriage (e.g., previous relationships, observations of other people's relationships, mass media portrayals of relationships), whereas other assumptions develop from specific experiences over time *within* the marriage.

Whereas numerous studies have been conducted investigating the role of attributions in marriage, few studies have attempted to explore the types of assumptions that spouses have about marriage in general or their particular marriage. Epstein and Eidelson have developed the Relationship Belief Inventory (RBI; Eidelson and Epstein, 1982; Epstein and Eidelson, 1981), which assesses a selected set of marital assumptions. They found that the more that an individual believed that spouses cannot change relationships, the more distressed the person was about the current relationship. They also found that the more an individual believed that spouses cannot change relationships and the more the person believed that disagreement is destructive to the relationship, the more the person preferred individual rather than marital therapy, and the lower the person's estimate (expectancy) that his or her own marital problems would improve with treatment. The association between marital distress and spouses' assumptions assessed by the RBI also has been found in subsequent investigations (e.g., Epstein *et al.*, 1987; Fincham and Bradbury, 1987b; Huber and Milstein, 1985).

Once spouses develop assumptions about the partner and the marriage, these assumptions are likely to influence other cognitions. Their assumptions are likely to influence what events they focus on and notice, their attributions for events that they do notice, and their predictions about what is likely to occur in the future.

Standards

In addition to making assumptions about the way that they believe things actually are, individuals also have standards for how things *should be*. In the marital domain, spouses have numerous standards for how a husband should behave, how a wife should behave, and what their overall relationship should be like. Although both assumptions and standards can be viewed as cognitive schemata because they are relatively stable cognitive structures used by individuals to categorize life experiences (Seiler, 1984), differentiating between them is important. Whereas assumptions provide the individual with information about characteristics of intimate relationships and factors that influence partners' behaviors, standards involve the important function of providing a basis for evaluating the acceptability of each partner's behavior. Thus, marital distress can result when a partner's standards for how the relationship should be do not match that person's assumptions about how the relationship actually operates.

Epstein and Eidelson's (1981) RBI currently is the only established validated measure of relationship standards. In particular, the RBI assesses two extreme standards that often are observed in clinical contexts. First, the "mind reading is expected" subscale assesses the extent to which each individual believes that partners should know what each other is feeling and thinking without there being any direct communication about the thoughts and feelings. Second, the "sexual perfectionism" subscale assesses the extent to which the person believes that sexual behavior should always be trouble free and result in feelings of euphoria. Eidelson and Epstein (1982) found that endorsement of these two standards is correlated with greater marital discord.

At the same time, other findings indicate that the extremeness of relationship standards is not necessarily associated with marital discord.
Baucom *et al.* (1990a) have recently developed a new self-report measure to
assess relationship standards, the Inventory of Specific Relationship Standards (ISRS). Based on data from a community sample of couples, Epstein
et al. (1991) found that the more strongly spouses held relationship standards emphasizing togetherness and personal investment in one's marriage, the greater their marital satisfaction. Even extreme endorsement of
such standards was not associated with distress. In fact, the strongest
predictor of marital distress was the degree to which the individual reported that he or she was dissatisfied with the way in which the standards
were being met in the marriage.

These findings appear to reflect the important difference between (1)
holding a relationship standard per se and (2) the cognitive and emotional
responses when a standard is violated. That is, holding high relationship
standards that stress intimacy between the partners and investment in the
relationship might encourage a spouse to work hard to make the relationship succeed by engaging in loving acts and accomplishing chores for the
relationship. Even though some of the relationship standards might be
unrealistically high, they might provide the impetus for developing a caring, loving relationship. What might be critical is the individual's reaction
if the standards are not fully met. If the spouse accepts that the relationship
is not perfect but still has provided a great deal of gratification, then the
high standards might have served him or her well. On the other hand, if
the individual becomes extremely upset when the standards are not met,
then these standards might become a liability for the marriage. Rational–
emotive therapists (e.g., Ellis and Dryden, 1987; Wessler and Wessler, 1980)
have noted how individuals' positive or negative evaluations of the violation of standards influence the levels of distress they experience. Clinical
observations of distressed couples commonly provide examples of how
spouses become upset when they demand that their personal standards
be met and realize that this occurrence is unlikely. Given that Epstein *et
al.*'s (1991) findings were based on community rather than clinic couples,
the sample might include spouses who are less harsh when their standards
are not met. At the least, the findings suggest that the role of standards in
marital discord is more complicated than previously thought.

Cognition within a Marital System

The discussion thus far has focused almost exclusively on the relation
between a specific cognition of one spouse and that person's satisfaction
with the relationship. However, given (1) that a marital relationship

involves two persons, (2) that we have identified five types of cognition that are of importance, and (3) that cognition, behavior, and emotion are all relevant to marital functioning, then the number and complexity of relations among these variables can become staggering. For example, within a given individual, the relations among the different cognitions are of importance. How do a spouse's attributions for a behavior ("He did it because he is thoughtless") influence that person's tendency to attend selectively to the partner's behavior in the future, in this example, perhaps selectively focusing on "thoughtless" behavior to the exclusion of thoughtful, loving acts?

Second, considering a single individual and a single cognitive variable (e.g., attributions), how does cognition regarding one's *own* behaviors interact with cognition regarding one's partner's behaviors in impacting marital satisfaction? Several studies have investigated this issue (e.g., Fincham *et al.*, 1987; Kyle and Falbo, 1985; Orvis *et al.*, 1976). After reviewing this body of literature, Bradbury and Fincham (1990) concluded that satisfied partners make similar attributions for their own and their partners' behavior, or they might actually make more positive attributions for their partners' behaviors relative to their own behavior. However, distressed spouses make more negative attributions for their partners' behaviors compared to the attributions they make for their own behaviors.

As a third example, within a given individual and considering a single cognitive variable, the relation between that cognition and subsequent behavior is of importance. Bradbury and Fincham (1992) obtained spouses' attributions for a major marital problem and then asked the partners to discuss that same problem. Even after controlling for level of marital satisfaction, they found that spouses who attributed the problem more to the partner's intent demonstrated higher rates of negative communication during the conversation. Although studies such as this do not identify the direction of causality between spouses' cognitions and their marital communication, they point to the importance of studying the cognition–behavior link.

These examples illustrate the interrelations among spouses' cognitions, behavior, and affect that exist when even small pieces of the broader picture are examined. Attempting to understand how all of these variables fit together and change over time as the couple continues to interact is clearly a challenging task. Future empirical efforts to unravel the complex interplay of cognition, behavior, and affect in the development of marital problems must be guided by theoretical models that take all of these components into account. The following is a description of the theoretical models that have formed the bases for existing research on cognition in marriage, as well as an outline of a broader model that includes causal links among the various types of cognitions described above, the spouses' affective responses to each other, and the couple's behavioral interactions.

MODELS AND EMPIRICAL FINDINGS CONCERNING COGNITION IN COUPLE RELATIONSHIPS

Partners' cognitions about their relationships have long been considered important determinants of marital quality and influences on relationship dysfunction across diverse theoretical orientations. For example, psychodynamic approaches have emphasized how individuals' responses to their current partners can be distorted by intrapsychic cognitive structures (e.g., introjects) and processes (e.g., projective identification) (cf. Baruth and Huber, 1984; Meissner, 1978), and it is assumed that interventions that foster insight into each person's historical material will reduce partners' distorted views of each other. Furthermore, it is assumed that the shift toward perceiving one's partner in an undistorted manner will reduce negative emotional and behavioral responses toward him or her. Approaches that apply systems theory concepts to family problems vary in the degree to which they take intrapsychic phenomena into account, but the reframing and relabeling interventions commonly used by structural and strategic family therapists (e.g., Todd, 1986) are based on the idea that individuals' emotional and behavioral responses to each other's behavior are influenced by their views of the behavior.

Unfortunately, the cognitive factors involved in various theoretical approaches to marital problems often have not been defined clearly enough and operationalized in ways that permit empirical tests of the models. An exception to this problem has been the rapidly growing theoretical, empirical, and clinical cognitive–behavioral literature on marriage. As is the case with the behavioral field as a whole, many of the earlier writings on behavioral marital therapy (BMT) (e.g., Jacobson and Margolin, 1979; O'Leary and Turkewitz, 1978; Stuart, 1969, 1980; Weiss, 1978) acknowledged the reciprocal influences between cognition and behavior, and they identified the types of cognition (negative trait attributions, unrealistic expectations) that the marital therapist should be prepared to "restructure." However, the specific roles of particular cognitive variables in an overall model of marital functioning remained fairly vague in these presentations. Most commonly, attributions were seen as mediating spouses' responses to each other's overt behaviors, as when one spouse produces a behavior requested by the partner, and the partner then discounts it as being due to pressure from the therapist rather than a reflection of genuine caring. The distress and negative behavior (coercion, withdrawal) that can occur when a partner's behavior does not meet one's standards also was emphasized in the literature, and therapeutic strategies for altering spouses' unrealistic standards were described. The cognitive factors were integrated into the behavior exchange model that underlies BMT, in that a partner's acts would be experienced as costs rather than benefits if they were attributed to negative causes or were judged to be inadequate when compared to the "template" of one's standards for the marriage. The cognitive factors themselves were not isolated in empirical studies, which assessed behavioral correlates of marital distress and evaluated the efficacy of behavioral treatments (see reviews by Baucom and Epstein, 1990; Weiss and Heyman, 1990).

The secondary role given to marital cognitions may be viewed in light of the enthusiasm for the emerging behavioral field, the encouraging results of initial BMT outcome studies, and the absence of validated measures of cognition that could be used in research. Consequently, although cognitions were considered important, little attention was paid to questions such as (1) whether cognition could cause the development of couples' behavioral problems; (2) how problematic marital cognition is formed; (3) how different types of cognition (e.g., attributions, standards) are related to one another; and (4) how much changes in behavior can produce changes in cognition, and vice versa (these are basic questions facing those who study the other kinds of psychological problems discussed in other chapters of this book).

As Fincham *et al.* (1990b) noted, there has been a marked increase in attention to cognitive (as well as emotional) factors in marriage, due to an "interface" between social and clinical psychology, the development of a multidisciplinary science of close relationships, research on links between affect and cognition, and the rapid growth of cognitive science. Furthermore, the "cognitive revolution" in psychology has been reflected in the growing influence of cognitive therapies (cf. Dobson, 1988). Although approaches such as Beck's cognitive therapy (e.g., Beck et al., 1979) and Ellis's rational–emotive therapy (e.g., Ellis and Dryden, 1987) initially were developed to address problems at the level of the individual, they have been applied increasingly to problems in couple and family relationships (Beck, 1988; Ellis *et al.*, 1989).

Although the confluence of these various trends has produced considerable clinical and research activity focused on the cognitions involved in marital problems, few writers have presented specific conceptual models in which the interplay of behavior, affect, and cognition is outlined. In the following sections, we review the models of marital cognition presented in the clinical and theoretical/research literatures, noting the basic assumptions that each model seems to include concerning the questions described above (e.g., what types of cognitions play roles in marital discord; what causal relations exist among cognitions, emotions, and behaviors). After summarizing research findings relevant to existing theoretical models, we describe a model that integrates concepts from existing models and discuss treatment implications.

Clinical Models of Marital Cognition

Ellis's Rational–Emotive Model

In the clinical realm, Ellis *et al.* (1989) acknowledge that cognition, affect, and behavior all interact, and they suggest that rational–emotive therapy (RET) with couples is a "systems-oriented" model. Their text, however, describes the traditional linear ABC model in which irrational thinking mediates a spouse's emotional and behavioral responses to a partner's behavior. The model of relationship dysfunction is essentially a combination of two individuals' extreme responses to each other's behavior, based on demanding "shoulds" or standards, a dire need for love, low frustration tolerance, and extreme negative evaluations when standards are not met. Each person's irrational responses to his or her partner then become the environmental stimuli or activating events (the A component of the model) that are perceived and negatively evaluated by the partner. Although Ellis *et al.* (1989) do not differentiate among types of cognitions involved in the B component of their model (in fact, some of their examples appear to be attributions and others standards), Wessler and Wessler's (1980) elaboration of the RET model includes the individual's selective perception of events and inferences within the activating event component.

The RET model focuses on stable cognitions that an individual brings to interactions with a partner, and it is assumed that it is the irrationality of an individual's beliefs, rather than the objective negativity of a partner's behavior, that creates severe disturbance (as opposed to dissatisfaction). Wessler and Wessler (1980) note that life events, such as the death of a beloved spouse, can produce intense emotional upset in the absence of irrational thinking, but destructive consequences such as escalating exchanges of aversive behavior between spouses are likely to result when extreme standards and evaluations are applied to events. The origins of irrational thinking are assumed to be earlier life experiences, including growing up in a society that fosters unrealistic romantic notions of intimate relationships through movies, love songs, and other mass media. Furthermore, Ellis *et al.* (1989) argue that each individual interprets life experiences in an idiosyncratic manner and constructs his or her own irrational belief system; however, the factors that differentiate individuals who develop irrational beliefs from those who do not are not specified in the model.

Ellis *et al*. (1989) note that they use behavioral interventions such as assertiveness training to alter spouses' current experiences and thereby counteract long-standing irrational beliefs. However, even though the model allows for behavior change leading to cognitive change, the primary path to change is the cognition-to-behavior link.

Beck's Cognitive Model

Beck's (1976; Beck *et al*., 1979) cognitive model of individual psychopathology has been applied to marital problems in a manner similar to the RET approach. As in RET, it is assumed that each spouse brings to the relationship basic beliefs (schemata) about the self and about intimate relationships (Beck, 1988; Dattilio and Padesky, 1990). These schemata (which may be conscious or beyond awareness) are developed through prior life experiences and "constitute the basis for coding, categorizing, and evaluating experiences during the course of one's life" (Dattilio and Padesky, 1990, p. 7). In terms of our typology of cognitions, the schemata include both assumptions about how partners and marriages *are* and standards about how they *should be*.

In Beck's model, the behavior of one spouse activates the partner's underlying schemata relevant to the situation, eliciting stream-of-consciousness "automatic thoughts," with associated emotional and behavioral responses. The individual's automatic thoughts commonly include inferences (in our typology, attributions and expectancies) that may be arbitrary and inaccurate, especially when based on inappropriate or extreme schemata. For example, a spouse with an underlying assumption, "people who care about each other go out of their way to initiate time together" may make an attribution that his or her partner is uncaring whenever the partner becomes absorbed in individual pursuits and fails to initiate shared activities. By focusing extensively on perceptual biases and faulty inferences in spouses' automatic thoughts, as well as underlying schemata, Beck's model tends to address a greater range of the cognitions in our typology than does the RET model. The model also differentiates between preexisting schemata that a spouse brings to the current relationship and schemata *specific to the relationship*, which develop from the couple's trial-and-error interactions with each other. Beck (1988) describes how an individual's trait attributions about a partner (e.g., "He likes to see me suffer"), which are based on inferences from repeated negative behavioral interactions, become crystallized into overgeneralized "frames" that shape future perceptions and inferences about the partner.

Although Beck's model commonly has been interpreted as focusing on linear causality, in which distorted or extreme thinking produces individual and relationship problems, Dattilio and Padesky (1990) note that the model also takes into account the impacts of affect and behavior on the individual's thinking. For example, the therapeutic procedure of assisting clients in designing "behavioral experiments," whereby the validity of an inference or underlying schema is tested *in vivo* is based on the idea that behavioral data can change cognitions. Consequently, although cognitive therapists who work with couples tend to emphasize cognitive interventions, they also spend time working with couples' problematic communication patterns that exacerbate conflict. Nevertheless, the literature on cognitive therapy with couples often does not seem to capture the extent to which marital dysfunction is maintained by ingrained negative behavioral exchanges, such as the escalating coercive exchanges identified in sequential analyses of couple interaction (e.g., Revenstorf *et al.*, 1984). These behavioral exchanges may occur in an "automatic" or overlearned manner, with little or no cognitive processing, and may require behavioral rather than cognitive intervention.

Social Cognition Models Applied to Marriage

It is artificial to separate clinically derived models of marital cognition from models that have been generated primarily from theory and research in the areas of social and cognitive psychology, because clinical theoreticians such as Beck have been influenced significantly by, and contributed to, basic research on social cognition, and many of the basic researchers in the field are practicing marital therapists as well. However, for the sake of clarity, the following models are grouped in this section because their roots have been primarily in basic psychological theory and research.

Doherty's Attribution–Expectancy Model

Doherty (1981a,b) describes a cognitive model of family conflict that focuses on attributions that family members make about the causes of relationship events and the expectancies they have concerning their abilities to solve relationship problems. Doherty's model is based on attribution theory (Kelley, 1973) and social learning theory (e.g., Bandura, 1977). In the model, the degrees to which an individual attributes the causes of family conflicts to particular sources (e.g., self vs. other family members, positive vs. negative intent, stable vs. unstable sources, voluntary vs. involuntary behavior, and global vs. specific sources) combine or interact with efficacy expectancies to determine how the person responds to conflict. For example, an individual who sees his or her partner as the source of a marital problem (rather than the self or factors outside the relationship), and views the partner's negative behavior as voluntary and based on malicious intent, is likely to exhibit blaming attitudes and behavior, focusing any change efforts on the other person. When negative partner behavior is attributed to global, stable, negative sources, the individual is likely to have low efficacy expectancies about improving the problem and will be more likely to exhibit learned helplessness responses (e.g., giving up rather than sustaining problem-solving efforts). Thus, Doherty (1981b) suggests that "while efficacy is proposed to predict persistence and helplessness effects, attributions influence both the direction and the affective valence of the individual's problem-solving attempts" (p. 39). Although Doherty notes that ongoing behavioral interactions among family members influence each person's attributions and expectancies, his model emphasizes the "cognition influences emotion and behavior" causal direction.

Drawing on social learning theory (e.g., Rotter et al., 1972), Doherty (1981b) suggests that the attributions and efficacy expectancies in his model can exist either in a situation-specific manner, or as generalized cognitive "sets." Based on an individual's past experiences in intimate relationships, he or she develops generalized attributions and efficacy expectancies (e.g., the expectancy that chronic marital conflicts are impossible to resolve). Although not directly stated in Doherty's discussion, it appears that these generalized cognitions may develop from past experiences either in a person's previous relationships or over time in the current one. They tend to exist as stable individual differences or styles that the person applies to specific conflict situations, although new experiences in the marriage may alter them. Doherty does not refer to such stable cognitive sets as schemata or cognitive structures, but they appear to fit into that category, primarily as basic assumptions about partners and close relationships. In fact, Baucom et al. (1989b) found that consistent attributional styles can be identified, and that the degree to which a spouse applies such a style across judgments of various partner behaviors is correlated with his or her level of marital distress.

Whereas Doherty's (1981b) model accounts for the development of individual differences in generalized attributions and expectancies, in terms of prior relationship experiences, there are few hints in the model about factors that would lead an individual to apply varying attributions and expectancies to a partner's behavior from one situation to another. In fact, little attention has yet been paid to determinants of situation-specific attributions. Baucom (1987) has argued that variability in spouses' attributions for relationship events stems at least in part from the variety of functions that attributions can serve. Based on a review of attribution studies, he notes that attributional activity is likely to be elicited when one's partner behaves in unexpected and novel ways, and when the behavior is aversive or important to the observing spouse. Among the reasons that Baucom identifies why spouses make attributions about each other's behavior are: (1) to achieve a sense of intimacy through understanding one's partner; (2) to identify causes of a partner's negative behavior so that one can take steps to change it; (3) to reduce disappointment and distress by making the partner's behavior predictable even if negative; (4) to reduce distress by attributing potentially upsetting partner behavior to a more benign cause (e.g., a partner forgot one's birthday because of situational job stress rather than due to lack of caring); (5) to protect or enhance oneself (e.g., blaming a partner for a relationship problem in order to maintain one's own self esteem); and (6) to maintain or enhance one's positive view of the partner or relationship. An example of how a spouse may overtly express a global trait attribution in order to motivate a partner to change would be, "You spend so much time on your work because you don't care about me. If you really cared, you would set aside more time for me."

Similar to Doherty (1981b), Baucom (1987) suggests that an individual's attributions, as well as his or her expectancies about a partner's future behavior, are likely to be shaped by the generalized beliefs (i.e., assumptions) about close relationships, which are developed through prior life experiences. Again, the theoretical link between stable schemata and situational inferences appears to be important.

Arias and Beach's (1987) review of basic attribution theory and research in social psychology, and its implications for the study of marital attributions, noted the general tendency for people to make dispositional attributions for others' behavior, and they identified several factors that influence the likelihood that such attributions will be made. For example, an observer is more likely to see an actor's behavior as intentional when he or she is aware that the actor had alternative behaviors available that may have had the same outcome. Thus, attributional cognitive mediation models of marital interaction clearly are becoming more sophisticated, especially as theoreticians and researchers are integrating concepts from the clinical and basic research fields.

The links among causal attributions, efficacy expectancies, and helplessness responses described by Doherty (1981a,b) closely parallel Abramson et al.'s (1978) attributional model of learned helplessness in depression. Based on the prominent status of attribution theory in psychology, the notable parallels between learned helplessness in depression and in marital distress (Epstein, 1985), and the fact that Doherty's model provided a testable set of hypotheses concerning marital cognition, Doherty's papers played a significant role in stimulating a large number of studies of distressed and nondistressed couples' attributions. In general, the cognitive model tested in the research studies (which are reviewed later) has been a linear unidirectional one in which attributions mediate spouses' affective and behavioral responses to each other's positive or negative behavior. Perhaps because attributions have been "center stage" in psychology during the past two decades, efficacy expectancies have until recently received minimal attention from marital researchers.

Fincham and Bradbury's Revised Attribution–Efficacy Model

Fincham and Bradbury (1987a) presented an attribution–efficacy model of cognition in marital conflict that was a revision of Doherty's model. First, they expanded the attributional component by differentiating between *causal* attributions (concerning the source of an event) and *responsibility* attributions (that involve accountability and intentionality). Second, they added to Doherty's model spouses' judgments about each other's capacities to foresee potential problems, to identify alternative behaviors that can avoid conflict, and to engage in the alternative responses. Third, they proposed a causal path in which causal attributions, responsibility criteria (e.g., intent), and capacities for pursuing alternative behavior all influence responsibility attributions (who is held responsible for conflict), which in turn influence blame judgments.

Concerning efficacy expectations (i.e., expectancies), Fincham and Bradbury's (1987a) revision of Doherty's model attempted to remove intention from the efficacy construct by restricting it to the belief that one can master the behaviors needed to produce a particular outcome, independent of one's intention to perform those acts. They also expanded Doherty's focus on expectancies that the dyad can influence conflict, adding expectancies about each partner's individual efficacy. Furthermore, they questioned whether attributions impact directly on helplessness or whether (as in learned helplessness theory) efficacy expectancies mediate their influence on helplessness. Finally, Fincham and Bradbury disagreed with Doherty's proposal that individuals with high efficacy expectancies focus their change efforts on the perceived causes of relationship conflicts, arguing instead that such efforts will be directed toward the most easily influenced sources.

As noted above, models of marital attribution have stimulated a sizable number of empirical studies, and reviews of that literature (e.g., Baucom and Epstein, 1990; Bradbury and Fincham, 1990; Thompson and Snyder, 1986) indicate considerable consistency in results supporting hypothesized associations between both causal and responsibility attributions and levels of marital satisfaction. These correlational studies suggest that attributions are salient components of spouses' phenomenological experiences of their marital relationships, but they do not provide information about the degree to which attributions produce levels of satisfaction, or vice versa. Fincham and Bradbury (1987b) took a step toward testing causality by conducting a longitudinal study in which marital satisfaction and spouses' attributions for marital problems were assessed at two points, twelve months apart. They found that *for wives*, both causal and responsibility attributions at time 1 predicted satisfaction level at time 2, but satisfaction at time 1 did not predict the time 2 attributions for either sex. Because both sexes' attributions were associated with level of current satisfaction at both points, Fincham and Bradbury speculate that "husbands' attributions may simply reflect their marital satisfaction, whereas wives' attributions actually influence their marital satisfaction over time" (p. 515). Because the study did not involve actual experimental mainpulation of variables, it does not address the causal question directly, but it is an improvement over concurrent correlational studies.

Fincham and Bradbury (1987a) used path analyses to test their attribution–efficacy model, assessing the associations of causal attributions, responsibility attributions, and efficacy expectancies with spouses' responses to marital conflict (e.g., blaming the partner; letting conflict in one area of one's relationship generalize to other areas). They found some initial support for the idea that both types of cognitions affect spouses' handling of conflict, but they note that the stronger role of the attributional variables may have been due to inadequate operationalization of efficacy expectancies. This is another encouraging example of an advance in design and methodology, but the need for further conceptual clarification and development of more refined assessment instruments in the marital cognition field is clear.

Schema Theory and Beliefs

Arias and Beach (1987) note that increasing attention has been paid in the field of social cognition to the study of the schema, a fairly stable "set of rules or a naive theory" (p. 116) held by an individual, which guides his or her attention to particular stimuli in the environment and shapes the types of inferences the person makes from an observed characteristic to unobserved ones. Because schemata influence perceptions of events and inferences concerning those events that are noticed, people tend to seek and find information that confirms their existing schemata. Based on social cognition research findings concerning this self-fulfilling characteristic of schemata, Arias and Beach propose that a spouse who holds a particular schema concerning a partner (e.g., "she's easily irritated") may behave in a defensive manner that elicits the irritated behavior that he expects.

Arias and Beach (1987) describe four types of schemata that are particularly relevant in marital relationships: (1) schemata concerning particular others (e.g., the person's own spouse); (2) self-schemata; (3) schemata concerning particular roles (e.g., husband, wife); and (4) schemata about interactions in particular social situations (e.g., reuniting after being apart all day). Nisbett and Ross (1980) divide schemata into the two broad categories of *personae*, which include characteristics and typical behaviors of particular people, or persons who occupy certain roles (which includes the first three of the types of schemata identified by Arias and Beach), and *scripts*, which involve sequences of events in social contexts (Arias and Beach's fourth type). According to Turk and Speers (1983), scripts also include estimates of probabilities that specific events will occur.

Baucom and Epstein (1990) note that the characteristics of an individual's personae and scripts can be based on a variety of sources, such as the person's own past life experiences, mass-media depictions of interpersonal relationships, and the person's imagination. Some personae and scripts are widely shared within a culture, whereas others are relatively idiosyncratic. As fairly stable cognitive structures, what various personae and scripts have in common is that they influence people's perceptions and inferences. Thus, for example, if a particular man's persona about the "wife" role includes characteristics such as "emotionally supportive, giving, affectionate, and loyal," when considering women he dates as potential mates, he is likely to pay close attention to the degree to which each woman exhibits behaviors suggestive of such traits. Furthermore, if this man marries a woman who appears to fit the persona well, he may become quite distressed if some aspect of her behavior at a future time does not "fit" the persona well, because he may make inferences that if his partner may not possess characteristic A of the persona, she may not possess any of the other characteristics that he associates with it. Consistent with basic schema theory, Baucom and Epstein propose that the inferences involved in spouses' attributions and expectancies about each other tend to be influenced by the intercorrelations among characteristics in their schemata.

As described earlier, the assumption that relatively stable schemata underlie momentary perceptual and inferential processes is a key component of Beck's (1976; Beck *et al.*, 1979) cognitive model of emotional disorders such as depression. In a number of studies (e.g., Dykman *et al.*, 1991; Hammen *et al.*, 1985, 1989; Miranda *et al.*, 1990), schemata that have been operationalized in terms of questionnaire measures of dysfunctional beliefs, general personality styles (e.g., autonomy, sociotropy), and self-concept have been found to be associated with depression. Furthermore, there is evidence that remitted depressed patients are more likely to relapse if they have residual "depressive" schemata (Eaves and Rush, 1984). Segal *et al.* (1992) found that life events are especially likely to elicit depression if they are relevant to the themes of an individual's depressive schemata, that is, there is "event–schema congruence." For example, Segal *et al.* found that if an individual's symptoms of depression had abated but his or her score on a measure of self-criticism concerning performance remained high, the person was especially likely to relapse if subsequently exposed to life events that involved performance problems. Such findings do not identify causality, but they are consistent with the concept of life events activating stable schemata associated with a particular affective response. This congruence aspect of schema theory has not yet been addressed in the area of marital distress, but it seems highly relevant.

Marital research related to schemata has as yet been limited, but the initial results indicate that particular types of assumptions and standards are associated with relationship distress. As described earlier, studies with the Relationship Belief Inventory (RBI; Eidelson and Epstein, 1982) have demonstrated that adherence to potentially unrealistic assumptions and standards is associated with greater marital distress. In addition, Jones and Stanton (1988) compared the ability of the *similarity* and the *content* of spouses' beliefs about marriage to predict marital distress. The congruency and content models, as well as a model combining both effects, were compared by administering the RBI, a scale assessing individually oriented irrational beliefs based on Ellis's RET model, and four marital satisfaction indices to a sample of community couples. Consistent with Epstein and Eidelson's (1981) findings, scores on the RBI were better predictors of marital distress than were those on the measure of general irrational beliefs, that is, the match between the content of the belief (schema) and the life event is important. Furthermore, for both sexes, greater perceived similarity in their relationship beliefs was correlated with greater satisfaction, whereas actual similarity between partners' beliefs, as well as accurate perception of each other's beliefs, was not associated with level of satisfaction. This finding is comparable to Epstein *et al.*'s (1991) finding that spouses' satisfaction with how their standards are met in their relationship is a much stronger predictor of marital satisfaction than the actual degree of discrepancy between partners' standards. Finally, in regression analyses that used both RBI spouse similarity scores and individual RBI self-ratings to predict distress, Jones and Stanton (1988) found that degree of adherence to dysfunctional beliefs was a significant predictor but similarity between spouses was not.

In Fincham and Bradbury's (1987b) longitudinal study, which was described earlier, spouses' causal attributions, responsibility attributions, and relationship beliefs all were significantly correlated in the expected direction with level of marital satisfaction at time 1, but only the attribution scores at time 1 predicted level of satisfaction twelve months later. Fincham and Bradbury conclude that their results are consistent with a model in which relationship beliefs shape attributions, which then impact satisfaction. However, as Fincham and Bradbury note, the results can only be considered preliminary and not a strong test of a causal model. Nevertheless, their study indicates the need to study marital cognition in a multivariate manner, attempting to test which types of cognitions have direct and indirect effects on spouses' satisfaction *and behavior* concurrently and over time.

Initial outcome studies assessing the effects of adding a cognitive restructuring component to behavioral marital therapy have raised as many questions as they have answered about links between spouses' cognitions and their behaviors. In two studies by Baucom and his associates (Baucom and Lester, 1986; Baucom *et al.*, 1990b), six weeks of cognitive restructuring (focused on causal attributions and unrealistic beliefs) followed by six weeks of BMT (problem solving, communication, and contracting) produced comparable but not greater improvement in marital satisfaction than twelve weeks of BMT. Within treatment conditions, in both studies the combination treatment produced significant decreases in RBI scores for both sexes, whereas BMT alone produced significant decreases on the RBI for females but not for males. Baucom *et al.* (1990b) raise a number of cautions against concluding at this point that cognitive interventions add nothing to BMT, but for the purpose of the present discussion, the finding that at least for females the behaviorally oriented treatment produced cognitive changes is of interest. Again, there is a parallel with results from research on depression, where treatments other than cognitive restructuring (e.g., medication) have been found to reduce negative cognitions. In the case of marital treatments, because BMT sessions traditionally do attend to spouses' cognitions about their behavioral interactions, more "pure" tests of the causal relation between marital behavior and cognition remain to be conducted.

Bradbury and Fincham's Contextual Model

Bradbury and Fincham (1991) note that Raush *et al.*'s (1974) work on marital communication had a significant impact on marital research, with its emphasis on observational coding of couple interaction rather than reliance on self-report measures. However, the theoretical model underlying Raush *et al.*'s work, which focused on object relations schemata, has received much less attention, perhaps due to the fact that marital interaction research in the 1970s and 1980s was conducted primarily by researchers with behavioral rather than psychodynamic orientations. As Bradbury and Fincham note, the mediational approach pursued by Raush *et al.* was a forerunner of the current interest in cognitive and affective factors in couple interaction, but its object relations schemata were not operational-ized and included in tests of the theoretical model. In fact, Raush *et al.'s* (1974) definition of object relations schemata as organizing structures that develop from prior experiences with other people and "organize images of oneself and others and the relations between oneself and others" (p. 49) seems remarkably similar to current definitions of schemata offered by cognitive theorists.

As in other cognitive models of couple interaction, Bradbury and Fin-cham's (1988, 1991) contextual model posits a circular process in which one partner's behavior is processed by the other partner, leading to emotional and behavioral responses on the latter's part; these responses then are processed by the former partner, leading to his or her own emotional and behavioral responses, and so on. The processing includes attending to the stimuli from the other person, identifying their qualities (whether they are positive or negative, expected or unexpected, and personally significant or insignificant), and choosing among response alternatives. The contextual model goes further, however, by identifying two major classes of variables that can influence each spouse's processing of the other's overt behavior. On one hand, *proximal context* variables include transient thoughts and emotions, usually elicited by recent prior events in the couple's interactions (e.g., memories and emotional responses to a partner's preceding actions). This subjective state is likely to influence the cognitive processing of the current partner behavior, including what aspects of the behavior are noticed.

On the other hand, *distal context* variables are relatively stable psycholog-ical characteristics of each spouse [e.g., personality traits; standards about the characteristics of a close relationship; cognitive representations (as-sumptions in our typology) of self, partner, or relationship]. Thus, the proximal context consists of labile thoughts and emotions that are elicited by specific stimuli in the here-and-now, whereas the distal context involves schemata that operate across many situations in a couple's interactions.

Bradbury and Fincham also propose that the proximal and distal context variables exert mutual influences on each other, such that the stable dis-tal factors influence the immediate thoughts and feelings experienced in the current interaction, and in turn the proximal thoughts and feelings can alter more stable aspects of the individual. For example, attributions formed about a partner's behavior in a specific situation are likely to be shaped by the observing spouse's long-standing assumptions about the partner's personality and motives. On the other hand, the relatively stable assumptions about the partner can be modified by new attributions elicited by the partner's behavior in a particular situation. In their research on their contextual model, Bradbury and Fincham (1988) operationalized the distal context with measures of sex roles and unrealistic relationship beliefs, whereas the measures of the proximal context included scales assessing causal and responsibility attributions. However, Bradbury and Fincham (1991) also noted that attributions can exist as relatively stable "styles" as well as situation-specific inferences.

Bradbury and Fincham (1988) used multiple-regression analyses to test alternative configurations of the contextual model, in which (1) proximal variables (causal and responsibility attributions) mediate the relationship between distal variables (sex roles and relationship beliefs) and marital satisfaction, and (2) proximal and distal variables have independent effects on satisfaction. The results, showing unique prediction of satisfaction by responsibility attributions and femininity sex role scores, supported the latter alternative, although Bradbury and Fincham do not rule out the possibility that attributions *partly* mediate the impact of distal variables on satisfaction.

A final component of the contextual model involves appraisals that spouses make just before and after an interaction, of either a marital or nonmarital focus. Bradbury and Fincham (1991) suggest that these appraisals influence and are influenced by the proximal and distal contexts. Unfortunately, the characteristics of the appraisals (i.e., whether they are evaluative judgments, attributions, expectancies) are unclear in the description of the model. If they are restricted to qualitative appraisals of the marriage (e.g., that it is a hurtful and unsupportive relationship), then it is unclear how the model encompasses the attributions and expectancies that a spouse makes *after* observing a partner's behavior.

In spite of some ambiguities in Bradbury and Fincham's (1988, 1991) contextual model, it has made a significant contribution to the conceptualization of cognitive factors in marital interaction, especially in its integration of transient and stable forms of cognition that can simultaneously influence an individual's processing of a partner's behavior. It captures the complexity of cognitive processing in a dyadic interaction, where, for example, an inference about the intentions behind a partner's current aversive act is likely to be influenced by stable assumptions about ways in which people express caring, attributions about causes of the partner's previous pleasant or unpleasant acts, anger about the previous behavior, and an overall appraisal of the marriage as a deteriorating relationship.

SUMMARY OF MODELS OF MARITAL COGNITION

There is considerable overlap among the various marital cognition models derived from clinical and social cognition bases. The most common components of the models fall into the distal and proximal context categories described by Bradbury and Fincham (1988). The models vary in the degree to which they include both types of cognitive variables (e.g., the RET model emphasizes stable beliefs, whereas Bradbury and Fincham's contextual model appears to weight distal and proximal cognitions equally). Although the large majority of empirical studies of marital cognition have been based on attribution models, there is increasing interest in assessing and studying the role of schemata. Parallel research on cognition in depression, as well as existing findings concerning an association between marital distress and unrealistic relationship assumptions and standards (e.g., Eidelson and Epstein, 1982), suggests that this can be a fruitful line of inquiry. Testing the event–schema congruence model that has been supported in depression seems to be an important direction for future marital research.

All of the models that we have reviewed include at least some of the five types of cognitions in our typology (selective perception, attributions, expectancies, assumptions, standards), even though the labels for these variables may differ. In general, however, the models do not fully differentiate them and indicate their interrelations, as well as their reciprocal effects with spouses' emotional and behavioral responses toward each other. Consequently, Fig. 10.1 presents a model that outlines the relations among the five types of cognition, behaviors, and affective responses. The model takes into account prior models, as well as clinically derived concepts such as spouses' "negative tracking" of each other's displeasing behaviors (Jacobson and Margolin, 1979) and "sentiment override" in which a spouse's preexisting general "affective–cognitive representation" of the partner influences his or her perceptions of the partner's current behavior more than the behaviors themselves do (Weiss, 1984).

In Fig. 10.1, note that both preexisting general schemata (assumptions and standards about human behavior and close relationships, developed from prior life experiences) and schemata that the individual develops about the current relationship because of interactions with the partner are activated when the partner exhibits specific actions relevant to the content of the schemata. The schemata in turn predispose the individual to notice events in the current relationship selectively. There also is an interplay between an individual's preexisting general relationship schemata and those that he or she develops within the current marriage. On one hand, long-standing assumptions and standards commonly will shape those applied to the present relationship, and on the other hand, idiosyncratic assumptions and standards arising from one's interactions with a particular partner can become generalized into broader schemata about relationships.

Both types of schemata, when activated by a relationship event, can shape the individual's inferences about the event, including attributions concerning its determinants and expectancies about its future consequences.

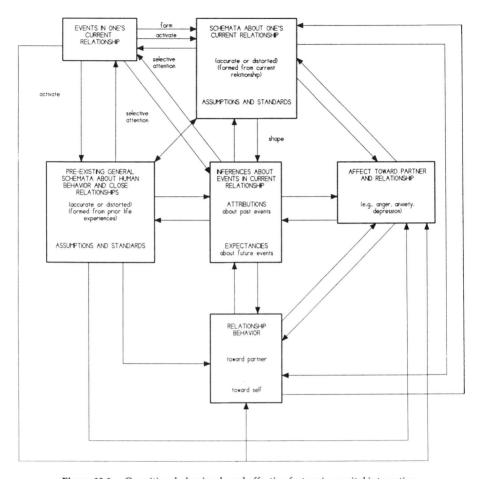

Figure 10.1.   Cognitive, behavioral, and affective factors in marital interaction.

In turn, current attributions and expectancies can modify the person's schemata, although it may take a considerable amount of new information to alter longstanding assumptions and standards.

Schemata (assumptions and standards) can have a direct impact on a spouse's affective and behavioral responses to partner behavior when the individual perceives, and evaluates as good or bad, some degree of match or mismatch between the partner's actions and the internalized "template" (as proposed in the RET and Beck models). In turn, an individual's attributions, expectancies, assumptions, and standards about the marriage also can be shaped by perceptions of his or her own behavioral and affective responses to the partner, self, and relationship. For example, in an initial therapy session, one couple described a pattern in which the husband would pursue the wife, seeking more time together, whereas the wife would withdraw. The wife reported that, "at times when he wants more from me, I become tense and really feel little warmth toward him." As she reported those emotions, her demeanor changed, and when the therapist asked about it, she replied,

> "I feel sad right now, because those feelings that I get just don't seem like normal feelings of someone who is in love with her husband. My mother thinks that since my father died when I was in my teens I put up a wall to protect myself from getting too attached to a man, and maybe she's right [assumption]. I think that when I feel tense when Joe approaches me, it is my wall going up [attribution]." When the therapist asked whether she could turn and tell her husband more about these thoughts and emotions rather than directing her comments to the therapist, she responded, "I'm afraid that if I look him in the eye, I'll shut off my feelings and not be able to say anything" [expectancy].

Consistent with Bradbury and Fincham's (1988) findings, the model indicates that attributions and expectancies elicited by relationship events not only act as mediators between distal variables (e.g., schemata) and satisfaction but also can have direct effects on marital satisfaction. As Baucom (1987) noted, attributional activity is more likely to occur when events in a relationship are unexpected, novel, or important to the observer. The same conditions might be expected to elicit an individual's tendency to form expectancies about future relationship events. An important question for cognitive assessment is whether a spouse's attributions have developed into a stable distal attributional "style" (i.e., schema) that is applied to varied partner behaviors in a stereotyped manner.

This model is not intended to supplant any of the models we have reviewed; rather, it is presented as a means of integrating concepts from those models while emphasizing the differentiation of the five types of cognitions that may interact in complex ways as spouses process information about their relationship.

CLINICAL IMPLICATIONS AND FUTURE DIRECTIONS

The growing complexity of models being offered to account for cognitive influences in marital interactions, as well as the growing body of empirical findings, have a number of implications for both clinical practice and future research in the area. First, there are clear conceptual grounds for differentiating several types of cognitive structures and processes that can play different roles in marital conflict, and the initial research findings tend to indicate that investigators have had some success in measuring these different variables. Consequently, it is important that clinical assessments and interventions take into account the variety of cognitions that may be influencing a couple's problems. Baucom *et al.* (1990b) stressed that future research comparing the efficacy of cognitive and behavioral marital treatments should take into account the matching of client needs and the foci of interventions. Not only might such matching be on the basis of the distinction between the cognitive and behavioral components of clients' problems, but they also may lead to cognitive interventions tailored to issues with specific types of cognitions in a particular couple.

Second, at this point the conceptual models for understanding marital cognition are much more advanced than the methods for assessing the key variables. As noted elsewhere (e.g., Baucom and Epstein, 1990; Fincham *et al.*, 1990b), the RBI has been the sole measure of relationship schemata used in marital studies, and the range of its subscales is quite limited. There has been a tendency for marital attribution researchers to devise their own scales for their studies, resulting in a lack of standardized instruments and difficulty for those who wish to compare studies. Recently there has been notable progress in the development of validated scales for assessing standards (Epstein *et al.*, 1991) and attributions (Fincham and Bradbury, 1992; Pretzer *et al.*, 1991). There is much work to be done, however, if researchers and clinicians are to have at their disposal a battery of instruments for assessing spouses' perceptions, attributions, expectancies, assumptions, and standards concerning their relationships.

Furthermore, a number of writers (e.g., Arias and Beach, 1987; Fincham *et al.*, 1990b) have stressed that existing methods for assessing spouses' cognitions have tapped conscious cognitions that an individual is willing to report or endorse on a standard questionnaire. Other methods for assessing cognitive processes and structures (e.g., reaction time when particular conceptual stimuli are presented; memory for schema-relevant and -irrelevant words) have not yet been applied in the marital field. Measuring the rapid processing of information that occurs in an ongoing couple interaction is a challenging task, but efforts toward that goal will be important if marital researchers are to test their conceptual models adequately.

Spouses' emotions are also becoming more prominent components of models guiding research and clinical practice (Baucom and Epstein, 1990). Consequently, there is a need for the development of more refined assessment of spouses' affective responses to each other. Researchers have tended to measure spouses' self-reports of global positive versus negative emotion regarding particular aspects of their interaction, such as being alone with each other (O'Leary *et al.*, 1983), or their positive versus nega-tive affect experienced while watching a videotape replay of a specific interaction with their partner (Gottman and Levenson, 1985). Typically there is no systematic assessment of specific emotions such as anger, anxi-ety, and sadness or depression in studies of marital conflict. One notable exception is Gottman and Levenson's (1986) behavioral coding of specific affects using facial expression cues and "cultural informant" coding, wherein individuals selected as skilled in judging emotions in a culture code each spouse's speech units into specific emotion categories, using context, verbal content, and nonverbal behavior cues. Just as the field is moving toward more differentiated assessment of cognitive variables, re-searchers can facilitate the testing of complex models of marital interaction by pursuing more refined measurement of partners' emotional responses. Such an approach to assessment would assist in the testing of concepts such as sentiment override and cognitive specificity in emotion (i.e., that particular content of cognitions elicits particular affective responses). As-sessment of global "distress" certainly gives the researcher or clinician significant information about the status of a couple's relationship, but it does not provide the fine-tuned data needed for specific therapeutic interventions.

The field of marital research and associated advances in clinical inter-ventions have developed rapidly in recent years, and the increased atten-tion to cognitive and affective factors holds considerable promise for increasing understanding of how intimate relationships function. The challenges that lie ahead involve refining theoretical models and devising methods for assessing the variables that affect the quality of couples' lives together.

REFERENCES

Abramson, L. Y., Seligman, M. E. P., and Teasdale, J. (1978). Learned helplessness in humans: Critique and reformulation. *Journal of Abnormal Psychology, 87*, 49–94.

Arias, I., and Beach, S. R. H. (1987). The assessment of social cognition in the context of marriage. In K. D. O'Leary (Ed.), *Assessment of marital discord* (pp. 109–137). Hillsdale, NJ: Erlbaum.

Bandura, A. (1977). *Social learning theory*. Englewood Cliffs, NJ: Prentice-Hall.

Baruth, L. G., and Huber, C. H. (1984). *An introduction to marital theory and therapy*. Monterey, CA: Brooks/Cole.

Baucom, D. H. (1987). Attributions in distressed relations: How can we explain them? In S. Duck and D. Perlman (Eds.), *Heterosexual relations, marriage and divorce* (pp. 177–206). London: Sage.

Baucom, D. H., and Epstein, N. (1990). *Cognitive–behavioral marital therapy*. New York: Brunner/Mazel.

Baucom, D. H., and Lester, G. W. (1986). The usefulness of cognitive restructuring as an adjunct to behavioral marital therapy. *Behavior Therapy, 17*, 385–403.

Baucom, D. H., Epstein, N., Sayers, S., and Sher, T. G. (1989a). The role of cognitions in marital relationships: Definitional, methodological, and conceptual issues. *Journal of Consulting and Clinical Psychology, 57*, 31–38.

Baucom, D. H., Sayers, S. L., and Duhe, A. (1989b). Attributional style and attributional patterns among married couples. *Journal of Personality and Social Psychology, 56*, 596–607.

Baucom, D. H., Epstein, N., Rankin, L. A., and Burnett, C. K. (1990a). *New measures for assessing couples' standards*. Paper presented at the annual meeting of the Association for Advancement of Behavior Therapy, San Francisco.

Baucom, D. H., Sayers, S. L., and Sher, T. G. (1990b). Supplementing behavioral marital therapy with cognitive restructuring and emotional expressiveness training: An outcome investigation. *Journal of Consulting and Clinical Psychology, 58*, 636–645.

Beck, A. T. (1976). *Cognitive therapy and the emotional disorders*. New York: International Universities Press.

Beck, A. T. (1988). *Love is never enough*. New York: Harper & Row.

Beck, A. T., and Emery, G. (1985). *Anxiety disorders and phobias: A cognitive perspective*. New York: Basic Books.

Beck, A. T., Rush, A. J., Shaw, B. F., and Emery, G. (1979). *Cognitive therapy of depression*. New York: Guilford Press.

Bradbury, T. N., and Fincham, F. D. (1988). Individual difference variables in close relationships: A contextual model of marriage as an integrative framework. *Journal of Personality and Social Psychology, 54*, 713–721.

Bradbury, T. N., and Fincham, F. D. (1990). Attributions in marriage: Review and critique. *Psychological Bulletin, 107*, 3–33.

Bradbury, T. N., and Fincham, F. D. (1991). A contextual model for advancing the study of marital interaction. In G. J. O. Fletcher and F. D. Fincham (Eds.), *Cognition in close relationships* (pp. 127–147). Hillsdale, NJ: Erlbaum.

Bradbury, T. N., and Fincham, F. D. (1992). Attributions and behavior in marital interaction. *Journal of Personality and Social Psychology, 63*, 613–628.

Christensen, A., and Nies, D. C. (1980). The Spouse Observation Checklist: Empirical analysis and critique. *American Journal of Family Therapy, 8*, 69–79.

Christensen, A., Sullaway, M., and King, C. (1983). Systematic error in behavioral reports of dyadic interaction: Egocentric bias and content effects. *Behavioral Assessment, 5*, 131–142.

Dattilio, F. M., and Padesky, C. A. (1990). *Cognitive therapy with couples*. Sarasota, FL: Professional Resource Exchange.

Dobson, K. S. (Ed.). (1988). *Handbook of cognitive-behavioral therapies*. New York: Guilford Press.

Doherty, W. J. (1981a). Cognitive processes in intimate conflict: I. Extending attribution theory. *American Journal of Family Therapy, 9*(1), 5–13.

Doherty, W. J. (1981b). Cognitive processes in intimate conflict: II. Efficacy and learned helplessness. *American Journal of Family Therapy, 9*(2), 35–44.

Dykman, B. M., Horowitz, L. M., Abramson, L. Y., and Usher, M. (1991). Schematic and situational determinants of depressed and nondepressed students' interpretation of feedback. *Journal of Abnormal Psychology, 100*, 45–55.

Eaves, G., and Rush, A. J. (1984). Cognitive patterns in symptomatic and remitted unipolar major depression. *Journal of Abnormal Psychology, 93*, 31–40.

Eidelson, R. J., and Epstein, N. (1982). Cognition and relationship maladjustment: Development of a measure of dysfunctional relationship beliefs. *Journal of Consulting and Clinical Psychology, 50*, 715–720.

Ellis, A., and Dryden, W. (1987). *The practice of rational-emotive therapy*. New York: Springer.

Ellis, A., Sichel, J. L., Yeager, R. J., DiMattia, D. J., and DiGiuseppe, R. (1989). *Rational-emotive couples therapy*. New York: Pergamon.

Epstein, N. (1985). Depression and marital dysfunction: Cognitive and behavioral linkages. *International Journal of Mental Health, 13* (3–4), 86–104.

Epstein, N., and Eidelson, R. J. (1981). Unrealistic beliefs of clinical couples: Their relationship to expectations, goals and satisfaction. *American Journal of Family Therapy, 9*(4), 13–22.

Epstein, N., Pretzer, J. L., and Fleming, B. (1987). The role of cognitive appraisal in self-reports of marital communication. *Behavior Therapy, 18*, 51–69.

Epstein, N., Schlesinger, S. E., and Dryden, W. (Eds.). (1988). *Cognitive–behavioral therapy with families*. New York: Brunner/Mazel.

Epstein, N., Baucom, D. H., Rankin, L. A., and Burnett, C. K. (1991). *Relationship standards in marriage: Development of a new measure of content-specific cognitions*. Paper presented in the symposium "Taking a Broader View of Marital Cognitions" (R. L. Weiss, Chair), at the annual meeting of the Association for Advancement of Behavior Therapy, New York.

Fincham, F. D., and Bradbury, T. N. (1987a). Cognitive processes in close relationships: An attribution-efficacy model. *Journal of Personality and Social Psychology, 53*, 1106–1118.

Fincham, F. D., and Bradbury, T. N. (1987b). The impact of attributions in marriage: A longitudinal analysis. *Journal of Personality and Social Psychology, 53*, 510–517.

Fincham, F. D., and Bradbury, T. N. (1992). Assessing attributions in marriage: The Relationship Attribution Measure. *Journal of Personality and Social Psychology, 62*, 457–468.

Fincham, F. D., Beach, S. R. H., and Baucom, D. H. (1987). Attribution processes in distressed and nondistressed couples: 4. Self-partner attribution differences. *Journal of Personality and Social Psychology, 52*, 739–748.

Fincham, F. D., Bradbury, T. N., and Beach, S. R. H. (1990a). To arrive where we began: A reappraisal of cognition in marriage and marital therapy. *Journal of Family Psychology, 4*, 167–184.

Fincham, F. D., Bradbury, T. N., and Scott, C. K. (1990b). Cognition in marriage. In F. D. Fincham and T. N. Bradbury (Eds.), *The psychology of marriage* (pp. 118–149). New York: Guilford Press.

Gottman, J. M., and Levenson, R. W. (1985). A valid procedure for obtaining self-report of affect in marital interaction. *Journal of Consulting and Clinical Psychology, 53*, 151–160.

Gottman, J. M., and Levenson, R. W. (1986). Assessing the role of emotion in marriage. *Behavioral Assessment, 8*, 31–48.

Hammen, C., Marks, T., Mayol, A., and deMayo, R. (1985). Depressive self-schemas, life stress, and vulnerability to depression. *Journal of Abnormal Psychology, 94*, 308–319.

Hammen, C., Ellicott, A., and Gitlin, M. (1989). Vulnerability to specific life events and prediction of course of disorder in unipolar depressed patients. *Canadian Journal of Behavioral Science, 21*, 377–388.

Heider, F. (1958). *The psychology of interpersonal relations*. New York: Wiley.

Holtzworth-Munroe, A., and Jacobson, N. S. (1985). Causal attributions of married couples: When do they search for causes? What do they conclude when they do? *Journal of Personality and Social Psychology, 48*, 1398–1412.

Huber, C. H., and Milstein, B. (1985). Cognitive restructuring and a collaborative set in couples' work. *American Journal of Family Therapy, 13*(2), 17–27.

Jacobson, N. S., and Margolin, G. (1979). *Marital therapy: Strategies based on social learning and behavior exchange principles*. New York: Brunner/Mazel.

Jacobson, N. S., and Moore, D. (1981). Spouses as observers of the events in their relationship. *Journal of Consulting and Clinical Psychology, 49*, 269–277.

Jones, E. E., and Davis, K. (1965). From acts to dispositions: The attribution process in personal perception. In L. Berkowitz (Ed.), *Advances in experimental social psychology* (Vol. 2, pp. 219–266). New York: Academic Press.

Jones, M. E., and Stanton, A. L. (1988). Dysfunctional beliefs, belief similarity, and marital distress: A comparison of models. *Journal of Social and Clinical Psychology, 7*, 1–14.

Kelley, H. H. (1973). The processes of causal attribution. *American Psychologist, 28*, 107–128.

Kyle, S. O., and Falbo, T. (1985). Relationships between marital stress and attributional preferences for own and spouse behavior. *Journal of Social and Clinical Psychology, 3*, 339–351.

Meissner, W. W. (1978). The conceptualization of marriage and family dynamics from a psychoanalytic perspective. In T. J. Paolino and B. S. McCrady (Eds.), *Marriage and marital therapy: Psychoanalytic, behavioral and systems theory perspectives* (pp. 25–88). New York: Brunner/Mazel.

Miranda, J., Persons, J. B., and Byers, C. N. (1990). Endorsement of dysfunctional beliefs depends on current mood state. *Journal of Abnormal Psychology, 99*, 237–241.

Nisbett, R., and Ross, L. (1980). *Human inference: Strategies and shortcomings of social judgment.* Englewood Cliffs, NJ: Prentice-Hall.

O'Leary, K. D., and Turkewitz, H. (1978). Marital therapy from a behavioral perspective. In T. J. Paolino and B. S. McCrady (Eds.), *Marriage and marital therapy: Psychoanalytic, behavioral and systems theory perspectives* (pp. 240–297). New York: Brunner/Mazel.

O'Leary, K. D., Fincham, F., and Turkewitz, H. (1983). Assessment of positive feelings toward spouse. *Journal of Consulting and Clinical Psychology, 51*, 949–951.

Orvis, B. R., Kelley, H. H., and Butler, D. (1976). Attributional conflict in young couples. In J. Harvey, W. Ickles, and R. Kidd (Eds.), *New directions in attributional research* (Vol. 1, pp. 353–386). Hillsdale, NJ: Erlbaum.

Pretzer, J., Epstein, N., and Fleming, B. (1991). The Marital Attitude Survey: A measure of dysfunctional attributions and expectancies. *The Journal of Cognitive Psychotherapy: An International Quarterly, 5*, 131–148.

Raush, H. L., Barry, W. A., Hertel, R. K., and Swain, M. A. (1974). *Communication, conflict and marriage.* San Francisco: Jossey-Bass.

Revenstorf, D., Hahlweg, K., Schindler, L., and Vogel, B. (1984). Interaction analysis of marital conflict. In K. Hahlweg and N. S. Jacobson (Eds.), *Marital interaction: Analysis and modification* (pp. 159–181). New York: Guilford Press.

Robinson, E. A., and Price, M. G. (1980). Pleasurable behavior in marital interaction: An observational study. *Journal of Consulting and Clinical Psychology, 48*, 117–118.

Rotter, J. B. (1954). *Social learning and clinical psychology.* Englewood Cliffs, NJ: Prentice-Hall.

Rotter, J. B., Chance, J., and Phares, E. J. (1972). *Applications of a social learning theory of personality.* New York: Holt, Rinehart & Winston.

Segal, Z. V., Shaw, B. F., Vella, D. D., and Katz, R. (1992). Cognitive and life stress predictors of relapse in remitted unipolar depressed patients: Test of the congruency hypothesis. *Journal of Abnormal Psychology, 101*, 26–36.

Seiler, T. B. (1984). Developmental cognitive theory, personality, and therapy. In N. Hoffmann (Ed.), *Foundations of cognitive therapy: Theoretical methods and practical applications* (pp. 11–49). New York: Plenum.

Seligman, M. E. P. (1975). *Helplessness: On depression, development, and death.* San Francisco: Freeman.

Stuart, R. B. (1969). Operant interpersonal treatment for marital discord. *Journal of Consulting and Clinical Psychology, 33*, 675–682.

Stuart, R. B. (1980). *Helping couples change: A social learning approach to marital therapy.* New York: Guilford Press.

Thompson, J. S., and Snyder, D. K. (1986). Attribution theory in intimate relationships: A methodological review. *American Journal of Family Therapy, 14*, 123–138.

Todd, T. C. (1986). Structural-strategic marital therapy. In N. S. Jacobson and A. S. Gurman (Eds.), *Clinical handbook of marital therapy* (pp. 71–105). New York: Guilford Press.

Turk, D. C., and Speers, M. A. (1983). Cognitive schemata and cognitive processes in cognitive–behavioral interventions: Going beyond the information given. In P. C. Kendall (Ed.), *Advances in cognitive–behavioral research and therapy* (Vol. 2, pp. 1–31). New York: Academic Press.

Weiss, R. L. (1978). The conceptualization of marriage from a behavioral perspective. In T. J. Paolino and B. S. McCrady (Eds.), *Marriage and marital therapy: Psychoanalytic, behavioral and systems theory perspectives* (pp. 165–239). New York: Brunner/Mazel.

Weiss, R. L. (1984). Cognitive and behavioral measures of marital interaction. In K. Hahlweg and N. S. Jacobson (Eds.), *Marital interaction: Analysis and modification* (pp. 232–252). New York: Guilford Press.

Weiss, R. L., and Heyman, R. E. (1990). Observation of marital interaction. In F. D. Fincham and T. N. Bradbury (Eds.), *The psychology of marriage: Basic issues and applications* (pp. 87–117). New York: Guilford Press.

Wessler, R. A., and Wessler, R. L. (1980). *The principles and practice of rational-emotive therapy.* San Francisco: Jossey-Bass.

Cognition in the Psychopathology of Youth and Implications for Treatment

Philip C. Kendall and Jennifer P. MacDonald

Temple University

Researchers and clinicians recognize that the cognitive activities of the subject/client are central to the development, assessment, and treatment of psychopathology. Considerable time and effort has been expended to examine the role of cognition in adult psychopathology (see other chapters in this volume), and although studies with children have been fewer, increasing research efforts are being directed specifically toward investigating the role of cognition in child and adolescent psychopathology and its treatment (Kendall, 1991). This chapter examines the current theoretical and empirical status of cognition in child psychopathology. First, theoretical perspectives are described and considered; second, a review of the research on several illustrative child/adolescent disorders (i.e. Attention-Deficit Hyperactivity Disorder (ADHD), depression, anxiety, aggression) is presented and discussed.

A THEORETICAL MODEL FOR CONSIDERING COGNITION IN YOUTH

The cognitive–behavioral model is a rational amalgam: a purposeful attempt to preserve the positive features of the behavioral approaches, while also working to incorporate into a model the cognitive activity and information-processing factors of the individual (Kendall and Hollon, 1979). The cognitive–behavioral model considers the role of affect, while also recognizing the importance of the social context (e.g., family). Thus, a cognitive–behavioral model of psychopathology in youth represents an integrated consideration of various aspects of the child's environment, both internal and external. The model is not concerned with uncovering unconscious early trauma or with the biological or neurological aspects of psychopathology. Although it is recognized that these and other influences exist, the present focus is on the cognitive functioning of the target youth with specific psychological difficulties. As a result, other components of the cognitive–behavioral approach are given less emphasis. It is important for the reader to note, however, that the discussion of cognition is only a portion of an integrated and comprehensive cognitive–behavioral model (Kendall, 1985, 1991).

Cognitive Constructs

Before examining studies of cognitive functioning in specific childhood psychopathologies, it is useful to consider the theoretical model of information processing that guides the approach. For some time, cognition and cognitive processes were viewed as inaccessible by many mental health professionals. Yet, increasingly, theorists are proposing taxonomic systems to describe the "unseen" cognitive mechanisms that influence information processing, and ultimately, behavior. One such classification system describes cognition not as a singular construct, but one that is conceptually divided into four elements: (1) cognitive structures; (2) cognitive content (or propositions); (3) cognitive operations (or processes); and (4) cognitive products (Ingram and Kendall, 1986, 1987; Kendall, 1985, 1991; Kendall and Ingram, 1987, 1989).

Cognitive structures can be described as the manner in which information is internally organized and represented in memory, similar to the hardware of a system of indexing and filing. These structured memories are based on the individual's history of experiences in the world. After repeated experiences within a social context involving certain behavioral events, the individual develops a set of anticipated experiences that are represented in the cognitive structures (Kendall and Braswell, 1982a).

The cognitive schema (the union of cognitive content and structure) has been the focus of much research, particularly with adult depressive disorders (Beck, 1967; Ingram, 1984), and recently in the study of adult anxiety (e.g., Ingram and Kendall 1986). The schema forms a unique frame of reference from which each individual constructs his or her own personal view of himself or herself, others, the environment, and the world. Schemata have been compared to "filters" (Meichenbaum *et al.*, 1985) or "templates" (Kendall, 1985), because the schema "filters" information for the individual, affecting what the individual attends to, perceives, recalls, and believes is important. Thus, the individual derives meaning, and his or her interpretation of the world, through the schemata.

Cognitive content (a.k.a. propositions) can be described as the information or content that is actually stored or represented in the cognitive structures. Cognitive operations, or processes, refer to the procedures or functions that the cognitive system utilizes to operate (e.g., the input, processing, and output of information). In other words, cognitive processes refer to the manner in which the individual perceives and interprets experiences. Lastly, cognitive products are the thoughts/cognitions that result from the interaction between information and the cognitive system of structures, content, and processes. Cognitive products are, for instance, the attributions that each individual uniquely assigns to his or her experience with the world.

The four components of this system are assumed to operate in a reciprocal and multidirectional fashion. Cognitive content, processes, and products interact in a manner unique to an individual as he or she attempts to make sense of experiences and events. Of particular importance for the present chapter, any or all of these components may be implicated in a specific type of psychopathology, and each component should be taken into account when planning disorder-specific therapeutic interventions.

Distinguishing Cognitive Deficiencies from Cognitive Distortions

There is an additional distinction that becomes important when examining the role of cognition in the psychopathology of youth. This distinction differentiates types of cognitive difficulties that are useful in describing and differentiating various disorders of childhood. The distinction is between cognitive deficiencies and cognitive distortions (Kendall, 1985, 1991). Cognitive *deficiencies* describe a lack of or insufficient amount of cognitive activity in situations where mental activity would be useful or beneficial to the individual's adjustment. This lack of cognitive activity can be seen in the absence of problem solving, perspective taking, and planning, for example, and is associated with a lack of verbal mediation and lack of self-control as well (Fuhrman and Kendall, 1986). Cognitive *distortions*, on the other hand, refer not to a lack of cognitive activity, but to an active but "crooked" thinking process. Cognitive processing is occurring, but the thinking is in some way distorted. For example, distortions can

Table 11.1 Number of Studies Identifying Cognitive Distortion or Cognitive Deficiency in Childhood Psychopathology[a,b]

Disorder	Cognitive Dysfunction	
	Distortion	Deficiency
Anxiety	6	0
Depression	9	0
ADHD	0	9
Aggression	23	27

[a]For a list of the specific articles included in the table, address correspondence to either author at the Department of Psychology, Temple University, Philadelphia, PA 19122.
[b]To tabulate studies for this table, a detailed, systematic review of the literature was undertaken for the period 1970–1991. This review included a computer literature search (Psych Lit) of titles of articles related to cognition and the specific target disorders, and a survey of journals known to publish studies that address the target content (i.e., *Journal of Consulting and Clinical Psychology, Journal of Abnormal Psychology, Cognitive Therapy and Research, Journal of Abnormal Child Psychology, Journal of Clinical Child Psychology, Child Development*). Studies identified by the computer search and/or journal search were then examined more carefully. Follow-up on the work of specific authors known to pursue the area of cognition and childhood psychopathology was also done. Although direct comparisons/tests exist, the present tally does not imply that all studies were a direct test of the presence of either distortions or deficiencies.

refer to an exaggeration of threat to the self, underappraisal of personal abilities, or misperceptions of the demand in the environment.

The distinction between deficient and distorted processing of information can be linked to the behavioral distinction between undercontrolled (or externalizing) disorders versus overcontrolled (or internalizing) disorders (cf. Achenbach, 1966). For example, undercontrolled, externalizing, or acting-out problems such as Attention-Deficit Hyperactivity Disorder (ADHD) involve cognitive deficiencies including a lack of self-control and a failure to employ mediational skills—basically, acting without thinking. In contrast, overcontrolled (or internalizing) psychopathologies such as depression, withdrawal, or anxiety involve cognitive distortions, such as negative self-evaluations and misinterpretation of environmental demands. Aggression (e.g., Conduct Disorder) is an example of a disorder of youth that involves *both* deficiencies and distortions in cognition. A tally of studies that have addressed the nature of cognitive dysfunction in various child psychopathologies (see Table 11.1) reveals strong support for the cognitive and behavioral associations suggested here.

It is the position of the authors that there are several important social and cognitive information-processing factors that must be considered as we seek to understand the role of cognition in childhood psychopathology, and that the differentiation of cognitive deficiencies and cognitive distortions is one of the more useful guides. Indeed, the distinction has been evident in the literature for over a decade, used by numerous authors, and examined directly in empirical research. The distinction has utility not only in understanding the nature of childhood disorders, but also in the development and implementation of disorder-specific treatment strategies. With this distinction in mind, and with a focus on both the nature of psychopathology and the implementation of psychological therapy, we turn now to a separate consideration of the role of cognition in four psychological disorders of youth: ADHD, Depression, Anxiety, and Aggression.

CHILDHOOD DISORDERS INVOLVING COGNITIVE DISTORTIONS

Cognitive Distortions in Childhood Depression

It is proposed that the nature of the cognitive disturbance in children with internalizing disorders such as depression and anxiety is related to cognitive distortions rather than cognitive deficiencies. As mentioned, cognitive distortions involve active and sufficient cognitive activity, yet the thinking process is distorted and maladaptive.

As is true of several of the symptoms of depression (Kashani *et al.*, 1981; Kovacs and Beck, 1977), the cognitive distortions found in depressed children are similar to those seen in depressed adults. Cognitive models of adult depression, such as those posited by Beck (1967) and Rehm (1977), (see also Alloy, 1988), stress the role of negative self-perceptions in the development and continuation of adult depression. Similarly, negative self-evaluation is a common distortion seen in depressed children.

Studies have shown these distortions to be characteristic of a variety of populations of depressed children, including outpatient diagnosed children, nonclinical samples, and inpatient groups. Leitenberg *et al.* (1986) developed the Children's Negative Cognitive Error Questionnaire (CNCEQ) to measure in children the four types of cognitive errors proposed by Beck's adult model. The CNCEQ, modeled after Lefebvre's Adult Cognitive Error Questionnaire (Lefebvre, 1980, 1981), presents descriptions of hypothetical situations or events followed by a statement about the event that reflects one of the four types of cognitive errors (catastrophizing, overgeneralizing, personalizing, or selective abstraction). Overall, children from a normal sample did not endorse any of the four errors as being similar to their own thoughts when they imagined experiencing the events described. However, children who self-reported depression on the Children's Depression Inventory (CDI; Kovacs, 1981), endorsed each of the four errors significantly more often than did their nondepressed peers.

A recent study by Kendall *et al.* (1990b) was designed specifically to assess whether childhood depression was associated with cognitive distortion or cognitive deficiency. Children in Grades 3–6 [diagnosed as depressed by the Schedule for Affective Disorders and Schizophrenia for School-Age Children (K-SADS), Puig-Antich and Ryan, 1986; and the Children's Depression Inventory, Kovacs, 1981] showed distortions in cognition, but did not demonstrate a cognitive deficiency when compared to nondepressed children. The depressed children, showing their bias toward negative self-evaluation, evaluated themselves significantly more negatively than did their nondepressed peers. To determine if the depressed children were lacking in ability and their ratings were simply a reflection of reality, the depressed children's self-ratings were then compared to ratings by a teacher who knew them well. The teacher's blind ratings showed no significant difference between the evaluations of depressed and nondepressed children, thus supporting the notion that the depressed children's cognitive views regarding their own abilities were not realistic, but distorted. The depressed children did not, however, differ from the nondepressed children on a measure of problem-solving style that taps cognitive deficiencies, indicating that the depressed children evidenced distortions but not deficiencies.

Several studies reported cognitive distortions in nonclinical populations of children. Kaslow *et al.* (1984) found distortion in self-appraisal to be evident across a wide age range of depressed private-school youngsters. First, fourth, and eighth graders who were classified as depressed according to the CDI, evaluated their performance more negatively than did the nondepressed children. Depressed children estimated that their drawings were not as well done, that it took them longer to complete the tasks, that their performance was worse than that of other children, and that they correctly copied fewer designs.

Depressed children from another nonclinical population were reported to show similar distortions in their evaluations of their own abilities (McGee *et al.*, 1986). Children that self-reported depression on the CDI evaluated their own general self-worth and academic capabilities significantly less favorably than did their nondepressed peers. The finding that depressed children did not score significantly lower on the Wechsler Intelligence Scale for Children (WISC-R; Wechsler, 1974), points to a relationship between depressive symptomatology and distortions in self-perception, rather than a relationship between depression and actual performance.

Despite similar task performance and achievement levels, public-school children scoring as depressed on the CDI evaluated themselves more negatively than their peers evaluated themselves (Meyer *et al.*, 1989). Depressed children also evaluated themselves more negatively than they evaluated their peers, whereas the nondepressed children did not devalue themselves in comparison to their peers.

The relationship between cognitive distortion and depression has been found to be evident in clinical populations of inpatient children as well. Haley *et al.* (1985) used the Cognitive Bias Questionnaire for Children (CBQC; Haley *et al.*, 1985) to study the cognitive distortions of inpatient children who were diagnosed as depressed. This questionnaire was developed, as was its adult counterpart (Cognitive Bias Questionnaire; Krantz and Hammen, 1979), following Beck's (1967) view that depressed individuals interpret the world through cognitive distortions, such as a negative view of self. Depressed children in the Haley *et al.* study did indeed demonstrate this self-appraisal distortion, whereas the nondepressed children in the study did not.

Asarnow and Bates (1988) demonstrated that inpatient depressed children exhibited cognitive distortions regarding self-evaluations. Children diagnosed with depression reported lower perceptions of their general self-worth, scholastic competence, athletic abilities, and physical appearance. They reported negative self-perceptions across a wider variety of domains than did nondepressed inpatient children in the study. These depressed children were in reality no less competent than their nondepressed counterparts on objective measures of IQ, achievement, and social status (see Asarnow, 1988, for a replication).

In summary, the nature of the cognitive difficulty involved in childhood depression relates to distortions in cognitive information processing, rather than to deficiencies in processing. Across various populations of depressed children, results indicate that depressed youngsters evaluate themselves, their performance, and their self-worth more negatively than do their nondepressed peers, and also more negatively than an objective evaluator, such as an educator. Although this cognitive distortion, or bias, has been consistently documented, cognitive deficiencies have not been reported to exist in depressed youngsters.

Cognitive Distortions in Childhood Anxiety

The role of cognitive functioning in childhood anxiety has not yet been as widely researched as the role of cognition in childhood depression. In 1988, a review by Francis concluded that "no definitive statements about the cognitions of anxious children can be made" (p. 276). Recently, however, research efforts are being directed toward the identification and understanding of cognitive disturbances in anxious children (see Kendall *et al.*, 1992ab). One model suggests that anxious children's cognitive processing is characterized by cognitive distortions. Specifically, anxious children appear to be preoccupied with unrealistic concerns about evaluation by themselves and others, and about the likelihood of severe negative consequences. In other words, they misinterpret the demands of the environment and their own abilities, and catastrophize about future consequences and results.

In part, notions about anxiety disorders in youth parallel the research on cognitive characteristics of adult anxiety. As early as 1962, Ellis described the tendency of anxious adults to "catastrophize," or exaggerate and overemphasize the worst possible outcome of a situation. From clinical observation, Beck (1976) concluded that anxiety causes adults to misinterpret both environmental and internal cues in a way that serves to increase their anxiety. It has also been noted that anxious adults have a biased view of the degree of danger associated with a given situation, and of their own vulnerability as well (Beck and Emery, 1985). Both theory and empirical findings (see also Barlow, 1988) support the notion that anxious adults show biases or misinterpretations as they process information (Mueller and Thompson, 1984; Smith *et al.*, 1983; Himle *et al.*, 1982; Gormally *et al.*, 1981).

Much of the existing literature on anxious children's cognition involves nonclinical samples of youth with specific fears, rather than children diagnosed with anxiety disorders. Nevertheless, this literature lends support for the existence of cognitive distortion in childhood anxiety. In two studies, Zatz and Chassin (1983, 1985) examined the cognition of test-anxious public-school children. The first study showed test-anxious children to exhibit more task-debilitating cognitions than non-test-anxious children. These cognitions included unfavorable social comparisons and unfavorable self-evaluations, such as "Everyone usually does better than me," "I am too dumb for this," "I don't do well on tests like this," and "I'm doing worse than the others." The anxious children who experienced such negative cognition did not significantly differ in ability from the nonanxious children in actual ability on performance measures such as anagrams, coding, and achievement tests. Thus, the test-anxious children were distorted in their perception of their own abilities (Zatz and Chassin, 1983). The second study ruled out the possibility of actual school ability affecting the anxious children's views of themselves. The findings of the first study were replicated, yet under natural test-taking conditions rather than during an analog testing situation. Again, test-anxious children demonstrated negatively distorted views of their own abilities.

Prins (1985) examined cognitive processing in children from a nonclinical population before they experienced an anxiety-provoking dental situation. The research looked at children's self-speech and the regulation of that self-speech. The self-speech of the children with the highest dental anxiety was found to be more negative than the self-speech of children with lower dental anxiety. Often, the thoughts of the highly dental-anxious children related to the threat of pain, such as "I think something bad is going to happen." Prins (1986) then examined the self-speech of children involved in an anxiety-provoking diving task. Again, children with the highest anxiety showed a tendency toward self-speech that was preoccupied with the threat of being hurt. The anxious children misinterpreted the situation as more dangerous than it actually was, with cognitions such as, "Oh. . . . I'll fall hard," "Maybe my head will hit the bottom," and "It'll go wrong again."

Meichenbaum (1977) has suggested that self-speech primarily influences three attentional and appraisal processes: appraisal of the aversive event, attribution of the arousal, and judging one's own competence to cope effectively with the aversive situation. Our cognitive distortion model suggests that, for anxiety-disordered youth, distortion would occur in all three of these processes. For instance, the above studies show distortions in the areas of appraisal of the situation and judging one's own competence.

Studies examining cognitive distortion in clinical samples of anxious children are few. In one study, Ronan et al. (1993) developed a questionnaire [Children's Anxious Self-Statement Questionnaire (CASSQ)] to assess the self-talk of anxiety-disordered and nonanxious children (depressotypic self-talk was also studied). Preliminary reliability and validity analyses indicate that the measure differentiates between anxious and nonanxious clinic children between the ages of 8 and 15 (Ronan et al., 1993). For example, on the CASSQ, anxious children score higher on a factor labeled Negative Self-Focused Attention than do nonanxious children. Given the association between negative self-statements and other disorders, such as depression, and the high correlation between anxiety and depression in children (Brady and Kendall, 1992), it is worth noting that the observed differences were specific to anxiety.

In summary, research on cognitive disturbance in anxious children has largely involved nonclinical samples and investigations of specific fears. Studies involving children diagnosed with anxiety disorders are rare, pointing out the need for increased efforts in this area. Nonetheless, the findings to date suggest that the self-speech of children with specific fears, of children exposed to an anxiety-provoking situation, and of those receiving an anxiety disorder diagnosis contains a tendency to distort: to focus on self-evaluation and to perceive increased threat in the environment.

Therapy for Disorders Involving Cognitive Distortions

Description of Procedures

To date, most of the therapy applied to children has focused on treating externalizing difficulties and cognitive deficiencies, such as those that are evident in ADHD (Barkley, 1990) and impulsive behavior (Kendall and Braswell, 1993). However, the application of treatments to target distortions such as those that are evident in anxiety and depression has been suggested (e.g., Graziano *et al.*, 1979a; Wells and Vitulano, 1984), and interest in pursuing interventions is growing.

A cognitive–behavioral approach to treating the cognitive difficulties involved in internalizing disorders such as depression and anxiety would be distinct from the approach to externalizing disorders because of the difference in the nature of the cognitive dysfunction. With depressed or anxious children, the goal is to identify the distorted processing, to aid the child in the modification of the distorted thinking, and to teach the children new "coping" processing styles (Kendall *et al.*, 1992a,b). There are some components of cognitive–behavioral treatment for children with internalizing disorders that are generic — they do not directly target cognitive distortions — and these components will not be discussed here. For more comprehensive descriptions of cognitive–behavioral treatment programs for depressed and anxious children see Kendall *et al.* (1992a,b), Kendall *et al.* (1992b), and Stark *et al.* (1991).

The goal of intervention at a cognitive level with childhood depression and anxiety is to identify and modify maladaptive cognitions or self-talk in order to promote realistic, adaptive, and "coping" focused thinking. Cognitively based therapies in general believe that maladaptive thinking plays a large role in the development and maintenance of maladaptive emotions and behavior, and that the alteration of distorted or faulty cognitive processing can lead to positive behavioral and affective change. This approach has been called "cognitive restructuring" (with adults; e.g., Goldfried, 1979) and "building a coping template" (Kendall *et al.*, 1992a,b).

Cognitive restructuring techniques attempt to modify the client's thinking by targeting the assumptions and attitudes that underlie the client's thoughts (Meichenbaum, 1977). Stark *et al.* (1991) describe how children can be taught to be their own "Thought Detectives" by identifying maladaptive thoughts, looking for evidence, and examining alternative explanations.

Identifying "thoughts" can be a difficult task for children, as they may be unaware that they have internal thoughts, or that these thoughts can be modified. Kendall *et al.* (1992a,b) describe a way to help children identify their thoughts. Children can be shown cartoon figures with empty "thought bubbles," and asked "what might be in that child's thought bubble?" The therapist can begin with neutral cartoon situations, and move toward portrayals that are more salient for the child, such as gradually moving toward cartoons depicting anxiety for the anxious client (see the Coping Cat Workbook, Kendall, 1990; Therapist's Treatment Manual, Kendall et al., 1989). In the Kendall et al. (1992a) cognitive–behavioral treatment of childhood anxiety disorders, children are taught to correct distorted thinking by following four steps when coping with anxiety-provoking situations. The steps, spelling out the acronym "FEAR," include: (1) Feeling frightened? (recognizing the anxiety or fear and somatic reactions); (2) Expecting bad things to happen? (recognizing the anxious self-talk); (3) Actions and attitudes that can help? (developing coping strategies); and (4) Results and rewards (self-evaluation and self-reward). The second step (expecting bad things to happen) focuses directly on anxious cognitive processing, helping the child to identify and examine negative, unrealistic, or catastrophic expectations of situation outcomes.

When looking for "evidence," the therapist and child evaluate the data that the child feels would be necessary to support a distorted thought, and then compare the evidence that actually exists. For example, with a depressed child who negatively evaluates his or her abilities, the child and therapist would explore what evidence would be necessary to show that the child was incompetent or incapable, and would then decide if that evidence actually did exist. Eventually, the child gathers evidence for a newly developed, more adaptive view, such as one in which he or she evaluates himself or herself in a more realistic manner. Generating and examining alternative interpretations is similar to looking for evidence, in that the child and therapist work together to more realistically evaluate the situation. They discuss explanations and interpretations other than the maladaptive ones that have been causing distress for the child.

Kendall et al. (1992a) describe "building a coping template" as a process with the goals of (1) removing the child's characteristic ways of misinterpreting events and (2) building a frame of reference for the child that includes strategies for coping. Perceptions of distress are not expected to vanish altogether, but by building coping strategies into the child's new way of looking at the world, formerly upsetting situations will be viewed in light of coping strategies that the child has within his/her repertoire.

Self-evaluation is a significant cognitive distortion for both anxious and depressed children and can be stressed in any of the above processes. The important concept is to alter the child's negatively biased view of him/herself. Helping the child to reward him/herself for progress during the therapy is a good way to directly emphasize the reality of accomplishment for the child, and to challenge maladaptive self-evaluation as it is occurring.

Self-monitoring, recommended by Stark *et al.* (1991), can be used throughout treatment to aid in attending to and modifying cognition. Unlike the externalizing child, depressed and anxious children do not need to be taught how to self-monitor — they do this already! Instead, they do need to be taught what to self-monitor, and in which direction to redirect their attention. Children are often urged to monitor the events that could refute their distorted thinking. For example, a depressed child may be asked to monitor examples of personal success, and a separation-anxious child may be asked to self-monitor times when he/she was safe without a parent.

Finally, modeling aids the child in his or her understanding of the coping processes. The therapist models the identification and modification of maladaptive thoughts as an example for the child. Modeling is especially useful with younger children who may have a more difficult time grasping the concepts or for older children who feel self-conscious about the tasks.

Outcome Studies of Depressed Children

Only a handful of treatment outcome studies evaluating the efficacy of treatments for depression in children have been reported. The studies that have been done have generally used "depressed" children selected from schools. Whether these results generalize to clinical samples requires further research. However, the majority of studies show promising results for the efficacy of cognitive–behavioral techniques in the treatment of childhood dysphoria/depression.

An early investigation reported that children (Grades 5 and 6), who received a cognitive restructuring treatment in which they were taught to identify and change maladaptive thoughts, showed improvement between pre- and posttreatment on self-report measures of depression (Butler *et al.*, 1980). Reynolds and Coats (1986) also reported that adolescents who received a cognitive–behavioral treatment moved from a moderate level of depression at pretreatment to nondepressed levels at posttreatment. In fact, at follow-up, none of the adolescent subjects in the cognitive–behavioral condition showed clinically relevant levels of depression.

An adaptation of Rehm's self-control treatment (Rehm *et al.*, 1987) was used to teach depressed children to evaluate their performances more realistically and to self-monitor in a more adaptive manner. This treatment was compared to a behavioral problem-solving condition. Children in the self-control condition reported significantly less depression. When compared to traditional counseling, cognitive–behavioral therapy again proved to be significantly better able to reduce depression in youngsters (Stark *et al.*, 1991). Techniques utilized in this treatment included self-monitoring, self-evaluation, and cognitive restructuring.

Outcome Studies of Anxiety in Children

Currently, there are precious few research evaluations of the efficacy of therapy for childhood anxiety disorders. There are, however, emerging studies that indicate that a cognitive–behavioral treatment has merit. For instance, although the majority of the literature focuses primarily on the treatment of specific fears such as nighttime fears, dental or medical fears, and evaluation anxiety, there are several clinical case studies describing applications of cognitive–behavioral therapy with anxious youngsters and at least one randomized clinical trial with anxiety-disordered youth. The studies show promising results, though more research needs to be done.

Cognitive–behavioral therapy for children's nighttime fears appears to have a positive effect. Children who were taught to use positive self-statements, positive imagery, and positive self-talk showed greater tolerance for being alone in a dark room (Kanfer *et al.*, 1975) and accomplished the goal of spending ten consecutive "fearless nights within a three to nineteen week period" (Graziano *et al.*, 1979b). Graziano and Mooney (1980) found significant improvement in children given a cognitive–behavioral intervention over a control group, and all six children in Giebenhain and O'Dell's (1984) study reached the goal of sleeping with only a night light.

Similar results have been found for the cognitive–behavioral treatment of dental fears (Siegel and Peterson, 1980, 1981; Peterson and Shigetomi, 1981). Intervention for children facing repeated or extremely painful medical procedures has been efficacious (Elliot and Olson, 1983; Dahlquist *et al.*, 1985; Jay *et al.*, 1985). In several cases children undergoing harsh medical treatments were instructed to create a "heroic scenario" (Elliot and Olson, 1983) and to reinterpret facing the procedure in the context of being a hero.

Several studies have examined the use of cognitive–behavioral therapy in the treatment of children's and adolescent's evaluation anxiety. With test-anxious adolescents, a cognitive modification procedure that included the identification and modification of inappropriate cognitive responses was shown to be more effective at reducing test anxiety than systematic desensitization (Leal *et al.*, 1981). Some studies, however, have not shown such positive results (Stevens and Pihl, 1983; Fox and Houston, 1981).

Promising results regarding the efficacy of cognitive–behavioral treatments with more generalized anxiety disorders were found by Kane and

Kendall (1989). Four children diagnosed with Overanxious Disorder were treated individually with a 16- to 20-session cognitive–behavioral treatment. The treatment focused on four major components: (1) recognizing anxious feelings and somatic reactions to anxiety; (2) clarifying cognitions in anxiety-provoking situations, and examining unrealistic or negative attribution or expectations; (3) developing a plan to help cope with the situation, modifying anxious self-talk into coping self-talk and determining what actions might be effective; and (4) evaluating the success of the coping strategies, with self-reward when appropriate. All children showed improvement on parent, independent clinician, and self-report measures. Two youngsters maintained their gains by both parent and self-report, while two children maintained their gains by self-report alone at 3-month follow-up. These data suggest that cognitive–behavioral therapy can be a viable treatment option for children with anxiety disorders.

The results of a randomized clinical trial of the effectiveness of a 16-week cognitive–behavioral treatment program for anxiety-disordered youth showed promising results (Kendall, 1993). Children referred to the Child and Adolescent Anxiety Disorders Clinic (CAADC) at Temple University who met criteria for an anxiety disorder diagnosis based on the Anxiety Disorders Interview Schedule for Children (ADIS-C; Silverman, 1987) were assigned randomly to a wait-list or treatment condition. Multiple-method assessments (e.g., parent and teacher reports, behavioral observations, self-report) at pre- and posttreatment were employed. Treated children showed significant differences from wait-list children on self-report measures (of both symptoms and coping ability) and parent report. Pretreatment and posttreatment diagnostic interviews also showed promising results on both parent and child report (64% of treated cases did not meet criteria for an anxiety diagnosis at posttreatment, compared to all but one of the subjects in the wait-list children). At 1-year follow-up, means for the treated cases were compared to their posttreatment scores. Nonsignificant results indicate that the early documented treatment-produced changes were maintained at 1-year follow-up. Thus, the analyses of a randomized clinical trial support the utility of cognitive–behavioral interventions with anxiety-disordered children and lend support to the notion of a cognitive component in childhood anxiety.

CHILDHOOD DISORDERS INVOLVING COGNITIVE DEFICIENCIES

Attention-Deficit Hyperactivity Disorder

The nature of the cognitive disturbance involved in externalizing disorders such as ADHD differs from the cognitive disturbance found in depression and anxiety. In contrast to the cognitive distortion or misguided information processing of children with internalizing disorders, children with ADHD show cognitive deficiencies, or a lack of sufficient cognitive activities such as problem solving and planning abilities.

That children with ADHD often act without thinking is generally accepted and has been widely researched for several decades. However, the names for the disorder have changed over the years, as has the specific focus of the disorder. Early on, the broad term "Minimal Brain Dysfunction" (MBD) was used to describe children with combinations of a large number of symptoms, including learning problems, aggression, inattention, and impulsivity (Clements and Peters, 1962). In the 1960s and 1970s, the narrower terms of "hyperactivity" and "hyperkinesis" were used to refer to children with an impulsive and overactive behavioral style. By 1980, sustained attention was seen as the primary symptom, and the disorder was labeled "Attention-Deficit Disorder" (ADD; American Psychiatric Association, 1980). DSM-III-R listed ADHD as one of the disruptive Behavior Disorders. Many studies have been reported using ADD, ADHD, and variously labeled youth of varying degrees of psychopathology. Some studies have used clinical samples, whereas others have used children who vary on the dimensions of interest, but who may or may not qualify for a disorder. For purposes of simplicity in this chapter, when a general or all-encompassing term is needed, hyperactivity or impulsivity will be used.

Although the labels and in a sense the conceptualization of the disorder have changed several times, the children represented nevertheless have many essential features in common. Douglas and Peters (1979) trace the difficulties of hyperactive children to *deficiencies* in the "mechanisms that govern (a) sustained attention and effort, (b) inhibitory control, and (c) the modulation of arousal levels to meet task or situational demands" (p. 67). Barkley (1990) has discussed the "Holy Trinity" of ADHD symptoms, two of which (inattention and impulsivity) are cognitively related. Recently, ADHD has been summarized as a style that shows *deficiencies* in higher order problem solving, in modulation of behavior to match environmental demands, and in overall self-regulation (Hinshaw and Erhardt, 1990; Whalen, 1989; Douglas *et al.*, 1988).

Numerous studies document the cognitive deficiencies that are found in hyperactive and impulsive children (see Barkley, 1990). A considerable amount of research demonstrates that hyperactive children are deficient in their ability to sustain and maintain attention to tasks (e.g., Zentall, 1985; Douglas, 1983; Barkley and Ullman, 1975; Routh and Schroeder, 1976). Studies have attempted to specify which situations and tasks are particularly difficult on the attentional capacity of these children. For example, this attentional deficiency has been reported to be seen most dramatically in situations involving dull repetitive tasks, such as homework and chores (Luk, 1985; Milich et al., 1982; Ullman et al., 1978; Zentall, 1985). Research focusing on distracter tasks has found that hyperactive children encounter the most difficulty in focusing attention when distracters are integrated into the particular task (Ceci and Tishman, 1984; McIntyre et al., 1978), or when the distracters are especially appealing (Radosh and Gittelman, 1981; Rosenthal and Allen, 1980). Investigations of the auditory attention of hyperactive children reveals difficulties in selective attention (Loiselle et al., 1980; Peters, 1977). Pearson et al. (1991) reported that impulsive hyperactive children were unable to allocate attention during complex tasks, whereas their nonhyperactive peers were able to do so.

Research has supported the notion that the cognitive functioning of hyperactive children is characterized by an inability to cognitively mediate their behavior, an impulsive, nonreflective style of approaching cognitive tasks, and disorganized problem solving. They have difficulty activating and following careful and planned cognitive processing. Their lack of forethought and planning often has a negative effect on their performance, especially on more complex problem-solving tasks.

Douglas (1980) summarized the cognitive difficulties of ADHD youngsters as an inability to "stop, look, and listen," and considers this inability to be the most important symptom of the disorder. She describes how these children are "unable to keep their own impulses under control in order to cope with situations in which care, concentrated attention or organized planning are required" (Douglas, 1980). Douglas and her colleagues reached these conclusions after comparing hyperactive and normal children on close to 150 variables, including parent and teacher ratings, academic measures, psychological and neurological tests, laboratory measures of vigilance, and reaction time (Douglas, 1972, 1974).

The problem of cognitive impulsivity has often been empirically measured as a pattern of rapid and inaccurate responses to tasks (Brown and Quay, 1977; Parry, 1973), such as Kagan's Matching Familiar Figures Test (MFFT; Kagan, 1966). The MFFT evaluates a child's cognitive tempo as reflective or impulsive, and quality performance often requires that children delay responding until all alternatives have been examined. Hyperactive and impulsive children have considerably more difficulty using problem-solving strategies and inhibiting responses on this task than do nonhyperactive children (e.g., Homatidis and Konstantareus, 1981). Hyperactive children exhibit short response latencies and high error rates (Campbell et al., 1971)—impulsive responding without thinking through all alternatives (Cohen et al., 1971; Firestone and Douglas, 1975). Inefficient search strategies (Douglas and Peters, 1980) and inefficient problem-solving skills (Tant and Douglas, 1982) have also been noted as characteristic of hyperactive youngsters.

Therapy for Impulsive/Hyperactive Youth

Description of Procedures   The most widely used treatment for hyperactivity is psychostimulant medication. The positive short-term clinical effects for stimulant medication have been consistently documented (Rapport and Kelly, 1990; Gadow, 1985, 1991; Douglas *et al.*, 1986; Rapport *et al.*, 1986; Klein *et al.*, 1980; Barkley, 1990). However, there are several limits to the use of stimulant medication. For example, some children do not respond to the medication and medication often appears to have little effect on cognitive reasoning, problem solving, and learning, thus leaving the children with skills deficits that require additional attention (Barkley, 1990; Campbell, 1976). Medication may not facilitate interpersonal skills or appropriate social responses (Hinshaw *et al.*, 1984; Pelham and Bender, 1982), and the gains made while on medication are not often maintained upon termination of the stimulant treatment (Barkley, 1990; Hechtman *et al.*, 1984; Gittelman-Klein *et al.*, 1976). Furthermore, the possibility of side effects, whether mild or severe, short term or long term (Barkley, 1990; Barkley *et al.*, 1990), often leads to resistance or hesitance from parents. Therefore, although medications are useful for many ADHD youth, their use remains controversial, and there is a strong need to develop and evaluate alternative or adjunct intervention procedures that can help these youngsters to more effectively cope with their environment.

Cognitive–behavioral therapy has been and continues to be one of the interventions that has been widely researched. Although the behavioral manifestations of hyperactivity are quite problematic, as mentioned before, many theorists believe that the cognitive deficits, such as the inability to "stop, look and listen," are the essence of the disorder (Douglas, 1980). Whalen *et al.* (1985) noted that cognitive–behavioral treatments provide "an ideal conceptual match to the core problems" (p. 392) of hyperactivity.

Following the work of Douglas came the direct application of cognitive–behavioral strategies to the particular deficiencies exhibited by the hyperactive/impulsive child. Hinshaw and Erhardt (1991) described Douglas's theoretical and empirical efforts as the beginning of the "modern era" of cognitive–behavioral applications with impulsive and hyperactive children, and to a large extent, current theories about cognitive deficiencies in these children follow from Douglas's theories. Cognitive–behavioral interventions with impulsive/hyperactive children seek to address cognitive deficiencies and to establish more adaptive, efficient modes of responding (e.g., Braswell and Bloomquist, 1991; Kendall and Braswell, 1985, 1993). With a focus on self-control skills, self-guidance, and reflective problem-solving strategies, the treatment strives for the child to internalize control skills needed to overcome deficiencies in thinking and to regulate his/her own behavior.

Teaching a thoughtful problem-solving process is a significant component of cognitive–behavioral treatments for hyperactive/impulsive children, for it focuses directly on the problem-solving "deficiencies" evident in the disorder. Self-instructions or self-directed statements can provide a thinking strategy for these children and can serve to guide them through the process of problem solving. This internalized speech (self-talk) can help the child to (1) recognize that a problem exists and identify its features; (2) initiate a strategy that moves toward a solution to the problem; (3) consider all options; and (4) take action in the chosen manner (Kendall and Braswell, 1993).

A typical sequence of the problem-solving training would be as follows: (1) the therapist models task performance and talks out loud while the child observes; (2) the child performs the task, instructing himself or herself out loud; (3) the therapist models task performance while whispering the self-instructions; (4) the therapist performs the task using covert self-instructions with pauses and behavioral signs of thinking; and finally (5) the child performs the task using covert self-instructions. A slightly different sequence offered by Hinshaw and Erhardt (1991) is a variation of a program introduced by Meichenbaum and Goodman (1971). The steps are as follows: (1) the therapist performs the task while talking out loud about the nature of the problem and the strategies he or she will employ; (2) the child then performs the task while talking out loud in a similar manner with overt external guidance from the therapist; (3) the child then performs the task while instructing himself or herself out loud; (4) the child again performs the task, yet this time whispers the instructions; and finally (5) the child performs the task while using private speech to guide behavior. An example of the use of verbalized self-talk with the task of completing arithmetic problems can be seen in Table 11.2.

Hinshaw and Erhardt (1991) support the use of self-evaluation with hyperactive children. By explicitly training the children to establish goals and standards for their behavior, and then aiding them in comparing their own performance to those standards, impulsivity and the lack of careful checking of work and performance (Douglas, 1980) can be reduced. Hinshaw and Erhardt (1991) described a process for teaching children in a group to self-monitor and self-evaluate through an activity called "The

TABLE 11.2 Example of the Use of Verbalized Self-Talk with an Impulsive Child Doing Arithmetic

O.K., what is it that I have to do? I need to answer these math problems. I'll need to go slowly and carefully. I'll need to check the plus and minus signs, and I'll need to check over my work. Now, here's the first problem, 14 + 3. It's a "plus" problem. I know that, it's 17. I'll write that down carefully. Wait, before I go on, I'll check myself. 14 + 3 . . . right, do the 1s column first, there's 7: the 10s column is a 1 . . . 17 is the answer. Great, I'm doing O.K. so far. Remember to keep going slowly. Next problem: 35 − 19. This one looks tougher . . . right, it's a minus sign. So, first, I have to take away the numbers in the 1s column. But look, 9 is bigger than 5, so I'll borrow from the 3. Now, 15 − 9, that's 6. I'll write that here. What's next? Right, subtract the 10s column. 3 − 1 is 2; I'll write that here. So 26 is the answer. I'll check by adding the number to the lower number. Wait a minute, that's not right! Don't worry, I'll check it carefully. Whoops, I must have forgot to change the 3 to a 2 when I borrowed. That's O.K., I can erase my answer and do it right. 2 − 1 is 1, so the answer is 16. Let's see if that checks. Good. Wow, even if I make a mistake, I can check it and make it right. Now I've finished. Nice job!

Match Game" (Hinshaw *et al.*, 1981). The therapist (or leader) announces, discusses, and models a behavioral criterion, such as paying attention. Each child attempts to match the 5-point rating that the teacher will give to him or her. The children announce out loud and discuss the rationale for their personal ratings, and then the leader does the same. The children receive points for their matches.

Numerous experiences with self-monitoring and self-evaluation, when guided by the therapist, can help children to become more reflective, and can aid in the reversal of the impulsive, careless, disorganized, and inconsistent style of these youngsters. Often, the practice of self-monitoring is done on an ongoing basis, and children are given opportunities and encouragement to be self-monitoring while performing other tasks. An example of the application of self-monitoring practice is offered by Hinshaw *et al.* (1981). The therapist and child together choose a target, such as paying attention. The therapist and child then discuss what it means to pay attention, and the therapist models good and bad examples of paying attention. This step establishes clear behavioral standards for the behavior and is crucial for the child. The self-evaluation "Match Game" (Hinshaw *et al.*, 1981) is then employed, to help the child to rate how well he or she was able to meet the behavioral criterion. The Match Game procedure is also used at the end of each of the 20 sessions in the second edition of the *Stop and Think Workbook* (Kendall, 1992a), a series of tasks, in workbook format, for use in training impulsive youth to learn self-control.

Outcome Studies of Youth with Cognitive Deficiencies

Studies evaluating the efficacy of treatment for hyperactivity are numerous. For example, cognitive–behavioral approaches have been evaluated on their own, in comparison to psychostimulant medication treatments, and in conjunction with stimulant medication treatments. For a detailed review the reader is referred to Abikoff (1985, 1987) and Abikoff and Klein (1992). Given this chapter's focus on cognition, a brief review of cognitive–behavioral treatment for hyperactivity/impulsivity will be provided with an emphasis on changes in cognitive functioning that emerge from treatment outcome research.

Cognitive–behavioral interventions have been found to be quite successful with samples of moderately impulsive or undercontrolled children (Kendall and Braswell, 1982b; Schleser *et al.*, 1983). Results achieved with more severely ADHD children, however, are more limited. Studies have documented improvement in the performance of hyperactive children of the MFFT and similar tests of vigilance and impulsivity after cognitive or cognitive–behavioral treatment strategies were employed (Brown, 1980; Brown *et al.*, 1985; Douglas, 1975; Moore and Cole, 1978; Kirby, 1984; Weithorn and Kagan, 1979). Qualitative improvement on the Porteus Mazes has been documented, suggesting that cognitive training helps impulsive children to plan the careful responses needed to perform well on this task (Abikoff, 1985).

Despite these cognitive gains, it is generally agreed that the original hope that cognitive–behavioral interventions for hyperactive children would solve "all the problems" of treatment maintenance and generalization to the home and school setting was not fulfilled (Braswell and Bloomquist, 1991). Various problems regarding the improper implementation of the treatments have been specified as concerns. For example, Abikoff (1985) has noted that training tasks often have little overlap with the outcome measures and that the length of training procedures has been too brief. Braswell and Kendall (1988) point out that some studies have not taken full advantage of behavioral contingencies—they should be employed routinely to reinforce learning the problem-solving skills and appropriate behavior, and to discourage undesired behavior. Prior treatment outcome studies have also failed to utilize parents or classroom teachers in the training procedures and implementation (Braswell and Bloomquist, 1991). Cognitive deficiencies, a central feature of the disorder, do seem to be improved with proper application of cognitive–behavioral therapy. However, additional research is needed to fully evaluate the effectiveness of cognitive–behavioral intervention for hyperactivity.

CHILDHOOD DISORDERS INVOLVING BOTH
DISTORTIONS AND DEFICIENCIES

Aggression in Youth

Aggression is one example of a childhood disorder in which youth have been found to exhibit both cognitive deficiencies and cognitive distortions. The difficulties are primarily evident in interpersonal situations, and thus the cognitive difficulties of the aggressive child have been labeled "social–cognitive" difficulties (Lochman *et al.*, 1991b). This social–cognitive theory has been based in part on Novaco's (1978) conceptualization of anger arousal in adults, and on Dodge's social information processing model (1986).

The reaction of the aggressive child to a potentially anger-arousing stimulus is believed to be due not to the reality of the event itself, but due to the child's personal appraisal of the situation (Lochman *et al.*, 1991b). In other words, following the deficiency/distortion model, the child's aggressive reaction is not based entirely on the factual aspects of the situation, but is largely affected by a deficiency in assessing the situation and the distorted manner in which he/she processed the social information.

Cognitive Deficiencies in Aggression in Youth

The social–cognitive deficiencies of aggressive children fall largely into two categories: (1) cue utilization (labeled a "cue utilization deficiency" by Milich and Dodge, 1984) and (2) problem-solving difficulties. Dodge's (1986) social-information processing view of aggression proposes a 5-step cognitive process as the antecedent to aggression. Deficiencies occurring during the first step (the perception and decoding of environmental cues) are related to cue utilization, while deficiencies occurring during the last three steps in the sequence (searching for a possible response, deciding on which response is appropriate, and enacting the chosen response) relate to problem solving (Gouze, 1987; Kendall *et al.*, 1991). The second step (the development of expectations of the behavior of others based on attributions of hostile intent) relates more to cognitive distortions, which will be discussed later in this section.

Aggressive children utilize cues inefficiently by failing to attend to relevant cues, selectively attending to hostile cues, and attending to later cues more effectively than those presented earlier. When scanning their social environment for cues, aggressive children characteristically do not attend to all relevant cues before making a social judgment. They respond more quickly and with less attention to relevant cues than do nonaggressive children (Dodge and Newman, 1981). In fact, Dodge and Newman found that nonaggressive children chose to listen to 40% more cues before making a decision. Dodge and Tomlin (1987) found aggressive youngsters to differ from nonaggressive children in their use of relevant benign cues in the interpretation of peers' behavior.

In addition to responding inefficiently to relevant cues, aggressive children have also been found to attend to, encode, and retrieve more cues with hostile connotations than do nonaggressive children (Dodge *et al.*, 1986; Lochman, 1989, Milich and Dodge, 1984). Gouze (1987) has likened this attentional bias to traditional notions of selective attention, that is, the tendency to focus on or select out certain aspects of the environment from competing cues (Swets and Kristofferson, 1970). Gouze (1987) found that aggressive boys paid more attention to aggressive social interactions (such as fighting), than to nonaggressive interactions. In addition, Dodge and Frame (1982) reported that aggressive children exhibit "selective recall" during both free recall and recognition. Although aggressive children in this study did not appear to attend more to hostile cues, they showed a high rate of responding with intrusions into recall, remembering social cues that had not actually occurred.

Lastly, aggressive children have been shown to have a recency bias in their utilization of cues (Dodge and Tomlin, 1983). These children are more likely to use the last cue that was presented in their evaluation of a social situation instead of evaluating all cues available (Milich and Dodge, 1984), and to recall significantly fewer relevant primacy cues than nonaggressive peers (Dodge & Tomlin, 1987).

The social problem-solving deficiencies exhibited by aggressive children involve their understanding of solutions to problems and consequences for aggressive actions. Early researchers concluded that aggressive children generate a fewer number of solutions to social problems than do nonaggressive children. In some of the first studies on this topic, Spivack and Shure (1974) found that preschool children identified by teachers as aggressive generated fewer solutions to hypothetical situations involving peer and parent interpersonal conflict. These findings were replicated regarding solutions to peer problems generated by elementary school children (Richard and Dodge, 1982), high-school students (Slaby and Guerra, 1988), and boys with adjustment problems that included aggression (Asarnow and Callan, 1985). However, findings have been equivocal regarding the number of solutions generated by aggressive boys, and some studies have failed to support Spivack and Shure's conclusions (Deluty, 1981; Enright and Sutherfield, 1980; Gouze, 1987).

Rather than a deficiency in the quantity of solutions generated, a deficiency in the quality and content of solutions has been posited to characterize the cognitive functioning of aggressive children. According to

Lochman *et al.* (1985), aggressive children have a marked paucity in the range and types of solutions they consider in solving social problems. Aggressive children tend to come up with a greater number of aggressive or incompetent solutions to problematic social situations. Milich and Dodge (1984) have called this tendency of aggressive children to generate more aggressive and less efficient solutions a "response decision bias." Gouze (1987) found that aggressive preschoolers provided aggressive solutions to hypothetical social dilemmas significantly more often than did nonaggressive preschoolers. Aggressive children also tended to provide an aggressive solution as their first solution. Boys in Grades 2–6 who were rated as aggressive by their teachers were more likely to suggest aggression as a first solution to a wide variety of social dilemmas and more likely to suggest physical aggression as a solution to peer provocation than were nonaggressive boys from the same sample (Walters and Peters, 1980). Deluty (1981), Asarnow and Callan (1985), and Richard and Dodge (1982) have reached similar conclusions regarding the social problem-solving solutions of aggressive youngsters.

Not only do the social solutions suggested by aggressive children tend to be aggressive in nature, they are also socially inappropriate and incompetent in other ways. Several studies show aggressive children to be prone to suggest bribery and manipulation or agonistic strategies in social interactions (Rubin and Clark, 1983; Rubin *et al.*, 1987).

Aggressive children have been found to generate a lesser number of verbal solutions and a greater number of nonverbal, direct-action solutions than nonaggressive children. Lochman and Lampron (1986) reported that aggressive youngsters in Grades 4 and 5 plan to use less verbal assertion to resolve peer conflict than nonaggressive youngsters, and plan to use more direct-action strategies to handle teacher criticism. These tendencies were markedly more pronounced in hostile situations than in situations where intent was ambiguous. Similar conclusions were reached by Lochman *et al.* (1989b). However, when aggressive children were given a multiple-choice format from which to choose their solutions to social dilemmas, they chose to use more verbal assertion and less direct action. The authors believe that the multiple-choice format interferes with the aggressive child's pattern of responding with the most salient and automatic response.

Cognitive Distortions in Aggression in Youth

As with cognitive deficiencies, the cognitive distortions evident in aggressive children have mostly to do with social and interpersonal situations, and interpretations of others' behavior. Aggressive children tend to interpret others' intentions as hostile and to expect aggression from others much more often than do nonaggressive children. The tendency to "assume the worst" regarding others' intentions has been referred to as a "hostile attributional bias" (Milich and Dodge, 1984). This has been found in a variety of situations for children of varying ages.

Dodge and Tomlin (1987) found that youngsters in Grades 6–8 identified as aggressive through sociometric procedures demonstrated a bias toward attributing hostile intent to a hypothetical child in a negative-outcome situation. Although subjects were presented with equally plausible hostile and benevolent explanations for the hypothetical child's behavior, aggressive children were significantly more likely to assume that hostile intentions were directing the behavior of the hypothetical child than were nonaggressive children.

With children from Grades 2–3 and 5–6, who were chosen as aggressive or nonaggressive by teacher ratings, Guerra and Slaby (1989) presented hypothetical stories in which a peer's behavior was ambiguous in intent, yet was standing in the way of the subject obtaining a desired object. For example, the subject is told that he or she forgot his or her lunch, and the peer that is sitting next to the subject refuses to give the subject the uneaten lunch that is being thrown away. Children rated as aggressive were significantly more likely to attribute hostile intent to the peer, and to perceive the peer as an adversary than were nonaggressive children. Similar results were also found by Asarnow and Callan (1985) with children in Grades 4–6 chosen as aggressive through sociometric methods.

Aggressive children distort ambiguous social cues and interpret situations as hostile, yet Waas (1988) found that when provided with accurate social information, aggressive children did not differ from nonaggressive children in their interpretation of social situations. Dodge and Frame (1982) also concluded that aggressive children were able to interpret clearly positive hypothetical social situations without a hostile bias, but were not able to do so for ambiguous stories. In other words, aggressive children do not exhibit cognitive distortions in situations that do not involve aggression.

Nasby et al. (1980) reported that aggressive children interpret the intent of hypothetical peers to be aggressive even when the situation realistically deserves a more positive interpretation. Ten- to sixteen-year-old boys in a residential treatment center diagnosed as aggressive by the Behavior Problem Checklist (Peterson, 1961) identified photographs as aggressive or negative, when the affect in the photographs was ambiguous and when the affect was clearly positive. The likelihood of the children to infer hostility became more marked as aggressiveness increased.

Several studies have examined the social cognitions of aggressive youngsters in actual interpersonal interactions rather than through the presentation of hypothetical situations. Dodge and Somberg (1987) reported that aggressive children not only exhibited a bias toward interpreting peers' behavior as hostile, but this tendency became more pronounced when subjects heard a confederate peer say that he was going to "get into a fight" with the subject. Using audiotapes of peers with either hostile intent, benevolent intent, or ambiguous intent, where the subjects believed that a peer was actually talking in another room, Dodge (1980) found that aggressive children did not show a bias toward hostile attributions when the peer's intent was benevolent, but did show this bias when the intent was ambivalent. These results from an actual situation are in agreement with Waas's (1988) findings that aggressive children do not distort when given correct social information in hypothetical situations.

It appears that, when lacking information, aggressive children not only distort the amount of aggressiveness and hostility in the actions of their peers, but they also distort the degree of their own aggression (Lochman, 1987). Fourth and Fifth Grade aggressive children not only demonstrated a tendency to perceive hostility in their peers during dyadic interactions, but they also tended to underestimate and minimize their own aggression toward their peer.

Aggressive subjects were more likely than their nonaggressive peers to predict that an unknown peer on a video would behave in an aggressive manner toward the subject (Dodge and Frame, 1982). It appears then, when studies are collected and integrated, that aggressive children do not view the world in general as hostile, but believe that others will be hostile to them in particular, reflecting a somewhat paranoid view of social situations.

In summary, aggressive children appear to exhibit both cognitive deficiencies and cognitive distortions in their evaluation of social situations. Their deficiencies occur in the utilization of both relevant and hostile cues, and in generating and choosing solutions to social problems. The cognitive distortions of aggressive youth center around their hostile attributional bias, or the tendency to distort both the aggressive intent of peers and the degree of their own aggression.

Treatment of Aggression in Youth

Description of Procedures Cognitive–behavioral therapy addresses both the deficient and the distorted social–cognitive processes in aggressive children. Because aggressive children are similar to hyperactive children in that they have been shown to react impulsively, failing to examine all possibilities or cues in a given situation, techniques to modify these cognitive deficiencies resemble those used for impulsivity/hyperactivity.

Self-directed problem-solving training is used to increase verbal mediation strategies that regulate social behavior. Through self-talk, children are helped to realistically identify a social dilemma, evaluate available information, assess alternative solutions, predict outcomes, and finally choose and follow a plan of action. This can help to inhibit the aggressive child's tendency toward fast, aggressive action and aid the child in recognizing and exploring social information and attributional alternatives that were previously overlooked.

With the goal of independent regulation of behavior in mind, aggressive children are also instructed in cognitive self-control strategies. Through both discussion and practice in increasingly more provoking situations, children are encouraged to develop a repertoire of coping statements and strategies that will help them in social situations. In developing this repertoire, children are taught to pay attention to environmental triggers of anger, and to anger-enhancing and anger-reducing cognitions.

The cognitive–behavioral approach addresses the cognitive deficiencies of aggressive children by focusing specifically on their difficulties in finding appropriate solutions to social dilemmas. Direct action is discouraged, and verbal solutions such as negotiation and discussion are stressed. The need for appropriate back-up solutions is also stressed to the children (Lochman et al., 1991b). In other words, the children are provided with a model for responding to social conflicts that they can refer to with their coping self-talk, and use in conjunction with their own repertoire of strategies.

Self-evaluation and social perspective-taking skills aid in the modification of the aggressive child's hostile distortions. Perspective-taking exercises are designed to improve the child's ability to more readily recognize the thoughts and intentions of others (cognitive perspective taking), and to enhance their understanding of the feelings of others (affective perspective taking) (Lochman et al., 1991b). A typical perspective-taking exercise would involve the child's examination of an ambiguous photograph, and a subsequent discussion about the child's perspective, and other perspectives as well. A self-evaluation exercise may involve the child's reexamination of a recent past interval of time or past situation and his or her consideration of the feelings of the various people involved. This retrospective look at how each person felt, thought, and behaved can heighten the aggressive child's sensitivity to the feelings of others in his or her social environment (Kendall et al., 1991).

Homework, or at-home journal activities may not be a sought-after activity for aggressive children, and their follow-through with these tasks has historically been poor. Nevertheless, this involvement in therapeutic activities while outside the therapeutic situation is a beneficial component of the cognitive–behavioral treatment program (Kendall *et al.*, 1991). At-home assignments provide real-life examples of problematic social situations and allow for practice in the child's environment, as well as affording the child the opportunity to earn rewards. Framing these assignments as "Show That I Can Tasks" (STIC Tasks; Kendall *et al.*, 1989) may increase compliance with aggressive children.

Outcome Studies with Aggressive Youth   The scope of this chapter does not permit a detailed review of all treatment outcome studies with aggressive youth. For a detailed review, the reader is directed to Kazdin (1987a), Lochman (1990), Lochman *et al.* (1991a), and McMahon and Wells (1989). Provided instead is a brief review with special emphasis on recent empirical findings.

Several early studies concluded that aggressive behavior in children could be altered by cognitive–behavioral therapy. Robin *et al.* (1976) found reductions in aggressive classroom behavior in children treated with imagery and social problem-solving training. Lochman *et al.* (1981) used an early form of what is now a more detailed anger-coping program with aggressive Second and Third Grade children. The children showed improvement on teachers' daily ratings of aggressive behavior. Several studies reported mixed results, finding improvements on some behavioral measures, but not on others. For example, Kettlewell and Kausch (1983) found that treated children showed improvements in self-reported anger, time-out restrictions, coping self-statements, and generation of solutions to problems, but showed no improvement on counselor- or peer-rated aggression. Garrison and Stolberg (1983) found only modest improvements in teacher-observed aggression, and Foreman (1980) found a response-cost technique to be effective in reducing teacher-rated aggression. Recently, Coie *et al.* (1990) treated three cohorts of children with a combination of cognitive–behavioral techniques and social-skills training. Cognitive–behavioral treatment did not show positive effects for two of the cohorts, yet it did for the third.

Several programmatic research efforts have shown more definitive treatment effects. Using their cognitive–behavioral anger-coping program, Lochman *et al.* (1984) found that elementary-school boys showed reductions in aggressive off-task behavior and in parents' ratings of aggression. The behavioral improvements seen in this study have been replicated elsewhere (e.g., Lochman and Curry, 1986; Lochman *et al.*, 1989a).

Kazdin *et al.* (1987a) reported reductions in parents' and teachers' ratings of the aggression of inpatient children following a problem-solving, skills-training program (combining the Kendall and Braswell, 1985, and Spivack and Shure, 1974 programs). Positive results were seen at posttest and at 1-year follow-up. These results were replicated when parent behavioral management training was added (Kazdin et al., 1987b), and with children in both outpatient and inpatient settings (Kazdin et al., 1989).

Recently, Kendall et al. (1990a) assessed a 20-session cognitive–behavioral treatment based on a program by Kendall and Braswell (1985) in comparison with the therapy currently used at a psychiatric hospital (i.e., supportive and insight oriented). Subjects were 6- to 13-year-old black and hispanic youth diagnosed as conduct disordered based on the Diagnostic Interview for Children (DICA; Herjanic and Reich, 1982). Results indicated the superiority of cognitive–behavioral therapy as measured by teacher ratings (of self-control and prosocial behavior) and self-report (of perceived social competence), though not all measures evidenced gains. The difference between the percentage of children who moved from deviant to within the nondeviant range of behavior was significantly higher for the cognitive–behavioral program, supporting the clinical utility of the treatment.

As is the case with most populations of highly aggressive children (see Kendall and Braswell, 1993; Kazdin, 1987b), lack of treatment generalization and lack of maintenance effects appear to be evident. Lack of maintenance was seen, for example, in the Kendall et al. (1990a) study after examination of 6-month follow-up data. Kendall et al. (1991) thus raise the important question of how best to modify cognitive–behavioral treatments for aggressive youth in order to insure that positive effects last beyond the confines of an effective operative program. Copeland (1981, 1982) and Kendall and Braswell (1985) advocate both the identification of change-producing or "active" ingredients in empirically documented treatment programs and the examination of individual factors that may affect the results of a therapeutic modality. The treatment approach could then be altered based on general findings and adjusted according to a child's particular situation.

Kendall et al. (1990a) researched the issue of the effects of individual characteristics on treatment outcome. Results indicated a significant relationship between various subject characteristics (self-reported verbal aggression, suspicion, and resentment) and poorer treatment outcome as measured by teacher report of behavioral changes. Additionally, children with a more internalized attributional style and those who perceived more active parental management in the family evidenced more behavioral improvement after the cognitive–behavioral intervention.

Thus, cognitive–behavioral therapy appears to be beneficial in treating aggressive youth, yet additional research is needed to address such issues as the utility of longer term interventions, the use of booster sessions, the effects of parental involvement in treatment, and the use of a family-based cognitive–behavioral approach.

THE BROADER PICTURE[1]

It might mistakenly be assumed that the "Cognitive–Behavioral" title implies the neglect of other factors operating in the development and treatment of child and adolescent psychopathology. However, the cognitive–behavioral approach actually integrates cognitive, behavioral, affective, and social components (Kendall, 1985, 1991; Kendall and Braswell, 1993). It does not ignore or deny the influence of affective states of the individual or the larger social context in which the organism is functioning. In fact, the cognitive–behavioral analyses and treatment of disorders of youth represents an integrationist perspective, considering both the internal and external environment of the child.

In accordance with the broader view of the cognitive–behavioral model, it is important to stress that cognitive factors are not assumed to be the *sole* source of explanation for all psychological disorders in youth. Cognition plays an important role in many forms of childhood psychopathology, yet it interacts with additional other factors. In some disorders, cognition may be much less influential. Nevertheless, as we have seen, cognitive factors do play a meaningful role in many of the prevalent disorders.

For youth, the centrality of the social/interpersonal context is unmistakable. Successful and fulfilling peer relationships are crucial for the healthy adjustment of children (Hartup, 1983). Examining peer relationships and social environments, such as school, may reveal information that is not available from an examination of specific symptoms. For example, aggressive children are deficient in their skills for processing social information, and they distort interpersonal cues. Here the interaction of cognitive style with peer interaction is a useful way to examine the development of the disorder, and to provide effective intervention strategies.

Several difficulties in childhood and adolescence can be better understood by examining the influence of peer-group membership and peer pressure. For example, many health-related behaviors such as substance abuse, smoking, and eating disorders are influenced by peers. Furthermore, the interaction between cognitive style and peer relationships may also extend into the realm of peer pressure. For example, children with aggressive tendencies and a peer group that acts out with aggressive or delinquent acts may be unable to generate alternative actions in social situations, and consequently follow along with the delinquent actions of the group.

[1]It should be noted that cognitive functioning has been studied in, and the cognitive–behavioral model has been applied to, other childhood disorders such as learning disabilities (Wong *et al.*, 1991) and anorexia (Fairburn *et al.*, 1986; Garner and Bemis, 1985).

The important role of the family in the life of a child need not be debated, for it is in this social environment that children learn many of the rules and patterns for their later social interactions. However, research concerning the interaction of familial contributions and child cognitive functioning to child psychopathology is far from extensive and further investigation is certainly needed. There are particular disorders for which familial influence has been investigated. Stark *et al.* (1991) suggested that the dysfunctional cognitions and behaviors exhibited by depressed youngsters are often produced and maintained by patterns in family functioning. They believe in the importance of involving the child's family in treatment procedures, helping the family to develop new family rules and modes of communication that may contribute to the child's modification of depressive thinking and behavior. In addition, certain childhood issues are considered to be even more strongly related to familial history or interaction patterns, such as difficulties related to divorce, incest, abuse or neglect, and acting-out behavior that is affected by parenting style (Patterson, 1982, 1986). More specifically, Patterson stresses the primacy of familial socialization processes in the development and maintenance of conduct-related behavior problems in childhood, focusing on the coercive and controlling styles that are learned and reinforced by both parent and child. Braswell (1991) and Braswell and Bloomquist (1991) make an argument for the involvement of families in cognitive–behavioral therapy for ADHD, and Kendall *et al.* (1992a) argue for familial involvement in the treatment of anxiety-disordered youth. Research is needed to take apart the disturbed child's maladaptive thinking from familial incentives that are maladaptive as well. A cognitive–behavioral analysis of family factors in child and adolescent psychopathology is welcomed.

ACKNOWLEDGMENT

Preparation of this review was facilitated by research Grant MH 44042 from the national Institute of Mental Health awarded to Philip C. Kendall.

REFERENCES

Abikoff, H. (1985). Efficacy of cognitive training interventions in hyperactive children: A critical review. *Clinical Psychology Review, 5*, 479–512.
Abikoff, H. (1987). An evaluation of cognitive–behavior therapy for hyperactive children. In B. B. Lahey and A. E. Kazdin (Eds.), *Advances in clinical child psychology* (Vol. 10, pp. 171–216). New York: Plenum.
Abikoff, H. and Klein, R. G. (1992). Attention-Deficit Hyperactivity and Conduct Disorder: Comorbidity and implications for treatment. *Journal of Consulting and Clinical Psychology, 60*, 881–892.

Achenbach, T. M. (1966). The classification of children's psychiatric symptoms: A factor analytic study. *Psychological Monographs, 80* (Whole No. 615).

Alloy, L. B. (Ed.). (1988). *Cognitive processes in depression.* New York: Guilford Press.

American Psychiatric Association (1980). *Diagnostic and Statistical manual of mental disorders* (3rd ed.). Washington, D.C.: American Psychiatric Association.

Asarnow, J. R. (1988). Peer status and social competence in child psychiatric inpatients: A comparison of children with depressive, externalizing and concurrent depressive and externalizing disorders. *Journal of Abnormal Child Psychology, 16,* 151–162.

Asarnow, J. R., and Bates, S. (1988). Depression in child psychiatric inpatients: Cognitive and attributional patterns. *Journal of Abnormal Child Psychology, 16,* 601–615.

Asarnow, J. R., and Callan, J. W. (1985). Boys with peer adjustment problems: Social–cognitive processes. *Journal of Consulting and Clinical Psychology, 53,* 80–87.

Barkley, R. A. (1977). A review of stimulant drug research with hyperactive children. *Journal of Child Psychology and Psychiatry, 18,* 137–165.

Barkley, R. A. (1990). *Attention deficit hyperactivity disorder: A handbook for diagnosis and treatment.* New York: Guilford Press.

Barkley, R. A., and Ullman, D. G. (1975). A comparison of objective measures of activity and distractibility in hyperactive and nonhyperactive children. *Journal of Abnormal Child Psychology, 3,* 213–244.

Barkley, R. A., McMurray, M. B., Edelbrock, C. S., and Robbins, K. (1990). The side effects of Ritalin: A systematic placebo controlled evaluation of two doses. *Pediatrics,* 184–192.

Barlow, D. (1988). *Anxiety and its disorders: The nature and treatment of anxiety and panic.* New York: Guilford Press.

Beck, A. T. (1967). *Depression: Clinical, experimental, and theoretical aspects.* New York: Harper & Row.

Beck, A. T. (1976). *Cognitive therapy and the emotional disorders.* New York: International Universities Press.

Beck, A. T. and Emery, G. (1985). *Anxiety disorders and phobias: A cognitive perspective.* New York: Basic Books.

Brady, E. U., and Kendall, P. C. (1992). Comorbidity of anxiety and depression in children and adolescents. *Psychological Bulletin, 111,* 244–255.

Braswell, L. (1991). Involving parents in cognitive–behavioral therapy with children and adolescents. In P. C. Kendall (Ed.), *Child and adolescent therapy: Cognitive–behavioral interventions* (pp. 316–351). New York: Guilford Press.

Braswell, L., and Bloomquist, M. L. (1991). *Cognitive–behavioral therapy with ADHD children: Child, family and school interventions.* New York: Guilford Press.

Braswell, L., and Kendall, P. C., (1988). Cognitive behavioral methods with children. In K. S. Dobson (Ed.), *Handbook of cognitive–behavioral therapies* (pp. 167–213). New York: Guilford Press.

Brown, R. T. (1980). *Modeling: A cognitive approach in ameliorating impulsivity in hyperactive children.* Paper presented at the annual meeting of the American Psychological Association, Montreal, Canada.

Brown, R. T., and Quay, L. C. (1977). Reflection-impulsivity of normal and behavior-disordered children. *Journal of Abnormal Child Psychology, 5,* 457–462.

Brown, R. T., Wynne, M. E., and Medinis, R. (1985). Methylphenidate and cognitive therapy: A comparison of treatment approaches with hyperactive boys. *Journal of Abnormal Child Psychology, 13,* 69–87.

Butler, L., Miezitis, S., Friedman, R., and Cole, E. (1980). The effect of two school-based intervention programs on depressive symptoms in preadolescents. *American Educational Research Journal, 17,* 111–119.

Campbell, S. B. (1976). Hyperactivity: Course and treatment. In A. Davids (Ed.), pp. 41–62. *Child personality and psychopathology: Current topics* (Vol. 3). New York: Wiley.

Campbell, S. B., Douglas, V. I., and Morgenstern, G. (1971). Cognitive styles in hyperactive children and the effects of methylphenidate. *Journal of Child Psychology and Psychiatry, 12*, 55.

Ceci, S. J., and Tishman, J. (1984). Hyperactivity and incidental memory: Evidence for attentional diffusion. *Child Development, 55*, 2192–2203.

Clements, S. C., and Peters, J. E. (1962). Minimal brain dysfunction in the school-aged child. *Archives of General Psychiatry, 6*, 185–197.

Cohen, N. J., Douglas, V. I., and Morgenstern, G. (1971). The effect of methylphenidate on attentive behavior and autonomic activity in hyperactive children. *Psychopharmacologia, 22*, 282–294.

Coie, J. D., Underwood, M., and Lochman, J. E. (1990). Preventing intervention with aggressive children in the school setting. In D. J. Pepler and K. H. Rubin (Eds.), *Development and treatment of childhood aggression*. Toronto: Erlbaum.

Copeland, A. P. (1981). The relevance of subject variables in cognitive self-instructional programs for impulsive children. *Behavior Therapy, 12*, 520–529.

Copeland, A. P. (1982). Individual difference factors in children's self-management: Toward individualized treatments. In P. Karoly and F. H. Karfer (Eds.), *Self-management and behavior change: From theory to practice*. New York: Pergamon.

Dahlquist, L. M., Gil, K. M., Armstrong, F. D., Ginsberg, A., and Jones, B. (1985). Behavioral management of children's distress during chemotherapy. *Journal of Behavior Therapy and Experimental Psychiatry, 16*, 325–329.

Deluty, R. H. (1981). Alternative thinking ability of aggressive, assertive, and submissive children. *Cognitive Therapy and Research, 5*, 309–312.

Dodge, K. A. (1980). Social cognition and children's aggressive behavior. *Child Development, 51*, 162–170.

Dodge, K. A. (1982). Social–cognitive biases and deficits in aggressive boys. *Child Development, 53*, 620–635.

Dodge, K. A. (1986). A social information processing model of social competence in children. In M. Perlmutter (Ed.), *Minnesota symposium on child psychology* (*Vol. 18*). Hillsdale, NJ: Erlbaum.

Dodge, K. A. and Frame, C. L. (1982). Social cognitive biases and deficits in aggressive boys. *Child Development, 53*, 620–635.

Dodge, K. A., and Newman, J. P. (1981). Biased decision making processes in aggressive boys. *Journal of Abnormal Psychology, 90*, 375–379.

Dodge, K. A., and Somberg, D. (1987). Hostile attributional biases among aggressive boys are exacerbated under conditions of threats to the self. *Child Development, 58*, 213–224.

Dodge, K. A., and Tomlin, A. (1983). *The role of cue utilization biases among aggressive children*. Unpublished manuscript. Cited in Milich, R., & Dodge, K. A. (1984). Social information processing in child psychiatric population. *Journal of Abnormal Child Psychology, 12(3)*, 471–490.

Dodge, K. A., and Tomlin, A. M. (1987). Utilization of self schemas as a mechanism of interpretational bias in aggressive children. *Social Cognition, 5*, 280–300.

Dodge, K. A., Petit, G. S., McClaskey, C. L., and Brown, M. M. (1986). Social competence in children. *Monographs of the Society for Research in Child Development, 51* (2, No. 213).

Douglas, V. I. (1972). Stop, look and listen: The problem of sustained attention and impulse control in hyperactive and normal children. *Canadian Journal of Behavior Science, 4*, 259–282.

Douglas, V. I. (1974). Sustained attention and impulse control: Implication for the handicapped child. In J. A. Swets and L. L. Elliott (Eds.), *Psychology and the handicapped child*. Washington, D.C.: U.S. Office of Education.

Douglas, V. I. (1975). Are drugs enough to treat the hyperactive child? *International Journal of Mental Health, 4*, 199–212.

Douglas, V. I. (1980). Treatment an training approaches to hyperactivity: Establishing internal or external control. In C. Whalen and B. Henker (Eds.), *Hyperactive Children: The social ecology of identification and treatment*. New York: Academic Press.

Douglas, V. I. (1983). Attentional and cognitive problems. In M. Rutter (Ed.), *Developmental neuropsychiatry* (pp. 280–328). New York: Guilford.

Douglas, V. I., and Peters, K. G. (1979). Toward a clearer definition of the attentional deficit in hyperactive children. In G. A. Hale and M. Lewis (Eds.), *Attention and the development of cognitive skills* (pp. 173–247). New York: Plenum.

Douglas, V. I., and Peters, K. G. (1980). Toward a clearer definition of the attentional deficit of hyperactive children. In G. A. Hall and M. Lewis (Eds.), *Attention and the development of cognitive skills* (pp. 173–247). New York: Plenum.

Douglas, V. I., Barr, R. G., Amin, K., O'Neill, M. E., and Britton, B. G. (1988). Dosage effects and individual responsivity to methylphenidate in attention deficit disorder. *Journal of Child Psychology and Psychiatry, 29*, 453–475.

Douglas, V. I., Barr, R. G., O'Neill, M. E., and Britton, B. G. (1986). Short term effects of methylphenidate on the cognitive, learning and academic performance of children with attention deficit hyperactivity disorder in the laboratory and in the classroom. *Journal of Child Psychology and Psychiatry, 29*, 191–211.

Elliot, C. H., and Olson, R. A. (1983). The management of children's behavioral distress in response to painful medical treatment for burn injuries. *Behavior Research and Therapy, 21*, 675–682.

Ellis, A. (1962). *Reason and emotion in psychotherapy*. New York: Stewart.

Enright, R. D., and Sutherfield, S. J. (1980). An ecological validation of social cognitive development. *Child Development, 51*, 156–161.

Fairburn, C. G., Cooper, Z., and Cooper, P. (1986). The clinical features and maintenance of bulimia nervosa. In K. D. Brownell and J. P. Foreyt (Eds.), *Handbook of eating disorders: Physiology psychology and treatment* (pp. 389–404). New York: Basic Books.

Firestone, P., and Douglas, V. I. (1975). The effects of reward and punishment on reaction times and autonomic activity in hyperactive children. *Journal of Abnormal Psychology, 3*, 201–216.

Foreman, S. G. (1980). A comparison of cognitive training and response cost procedures in modifying aggressive behavior in elementary school children. *Behavior Therapy, 11*, 594–600.

Fox, J. E., and Houston, B. K. (1981). Efficacy of self instruction ' training for reducing children's anxiety in an evaluative situation. *Behavior Research and Therapy, 19*, 509–515.

Francis, G. (1988). Assessing cognitions in anxious children, *Behavior Modification, 12*, 267–281.

Fuhrman, M. J., and Kendall, P. C. (1986). Cognitive tempo and behavioral adjustment in children. *Cognitive Therapy and Research, 10*, 45–51.

Gadow, K. D. (1985). Relative efficacy of pharmacological, behavioral and combination treatments for enhancing academic performance. *Clinical Psychology Review, 5*, 513–533.

Gadow, K. D. (1986). *Children and medication, Volume 1: Hyperactivity, learning disabilities, and mental retardation*. Boston: Little, Brown, & Co.

Gadow, K. D. (1991). Clinical issues in child and adolescent psychopharmacology. *Journal of Consulting and Clinical Psychology, 59*, 842–852.

Garner, D. M., and Bemis, K. M. (1985). Cognitive therapy for anorexia nervosa. In D. Garner and P. Garfinkel (Eds.), *Handbook of psychotherapy for anorexia nervosa and bulimia*. New York: Guilford Press.

Garrison, S. R., and Stolberg, A. L. (1983). Modification of anger in children by affective imagery training. *Journal of Abnormal Child Psychology, 11*, 115–130.

Giebenhain, J. E., and O'Dell, S. L. (1984). Evaluation of a parent-training manual for reducing children's fear of the dark. *Journal of Applied Behavior Analysis, 17*, 121–125.

Gittleman-Klein, R., Klein, D. F., Katz, S., Saraf, K., and Pollack, E. (1976). Comparative effects of methylphenidate and thioridazine in hyperactive children: I. Clinical results. *Archives of General Psychiatry, 33*, 1217–1231.

Goldfried, M. R. (1979). Anxiety reduction through cognitive–behavioral intervention. In P. C. Kendall and S. D. Hollon (Eds.), *Cognitive–behavioral interventions: Theory, research, and procedures*. New York: Academic Press.

Gormally, J., Sipps, G., Raphael, R., Edwin, D., and Varvil-Weld, D. (1981). The relationship between maladaptive cognitions and social anxiety. *Journal of Consulting and Clinical Psychology, 49*, 300–301.

Gouze, K. R. (1987). Attention and social problem solving as correlates of aggression in preschool males. *Journal of Abnormal Child Psychology, 15*(2), 181–197.

Graziano, A. M., and Mooney, K. C. (1980). Family self-control instruction for children's nighttime fear reduction. *Journal of Consulting and Clinical Psychology, 48*, 206–213.

Graziano, A. M., DeGiovanni, I. S., and Garcia, K. S. (1979a). Behavioral treatment of children's fears: A review. *Psychological Bulletin, 86*, 804–830.

Graziano, A. M., Mooney, K. C., Huber, C., and Ignasiak, D. (1979b). Self-control instruction for children's fear reduction. *Journal of Behavior Therapy and Experimental Psychiatry, 10*, 221–227.

Guerra, N. G., and Slaby, R. G. (1989). Evaluative factors in social problem solving by aggressive boys. *Journal of Abnormal Child Psychology, 17*(3), 277–289.

Haley, G. M., Fine, S., Marriage, K., Moretti, M., and Freeman, R. (1985). Cognitive bias and depression in psychiatrically disturbed children and adolescents. *Journal of Consulting and Clinical Psychology, 53*, 535–537.

Hartup, W. W. Peer relations. In P. Mussen (Ed.), *Handbook of child psychology*, (Vol. 4), 4th ed. New York: Wiley, 1983.

Hechtman, L., Weiss, G., Perlman, R., and Amsel, R. (1984). Hyperactives as young adults: Initial predictors of outcome. *Journal American Academy of Child Psychiatry, 31*, 557–567.

Herjanic, B., and Reich, W. (1982). Development of a structural psychiatric interview for children: Agreement between child and parent on individual symptoms. *Journal of Abnormal Child Psychology, 10*, 307–324.

Himle, D. P., Thyer, B. A., and Papsdorf, J. D. (1982). Relationships between rational beliefs and anxiety. *Cognitive Therapy and Research, 6*, 219–224.

Hinshaw, S. P., and Erhardt, D. (1990). Behavioral treatment of attention deficit-hyperactivity disorder. In V. B. Van Hasselt and M. Hersen (Eds.), *Handbook of behavior therapy and pharmacotherapy for children: An integrative approach*. New York: Plenum.

Hinshaw, S. P., and Erhardt, D. (1991). In P. C. Kendall (Ed.), *Child and adolescent therapy: Cognitive–behavioral procedures* (pp. 98–130). New York: Guilford Press.

Hinshaw, S. P., Henker, B., and Whalen, C. K. (1981). *Self-regulation for hyperactive boys: A training manual*. Unpublished manuscript, University of California at Los Angeles.

Hinshaw, S. P., Henker, B., and Whalen, K. (1984). Self-control in hyperactive boys in anger inducing situations: Effects of cognitive–behavioral training and of methylphenidate. *Journal of Abnormal Child Psychology, 12*, 55–57.

Homatidis, S., and Konstantareas, M. M. (1981). Assessment of hyperactivity: Isolating measures of high discriminant validity. *Journal of Consulting and Clinical Psychology, 49,* 533–541.

Ingram, R. E. (1984). Toward an information-processing analysis of depression. *Cognitive Therapy and Research, 8,* 443–447.

Ingram, R. E., and Kendall, P. C. (1986). Cognitive clinical psychology: Implications of an information processing perspective. In R. E. Ingram (Ed.), *Information processing approaches to clinical psychology* (pp. 3–21). New York: Academic Press.

Ingram, R. E., and Kendall, P. C. (1987). The cognitive side of anxiety. *Cognitive Therapy and Research, 11,* 523–537.

Jay, S. M., Elliott, C. H., Ozolins, M., Olson, R. A., and Pruitt, S. D. (1985). Behavioral management of children's distress during painful medical procedures. *Behavior Research and Therapy, 23,* 513–520.

Kagan, J. (1966). Reflection-impulsivity: The generality and dynamics of conceptual tempo. *Journal of Abnormal Psychology, 71,* 17–24.

Kane, M. T., and Kendall, P. C. (1989). Anxiety disorders in children: A multiple baseline evaluation of cognitive–behavioral treatment. *Behavior Therapy, 20,* 499–508.

Kanfer, F. H., Karoly, P., and Newman, A. (1975). Reduction of children's fears of the dark by competence-related and situational threat-related verbal cues. *Journal of Consulting and Clinical Psychology, 43,* 251–258.

Kashani, J. H., Husain, A., Shekim, W. O., Hodges, K. K., Cytryn, L., and McKnew, D. H. (1981). Current perspectives on childhood depression: An overview. *American Journal of Psychiatry, 138,* 143–153.

Kaslow, N. J., Rehm, L. P., and Siegel. (1984). Social–cognitive and cognitive correlates of depression in children. *Journal of Abnormal Child Psychology, 12,* 605–620.

Kazdin, A. E. (1987a). Treatment of antisocial behavior in children: Current status and future directions. *Psychological Bulletin, 102,* 187–203.

Kazdin, A. E. (1987b). *Conduct disorder in childhood and adolescence.* Beverly Hills, CA: Sage.

Kazdin, A. E., Colbus, D., and Rodgers, A. (1986). Assessment of depression and diagnosis of depressive disorders among psychiatrically disturbed children. *Journal of Abnormal Child Psychology, 14,* 499–515.

Kazdin, A. E., Bass, D., Siegel, T., and Thomas, C. (1989). Cognitive–behavioral therapy and relationship therapy in the treatment of children referred for antisocial behavior. *Journal of Consulting and Clinical Psychology, 57*(4), 522–535.

Kazdin, A. E., Esveldt-Dawson, K., French, N. H., and Unis, A. S. (1987a). Problem-solving skills training and relationship therapy in the treatment of anti-social child behavior. *Journal of Consulting and Clinical Psychology, 55,* 76–85.

Kazdin, A. E., Esveldt-Dawson, K., French, N. H., and Unis, A. S. (1987b). Effects of parent management training and problem-solving skills training combined in the treatment of antisocial child behavior. *Journal of the American Academy of Child and Adolescent Psychiatry, 26,* 416–424.

Kendall, P. C. (1985). Toward a cognitive–behavioral model of child psychopathology and a critique of related interventions. *Journal of Abnormal Psychology, 13,* 357–372.

Kendall, P. C. (1991). Guiding theory for therapy with children and adolescents. In P. C. Kendall (Ed.), *Child and adolescent therapy: Cognitive–behavioral procedures* (pp. 3–22). New York: Guilford Press.

Kendall, P. C. (1992a). *Stop and think workbook* (2nd ed.). Available from the author, Department of Psychology, Temple University, Philadelphia, PA 19122. The accompanying *Treatment manual* is also available from the author.

Kendall, P. C. (1990). *Coping cat workbook*. Available from the author, Department of Psychology, Temple University, Philadelphia, PA 19122. The accompanying *Treatment manual* is also available from the author.

Kendall, P. C. (1993). Treating anxiety disorders in youth: Results of a randomized clinical trial. *Journal of Consulting and Clinical Psychology, 61*, in press.

Kendall, P. C., and Braswell, L. (1982a). Cognitive–behavioral assessment: Model, measures, and madness. In J. Butcher and C. Spielberger (Eds.), (pp. 35–82). *Advances in personality assessment* (Vol 1). Hillsdale, NJ: Erlbaum.

Kendall, P. C., and Braswell, L. (1982b). Cognitive–behavioral self-control therapy for children: A components analysis. *Journal of Consulting and Clinical Psychology, 50*, 672–689.

Kendall, P. C., and Braswell, L. C. (1985). *Cognitive–behavioral therapy for impulsive children*. New York: Guilford Press.

Kendall, P. C., and Braswell, L. (1993). *Cognitive–behavioral therapy for impulsive children* (2nd ed.). New York: Guilford Press.

Kendall, P. C., and Hollon, S. D. (1979). Cognitive–behavioral interventions: Overview and current status. In P. C. Kendall and S. D. Hollon (Eds.), *Cognitive–behavioral interventions: Theory, research, and procedures* (pp. 1–13). New York: Academic Press.

Kendall, P. C., and Ingram, R. E. (1987). The future for cognitive assessment of anxiety: Let's get specific. In L. Michelson and M. Ascher (Eds.), *Anxiety and stress disorders: Cognitive–behavioral assessment and treatment*. New York: Guilford Press.

Kendall, P. C., and Ingram, R. E. (1989). Cognitive–behavioral perspectives: Theory and research on depression and anxiety. In P. C. Kendall and D. Watson (Eds.), *Anxiety and depression: Distinctive and overlapping features*. New York: Academic Press.

Kendall, P. C., Kane, M., Howard, B., and Siqueland, L. (1989). *Cognitive–behavioral treatment for anxious children: treatment manual*. Available from P. C. Kendall, Department of Psychology, Temple University, Philadelphia, PA 19122.

Kendall, P. C., Reber, M., McClear, S., Epps, J., and Ronan, K. R. (1990a). Cognitive–behavioral treatment of conduct disordered children. *Cognitive Therapy and Research, 14*, 279–297.

Kendall, P. C., Stark, K. D., and Adam, T. (1990b). Cognitive deficit or cognitive distortion in childhood depression. *Journal of Abnormal Child Psychology, 18*, 225–270.

Kendall, P. C., Ronan, K. R., and Epps, J. (1991). Aggression in children/adolescents: Cognitive–behavioral treatment perspectives. In D. Peplar and K. Rubin (Eds.), *Development and treatment of childhood aggression*. Hillsdale, NJ: Erlbaum.

Kendall, P. C., Chansky, T. E., Kane, M. T., Kim, R. S., Kortlander, E., Ronan, K. R., Sessa, F. M., and Siqueland, L. (1992a). *Anxiety disorders in youth: Cognitive–behavioral interventions*. Needham, MA: Allyn and Bacon.

Kendall, P. C., Kortlander, E., Chansky, T., and Brady, E. (1992b). Comorbidity of anxiety and depression in youth: Implications for treatment. *Journal of Consulting and Clinical Psychology, 60*, 869–880.

Kettlewell, P. W., and Kausch, D. F. (1983). The generalization of the effects of a cognitive–behavioral treatment program for aggressive children. *Journal of Abnormal Child Psychology, 11*, 101–104.

Kirby, E. A. (1984). *Durable and generalized effects of cognitive behavior modification with attention deficit disorder children*. Paper presented at the annual meeting of the American Psychological Association, Toronto, Canada.

Klein, D. F., Gittelman, R., Quitkin, F., and Rifkin, A. (1980). *Diagnosis and drug treatment of psychiatric disorders: Adults and children* (2nd ed.). Baltimore: Williams & Wilkins.

Kovacs, M. (1981). Rating scales to assess depression in school-aged children. *Acta Paedopsychiatrica, 46*, 305–315.

Kovacs, M., and Beck, A. T. (1977). An empirical clinical approach towards a definition of childhood depression. In J. Schulterbrandt and A. Raskin (Eds.), *Depression in children: Diagnosis, treatment, and conceptual models* (pp. 1–25). New York: Raven Press.

Krantz, S. E., and Hammen, C. L. (1979). Assessment of cognitive bias in depression. *Journal of Abnormal Psychology, 88,* 611–619.

Leal, L. L., Baxter, E. G., Martin, J. M., and Marx, R. W. (1981). Cognitive modification and systematic desensitization with test anxious high school students. *Journal of Counseling Psychology, 28(6),* 525–528.

Lefebvre, M. F. (1980). *Cognitive distortion in depressed psychiatric and low back pain patients.* Unpublished doctoral dissertation, University of Vermont, Burlington.

Lefebvre, M. F. (1981). Cognitive distortion and cognitive errors in depressed psychiatric and low back pain patients. *Journal of Consulting and Clinical Psychology, 49,* 517–525.

Leitenberg, H., Yost, L. W., and Carroll-Wilson, M. (1986). Negative cognitive errors in children: Questionnaire development, normative data, and comparisons between children with and without self-reported symptoms of depression, low self-esteem, and evaluation anxiety. *Journal of Consulting and Clinical Psychology, 54,* 528–536.

Lochman, J. E. (1987). Self and peer Perceptions and attributional biases of aggressive and nonaggressive boys in dyadic interactions. *Journal of Consulting and Clinical Psychology, 55(3),* 404–410.

Lochman, J. E. (1989). *Hardware versus software: Land of deficiency in social–cognitive processes of aggressive boys.* Paper presented at the first annual meeting of the Society for Research in Child and Adolescent Psychopathology, Miami.

Lochman, J. E. (1990). Modification of childhood aggression. In M. Hersen, R. Eisler, and P. M. Miller (Eds.), *Progress in behavior modification* (Vol. 25). Newbury Park, CA: Sage.

Lochman, J. E., and Curry, J. F. (1986). Effects of social problem solving training and self instruction training with aggressive boys. *Journal of Clinical Child Psychology, 15,* 159–164.

Lochman, J. E., and Lampron, L. B. (1986). Situational social problem solving skills and self esteem of aggressive and non-aggressive boys. *Journal of Abnormal Child Psychology, 14,* 605–617.

Lochman, J. E., Nelson, W. M., III, and Sims, J. P. (1981). A cognitive behavioral program for use with aggressive children. *Journal of Clinical Child Psychology, 13,* 527–538.

Lochman, J. E., Burch, P. R., Curry, J. F., and Lampron, L. B. (1984). Treatment and generalization effects of cognitive–behavioral and goal-setting interventions with aggressive boys. *Journal of Consulting and Clinical Psychology, 52,* 915–916.

Lochman, J. E., Lampron, L. B., Burch, P. R., and Curry, J. F. (1985). Client characteristics associated with treatment outcome for aggressive boys. *Journal of Abnormal Child Psychology, 13,* 527–538.

Lochman, J. E., Lampron, L. B., Gemmer, T. C., Harris, R., and Wyckoff, G. M. (1989a). Teacher consultation and cognitive–behavioral interventions with aggressive boys. *Psychology in the schools, 26,* 179–188.

Lochman, J. E., Lampron, L. B., and Rabiner, D. L. (1989b). Format differences and salience effects in social problem-solving assessment of aggressive and non-aggressive boys. *Journal of Consulting and Clinical Psychology, 18(3),* 230–236.

Lochman, J. E., White, K. J., Curry, J. F., and Rumer, R. (1991a). Antisocial behavior. In V. B. Van Hasset and D. J. Kolko (Eds.), *Inpatient behavior therapy for children and adolescents.* New York: Plenum.

Lochman, J. E., White, J. E., and Wayland, K. K. (1991b). Cognitive–behavioral assessment and treatment with aggressive children. In P. C. Kendall (Ed.), *Child and adolescent therapy: Cognitive–behavioral procedures* (pp. 25–65). New York: Guilford Press.

Loiselle, D. L., Stamm, J. S., Maitinsky, S., and Whipple, S. C. (1980). Evoked potential and behavioral signs of attentive dysfunctions in hyperactive boys. *Psychophysiology, 17*, 193–201.

Luk, S. (1985). Direct observations studies of hyperactive behaviors. *Journal of the American Academy of Child Psychiatry, 24*, 338–344.

McGee, R., Anderson, J., Williams, S., and Silva, P. A. (1986). Cognitive correlates of depressive symptoms in eleven year old children. *Journal of Abnormal Child Psychology, 14*, 517–524.

McIntyre, C. W., Blackwell, S. L., and Denton, C. L. (1978). Effect of noise distractibility on the spans of apprehension of hyperactive boys. *Journal of Abnormal Child Psychology, 6*, 483–492.

McMahon, R. J., and Wells, K. C. (1989). Conduct disorders. In E. J. Mash and P. A. Barkley (Eds.), *Treatment of childhood disorders* (pp. 73–134). New York: Guilford Press.

Meichenbaum, D. (1977). *Cognitive-behavior modification: An integrative approach.* New York: Plenum.

Meichenbaum, D., and Goodman, J. (1971). Training impulsive children to talk to themselves: A means of developing self-control. *Journal of Abnormal Psychology, 77*, 115–126.

Meichenbaum, D., Bream, L. A., and Cohen, J. S. (1985). A cognitive–behavioral perspective of child psychopathology: Implications for assessment and training. In B. McMahon and R. Peters (Eds.), *Childhood disorders: Behavioral–developmental approaches* (pp. 65–115). New York: Brunner/Mazel.

Meyer, N. E., Dyck, D. G., and Petrinack, R. J. (1989). Cognitive appraisal and attributional correlates of depressive symptoms in children. *Journal of Abnormal Psychology, 17*(3).

Milich, R., and Dodge, K. A. (1984). Social information processing in child psychiatric populations. *Journal of Abnormal Child Psychology, 12*, 471–490.

Milich, R., Loney, J., and Landau, S. (1982). The independent dimensions of hyperactivity and aggression: A validation with playroom observation data. *Journal of Abnormal Psychology, 91*, 183–198.

Moore, S. F., and Cole, S. D. (1978). Cognitive self-mediation training with hyperkinetic children. *Bulletin of the Psychonomic Society, 12*, 18–20.

Mueller, J. H., and Thompson, W. B. (1984). Test anxiety and distinctiveness of personal information. In H. M. van der Ploeg, R. Schwarzer, and C. D. Spielberger (Eds.), *Advances in test anxiety research* (Vol. 3, pp. 21–37). Hillsdale, NJ: Erlbaum.

Nasby, W., Hayden, B., and DePaulo, B. M. (1980). Attributional bias among aggressive boys to interpret unambiguous social stimuli as displays of hostility. *Journal of Abnormal Psychology, 11*, 257–272.

Novaco, R. W. (1978). Anger and coping with stress: Cognitive–behavioral interventions. In J. P. Foreyet and D. P. Rathjen (Eds.), *Cognitive–behavioral therapy: Research and application.* New York: Plenum.

Parry, P. (1973). *The effect of reward on the performance of hyperactive children.* Unpublished doctoral dissertation, McGill University, Montreal.

Patterson, G. R. (1982). *Coercive family process.* Eugene, OR: Castalia.

Patterson, G. R. (1986). Performance models for antisocial boys. *American Psychologist, 41*, 432–444.

Pearson, D. A., Lane, D. M., and Swanson, J. M. (1991). Auditory attention switching in hyperactive children. *Journal of Abnormal Child Psychology, 19*(4), 479–492.

Pelham, W. E., and Bender, M. E. (1982). Peer relationships in hyperactive children: Description and treatment. In K. Gadow and I. Bailer (Eds.), *Advances in learning and behavioral disabilities* (Vol. 1, pp. 365–436). Greenwich, CT: JAI Press.

Peters, K. G. (1977). *Selective attention and distractibility in hyperactive and normal children.* Unpublished doctoral dissertation, McGill University, Montreal.

Peterson, D. R. (1961). Behavior problems of middle childhood. *Journal of Consulting Psychology, 25,* 205–209.

Peterson, L., and Shigetomi, C. (1981). The use of coping techniques in minimizing anxiety in hospitalized children. *Behavior Therapy, 12,* 1–14.

Prins, P. J. M. (1985). Self-speech and self regulation of high- and low-anxious children in the dental situation: An interview study. *Behavior Research and Therapy, 23,* 641–650.

Prins, P. J. M. (1986). Children's self-speech and self-regulation during a fear provoking behavioral test. *Behavior Research and Therapy, 24,* 181–191.

Puig-Antich, J., and Ryan, N. (1986). *The schedule for affective disorders and schizophrenia for school-age children (6–18 years) — Kiddie SADS (K-SADS).* Unpublished Manuscript, Western Psychiatric Institute and Clinic, Pittsburgh.

Radosh, A., and Gittelman, R. (1981). The effect of appealing distractors on the performance of hyperactive children. *Journal of Abnormal Child Psychology, 9,* 179–189.

Rapport, M. D., and Kelly, K. L. (1990). Psychostimulant effects on learning and cognitive functioning in children with attention deficit hyperactivity disorder: Findings and implications. In J. L. Mateson (Ed.), *Hyperactivity in children: A handbook.* New York: Pergamon.

Rapport, M. D., DuPaul, G. J., Stoner, G., and Jones, J. T. (1986). Comparing classroom and clinic measures of attention deficit disorder: Differential, idiosyncratic, and dose–response effects of methylphenidate. *Journal of Consulting and Clinical Psychology, 54,* 334–341.

Rehm, L. P. (1977). A self-control model of depression. *Behavior Therapy, 8,* 787–804.

Rehm, L. P., Kaslow, N. J., and Rabin, A. S. (1987). Cognitive and behavioral targets in a self-control therapy program for depression. *Journal of Consulting and Clinical Psychology, 55,* 60–67.

Reynolds, W. M., and Coats, K. I. (1986). A comparison of cognitive–behavior therapy and relaxation training for the treatment of depression in adolescents. *Journal of Consulting and Clinical Psychology, 54,* 653–660.

Richard, B. A., and Dodge, K. A. (1982). Social maladjustment and problem solving in school aged children. *Journal of Consulting and Clinical Psychology, 50,* 226–233.

Robin, A. L., Schneider, M., and Dolnick, M. (1976). The turtle technique: An extended case study of self-control in the classroom. *Psychology in the Schools, 73,* 449–453.

Ronan, K. R., Kendall, P. C., and Rowe, M. (1993). *Negative affectivity in children: Development and validation of a self-statement questionnaire.* Manuscript submitted for publication.

Rosenthal, R. H., and Allen, T. W. (1980). Intratask distractibility in hyperkinetic and nonhyperkinetic children. *Journal of Abnormal Child Psychology, 8,* 175–187.

Routh, D. K., and Schroeder, C. S. (1976). Standardized playroom measures as indices of hyperactivity. *Journal of Abnormal Child Psychology, 4,* 199–207.

Rubin, K. H., and Clark, M. L. (1983). Preschool teachers' ratings of behavioral problems: Observational, sociometric, and social–cognitive correlates. *Journal of Abnormal Child Psychology, 11,* 273–285.

Rubin, K. H., Moller, L., and Emptage, A. (1987). The Preschool Behavior Questionnaire: A useful index of behavior in elementary school-age children. *Canadian Journal of Behavioral Sciences, 19,* 86–100.

Schleser, R., Meyers, A. W., Cohen, R., and Thackwray, D. (1983). Self-instruction interventions with non-self-controlled children: Effects of discovery versus faded rehearsal. *Journal of Consulting and Clinical Psychology, 51,* 954–955.

Siegel, L. J., and Peterson, L. (1980). Stress reduction in young dental patients through coping skills and sensory information. *Journal of Consulting and Clinical Psychology, 48*, 785–787.

Siegel, L. J., and Peterson, L. (1981). Maintenance effects of coping skills and sensory information on young children's response to repeated dental procedures. *Behavior Therapy, 12*, 530–535.

Silverman, W. K. (1987). *Anxiety Disorders Interview Schedule for Children (ADIS-C)*. Albany, New York: Center for Stress and Anxiety Disorders.

Slaby, R. G., and Guerra, N. G. (1988). Cognitive mediators of aggression in adolescent offenders. 1. Assessment. *Developmental Psychology, 24*, 580–588.

Smith, T. W., Ingram, R. E., and Brehm, S. S. (1983). Social anxiety, anxious self-preoccupation, and recall of self-relevant information. *Journal of Personality and Social Psychology, 44*, 1276–1283.

Spivack, G., and Shure, M. (1974). *Social adjustment of young children*. San Francisco: Jossey-Bass.

Stark, K. D., Rouse, L. W., and Livingston, R. (1991). Treatment of depression during childhood and adolescence: Cognitive–behavioral procedures for the family. In P. C. Kendall (Ed.), *Child and adolescent therapy: Cognitive–behavioral procedures* (pp. 165–208). New York: Guilford Press.

Stevens, R., and Pihl, R. O. (1983). Learning to cope with school: A study of the effects of a coping skill training program with test-vulnerable seventh grade students. *Cognitive Therapy and Research, 7*, 155–158.

Swets, J. A., and Kristofferson, A. B. (1970). Attention. *Annual Review of Psychology, 21*, 339–366.

Tant, J. L., and Douglas, V. I. (1982). Problem solving in hyperactive, normal, and reading disabled boys. *Journal of Abnormal Child Psychology, 10*, 285–306.

Ullman, D. G., Barkley, R. A., and Brown, H. W. (1978). The behavioral symptoms of hyperkinetic children who successfully responded to stimulant drug treatment. *American Journal of Orthopsychiatry, 48*, 425–437.

Waas, G. A. (1988). Social attributional biases of peer-rejected and aggressive children. *Child Development, 59*, 969–992.

Walters, J., and Peters, R. D. (1980). *Social problem solving in aggressive boys*. Paper presented at the annual meeting at the Canadian Psychological Association, Calgary.

Wechsler, D. (1974). *Manual for the Wechsler Intelligence Scale for Children — revised*. New York: Psychological Corp.

Weithorn, C. J., and Kagan, E. (1979). Training first graders of high-activity level to improve performance through verbal self-direction. *Journal of Learning Disabilities, 12*, 82–88.

Wells, K. C., and Vitulano, L. A. (1984). Anxiety disorders in childhood. In S. Turner (Ed.), *Behavioral theories and treatment of anxiety* (pp. 413–433). New York: Plenum.

Whalen, C. K. (1989). Attention-deficit hyperactivity disorder. In T. H. Ollendick and M. Hersen (Eds.), *Handbook of child psychopathology* (2nd ed., pp. 131–169). New York. Plenum.

Whalen, C. K., Henker, B., and Hinshaw, S. P. (1985). Cognitive–behavioral therapies for hyperactive children: Premises, problems and prospects. *Journal of Abnormal Child Psychology, 13*, 391–410.

Wong, B., Harris, K., and Graham, S. (1991). Academic applications of cognitive–behavioral programs with learning disabled students. In P. C. Kendall (Ed.), *Child and adolescent therapy: Cognitive behavioral procedures* (pp. 245–275). New York: Guilford Press.

Zatz, S., and Chassin, L. (1983). Cognitions of test anxious children. *Journal of Consulting and Clinical Psychology, 51*(4), 526–534.

Zatz, S., and Chassin, L. (1985). Cognitions of test anxious children under naturalistic test-taking conditions. *Journal of Consulting and Clinical Psychology, 53,* 393–401.

Zentall, S. S. (1985). Stimulus control factors in search performance of hyperactive children. *Journal of Learning Disabilities, 18,* 480–485.

Cognitive Deficits in Schizophrenia

Richard A. Steffy

University of Waterloo

It is safe to say that schizophrenic patients are impaired, relative to most others, in just about every psychological, social, and psychophysiological function imaginable. A century or more of keen clinical observation dating back to the work of Emil Kraepelin and Eugen Bleuler, and extending through the last half century of laboratory investigations, has documented differences in nearly all levels of psychological functioning. Clinician's attention has been directed mainly toward faults in thinking, emotional control, and interpersonal relating. Researchers have found weaknesses in attention, memory, thought, language, and other information processes (Chapman and Chapman, 1973; Cromwell, 1975; Neale and Oltmanns, 1980; Steffy and Waldman, in press). As might be expected, both anatomical and physiological irregularities also have been found to be abundant in schizophrenic individuals. Reduced metabolic and blood-flow functioning in frontal areas (Buchsbaum, 1990), enlarged ventricles (Johnstone *et al.*, 1989), temporal lobe asymmetries (Crow, 1990), and countless other observations of CNS and ANS differentiating features have become the subject of considerable interest in recent investigations. From a great volume of research, then, schizophrenic patients are seen to differ from normal controls and in many instances from other patients, no matter whether simple or complex functions are studied. Workers in our lab often

429

commented that schizophrenics seemed to show deficits on just about everything except shoelace tying, until lacing behavior, too, was reported to be faulty (Allen, 1987).

Although hundreds of studies report features differentiating schizophrenics from controls, for the most part this work has not clarified our understanding of schizophrenia because the differences reflected only *generalized deficits*, arising from pervasive inadequacies. For a test to document a *differential deficit* or specific dysfunction, it must show a greater level of deficit than observed on measures of general functioning. For example, one might wish to claim that schizophrenics have a specific visual information-processing (VIP) deficit (relative to control subjects) on the basis of weak performances that result from the laboratory presentation of distracting stimuli. To establish such a view, it would be necessary to show first of all that schizophrenic subjects tested on a nondistracted version of a VIP test have a normal range of scores, and then to ensure that the distracter stimulation used was not confounded with other demands for thinking or intellectual ability — demands that schizophrenic subjects are generally found less capable meeting than are controls. To ensure that schizophrenics are not shown as being different simply because of methodological artifact, Chapman and Chapman (1973) have set standards for the matching of the reliability and the discriminating power of items used to assess levels of an experimental factor. Although some would argue that matching of items is not the only corrective to confounds from generalized deficits — and may on occasion be a misleading approach when the matching on one variable unmatches on another variable (Knight, 1984) — nevertheless, the Chapmans' argument has sharpened our appreciation for what constitutes an adequate experimental difference in documenting specific performance deficits. Unfortunately, early research was less likely to be cautious about the source of deficit performance than was more recent work, so our review of the multifaceted and voluminous research of schizophrenic cognitive deficits has focused on the most cohesive and repeated trends in this domain.

The Importance of "Thought Disorder" Symptoms in Schizophrenic Diagnosis

The fact that schizophrenic patients have many diverse dysfunctions has also been reflected in the classification systems used to diagnose individual patients over the past century. Tables 12.1, 12.2, and 12.3 give representative diagnostic systems from North America, Europe, and empirical classification studies, respectively, all of which show breadth in the range of individual symptoms (thought, perception, motor, etc.) used to diag-

TABLE 12.1 Psychological Dysfunctions Reflected in Classification Systems: Standard American System

Psychological function	DSM-III (1990)	DSM-II (1968)
Thought content	Delusions (bizarre, somatic, grandiose, religious, nihilistic), delusions with incoherence	Thoughts known by others, sense of control by others, bizarre delusions, special meanings to everyday events, autistic thinking
Thought form	Incoherence	Thinking is vague, obscure, elliptical, expression is often incomprehensible, breaks and interpolations in speech
Affect	Blunted affect (accompanied by incoherence)	Mood is shallow or incongruous with situation
Motor	Catatonic or other disorganized behavior (with incoherence)	Inertia, negativism, stupor; catatonic reactions
Perceptual	Hallucinations with persecutory content. Auditory hallucinations about the self	Auditory hallucination. Irrelevant features seem unduly important

TABLE 12.2 Psychological Dysfunctional Reflected in Classification Systems: European System

Psychological function	Schneider (1959)	Langfeldt (1939)
Thought content	Audible thoughts, thought insertions, withdrawal, and broadcasting. Made volition	Delusions of being controlled; willpower, movement, verbalization, and feeling problems; thoughts broadcasted
Thought form		
Affect	Made feelings	
Motor	Somatic passivity	
Perceptual	Voices arguing, voices commenting, delusional percepts	Somatic hallucinations

TABLE 12.3   Psychological Dysfunctions Reflected in Classification Systems:
Empirically Defined System

Psychological function	WHO-12 Signs (1973)	Newmark *et al.* (1975)
Thought content	Delusions (widespread, bizarre, nihilistic) Thought transmittal	Autism, symbolism, delusions, magical thinking, paralogia, paleologic thinking
Thought form	Incoherent speech	Loose associations, incoherence, overinclusive thinking, neologisms, verbiageration, blocking, circumstantiality
Affect	Blunted affect	Flat affect, ambivalence, agitation
Motor		Stereotyped behavior
Perceptual		Hallucinations

nose schizophrenia. Despite the diversity, one class of symptoms, *thought disorder* (cognitive symptoms), stands out among all as the accepted major symptom of schizophrenia, although there remain serious definitional and measurement problems, for example:

1. As may be noted in the first two rows of the table, diagnostic systems consider both delusions (false beliefs, such as the notion that one has supernatural powers, that reflect a disturbance in the *content* of speech despite adequate syntax), and also problems of language structure (disturbance of the *form* of the language). The latter may include the use of neologisms (freshly coined words), words chosen because of rhyming features ("He sanged and hanged on the range"), and other faults that interfere with communications. Although these disturbances of content and form are both considered to be classic signs of "thought disorder," they are generally regarded as independent features. In fact, the content and form distinctions are congruent with the important distinction of "distortions" and "deficiencies" introduced by Kendall (1985, 1991) to separate cognitive pathologies that reflect dysfunctional from those of insufficient thinking processes.

2. Dysfunctional affect (typically witnessed as a flat, blunted, unresponsive quality to voice tone and facial expression, or occasionally as an overly emotional response to an event), attention and perceptual organization problems may better account for schizophrenic disturbance and outcome than thought-disorder disturbances (Knight *et al.*, 1979).

3. Distinguishing between impaired language and impaired thought has proven impossible; arguments continue in the literature about whether spoken language or thinking is the most appropriate system to study (Rochester and Martin, 1979).

4. Clinical indications of thought disorder have low levels of sensitivity. Many diagnosed schizophrenics do not show thought disorder either in natural language or on psychological measures (e.g., Bellak, 1979). Moreover, thought-disorder measures show weak specificity; diagnostic groups other than schizophrenia show flagrant signs of thought disorder (Harrow and Quinlan, 1985).

Despite these definitional problems, DSM-III-R places a heavy emphasis on thought-disorder symptoms to diagnose schizophrenia. The primary question of this chapter asks whether the long-standing investment in studies of thought disorder has fulfilled its promise.

Our account starts with a quick review of the classical positions advanced by Kraepelin and Bleuler. Their writings clearly set the stage for many hundreds of investigations into cognition — communication problems and inferred thought-disordered processes. The next section reports the product of much clinical and lab work during the past half century, seeking to clarify mechanisms underlying this important symptom complex. Current and "new frontier" concerns are then briefly described. This part of the story promises good progress, but it also shows the distance yet to travel, especially in the development of rehabilitative technologies described in the final portion of the chapter.

EARLY CONTRIBUTIONS

Emil Kraepelin (1856–1926)

Considered the "father of modern psychiatry," Emil Kraepelin made a profound contribution to the classification of the psychiatric disorders. After working in Wilhelm Wundt's Leipzig laboratory, Kraepelin developed his first volume of disease listings in 1883. From his clinical insights the diverse disorders of catatonia, paranoia, and hebephrenia were described to share similarities — particularly, a bad outcome — that allowed these previously separate syndromes to be grouped together as one disorder. By the time of his fifth edition, schizophrenia had been identified and labeled as a "dementing process" (*Verbloedungsprocesse*). Subsequently (in 1899), the label "dementia praecox" was chosen to characterize the early onset and the progressive deterioration (or dementia) that Kraepelin regarded to be the defining attributes of this disorder.

Kraepelin's definition of schizophrenia collected many diverse symptoms under one roof. In his eighth edition published in 1919 and translated into English by R. M. Barclay, Kraepelin had amassed 36 major categories of schizophrenic dysfunction, including a heavy investment in thought-disordered symptoms, which he considered of utmost importance in defining dementia praecox. His list of symptoms included thought deficits (e.g., problems in the train of thought, stereotyped thinking, thought constraint) along with problems of attention, perception, will, coordination, and other dysfunctions. In the fashion characteristic of his diligent personal style, Kraepelin illustrated each category with dozens of particular symptoms (replete with extensive behavioral descripters) that helped identify the dysfunction. His choice of descripters will stand forever as a monument to high-quality descriptive psychiatry. What Kraepelin did not provide was a clear idea about the mechanism underlying the disorder. He did, however, feel strongly that there was a single unifying neurobiological cause that underwrote all of the many symptomatic variations, a point of view he shared with Eugen Bleuler.

Eugen Bleuler (1857–1939)

A second major contribution to current definitions of schizophrenia came from the work of Eugen Bleuler. A contemporary of Kraepelin, Bleuler lived in Switzerland where he served as the director of the Borgholzli Clinic and had professorial rank at the University of Zurich, an appointment he took in 1898. Bleuler coined the term "schizophrenia" in 1911 in his text *Dementia Praecox or the Group of Schizophrenias* (translated into English in 1950), partly in dissatisfaction with the view of deterioration and early onset implicit in Kraepelin's dementia praecox label. In fact, it was Bleuler's writing about remitted schizophrenics that eventually led Kraepelin to rescind his conservative view that progressive deterioration occurred in all dementia praecox cases; Bleuler argued that at least 15% of schizophrenics recovered from the disorder.

To understand Bleuler's views of schizophrenia, it is helpful to recognize that for awhile he was a member of Freud's inner circle, working closely with Carl Jung (who Bleuler hired as an assistant physician in his Borgholzli clinic). Although Bleuler eventually broke off his association with both Freud and Jung, psychoanalytic theory permeated his ideas about schizophrenia, particularly the functional significance of symptoms. Bleuler boldly described mental faults and speculated on the possibility that some schizophrenic symptoms are compensatory mechanisms used essentially to help control confusion consequent to the breakdown. To amplify this view, Bleuler distinguished between "fundamental" and "accessory" symptoms. Fundamental symptoms were considered to be pathognomonic, but unfortunately, his list of fundamentals contained inferred, difficult-to-define features. The four he proposed, known as the four *As*, included disturbances of: (1) *association* (problems in the organization of thought); *affect* (indifference, moodiness, and inappropriate displays of emotion); *ambivalence* (an internal contradiction between impulses and thoughts); and *autism* (withdrawal from reality contact and a predominance of fantasy in thought). In contrast, Bleuler's list of accessory symptoms were observable behaviors such as delusional statements and hallucinatory reports. Bleuler gave them second-class status because they are found in other psychopathologies, and he regarded them to be coping or restitutive reactions to disorganization rather than core attributes.

Kraepelin and Bleuler's different approaches to classification led to different diagnostic practices. Kraepelin's atheoretical descriptive approach (linking diagnostic labels to clearly observable features) became foremost in the work of European psychiatry and persisted in subsequent classification schemes, primarily the positions of Langfeldt (1939) and Schneider (1959) (see Table 12.2). On the American continent, however, Bleuler's position was favored over Kraepelin's, possibly because of the acclaim given to Freud by American leaders such as G. Stanley Hall and Adolf Meyers. From a historical perspective, the American choice was quite costly. A reliance upon Bleuler's unobservable constructs (the four *As*) in diagnostic practice made the criteria for schizophrenia progressively more murky. In the first two editions of the Diagnostic Statistical Manual (DSM), the description of schizophrenia was impossibly vague, thereby contributing to the vastly increased use of the schizophrenic diagnosis in the United States in contrast to European practice.[1] In fact, when the diagnostic practices on the two continents were investigated, as expected, they were found to reflect quite different standards employed by their respective diagnosticians (Kuriansky *et al.*, 1974).

American psychiatry, in the 1970s, set into motion a fairly severe revision in its diagnostic manual to make the standards much more precise, reliable, and in line with the diagnostic practices in the International Classification of Diseases (ICD) used by European practitioners (Spitzer *et al.*, 1980). The current diagnostic system, DSM-III-R (American Psychiatric Association, 1987), is considered to be much more precise and reliable, and was designed to yield a substantially lower rate of schizophrenic diagnoses

[1]Solovay *et al.* (1987) considered the new availability of phenothiazine medications to have inflated schizophrenia diagnosis in this era. It can be reasoned that practitioners were drawn to using the label because the diagnostic label legitimized the use of these antipsychotic agents. The problem with this explanation, however, is that it does not explain why this dynamic occurred on the American and not the European continent.

than that of earlier systems (Strauss and Gift, 1977). The problems that may have resulted from profligate use of the schizophrenic label in research before DSM-III arrived are impossible to determine in retrospect, but one may suspect the validity of research using earlier DSM versions of schizophrenia because of the many different types of disturbance included in the label. Some investigators attempted to control population heterogeneity by using collateral measures of pathology (e.g., measures of chronicity, degree of withdrawal, process-reactive ratings, and various research-based classifications) as auxilliaries to the schizophrenic diagnosis, but most of the earlier work on schizophrenics' thought disorder must be viewed with some caution because of the imprecise diagnostic standards available at the time.

Bleuler's Concept of Schizophrenic Cognition

Bleuler was more adventuresome than Kraepelin in attempting to describe a mechanism (the concept of "broken associative threads") by which thought disorder occurred in schizophrenics. Based on the view that all ideas, their connections to words, and words' connections to sentences are interlinked in a neural network with individual "threads," Bleuler argued that a full array of connections is required for normal thinking. When for one reason or another the threads break, thinking becomes jumbled, shows excessive preoccupation with particulars, is governed by extraneous influences, and otherwise appears "schizophrenic" in quality. Bleuler departed from Freud in the development of this conception insofar as he shared Kraepelin's view that some type of neurobiological disease process would eventually be discovered to account for the broken associative threads.

The ideas advanced by Bleuler were naive and untestable in comparison to today's cognitive models, but they did inspire a series of investigations, built upon word-association test procedures. Bleuler felt that this task (asking people to give the first word that comes to mind in reply to stimulus words) was an appropriate pathway to explore loose association. His student, Carl Jung, had devised the word-association technique to investigate mental processes, and their mutual investment in this procedure was soon to be encouraged by a massive empirical study conducted by Kent and Rosanoff (1910). Kent and Rosanoff found that schizophrenic patients gave many more "individual" responses to stimulus words (defined as answers unique to a sample of 1000 normal subjects' responses). Other investigators also found that schizophrenics gave highly individualized responses (e.g., Dokecki et al., 1968); however, a number of investigators made it clear that the mere presence of idiosyncratic responses does not give experimental support to Bleuler's theories about "broken threads." Problems of mishearing the stimulus words (Moon *et al.*, 1968) and state variation (momentary anxiety, differential responding to instructional set, and the like) were found to confound the observed deviancy in schizophrenic answers (O'Brian and Weingartner, 1970). The word-association techniques simply did not have sufficient power to test the "broken threads" model of Bleuler's. In addition, more parsimonious explanations of schizophrenics' idiosyncratic responding were to be advanced in later research. Despite the shortcomings in this early work, the ball was now rolling, so to speak, and a heavy investment in theorizing and study of schizophrenic thought disorder followed over the next half century.

EMPIRICAL AND THEORETICAL DEVELOPMENTS

The major task facing any investigator of schizophrenic processes is the problem of inferring events in the head from either the patient's language production or response to various tests of language or problem-solving challenges. Workers in this area have taken quite creative tacks in approaching conceptual dysfunctions, including studies of delusional themes, deviant language use, and laboratory measures of cognitive dysfunctions and of related information processes.

The Study of Delusions

There has been a heavy representation of delusional symptoms in various diagnostic systems (see the weight given to them in Tables 12.1, 12.2, and 12.3), but the study of delusional behavior has been disappointing. Oltmanns and Maher (1988) recently commented, "Delusions may be among the most poorly understood phenomena in psychopathology." In a major review of delusional thinking in 1983, Winters and Neale found the lack of research into delusions surprising given that the World Health Organization (WHO) International Psychiatric Study of Schizophrenia, investigating definitions of schizophrenia across nine countries, found that delusional symptoms were generally found in over half of the schizophrenic patients (WHO, 1973). For example, delusions of reference (a sense that people are taking special notice of one's actions) were present in 67%, and delusions of persecution in 64%, of their sample of 306 schizophrenic patients.

Delusions are admittedly difficult to study. They are diagnosed with low levels of clinician agreement, are hard to distinguish from other varieties of beliefs and self deceptions, and are found in high proportions of many other diagnostic categories, for example, mood disturbances, conditions associated with substance abuse, and borderline personality disorders (Kendler *et al.*, 1983). One estimate indicates that 70 different disorders are known to be accompanied by delusional symptoms (Maher, 1988). Although elusive, they are an important feature of current diagnostic practice and deserve the increased experimental attention recently shown in some labs (Chapman and Chapman, 1988; George and Neufeld, 1985; Harrow *et al.*, 1988).

Earlier theories about schizophrenia range widely in their efforts to explain delusions. Classic psychoanalytic theory, for example, stated that paranoid delusions were projections of repressed homosexual impulses. Sullivan viewed delusions as mechanisms devised to save self-esteem or to provide a sense of personal security. Learning theorists in turn have tried to explain delusions in terms of avoidance responses, arising especially from fear of interpersonal encounters (Mednick, 1958). In support of this view, Shimkunas (1972) found that delusional themes increased (albeit to a nonsignificant degree) when schizophrenic patients were instructed to give self-disclosures, reflecting the possibility that delusional behavior derives from fears of interpersonal rejection.

Winters and Neale's (1983) excellent summary finds that the experimentation deriving from early theories generally had methodological flaws, but collectively gave some guidance to future trends. Theories about delusions tend to follow one of two major pathways. The predominant one centers on information-processing deficits, for example, a perceptual overload, as described by the creative research of Heilbrun (1975). The second approach views delusions as *motivated behavior*, essentially an attempt to make sense out of overwhelming experiences. In this approach, the delusional belief is considered to be a product of normal cognitive processes that are employed by patients to cope with experiences that are aversive or otherwise too difficult to assimilate (Maher, 1988; Shimkunas, 1972).

One variety of research capitalizes on the regular presence of a systematized delusional scheme in paranoid patients. George and Neufeld (1985) have reviewed studies showing perceptual cognitive style differences between paranoid and nonparanoid schizophrenics, and conclude that a "jump-to-conclusions" response strategy characterizes paranoid thinking. An especially graphic paranoid–nonparanoid difference was observed by McCormick and Broekema (1978) who required their subjects simply to identify slides of common objects presented initially out of focus and to give the confidence of their judgments. Nonparanoid schizophrenic and normal control subjects' accuracy improved and confidence increased as the pictures were systematically brought into focus. Paranoid schizophrenics, however, gave low-accuracy, high-confidence guesses from the start, and were slow to improve their accuracy as visibility was improved.

Other investigators paint a similar picture of the paranoid schizophrenic patient's impetuous, "my mind is made up" quality of response (Broga and Neufeld, 1981; Magaro, 1980).

Although the progress in understanding paranoid response styles has provided some understanding of delusions, until recently little direct study has occurred. As will be reviewed in later sections, new measures mapping dimensions of delusions and their change over time (Chapman and Chapman, 1988; Harrow *et al.*, 1988) and behavioral modification strategies (e.g., Lowe and Chadwick, 1990) offer special promise for better understanding of delusional beliefs.

Aberrant Language Production

Second only to delusional content, signs of disordered language rank highly in classification systems used to diagnose schizophrenia. Schizophrenics are notorious for their problems of communication clarity, with many statements characterized by vague, irrelevant language and loosely connected ideas (comparable to Bleuler's "loose associations"). Empirical investigations of language disorder, however, report only modest percentages of schizophrenic patients showing such disturbances of language. The WHO (1973) International Pilot Study of Schizophrenia, for example, noted that only about 10% of their large sample showed classic signs of language disturbance. Schizophrenic patients generally make sensible use of words and produce sentences with adequate grammatical structure (Rochester and Martin, 1979). Even those judged to be especially thought disordered by clinical judges rarely show dysfunctional language at the level of individual words, phrases, or sentences. Given that language faults are not typical of many schizophrenic patients, research practices recently have incorporated designs that contrast diagnostic (schizophrenic and other) groups with and without thought disorder (e.g., Harvey, 1983; Rochester and Martin, 1979).

Studies of language have relied on a variety of measures to assay segments of free speech (e.g., statements from a 5-minute tape recording of a "personal life experience") or open-ended verbalizations given to projective tests. These investigations include the search for clinical signs, receptivity to others' language, fine-grained linguistic analyses, and narrative speech. Reviews of each of these strategies follows.

Clinical Symptoms

From clinical investigations of patients dating back to the work of Bleuler and Kraepelin, lists of disordered-language behaviors (such as derailment, poverty of speech, tangential thinking, bizarreness, incoherence, pressure of speech) have been compiled into symptom ratings and checklists (e.g., the Thought, Language and Communication Scale (TLC) of Andreason, 1979). The first major inventory of thought-disordered symptoms was created by Rapaport *et al.* in 1945 (updated in 1968). It was constructed with the view that psychosis reflected a breakdown in "psychological distance," that is, too little or too great an influence from stimulus materials. Schizophrenic verbalizations (especially to projective tests) might show "distanciation" with a focus on irrelevancies or remote symbols (e.g., "this blot is the work of the Devil") or it might show a loss of perspective reflected in personal intrusions and emotional overresponse to the stimuli. Although this "too great and too little" distance distinction has found some support in recent multidimensional scaling efforts (Schuldberg and Boster, 1985), major efforts to codify thought-disorder signs came from refinements of Rapaport's system made by others.

Watkins and Stauffacher (1952) developed the Delta Index, an instrument that includes scaling of the severity of the deviant category listings, from Rapaport's inventory of speech-disturbance signs. The Delta Index reliably discriminated between schizophrenics and others (Powers and Hamlin, 1955), as did its successor, the Thought Disorder Index (TDI) created by Johnston and Holzman (1979). The TDI's latest version includes 23 thought-disorder categories with a 6-factor structure resolution, and has shown quite satisfactory interrater agreements and internal reliability. Harrow's Bizarre-Idiosyncratic Thinking Index (Harrow and Quinlan, 1985; Marengo *et al.*, 1986) also includes a large variety of thought-disordered statements, ranging from the most subtle to the most flagrant disturbances, allowing assessment of language-structure problems, content peculiarity, and intermixing of personal and task material. Harrow's scales intercorrelate well with each other, yield quite good reliability, and show adequate concurrent and predictive validity (Marengo *et al.*, 1986). These clinical symptom measures have been found sensitive to change in clinical status (Hurt *et al.*, 1983), are capable of distinguishing children at heightened risk for schizophrenia from controls (Arboleda and Holzman, 1985), and also show promise of good construct validity (Nuechterlein *et al.*, 1986).

It is worth noting, however, that although aggregate measures (summarizing across a variety of signs or global ratings) have shown adequate validity, individual indicators are rarely successful discriminators. Reilly *et al.* (1975), for example, found only "loose associations" and "communication gaps," among many individual signs, to yield significant group differences. Of further concern, many measures of thought disorder are not capable of discriminating among major psychiatric disorders (Johnston and Holzman, 1979; Harrow and Quinlan, 1985); some of the scales are more sensitive to bipolar (manic) than to schizophrenic disorders. Interesting work attempts to discriminate manic and schizophrenic patients. Solovay *et al.* (1987) report that manic patients' thought disorder is likely to show playful combinatory qualities, with flippant, energetic, and extravagant flavors to their speech. In contrast, schizophrenics tend to use fragmented statements with ill-defined referrents and frequent interpenetration of personal issues. Solovay and colleagues characterize schizophrenic thinking as revealing bewilderment and turmoil. For example, a 22-year-old female with a lengthy history of schizophrenic symptoms said, "They told me you would know about me. I don't know why you and Jimmy torture me this way. I don't know why you don't like me." Manics, however, are more colorful and playful in self-expression, for example, "Went to the dance and fish-fry last night, doc. Had a 'dancefrying' good time — gals flying around all over the place."

A somewhat different pathway to understanding thought disorder has been pursued by the team of Singer and Wynne (1965) investigating *communication deviance* (CD) signs in the language of relatives of schizophrenic patients. Their work focuses on the manner in which thought disorder is transmitted through the language style of parents rather than a documentation of patients' language disorder. Singer and Wynne believe that parents' failure to provide adequate indications of their meanings and adequate models as communicators may cause the bewilderment and language dysfunctions that appear in their offsprings' schizophrenic episodes. Their measures assess the degree to which a shared focus of attention is represented in the language habits of relatives of schizophrenic patients. This work has been rewarded with remarkably strong findings. Singer blindly matched offspring with parents in 41 out of 46 cases and separated schizophrenic, borderline schizophrenic, neurotic, and normal individuals [a finding repeatedly validated (Singer and Wynne, 1966a)], with many third variables (race, class, and the like) ruled out (Singer and Wynne, 1966b). Measures of CD and thought disorder were not found to be highly correlated (Johnston and Holzman, 1979) in schizophrenic patients, thus confirming Singer and Wynne's view that their measure is more germane to developmental influences rather than to manifest illness.

Measures of Language Receptivity

Possibly, schizophrenics talk in strange ways because they do not understand what others say to them, and they have their own personal language (Schwartz, 1982). To track this possibility, Hotchkiss and Harvey (1986) reviewed the "contextual constraint" and the "click paradigm" strategies used to test schizophrenic patients' capacity to understand language. In the contextual constraint studies, word groupings are devised to provide different approximations to good English sentences. Schizophrenics are found less able to recall all sentences — regardless of level of structure — than normals, but show improvement in recall of statements with greater approximation to real language proportional to normal subjects' improvement (Gerver, 1967; Truscott, 1970). A similar impression of schizophrenics' processing of language was obtained from the "embedded click" approach. In this task subjects are asked to listen to sentences in which click sounds are imposed at points before, during, or after clause boundaries (breaks in the discourse). The overall findings from this work suggest that schizophrenics made patterns of errors similar to normal subjects, that is, they tend to displace the sound of the click from within the clause toward the boundaries of the clause. Although schizophrenic communication problems may make them seem unreceptive to information, these findings suggest that their language impairment should not be attributed to an incapacity to understand others' statements.

Fine-Grained Linguistic Analysis

Linguists have searched a number of detailed language features (aspects of phonology, meaning, syntax, rules of grammar, etc.) in efforts to locate what is most perplexing to listeners about thought-disordered schizophrenic speech. As early as 1944, Fairbanks found that schizophrenic patients use significantly fewer different parts of speech and fewer different words in their expressions than do normals. A *type-token ratio* indexing the relationship between the number of different words (types) and the total number of words (tokens) used has repeatedly been found lower for schizophrenic patients across investigations, and especially so for speech-disordered subsamples (e.g., Manschreck *et al.*, 1981). These findings suggest that schizophrenics' language imparts less information than the language of others. A similar impression comes from the study of *object-subject ratios*. Maher *et al.* (1966) found the predicates of schizophrenic statements to include significantly more object nouns relative to subject nouns than other groups. Schizophrenic patients' high object/subject ratios reflected repetitive, superfluous, and otherwise wordy object clauses in their communications.

A number of investigators have used the *cloze technique* in which individual words are deleted from sentences in order to learn how easily normal readers or listeners can estimate what the missing word might be. Schizophrenic statements with words deleted by the experimenter are found less easy to complete by others (Cozlino, 1983).[2] The evidence from these linguistic analyses suggests that wordy and uninformative speech patterns regularly found in schizophrenic patients are a reliable feature of the disorder; however, it also shows that schizophrenics' understanding of speech is not the weak link in their language faults.

Linguistic Analyses of Narratives

Rochester and Martin, in their 1979 study of schizophrenic "Crazy Talk," made an extensive psycholinguistic analysis of several types of narrative speech samples to compare the language of thought-disordered (TD) schizophrenics, normal control subjects, and a group of diagnosed schizophrenic patients with no manifest thought-disorder symptoms (NTD). Although thought disturbances (form or content) are considered the primary diagnostic sign of a schizophrenic disorder, delusional thought and deficient language do not occur in all cases. Hallucinations (perceptual distortions), problems of affect, and other symptoms (American Psychiatric Association, 1987) permitted a diagnosis of the NTD schizophrenics used creatively in this study to disentangle TD symptoms from the schizophrenic disorder.

Unlike other psycholinguists (e.g., Chaika, 1974) who searched for aphasic speech signs (paraphrasias, neologisms, phonological distortions, etc.), or those who examined particular language scores (e.g., type-token ratios), Rochester and her colleagues focused on communication factors that make thought-disordered statements difficult to comprehend. Their work used both expert and lay judges instructed to evaluate individual statements in transcribed narratives. Rochester *et al.* (1977) found lay judges to be 75% accurate in designating "disruptive statements" that mental-health workers judged to be "thought-disordered," with a modest false-alarm rate of only 5% for normal subjects' statements. This accuracy is remarkable insofar as most of schizophrenic patients' individual phrases are adequately coined, with good syntax and clear meanings, even among those patients specially selected to show disorganized and confusing language. With this complexity in mind, Rochester and her colleagues have searched narratives to learn why schizophrenic language seems hazy, vague, and otherwise deficient. Three features were found to discriminate TD schizophrenics from others, namely, long interclause pauses, excessive

[2]Although this interesting technique uses normal judges to index the communication flaw, it is problematic because the results vary considerably with the verbal skill of the listener-judges (Hotchkiss and Harvey, 1986).

use of lexical clause connectors (from cohesion analyses), and weak clarity of references.

In Rochester and Martin's (1979) study, TD schizophrenics gave distinctively *long pauses* between clauses, suggesting that an organizational problem or a need to restablish their own attentional set after phrases had been completed might be responsible for the long pause durations. Consistent with these findings, Clemmer (1980) has shown that schizophrenics use greater numbers of hesitation phrases (e.g., "ah"s and "uh"s) than do normal subjects.

Rochester and Martin (1979) also examined the way in which schizophrenic patients tie their thoughts together within a narrative, using a cohesion analysis to study interconnections of speech elements. Rochester and Martin found that TD schizophrenics used fewer cohesive tie linkages (e.g., simple conjunctions like "and," "but," "so") than do normal control subjects, but make significantly greater use of *lexical cohesion*, particularly in an interview-based narrative. They tend to forge connections among their thoughts by repeating the same word or by liberal use of synonyms from sentence to sentence. They may, for example, rely heavily on words with similar roots: "I need my *strength*, I wish I had *stronger* arms. The *strongest* are the best." The TD schizophrenic's reliance on lexical connections is consistent with impressions of schizophrenic speakers as being more repetitive and making more concrete reference to the immediate situation than do other subjects.[3]

Finally, TD schizophrenic subjects in the Rochester and Martin (1979) study showed especially weak attention to *references*. As though they assume that their listeners had prior knowledge about the topic being expressed, the TD schizophrenics often neglected to identify "nominal groups" in their speech. They may, for example, use pronouns that are not linked explicitly to anybody's name or identity (e.g., "*they* make *it* very difficult!" with no clarification of who "they" are or what "it" is). Taken collectively, these three speech differences seem to reflect impairment in the goal direction of schizophrenic communicative efforts.

From this pattern of production difficulties Rochester and Martin (1979) have speculated on the role of attentional, organizational, and short-term memory deficits in schizophrenic language problems. Linking language to the well-documented information faults of schizophrenics has been suggested by others as well (e.g., Space and Cromwell, 1978; Maher, 1988).

---

[3]Recent studies, however, cast some doubt on the ability of lexical cohesion indices to distinguish among diagnostic groups (Harvey, 1983). Ragin and Oltmanns (1986) found that schizophrenics differed from manic and schizo-affective patients, but, contrary to Rochester and Martin's (1979) results, their schizophrenic sample gave fewer lexical cohesion responses than the other disturbed groups.

Although efforts to investigate information-processing faults in language-demanding tasks have been slow to develop (as will be noted in the next section) lately they have shown excellent progress, especially in various communication analogue procedures that have been developed.

Laboratory Investigations

Since the time of the first word-association tests (Kent and Rosanoff, 1910) a number of laboratory tasks have been devised in order to clarify the mechanisms underlying thought disorder. This research has for the most part been theory driven. Some of the older versions (the regression model and the loss-of-abstract-attitude model) evolved from the notion that schizophrenic thinking simply stems from a primitive or immature mind set, perhaps a derivative of a developmental disorder, or a regression during the psychotic episodes to an earlier level of functioning. Newer approaches are built on concepts of information processes central to schizophrenic dysfunctions.

Regression Models

Freud disavowed interest in serving schizophrenic patients, but some of his followers extended Freudian theory to focus on schizophrenics' primary process thinking (Rosen, 1953). Primary process thinking — typical of young children, dreams, and delirium — is characterized by loss of reality testing, arbitrary thought processes, symbolic distortions, substitution of thoughts, and other concepts elaborated in Freudian theory. Attempts to test the relevance of the regression hypothesis have compared adult schizophrenics and adult normals with children's norms on proverbs tests (Benjamin, 1964; Gorham, 1956), word-form tests requiring use of synonyms, homonyms, and antonyms (Burstein, 1961), and measures of cause-and-effect reasoning (e.g., Cameron, 1938). These studies found that children and schizophrenic patients are both less adequate than normal adults, but their tests of the regression hypothesis has not adequately controlled the many factors other than immature reasoning that differentiate children and schizophrenics. For example, schizophrenics' tendencies to insert personal material and their susceptibility to distracting influences make their problem solving seem limited (Wegrocki, 1940). In short, there is no compelling evidence for an age-specific lag or a reversal in functioning.

Loss of Abstract Attitude: Concrete Thinking

Interviewer: "And what brings you to the hospital?"
Patient: "Mr. Jones drove me in his car."

Interviewer: "No, I meant what problems did you have."
Patient: "There was no problem, he pulled up to the front door."

Clinicians recognize this conversation as typical of concrete or literal-minded thinking patterns often encountered in schizophrenic patients. Kurt Goldstein (1939) adopted the view that such concrete thinking is an index of a major fault in personality integration, an impairment he labeled a "loss in abstract attitude." With his background in neurology and psychiatry, Goldstein recognized this loss in both brain-damaged and schizophrenic patients. Goldstein initially believed that concreteness was a major fault of both types of disorders, although he eventually reported subtle ways in which these two populations differed, such as the schizophrenic patients' greater susceptibility to personal intrusions.

Goldstein's work departed from his contemporaries' emphasis on language dysfunctions, favoring instead a laboratory (object classification) task to study dysfunctional abstractions. The task Goldstein and Schaerer (1941) devised required sorting of a set of common objects (such as tools, kitchen utensils, matches, foods, etc.) into sensible categories. Schizophrenic performances could be characterized as "stimulus bound," depicting "an unreflective, volitional fault" that causes these patients to be unduly influenced by particular task features. This limitation makes it especially difficult for them to divide attention when two features need to be regarded concurrently, a point reinforced by modern investigation of information-processing deficits (e.g., Knight, 1984; Spring, 1985).

Goldstein's views were popular with clinicians and researchers alike in the 1940s and 1950s, but this work has been critiqued because of his use of vague concepts ("abstract attitude" and "conscious volition"), the nonstandardized way in which his tests were delivered to subjects, a low rate of deficit, and the presence of third variable (e.g., distraction) influences on the data (Chapman and Chapman, 1973). Nevertheless, investigations with psychometrically more sophisticated procedures have continued to show abstraction test differences between schizophrenic and control subjects, and also have found differences among schizophrenic subgroups (Harrow *et al.*, 1974; Tutko and Spence, 1962). Moreover, some work has made progress in clarifying the mechanism of concreteness. Miller (1967) contrasted a set of objects that could be appropriately sorted according to either of two features (e.g., the nature of the material used and the accepted use of the object) with a set designed around a single feature, in order to test the role of decision load in eliciting concrete thinking. He learned that schizophrenic patients were disadvantaged relative to normal controls when there was an extra requirement for managing conjoined features, a finding he interpreted to reflect a selective attention deficit rather than conceptual concreteness.

Information-Processing Deficits and Distortions

Although developmentally based theories of thought disorder seem descriptive of the immature thought patterns often observed in schizophrenic thinking, such views have little explanatory power, especially when the apparent primitivization results from excessive preoccupation with detail, selective attention difficulties, and problems of distraction. Because information-processing deficits have often been invoked to explain language or thinking disorder, it is not surprising that other theories of thought disorder attempted to build measures based upon notions of conceptual and perceptual faults.

Studies of Erroneous Logic

Measures of schizophrenic patients' reasoning capacities have been devised to study schizophrenic errors of logic.

> Hitler had a moustache.
> My boss has a similar-looking moustache.
> My boss is Hitler.

The logical fallacy of an undistributed middle term or sentence predicate (i.e., the moustache) is obvious in the above syllogism (an argument based on a major and minor premise followed by a conclusion). Clinicians' notice of distorted logic in schizophrenics propelled the modest syllogism into prominence through the efforts of E. Von Domarus (1944) and his advocate, Silvano Arieti (1955). In their view, the schizophrenic's primary cognitive deficit is a paralogical fault characterized by undue attention to the identity of predicates. In other words, conclusions are drawn and behaviors justified by simple observations of shared attributes. If, for example, some man harmed you, and John is a man, John may be considered dangerous, in a rather simple paralogical leap. Insofar as schizophrenic thinking often shows premature closure and weak logic, this Arieti–Von Domarus construction was given much credit by clinicians in the past. But research investigating its theoretical and practical utility has uniformly failed to confirm any discriminating power in syllogistic tasks. This may be because syllogistic reasoning is a fairly rare event in day-to-day discourse. Furthermore, when syllogisms are used in argument, it has been noted that normal subjects make a high rate of syllogistic errors (Gottesman and Chapman, 1960); consequently, syllogistic tests have shown little utility.

Overinclusive Thinking

Patient: "I'm on heavy drugs."
Interviewer: "Heavy drugs. What sort of drugs."
Patient: "LSD, heroin."
Interviewer: "Before you came here?"
Patient: "No, I got it from the doctor."
Interviewer: "The doctor gave you LSD?"
Patient: "He was giving me LSD. He was giving me speed . . . He was giving me grass . . . Acid."
Interviewer: "Why was he giving you these?"
Patient: "To drug me up."

Schizophrenic patients are known to use words with such imprecision that the chronic schizophrenic quoted in the above statement is seen to confuse all manner of street drugs with the medications that his psychiatrist prescribed. Clinicians have observed that schizophrenics regularly substitute words of similar meanings for each other and define their concepts in a broad and all-encompassing fashion. Cameron's (1938) theorizing and research has documented the importance of overinclusive thinking, especially among chronic, nonparanoid, and process-schizophrenic patients. Cameron's studies used a mixture of standardized test challenges to normal children and adults, brain damaged, and schizophrenic patients to document their different classificatory principles. He found that schizophrenics make special use of "cluster thinking" (tendencies to make tangential links between objects), "metanymic distortions" (words only approximately comparable to the meaning of the words intended), and "interpenetration of themes" (intrusion of personal meanings). Cameron noted that schizophrenic patients have considerable difficulties in their attentional focus and they regularly seem to broaden their categorizations to include instances that reach far beyond what normals can accept.

Cameron's work, much like Goldstein and Scherer's (1941) efforts, spawned a large number of investigations using various language-demanding and object-sorting tests (e.g., Epstein, 1953). The major empirical work on overinclusion was conducted by Robert Payne and his collaborators (Payne *et al.*, 1959) using a wide variety of tests (e.g., Proverbs, Object Sorting, Unusual Solutions). Their research showed not only the expected differences between schizophrenic patients and controls, but also yielded correlations between overinclusion measures and the occurrence of delusions. Although promising findings were reported, the measures of overinclusion also were noted to show weak intercorrelation (Payne and Hewlett, 1960), were unstable over time (Sturm, 1965), and more greatly reflected the verbosity of the subjects than a conceptual disability (Gathercole, 1965). Payne eventually critiqued the overinclusion concept, indicating that it was not adequate to the task of measuring schizophrenic deficit with precision (Payne, 1971). Others, however, carried on the study of overinclusive thinking, extending the tests and showing stable deficits in schizophrenics (Chapman, 1961). In a series of studies, both measures of overinclusion as well as measures of overexclusion were found by the Chapman team to be heavily dependent on the type of stimulus pull that the category label provided. That is, if subjects were supplied category labels with commonly accepted unambiguous meanings (recognizable to both normal and schizophrenic subjects), such labels had greater power than less clear labels to command an overinclusive response from schizophrenic patients. Despite Payne's own skepticism about the utility of these measures, his work continues to have stature. Problems of bandwidth in the sorting behavior of schizophrenics are regarded as a substantial conceptual difficulty for these patients.

A Study of the Biases (Distortions) in Schizophrenic Cognitive Behavior

The Chapman and Chapman (1973) theory of schizophrenic communication problems is built on the view that schizophrenic cognition is not qualitatively different in structure from thought patterns found in normal adults. They see schizophrenic thought as an excessive and an uncorrected expression of normal biases. When normal subjects are given an opportunity to free associate, or are tested in conditions where they have inadequate information, they, too, tend to show cognitive deficits. Research into categorizing behavior and verbal associations of normal subjects shows reliable biases, based, for example, on the recency of associations, the novelty of events, the familiarity of the object, and many other influences (Campbell, 1958). Consistent with these findings, Chapman and Chapman's (1973) classic text gives abundant evidence that normals and schizophrenics share preferences in the interpretation and use of words. For example, either group sorting an item such as a "rubber ball" would be inclined to identify the ball with other rubber items more so than with other round items. Although schizophrenic patients show biases and performances similar to normals if the words are viewed in isolation, when the bias is put into competition so that a weak (less probable) meaning of a word is the appropriate choice to solve a language problem, here is where normals and schizophrenics will differ. Normal subjects can make the switch to accept an overriding contextual meaning, whereas schizophrenic patients tend to endorse the same "strong meaning" choice. Exemplifying this point, the Chapmans note that if subjects are required to *pair the word* "gold" with a conceptually similar word given in a set of multiple choice items (e.g., table, steel, fish, house), normals will more often connect gold with another metal (such as "steel") as the appropriate conceptual category. Schizophrenics in turn, would be much more likely to select the alternative choice of "fish," because of the strongly established association in the word "goldfish." Similarly, with the requirement to find the correct multiple choice alternative that *defines the noun* "shoot," normals would be more inclined to accept the word "sprout" as the correct alternative, even though "rifle" or "gun" might be a higher associate in their vocabulary. Schizophrenics, however, will yield to the high association more often than normals and select the frequent connection (gold–fish or gun–shoot) in their answers.

Tests of the influence of preferred meanings in a variety of other language tasks (word associations, proverbs, etc.) have shown that schizophrenics tend to apply the "strong meaning" in an unreflective manner despite a context that may require the preferred meaning to be suppressed in favor of a less preferred, low-associate meaning. In the previously cited instance of a concrete response to the question "What brought you to the hospital?," the schizophrenic's literal interpretation reflects a focus upon "brought" meaning "conveyance," and therefore elicits an answer about a particular vehicle, Mr. Jones's car. The meaning intended by the questioner concerning the "causal factors leading to hospitalization" were obscure to that patient.

The Chapmans' theory is consistent with the various clinical and theoretical observations that various authors offer. It is likely that the "volitional weakness" described by Goldstein reflects the failure of schizophrenic patients to apply enough effort required to search word meanings for low-associative alternatives. The power of "similar predicates" in syllogistic reasoning tests is greater if the middle term is a term strongly associated with conclusions than if it is a weak associate (Gruber, 1965). The distinct advantage to the Chapmans' view over alternative explanations is that their position allows the prediction of which language episodes are most likely to show schizophrenics' conceptual faults. Their theory offers a substantial advance in documenting the conceptual dysfunctions of schizophrenics. However, their position does not provide explanations as to why schizophrenics are more inclined to use "strong" or "preferred meanings" in managing conceptual language demands. The Chapmans have suggested that schizophrenic disturbances might reflect underlying deficits in information processing. Some efforts to elucidate such deficits are described in the next section.

Direct Challenges of Schizophrenic Communications

Several laboratories have led the way in developing direct tests of communication processes in order to clarify information-processing deficits that may underlie schizophrenic thought and language problems.

Cohen's Referential Communication Task

A major boost in the understanding of pragmatic failures in schizophrenic communication comes from the referential communication task studies of Bertram Cohen and his colleagues. In their procedures, subjects are required to orally describe an object or word so that a listener would be able to choose it from among a set of like items. In one procedure, a subject's task is to invent a "clue word" that would signal to a listener which member of a pair of words had been chosen as a target (Cohen and Camhi, 1967). For example, the choice of the word "car" in the pair "car–automobile" could be signaled by the clue word "sports" because of the clue's association to the term "sportscar." Cohen *et al.* (1974) extended the clue procedure to elicit extensive speech segments by requiring subjects to describe colors of similar hues but with subtle physical differences in brightness, saturation, and the like. Similar to the Cohen and Camhi technique, speakers were given the task of describing one color chip within sets of multiple colors in a way that would allow a listener to know which particular color had been selected. Since the speakers were not allowed to give a simple location-based clue, a verbal invention (such as the clue, "robin's egg blue") was needed to describe one item in a particular set of blue-toned colors.

Cohen *et al.*'s (1974) findings showed first of all that schizophrenic listeners were not at all impaired relative to normal controls, a finding that confirmed the contextual constraint and click study findings showing adequate receiver qualities in schizophrenics' understanding of language. Schizophrenic speakers, however, communicated much less effectively than control subjects, giving clue words that were difficult for judges to use. Consistent with their model, these studies found schizophrenics able to generate associations (in a hypothesized "sampling stage"), but were less able (in a second "comparison stage" of processing) to edit out irrelevant utterances that would not be useful to the listener.

A test of several alternative models of processing was brought to a dramatic conclusion in the Cohen *et al.* (1974) report by an examination of verbatim accounts of schizophrenic speech elicited in the color-selection task. Although schizophrenics did not differ from normals on simple versions of the tasks, the more difficult demands (larger number of items and narrower differences in hue) yielded severely deficient scores on several performance indices. An especially impressive finding on the difficult versions was a marked deterioration in the quality of schizophrenics' statements, in some cases approaching "word salad" levels of speech, with loosely associated chains of language. Cohen summarized schizophrenics' quality of performance as a *perseverative-chaining deficit* in which self-editing breaks down. To illustrate the difference, Cohen quotes a normal patient describing a salmon-colored stimulus to say: "These are clay colors. They seem identical. But the one to talk about has more white in it." A schizophrenic patient viewing the same color reported:

> "Oy vehs mir: This is what a color is? This is what I have to talk about? This here? Such a color? Like a can of salmon. Maybe some vinegar. Eat." (B. D. Cohen, personal communication)

Cohen's findings of perseverative-chaining deficits clarifies the nature of various language faults (highly repetitive speech, large object–subject ratios, etc.) by indicating schizophrenics' failure to adequately strain their own language for irrelevant and loosely associated concepts. Like the previously cited object-sorting tests study with alternative choices (Miller, 1967) Cohen finds that thought-disordered language is especially likely to occur where a task requires shared attention. That is, when the speaker must concurrently generate associations, assess the listener's need, and test their own utterance for relevance, it is then that high levels of communication disturbance erupt.

Harrow's Study of Perspective Taking in Schizophrenics

Do schizophrenic and other thought-disordered patients know that their language habits are confusing and seem bizarre to their listeners? Harrow *et al.* (1989) addressed this question by asking patients (and controls) to make judgments about their own statements. Subjects were administered a proverbs test under several conditions, two of which fedback their statements for review, asking the subjects to rate their own clarity of communication. If the schizophrenics and other thought-disordered subjects were asked to rate their own statements immediately after having uttered them, they did not perceive their own comments to be thought disordered. If, however, they were later provided samples of their own best and worst proverbs answers to make a paired comparison, they were sensitive to the different qualities of the statements. Harrow found interesting the fact that schizophrenic patients were also sensitive to thought-disordered statements of other schizophrenics, so they were not generally ignorant about the quality of communication. The major finding of this investigation would lead one to suspect that schizophrenics are quite poor in monitoring their own immediate productions, a finding consistent with Cohen's documentation of self-editing problems.

Harvey's Studies of Reality-Monitoring Capacities in Schizophrenic and Other Psychiatric Patients

Problems that schizophrenics have in maintaining a perspective on their own language productions has been clarified by Harvey's (1985) investigation of patients' sensitivity to the different sources of information given during a memory task. In a *reality-monitoring paradigm* (Raye and Johnson, 1980), subjects were required to listen to a list of common words read alternately by male and female voices. In a second condition, subjects were themselves required to read words alternately out loud and quietly (covertly). On subsequent recognition tests, subjects were required to recognize which words had been presented to them (in a list mixing presented with nonpresented items) and then to name the source (one of the two speakers in the first "listen–listen" condition, or the overt or covert expression in the second "say–listen" condition). Harvey found both thought-disordered (TD) schizophrenic and TD manic speakers had memory problems distinguishing them from NTD and normal control subjects. TD manics had most problems discriminating between the two external sources, whereas TD schizophrenic patients were less accurate in discriminating what was said from what was thought in the "say–think" condition. In fact, both TD groups had a significantly greater tendency to erroneously report that they said stated words out loud that had only been given covert expression. Reminiscent of the reference problems characterizing schizophrenic speech, TD patients are seen in the reality-monitoring task to be unable to remember to say everything needed. Confusions about the occurrence of what was planned to say and what has actually been said may play a decisive role in making TD language seem incoherent.

Although Harvey's application of the reality-monitoring procedure has not stood up well in all subsequent research (Harvey *et al.*, 1990), it still seems a promising approach to clarify the information-processing deficit basic to thought disorders. The original finding blends well with the Cohen *et al.* (1974) and Harrow *et al.* (1989) studies and forecasts the spread of interest in information-processing faults that might underlie manifestations of language and thought disorders.

THE RESEARCH FRONTIER

As seen thus far, there has been considerable work in charting the cognitive difficulties found in schizophrenic patients. Major advances have been made in developing and refining instruments to measure free language (Communication Deviance, TDI, TLC, etc.), to capture specific language faults (such as weak use of references), and to create laboratory

communication tasks that reveal deficits underlying language disturbances. For the most part, this work has yielded reliable measures with
reasonable levels of concurrent validity, preparing the ground for much
needed attention to the interrelationships of diverse measures of thought
and language and their associations to other important factors, including
diagnosis, life history, treatment response, and outcome. But one area still
needing considerable foundation work prior to exploration of its external
validity is the definition and measurement of delusional thinking. A discussion of requirements in this domain begins the account of work to
be done.

Needed Refinements

Understanding Delusions

Although considered a major feature of schizophrenic patients' cognitive distortion, and enjoying an upsurge in attention among senior investigators in the field (Oltmanns and Maher, 1988), the place of delusions in
schizophrenic pathology is not well understood. Confusion results from
the fact that delusions are not found specific to schizophrenia and are
difficult events to measure. To improve understanding of delusions, investigators must address the following concerns.

1. There are many individual delusional themes (grandeur, persecution, reference, etc.) now treated as separate identifiable symptoms of
schizophrenia. For example, nine are listed in DSM-III-R and others in
diverse diagnostic systems (see Tables 12.1, 12.2, and 12.3), but the psychological relevance of particular delusional themes has not been established.
Some work shows possible connections between delusional content and
the personality of individual patients (Forgus and DeWolfe, 1974). Self-
theorists find that maladaptive self-evaluative habits, particularly those
used to manage self-discrepancies, can elicit delusional thinking on occasions when the self-system is challenged (Higgins and Moretti, 1988).
Research focused on the relevance of various types of delusional belief to
life adjustment needs to be pursued.

2. The stability of delusions requires examination. Harrow et al. (1988)
report little change after a month of hospitalization in any of three dimensions (conviction, perspective on the views of others, and emotional commitment) that he studied, but other reports suggest considerable variation
in conviction can occur (Sacks et al., 1974). A need for increased use of
situational analyses of delusional behavior is suggested by observations
that greater degrees of thought-disordered language result when schizophrenic patients talk about their psychotic experiences (Chapman and

Chapman, 1988). Exactly when and how often delusional themes emerge, and what factors operate in altering the degree of conviction with which they are held, seems critical to understanding their place among thought-disorder symptoms, and their relevance to social adjustment (Harrow *et al.*, 1988).

3. Investigations need to weigh the importance of correlated dimensions. DSM-III-R distinguishes between delusions that are congruent or incongruent with mood. Other clinically recognized distinctions include the presence of concurrent hallucinations and variations of the coherence (or structure) of the delusional belief. The importance of these features is unknown.

4. Foundation work investigating differences in belief between normal and psychopathological populations will be required to more clearly establish the boundary between normal "wild ideas" (including unpopular convictions) and delusions. A number of authors observe considerable error and bias in so-called normal populations' logic (Kahneman and Miller, 1986), findings which cast a normalizing light on the delusions of the mentally disturbed. Kihlstrom and Hoyt (1988) and Maher (1988) conclude that if normals and schizophrenics are both error prone, than the delusions probably do not reflect different capacities or defects, but rather result from the amount of "anomalistic experiences" that need to be assimilated and made sensible. With an abundance of unaccounted for and weird experiences (perhaps perceptual aberrations, autonomic surges, and other deregulated states), schizophrenics may need to more often invent explanations (such as believing that one's life circumstances are caused by the hostile intentions and malevolent actions of other people) to explain their personal discomfort. Normals may simply have less need for extreme explanations of life events because they have fewer anomalous moments.

5. The developmental course of delusions has been tracked by Chapman and Chapman's (1988) study of schizotypic university students. Many of this population report strange beliefs that become the basis for full-blown delusions. A careful sifting of schizotypic subject beliefs in the Chapmans' study encourages the view that early warning and intervention can follow from the study of prepsychotic cognitions, and such study would enable a clearer view of the developmental course of thought disturbance.

Establishing the Association between Measures of Language Disturbance

The association among diverse thought-disorder measures needs to be mapped. Studies have shown that some laboratory measures are correlated with clinician judgments of symptoms and language-demanding tasks

(Harvey and Serper, 1990; Johnston and Holzman, 1979; Nuechterlein *et al.*, 1986), but there is still much work to be done to establish the network of associations among diverse measures of delusional thought, aberrant language functioning, diagnostic signs of thought problems (derailment, closure problems, etc.), laboratory-measured deficits, and the various nuisance variables (I.Q., education, cultural patterns, etc.) that are known associates of adjustment. Such efforts would require well-diagnosed, large-scale samples and the development of causal models and other multivariate strategies.

Criterion Validation

Measures of thought disorder need to be associated to real-life events reflecting etiology, diagnostic categories, treatment responsivity, brain measures, and long-term outcome. Giving promise to the validity of thought-disorder measures, the TDI and various Rorschach indices have been found to intercorrelate (indicating convergent validity), and the TDI measure has been found to be independent of sex, ethnic background, socioeconomic status, race, premorbid status, and paranoid tendencies, indicating divergent validity (Johnston and Holzman, 1979). However, the exact sensitivity — and value — of the various measures of thought disorder for assessing the functioning of all schizophrenics is not fully appreciated. Some limitations have appeared, with the TDI being a significant discriminator of only chronic schizophrenics, with measures of overinclusion found sensitive only in samples of acutely disturbed schizophrenics (Payne, 1971), and with Harrow and Quinlan's (1985) measures of Bizarre and Idiosyncratic thinking predicting outcome only in a subsample of the most extremely language-disordered patients. These findings give notice that the various measures of language and thought impairment are not equivalent nor are they yet useful for differential diagnosis. Knight and his colleagues (Knight *et al.*, 1979) also question the value of thought-disorder indices for prognosis estimates. In a long-term follow-up study of first-break acute schizophrenic patients, measures of affect were more effective than measures of thought disorder in predicting affect and thought-disorder status 22 years later in a cross-lagged panel correlation design. Clearly, much basic work needs to be done to assess the utility of thought-disorder measures for different subtypes and for understanding their relevance to adjustment outcomes.

Understanding the Mechanisms of Thought Disorder

As noted in the chapter opening, major advances have come from investigations of basic information processing (IP) and brain functions. It is time now to turn our best IP and brain-science lab technologies to the effort to explain language/thought-disorder symptoms.

Information Processing Deficits

As repeatedly stated in previous sections, many authors have speculated about the role of information-processing (IP) deficits, such as lapses of focus and memory, weak sustained and selective attention, in the genesis of thought- and language-disorder symptoms. IP deficits in schizophrenia have been well studied over the past fifty years and have shown strong relationships to clinical phenomena, to differences within the schizophrenia spectrum, to prognosis, to functioning of nonaffected family members, and to genetic markers of vulnerability (Cromwell, 1975, in press; Spaulding and Cole, 1984; Steffy and Waldman, in press). Recent IP study developments have incorporated models of cognitive theorists (e.g., Posner, 1978) into the study of schizophrenic deficits. Nuechterlein and Dawson (1984), for example, identified nine processing links or stages (problems of detection, sensory storage, sustained focus, selective attention, short-term memory, etc.) that could potentially complicate schizophrenics' task performances. Knight (1984) has found short-term visual-integration deficits to be especially problematic in schizophrenic samples, and others have clarified the role of long-term memory deficits in chronic schizophrenic patients (Calev *et al.*, 1983). Current IP research is focused on the question of where in the information chain the schizophrenic patient is most vulnerable.

This work may provide a foundation to help clarify the nature of disturbed thought and language processes. Giving some encouragement to this view, recent work found schizophrenics' susceptibility to distraction as a particularly potent factor in accounting for laboratory language task (reality monitoring) performances and other indices of language weakness as well (Harvey *et al.* 1988). Asarnow and MacCrimmon (1982) found relationships between Span of Apprehension Test (selective attention) scores and a conceptual measure of associative intrusions.

The immediate question in efforts to link the IP and conceptual domains is "where to begin?" Several paths might be followed. It is, of course, impractical to think that all IP stages could be sampled concurrently with the full variety of thought-disorder indices. However, some improved understanding might come from the use of a standard battery of the most discriminating (IP) measures collected during new research into language and thought disturbances. Just as we now routinely collect information on symptom features, medication levels, IQ, age, sex, and other such factors, a battery of the most sensitive IP measures could regularly be made available for subject typing (e.g., the COGLAB battery of Spaulding *et al.*, 1981).[4]

Perhaps an equally productive approach can be found in feature analyses of language and conceptual tasks in order to recognize their pattern of information-processing demands. It is possible that complex communication tasks with high degrees of uncertainty concerning when to speak and what to say may be particularly difficult for schizophrenics with, for example, the most substantial selective-attention deficits, or language requirements in which much new information needs to be juggled might be a special problem for patients with short-term memory deficits. Lengthy communications might be most impaired for individuals with problematic sustained attention. Language tasks that require a close inspection of visual displays (e.g., reading aloud) may be most difficult for patients with greatest levels of perceptual organization problems. In this respect, Harvey *et al.*'s (1988) report of correlations between measures of distractability and language-processing requirements illustrates the utility of understanding individual differences connecting IP and conceptual domains. Space and Cromwell's (1978) report of dysfluencies on the Bannister Grid Test (appearing as an occasional "tuning out" or "micropsychotic" episode during testing) may further reflect upon the impact of specific attentional difficulties on particular conceptual demands.

Brain-Measure Correlates of Thought Disorder

During the 1990s (the "decade of the brain"), it is not surprising that considerable progress has been made in applying neuroscience technologies to the study of schizophrenia, a development waiting to be applied specifically to conceptual dysfunction. Current views of brain faults in schizophrenia implicate both cortical and subcortical portions of the brain. Gruzelier and Flor-Henry (1979) and others have found schizophrenics' neuropsychological test findings suggestive of left hemisphere impairments. The possibility of distinctive malfunctions in left hemisphere structures is given further weight by a variety of anatomical and physiological findings, for example, ventricular enlargements in the left temporal horn of lateral cerebral structures (Roberts and Crow, 1987) and greater left temporal lobe deficit in evoked response measures (Faux *et al.*, 1988). Although

---

[4]Spaulding *et al.*'s (1981) COGLAB contains an especially good set of measures (Reaction Time, Span of Apprehension, Continuous Performance Test, etc.) in an efficient package. Various IP measures have been shown to have quite good sensitivity and specificity. For example, Steffy and Waldman (in press) report that a combination of simple reaction-time measures is 75% accurate in diagnosing process schizophrenics, with errors in only 25% of psychiatric controls and 5% of normal controls. Holzman *et al.*'s (1974) report of data on eye-tracking measures shows equally good levels of discrimination.

neuropsychological understandings would make a left hemisphere, especially a temporal lobe, lesion a sensible correlate of the language and thought disturbances characteristic of schizophrenics, the picture of schizophrenic patients' central nervous system is not perfectly clear. Brain measurements do not regularly lateralize (e.g., Gur *et al.*, 1985) and when they do, the findings are sometimes in opposition. For example, increased fast-wave EEG patterns have been found in the temporal lobe by Flor-Henry (1983), whereas abnormally slow wave activity in temporal lobes have been observed by Abrams and Taylor (1979). Further questioning the hypothesis of a left hemisphere malfunction in schizophrenia, Venables (1984) reinterprets much of the evidence arguing for a left hemisphere deficit to indicate instead a right hemisphere fault. Venables' review argues that a failure in right hemisphere preattentive processes imposes too heavy a requirement on the left brain, requiring the left side to assume the work of both hemispheres and thereby straining its capacity to do left hemisphere tasks adequately.

Brain studies in schizophrenia have also implicated frontal lobe functioning, supported by brain-scan indications of hypofrontal functioning in cerebral blood flow, and to some degree in PET measures, as well (Weinberger and Berman, 1988). Neuropsychological evidence using measures sensitive to prefrontal cortical damage, such as the Wisconsin Card-Scoring Test, reliably yields deficit performances in schizophrenics (Goldberg and Weinberger, 1988).

Speculations about the relevance of abnormalities in subcortical anatomy and functioning abound in current literature. Views of hippocampal dysfunction, for instance, lend themselves easily to speculation about the weak memory evident in many schizophrenic language problems (evident in pauses, inadequate referrents, etc.) as well as in findings of memory impairment (Koh, 1978). One particularly promising linkage derives from evidence of dysregulation in schizophrenics' thalamus. Crosson and Hughes (1987) observed that the thalamus is a major crossroad in all brain action, and therefore it is a likely place to look for the cause of speech and language dysregulation. Multiple looping (entry and exit) of information through thalamic structures must occur efficiently to allow the integration of communication subroutines (linking communication goals, vocabulary selection, syntax, editing of language production, analysis of listener's response, etc.). Indeed, Oke and Adams (1987) may have found the "monkey wrench that spoils the works" in their histology reports of abnormal growth of dopaminergic tissue in 6 out of 7 autopsied brains of schizophrenic patients. Since dopamine tissues are not found in normal brains, this finding stands out as a particularly fascinating possible physical basis for disrupted speech and thought. It awaits validation with drug-naive schizophrenic individuals and nonschizophrenic thought-disordered samples.

These and other advances in the neurosciences present interesting pathways for future research, possibility allowing the link of various symptoms of thought and language dysfunction to anomalous functions in particular parts of the brain. Given the complexity of schizophrenia as we know it, more research into brain–behavior associations will need to occur before such linkages can be determined. The early findings give promise of separate pathways. It has been observed, for example, that individuals with clusters of positive symptoms (typically, the more flagrant signs of thought disorder, such as the report of delusions, are named "positive" because their presence suggests an energetic behavioral response to the disorder) make a much better response to treatment than those with predominantly "negative" symptoms. The latter reflect a defeatist, passive, giving-up behavioral pattern, featuring apathy and the lack of volition (Carpenter *et al.*, 1985). There are also indications of different neurological pathways. Negative symptoms tend to be associated with enlarged ventricles and cortical atrophy; patients with predominantly positive symptoms have been considered to have faults in dopaminergic tissues. Neuropsychological test results show negative symptoms to be more often associated with language-processing faults, whereas positive symptoms are linked to visual–spatial faults (Walker and Harvey, 1986). The exciting work detailing different neurodevelopmental pathways found in various schizophrenic patient groups has been recently reviewed by Walker (1991) and by Straube and Oades (1992).

This chapter is not the place for a full consideration of all the disordered biology and IP hypotheses that have been advanced, but the possibility of linking behavioral symptomatic disturbances to the insights of both experimental psychopathology and neuroscience is an exciting one that is just being opened for exploration. An equally exciting research area is the work of behavioral and cognitive therapists attempting to directly modify disturbed language and thought.

TREATMENT

Just about everything under the sun has been attempted as a treatment of schizophrenia: medications, megavitamins, convulsive therapies, brain surgery, group therapy, milieu therapy, psychoanalysis, remotivation therapy, LSD, art therapy, and a variety of behavioral approaches as well. Tranquilizers are, of course, the treatment of choice; approximately 70% of acutely disturbed schizophrenic patients show substantial levels of improvement after medication compared to approximately 25% of those receiving placebos (Davis *et al*. 1980), but the fact that there are high relapse rates, strong side effects, and little if no impact for many of those with negative symptoms makes behavioral treatments seem appealing. With medications held constant, a recent major study of the value of psycho-therapy for schizophrenic patients found that a behavioral approach, fea-turing a "Reality-Adaptive, Supportive" (RAS) strategy, assisted patients to achieve better work record, shorter length of hospitalization, and more improved interpersonal skills than those resulting from a psychodynamic-based treatment (Gunderson *et al*., 1984). Although a traditional psycho-dynamic approach helped self-perceptions and interpretations of daily events, overall, the specific life-skill oriented (RAS) approach showed the greater practical utility.

The value of Gunderson *et al*.'s (1984) RAS approach blends nicely with a large set of accomplishments arising from behavior modification ap-proaches (e.g., including token economies) that assist self-care and work behaviors. Operant approaches help patients to develop better social skills, active listening, clearer verbal utterances, and other basic social behaviors. Collectively, these works show that a variety of skills can be improved through behavioral technologies even with the most regressed patients (Anthony and Liberman, 1986; Paul and Lentz, 1977). These improvements in social behavior and reduction of deviance have led investigators to ask whether the behavior approaches can specifically reduce thought disorder.

Behavioral Treatments Directed toward Relieving Thought-Disorder Symptoms

Several dozen studies and case reports in the literature through the past two to three decades demonstrate the power of behavioral technologies for reducing delusional, bizarre, hallucinatory, and aggressive verbal habits of schizophrenic patients. Most of these studies have reported treatments with one or, at most, a few chronic and paranoid individuals with long-standing histories of delusional speech. Typically, these studies employ experimental controls for contingency of reinforcement, multiple base-line analyses, ABA designs, and use conversational prompts to elicit the pa-tients' most typical delusional themes (e.g., Alford, 1986; Bulow *et al*., 1979).

Most of the behavioral treatments resulted in short-term gains but only a few studies have found full generalization and long-term maintenance (Bulow *et al*., 1979; Foxx *et al*., 1988). In one instance, behavioral treatment was found effective in reducing delusional speech in the lab and general-ized to encounters with nurses on the ward, but showed no impact in reducing the patients' delusional statements in a private psychiatric interview (Wincze *et al.*, 1972). However, some evidence of sustained improvements has been reported. Nydegger's (1972) 20-year-old paranoid patient sustained a reduction in delusional talk, possibly because of his parents' continuing therapeutic effort with their son during aftercare. Belcher (1988) found aversive stimulation (enforced hallway walks) quite helpful in the long-term control of verbally abusive outbursts in a chronic schizophrenic male inmate of a nursing home.

Cognitive Behavioral Modification Strategies to Reduce Thought Disorder

Cognitive Behavioral Modification (CBM) approaches seem to have been successful in producing generalization across tasks and situations, and in yielding some sustained improvements over standardized behavioral strategies. Meichenbaum (1969) showed good effects decreasing the frequency of "sick talk" and increasing the level of proverb abstraction among schizophrenics. Subsequently Meichenbaum and Cameron (1973) investigated self-instructional (SI) training on various tests of attention. In one study a single training session led to improved Digit Symbol Substitution Test performance and distracted recall test performances. The 1973 paper also reported a second study in which extensive SI training effects were obtained on a structured interview and proverbs procedure, and this training generalized to scores on ink blot and distracted recall test scores that were not part of the training exercises. Meichenbaum's technique fostered new coping strategies by training subjects to analyze the demands of tasks with the use of cognitive rehearsal, planning, and self-focusing instructions. Modeling exercises were added to assist coping with frustration, and statements were practiced to help subjects maintain improvements.

More recent approaches include Alford's (1986) treatment program using reinforcement strategy plus repeated evaluations and reinterpretations of delusional beliefs in a 22-year-old male schizophrenic. This therapy led to decreased delusional statements, and also a reduction of the strength of the delusional conviction as noted in the patient's diary records. Moreover, the client had a reduced need for PRN medication. Hole *et al.*'s (1979) study found that an open discussion of delusions was helpful with their clientele. In that project, the therapist focused on the relevance of delusional beliefs to the clients' current experience, the patients' means of managing information inconsistent with their delusions, and the patients' opinions about any changes in the delusional belief that may have naturally occurred. Recently Lowe and Chadwick (1990) developed an intervention in which their subjects were guided to consider alternative views of their maladaptive beliefs. Subjects were initially given instructions on the way that rules and beliefs generally influence behavior. Following this preparation, they were asked to address their own maladaptive rules, and finally instructed how to monitor and evaluate various alternative beliefs. Five out of the six subjects showed remission from their delusions, sustained over a 6-month follow-up.

A potentially important feature of the CBM approach is a deliberate caution against denigrating or interpreting patients' delusions as symptomatic of "illness." Instead, clients are assisted to view delusions as explanations of life experiences and then to consider replacement beliefs, essentially a reattributional analysis like that devised by Johnson *et al.* (1977). Common to these treatments is an energetic effort to learn the patients' personal experiences that might have been fundamental to the delusional belief. The CBM strategies seem entirely consistent with Maher's 1988 theory, viewing delusional thinking as an effort to make sense out of unexplained personal experiences.

John Strauss (1989) has advanced similar ideas in arguing that disordered thought and language symptoms should not be seen as deficits or illness, but rather as efforts to cope with strange and overwhelming personal experiences. How schizophrenics manage to comprehend and cope with their psychotic episodes may be a resource that therapists can harness for work with their clientele. Strauss contends that many clever solutions have been devised by patients and ex-patients attempting to deal with personal distresses. His interviews with schizophrenic patients reveal various strategies to ignore, to reframe, and to withhold public disclosure of their delusions. Some patients seem to find that the recently popularized view of an organic etiology of schizophrenia is able to offer them a personal sense of relief. They seem to prefer the view that a brain fault, rather than a mysterious and/or externalized force, causes their distress. Other patients have found a refreshing temporal perspective in viewing their schizophrenia as analogous to physical disorders. In the words of one client:

> "When I start to feel weird, its time to call in sick and expect to stay home away from people for a week or two. Like in hayfever season, I know it's best to stay away from pollen and soon it will be better again." (R. A. Steffy, personal file)

This client showed a helpful insight about avoiding life stresses and the complications that result from his own secondary reactions to bouts of disturbance. Although his self-treatment may appear to require social withdrawal—a symptom often associated with a worsening condition—in his case it seems to involve a planned retreat rather than a slide into chronicity. Helpful to his effort is the conviction that the retreat to his room is a personally controlled therapeutic decision requiring only a temporary adjustment.

Strauss would agree that the insights of such patients may provide valuable guides for future CBM strategies. Engaging patients as experts in their own condition and major contributors to their outcome could become an important adjunct to cognitive treatment approaches. Recent evidence from family therapies attempting to develop better communications within the home have shown major successes in reducing relapse rates among ex-psychiatric patients (Falloon *et al.*, 1984). Insofar as delusional and bizarre language is one of the most important factors in rehospitalization, it is particularly important that our treatments be coordinated with home-care efforts to reduce patients' crazy talk. Although not all behavioral and CBM therapies have been successful in altering the strange language and beliefs of schizophrenics, these approaches, along with new insights about schizophrenics' personal coping efforts and improved ways to arrange the family life of these patients, are most encouraging developments.

CONCLUSION

Study of the language behavior and thought patterns over the past 100 years has confirmed Bleuler's and Kraepelin's view that cognitive difficulties are frequently observed in schizophrenic patients. However, the relevance of language/thought-disorder signs to understanding the nature of schizophrenic processes has been disappointing. Quantitative measurements, be they counts of clinical signs, evaluation of speech integrity, or laboratory challenges, find that not all schizophrenics show clear-cut conceptual disturbances, and find that many nonschizophrenic psychiatric (particularly bipolar and organic) disorders do show severe conceptual problems. Although some work has found specific patterns of thought-disordered language differentiating among diagnostic groups, (schizophrenics showing more intrusive errors, manic patients showing more flippant and playful qualities to their statements), as yet no clear fingerprint of the different disorders has been established.

Throughout the chapter we have taken note of investigators' frequently voiced opinion that information-processing (IP) deficits may be basic to schizophrenics' conceptual problems that are found in schizophrenics' language and thought, rather than a specific aphasialike disability. Some of the disturbances in language, for example could be considered a product of short-term memory or attentional problems in which the schizophrenic has wandered from his/her communication goal. Excessive pauses at phrase boundaries, inadequately specified references, and other such faults make it seem plausible that schizophrenics often lose track of what they intend to say. Similarly, delusional thinking might be a reflection of these patients' efforts to make sense out of complex and overwhelming experiences — perhaps an information-processing overload, an autonomic nervous system perturbation, or an organizational problem.

This reductionistic analysis of thought/language-disordered behavior is by no means proven, but has been a compelling alternative to workers in the field, and fortunately may permit a bridging of the gap between the IP and conceptual domains. In the text, we recommended that future investigations into conceptual functioning use an established battery of measures of IP deficits in order to begin the study of interrelations between the two levels of functioning. Verbal-task analysis might also allow explicit hypotheses about particular IP stage faults accounting for variation in thought-disorder symptoms.

Further penetration into the understanding of cognitive disturbances might come from the brain-mapping technologies currently on the research frontier. Neuropsychological and neurophysiological measures yielding signs of left temporal and frontal lobe difficulties might be especially informative in accounting for the variety of conceptual lab-measure deficits and clinical signs as well. Linkages across these domains must eventually occur in order for us to put the classic signs of thought disorder into full perspective. Polythetic measurement strategies (Corning and Steffy, 1979) are long overdue in our analysis of behavioral disorders. Too often our research imaginations have been limited to a simple study of the way that schizophrenics and nonschizophrenics differ on a particular behavioral index. In the future, comprehensive batteries of measures evaluating specific conceptual thoughts concurrently with IP and brain-function measures (and probably life-adjustment factors as well) will help to frame the big picture of schizophrenic disturbances. We forecast that the conceptual problems of schizophrenics will continue to be a major defining attribute; it is after all one of the major features that society uses to define the disorder and is a personally striking set of features. One can only hope that research efforts will soon allow thought and language symptoms to be measured with greater precision and with clearer understanding about their mechanisms and their relevance for personal adjustment. The treatments required for schizophrenic patients have made good progress. The behavioral technology shows particular promise in assisting cognitive disturbances. The CBM approach, with its focus on clients' needs and experiences and its effort to elicit problem-solving skills, may offer a valuable therapeutic component for schizophrenic patients' treatment. Cognitive treatments are especially flexible in admitting patient's current adaptive coping into their treatment package, and also may be able to expand the solutions devised by clients who continue in good remission.

REFERENCES

Abrams, R., and Taylor, M. A. (1979). Laboratory studies in the validation of psychiatric diagnosis. In J. Gruzelier and P. Flor-Henry (Eds.), *Hemisphere asymmetries of function in psychopathology*. Amsterdam: Elsevier-North Holland.

Alford, B. A. (1986). Behavioral treatment of schizophrenic delusions: A single-case experimental analysis. *Behavior Therapy, 17,* 637–644.

Allen, C. K. (1987). Occupational therapy: Measuring the severity of mental disorders. *Hospital and Community Psychiatry, 38,* 140–142.

American Psychiatric Association. (1987). *Diagnostic and statistical manual of mental disorders (2nd ed., 1968; 3rd ed. revised,* 1987). Washington, D.C.: American Psychiatric Association.

Andreason, N. C. (1979). Thought, language, and communication disorders: I. Clinical assessment, definition of terms, and evaluation of their reliability. *Archives of General Psychiatry, 36,* 1315–1321.

Anthony, W. A., and Liberman, R. P. (1986). The practice of psychiatric rehabilitation. *Schizophrenia Bulletin, 12,* 542–559.

Arboleda, C., and Holzman, P. D. (1985). Thought disorder in children at risk for psychosis. *Archives of General Psychiatry, 42,* 1004–1013.

Arieti, S. (1955). *Interpretation of schizophrenia.* New York: Brunner/Mazel.

Asarnow, R. F. and MacCrimmon, D. J. (1982). Attention information processing, neuropsychological functioning and thought disorder during the acute and partial recovery phases of schizophrenia: A longitudinal study. *Psychiatry Research, 7,* 309–319.

Belcher, T. L. (1988). Behavioral reduction of overt hallucinatory behavior in a chronic schizophrenic. *Journal of Behavior Therapy and Experimental Psychiatry, 19,* 69–71.

Bellak, L. (Ed.). (1979). *Disorders of the schizophrenic syndrome.* New York: Basic Books.

Benjamin, J. D. (1964). A method for distinguishing and evaluating formal thinking disorders in schizophrenia. In J. S. Kasanin (Ed.), *Language and Thought in Schizophrenia.* New York: W. W. Norton, 65–90.

Bleuler, E. (1950). *Dementia Praecox or the group of schizophrenias.* New York: International Universities Press (originally published in 1911).

Broga, M. I., and Neufeld, R. W. J. (1981). Multivariate cognitive performance variables and response styles among paranoid and nonparanoid schizophrenics. *Journal of Abnormal Psychology, 90,* 495–509.

Buchsbaum, M. S. (1990). Frontal lobes, basal ganglia, temporal lobes — three sites for schizophrenia. *Schizophrenia Bulletin, 16,* 377–389.

Bulow, H., Oei, P. S., and Pinkey, B. (1979). Effects of contingent social reinforcement with delusional chronic schizophrenic men. *Psychological Reports, 44,* 659–666.

Burstein, A. (1961). Some verbal aspects of primary process thought in schizophrenia. *Journal of Abnormal and Social Psychology, 62,* 155–157.

Calev, A., Venables, P. H., and Monk, A. F. (1983). Evidence for distinct verbal memory pathologies in severely and mildly disturbed schizophrenics. *Schizophrenia Bulletin, 9,* 247–264.

Cameron, N. (1938). Reasoning, regression and communication in schizophrenics. *Psychological Monographs, 50,* (1, Whole No. 221).

Campbell, D. T. (1958). Systematic error on the part of human links in communication systems. *Information and Control, 1,* 334–369.

Carpenter, W. T., Jr., Strauss, J. S., and Bartko, J. J. (1973). Flexible system for the diagnosis of schizophrenia: report from the WHO International Pilot Study of Schizophrenia. *Science, 182,* 1275–1278.

Carpenter, W. T., Jr., Heinrichs, D. W., and Alphs, L. (1985). Treatment of negative symptoms. *Schizophrenia Bulletin, 11*, 440–452.

Chaika, E. (1974). A linguist looks at "schizophrenic" language. *Brain and Language, 1*, 257–276.

Chapman, L. J. (1961). A reinterpretation of some pathological disturbances in conceptual breadth. *Journal of Abnormal and Social Psychology, 62*, 514–519.

Chapman, L. J., and Chapman, J. P. (1973). Problems in the measurement of cognitive deficit. *Psychological Bulletin, 79*, 380–385.

Chapman, L. J., and Chapman, J. P. (1988). The genesis of delusions. In T. F. Oltmanns and B. A. Maher (Eds.), *Delusional beliefs* (pp. 167–183). New York: Wiley.

Clemmer, E. J. (1980). Psycholinguistic aspects of pauses and temporal patterns in schizophrenic speech. *Journal of Psycholinguistic Research, 9*, 161–185.

Cohen, B. D., and Camhi, J. (1967). Schizophrenic performance in a word-communication task. *Journal of Abnormal Psychology, 72*, 240–246.

Cohen, B. D., Nachmani, G., and Rosenberg, S. (1974). Referent communication disturbances in acute schizophrenics. *Journal of Abnormal Psychology, 83*, 1–14.

Corning, W. C. and Steffy, R. A. (1979). Taximetric strategies applied to psychiatric classification. *Schizophrenic Bulletin, 5*, 194–305.

Cozlino, L. L. J. (1983). The oral and written productions of schizophrenic patients. In B. A. Maher and W. B. Maher (Eds.), *Progress in experimental personality research, volume 12*, New York: Academic Press.

Cromwell, R. L. (1975). Assessment of schizophrenia. *Annual Review of Psychology, 26*, 593–619.

Cromwell, R. L. (In press). A summary view of schizophrenia. *In* R. L. Cromwell and C. R. Snyder (Eds.), *Schizophrenia: Origins, Processes, Treatment, and Outcome*. New York: Oxford Press.

Crosson, B., and Hughes, C. W. (1987). Role of the thalamus in language: Is it related to schizophrenic thought disorder? *Schizophrenia Bulletin, 13*, 605–622.

Crow, T. J. (1990). Temporal lobe asymmetries as the key to the etiology of schizophrenia. *Schizophrenia Bulletin, 16*, 433–443.

Davis, J. M., Schaffer, C. G., Killian, G. A., Kinard, C. and Chan, C. (1980). Important issues in the drug treatment of schizophrenia. *Schizophrenia Bulletin, 6*, 70–87.

Dokecki, P. R., Polidoro, L. G., and Cromwell, R. L. (1968). The chronicity of premorbid adjustment dimensions as they relate to commonality and stability of word association responses in schizophrenics. *Journal of Nervous and Mental Disease, 146*, 310–311.

Epstein, S. (1953). Overinclusive thinking in a schizophrenic and a control group. *Journal of Consulting Psychology, 17*, 384–388.

Fairbanks, A. (1944). The quantitative differentiation of samples of spoken language. *Psychological Monographs, 56* (2, Whole No. 255), 19–38.

Falloon, I. R. H., Boyd, J. L., and McGill, C. W. (1984). *Family care of schizophrenia*. New York: Guilford Press.

Faux, S. F., Torello, M. W., McCarley, R. W., Shenton, M. E., and Duffy, F. H. (1988). P300 in schizophrenia: confirmation and statistical validation of temporal region deficit in P300 topography. *Biological Psychiatry, 23*, 776–790.

Flor-Henry, P. (1983). Determinants of psychosis in epilepsy: Laterality and forced normalization. *Biological Psychiatry, 18*, 1045.

Forgus, R. H., and DeWolfe, A. S. (1974). Coding of cognitive input in delusional patients. *Journal of Abnormal Psychology, 83*, 278–284.

Foxx, R. M., McMorrow, M. J., Davis, L. A., and Bittle, R. G. (1988). Replacing a chronic schizophrenic man's delusional speech with stimulus appropriate responses. *Journal of Behavior Therapy and Experimental Psychiatry, 19*, 43–50.

Gathercole, C. E. (1965). A note on some tests of overinclusive thinking. *British Journal of Medical Psychology, 38*, 59–62.

George, L., and Neufeld, R. W. J. (1985). Cognition and symptomatology in schizophrenia. *Schizophrenia Bulletin, 11*, 264–285.

Gerver, D. (1967). Linguistic rules and the perception and recall of speech by schizophrenic patients. *British Journal of Social and Clinical Psychology, 6*, 204–211.

Goldberg, T. E., and Weinberger, D. R. (1988). Probing prefrontal function in schizophrenia with neuropsychological paradigms. *Schizophrenia Bulletin, 14*, 179–184.

Goldstein, K. (1939). The significance of special mental tests for diagnosis and prognosis in schizophrenia. *American Journal of Psychiatry, 96*, 575–587.

Goldstein, K. and Scheerer, M. (1941). Abstract and concrete behavior: An experimental study with special tests. *Psychological Monographs, 53* (2, Whole No. 239).

Gorham, D. R. (1956). Use of the proverbs tests for differentiating schizophrenics from normals. *Journal of Consulting Psychology, 20*, 435–440.

Gottesman, L., and Chapman, L. J. (1960). Syllogistic reasoning errors in schizophrenia. *Journal of Consulting Psychology, 24*, 250–255.

Gruber, J. (1965). *The Von Domarus principle in the reasoning of schizophrenics.* Unpublished doctoral dissertation, Southern Illinois University.

Gruzelier, J. H., and Flor-Henry, P. (Ed.). (1979). *Hemisphere asymmetries of function in psychopathology.* Amsterdam: Elsevier-North Holland.

Gunderson, J. G., Frank, A. F., Katz, H. M., Vannicelli, M. L., Frosch, J. P., and Knapp, P. H. (1984). Effects of psychotherapy in schizophrenia: II. comparative outcome of two forms of treatment. *Schizophrenia Bulletin, 10*, 564–598.

Gur, R. E., Gur, R. C., Skolnick, B., Caroff, S., Obrist, W. D., Resnick, S. and Reivich, M. (1985). Brain function in psychiatric disorders. III. Regional cerebral blood flow in medicated schizophrenics. *Archives of General Psychiatry, 44*, 119.

Harrow, M., and Quinlan, D. (1985). *Disordered thinking and schizophrenic psychopathology.* New York: Gardner Press.

Harrow, M., Adler, D., and Hanf, E. (1974). Abstract and concrete thinking in schizophrenia during the prechronic phases. *Archives of General Psychiatry, 31*, 27–33.

Harrow, M., Rattenbury, F., and Stoll, F. (1988). Schizophrenic delusions: An analysis of their persistence, of related premorbid ideas, and of three major dimensions. In T. F. Oltmanns and B. A. Maher (Eds.), *Delusional beliefs* (pp. 184–211). New York: Wiley.

Harrow, M., Lanin-Kettering, I. and Miller, J. G. (1989). Impaired perspective and thought pathology in schizophrenic and psychotic disorders. *Schizophrenic Bulletin, 15*, 605–622.

Harvey, P. D. (1983). Speech competence in manic and schizophrenic psychoses: The association between clinically rated thought disorder and cohesion and reference performance. *Journal of Abnormal Psychology, 92*, 368–377.

Harvey, P. D. (1985). Reality monitoring in mania and schizophrenia. The association of thought disorder and performance. *The Journal of Nervous and Mental Disease, 173*, 67–73.

Harvey, P. D., and Serper, M. R. (1990). Linguistic and cognitive failures in schizophrenia. A multivariate analysis. *Journal of Nervous and Mental Disease, 178*, 487–494.

Harvey, P. D., Earle-Boyer, E. A., and Levinson, J. C. (1988). Cognitive deficits and thought disorder: A retest study. *Schizophrenia Bulletin, 14*, 57–66.

Harvey, P. D., Docherty, N. M., Serper, M. R., and Rasmussen, M. (1990). Cognitive deficits and thought disorder: II. An 8-month followup study. *Schizophrenia Bulletin, 16*, 147–1156.

Heilbrun, A. B. (1975). A proposed basis for delusion formation within an information-processing model of paranoid development. *British Journal of Social and Clinical Psychology, 14*, 63–71.

Higgins, E. T., and Moretti, M. M. (1988). Standard utilization and the social-evaluative process: vulnerability to types of aberrant beliefs. In T. F. Oltmanns and B. A. Maher (Eds.), *Delusional beliefs* (pp. 110–137). New York: Wiley.

Hole, R. W., Rush, A. J., and Beck, A. T. (1979). A cognitive investigation of schizophrenic delusions. *Psychiatry, 42,* 312–319.

Holzman, P. S., Proctor, L. R., Levy, L., Yasillo, J. J., Meltzer, H. Y., and Hurt, S. W. (1974). Eye-tracking dysfunctions in schizophrenic patients and their relatives. *Archives of General Psychiatry, 31,* 143–151.

Hotchkiss, A. P., and Harvey, P. D. (1986). Linguistic analyses of speech disorder in psychosis. *Clinical Psychology Review, 6,* 155–175.

Hurt, S. S., Holzman, P. S., and Davis, J. M. (1983). Thought disorder: The measurement of its changes. *Archives of General Psychiatry, 40,* 1281–1285.

Johnson, W. G., Ross, J. M., and Mastria, M. A. (1977). Delusional behavior: An attributional analysis of development and modification. *Journal of Abnormal Psychology, 86,* 421–426.

Johnston, M. H., and Holzman, P. S. (1979). *Assessing schizophrenic thinking.* San Francisco: Jossey-Bass.

Johnstone, E. C., Owens, D. G. C., Bydder, G. M., Colter, N., Crow, T. J., and Frith, C. D. (1989). The spectrum of structural brain changes in schizophrenia: Age of onset as a predictor of cognitive and clinical impairments and their cerebral correlates. *Psychological Medicine, 19,* 91–103.

Kahneman, D. and Miller, D. T. (1986). Norm theory: Comparing reality to its alternatives. *Psychological Review, 93,* 136–153.

Kendall, P. C. (1985). Cognitive processes and procedures in behavior therapy. In C. M. Franks, G. T. Wilson, P. C. Kendall, and K. D. Brownell (Eds.), *Annual review of behavior therapy: Theory and practice* (Vol. 10, pp. 123–163). New York: Guilford Press.

Kendall, P. C. (1991). Guiding theory for treating children and adolescents. In P. C. Kendall (Ed.), *Child and adolescent therapy: Cognitive–behavioral procedures* (pp. 3–24). New York: Guilford Press.

Kendler, K. S., Glazer, W. M., and Morgenstern, H. (1983). Dimensions of delusional experience. *American Journal of Psychiatry, 140,* 466–469.

Kent, H., and Rosanoff, A. J. (1910). A study of association in insanity. *American Journal of Insanity, 67,* 326–390.

Kihlstrom, J. F., and Hoyt, I. P. (1988). Hypnosis and the psychology of delusions. In T. F. Oltmanns and B. A. Maher (Eds.), *Delusional beliefs* (pp. 66–109). New York: Wiley.

Knight, R. A. (1984). Converging models of cognitive deficit in schizophrenia. In W. D. Spaulding and J. K. Cole (Eds.), *1983 Nebraska symposium on motivation, vol 31: Theories of schizophrenia and psychosis.* Lincoln: University of Nebraska Press.

Knight, R. A., Roff, J. D., Barrnett, J., and Moss, J. L. (1979). Concurrent and predictive validity of thought disorder and affectivity: A 22-year follow-up of acute schizophrenics. *Journal of Abnormal Psychology, 88,* 1–12.

Koh, S. D. (1978). Remembering of verbal materials by schizophrenic young adults. In S. Schwartz (Ed.), *Language and cognition in schizophrenia* (pp. 55–99). Hillsdale, NJ: Erlbaum.

Kraepelin, E. (1919). *Dementia Praecox and Paraphrenia* (translated by R. M. Barclay). Edinburgh: E. and S. Livingston. (Originally published in 1913).

Kuriansky, J. B., Deming, W. E. and Gurland, B. J. (1974). On trends in the diagnosis of schizophrenia. *American Journal of Psychiatry, 131,* 402–408.

Langfeldt, G. (1939). *The schizophrenic states.* Copenhagen: Munksgaard E.

Lowe, C. F., and Chadwick, P. D. J. (1990). Verbal control of delusions. *Behavior Therapy, 21,* 461–479.

Magaro, P. A. (1980). *Cognition in schizophrenia and paranoia: The integration of cognitive processes.* Hillsdale, NJ: Erlbaum.

Maher, B. A. (1988). Anomalous experience and delusional thinking: The logic of explanations. In T. F. Oltmanns and B. A. Maher (Eds.), *Delusional beliefs* (pp. 15–33). New York: Wiley.

Maher, B. A., McKean, K. O., and McLaughlin, B. (1966). Studies in psychotic language. In P. J. Stone, D. C. Dunphy, M. S. Smith, and D. M. Ogilvie (Eds.), *The general inquirer: A computer approach to content analysis* (pp. 469–503). Cambridge, MA: MIT Press.

Manschreck, T. C., Maher, B. A., and Ader, D. N. (1981). Formal thought disorder, the type–token ratio and voluntary motor movement in schizophrenia. *British Journal of Psychiatry, 139,* 7–15.

Marengo, J. T., Harrow, M., Lanin-Kettering, I., and Wilson, A. (1986). Evaluating bizarre-idiosyncratic thinking: A comprehensive index of positive thought disorder. *Schizophrenia Bulletin, 12,* 497–511.

McCormick, D., and Broekema, V. (1978). Size estimation, perceptual recognition, and cardiac rate response in acute paranoid and nonparanoid schizophrenia. *Journal of Abnormal Psychology, 87,* 385–398.

Mednick, S. A. (1958). A learning theory approach to research in schizophrenia. *Psychological Bulletin, 55,* 316–327.

Meichenbaum, D. (1969). The effects of instructions and reinforcement on thinking and language behavior of schizophrenics. *Behavior Research and Therapy, 7,* 101–114.

Meichenbaum, D., and Cameron, R. (1973). Training schizophrenics to talk to themselves: a means of development of self-controls. *Behavior Therapy, 4,* 515–525.

Miller, G. A. (1967). *The reinterpretation and prediction of "concrete" behavior in schizophrenia using the theory of restricted mediation.* Unpublished doctoral dissertation, Southern Illinois University.

Moon, A. F., Mefferd, R. B., Jr., Wieland, B. A., Pokorny, A. D., and Falconer, G. A. (1968). Perceptual dysfunction as a determinant of schizophrenic word associations. *Journal of Nervous and Mental Disease, 146,* 80–84.

Neale, J. M., and Oltmanns, T. F. (1980). *Schizophrenia.* New York: Wiley.

Neale, J. M., Oltmanns, T. F., and Harvey, P. D. (1985). The need to relate cognitive deficits to specific behavioral referents of schizophrenia. *Schizophrenia Bulletin, 11,* 286–291.

Newmark, C. S., Raft, D., Toomey, T., Hunter, W., and Mazzaglia, J. (1975). Diagnosis of schizophrenia: Pathognomonic signs or symptom clusters. *Comprehensive Psychiatry, 16,* 155–163.

Nuechterlein, K. H. and Dawson, M. E. (1984). Information processing and attentional functioning in the developmental course of schizophrenic disorders. *Schizophrenia Bulletin, 10,* 160–203.

Nuechterlein, K. H., Edell, W. S., Norris, M., and Dawson, M. E. (1986). Attentional vulnerability indicators, thought disorder, and negative symptoms. *Schizophrenia Bulletin, 12,* 408–426.

Nydegger, R. N. (1972). The elimination of hallucinatory and delusional behavior by verbal conditioning and assertive training: A case study. *Journal of Behavior Therapy and Experimental Psychiatry, 3,* 225–227.

O'Brian, J. P., and Weingartner, H. (1970). Associative structure in chronic schizophrenia. *Archives of General Psychiatry, 22,* 136–142.

Oke, A. F., and Adams, R. N. (1987). Elevated thalamic dopamine: Possible link to sensory dysfunctions in schizophrenia. *Schizophrenia Bulletin, 13,* 589–604.

Oltmanns, T. F., and Maher, B. A. (1988). *Delusional beliefs.* New York: Wiley.

Paul, G. L., and Lentz, R. (1977). *Psychosocial treatment of chronic mental patients*. Cambridge, MA: Harvard University Press.

Payne, R. W. (1971). Cognitive defects in schizophrenia: Overinclusive thinking. In J. Hellmuth (Ed.), *Cognitive studies, Vol. 2: Deficits in cognition* (pp. 53–89). New York: Brunner/Mazel.

Payne, R. W., and Hewlett, J. H. C. (1960). Thought disorder in psychotic patients. In H. J. Eysenck (Ed.), *Experiments in personality* (Vol. 2, pp. 3–104). London: Routledge & Kegan Paul.

Payne, R. W., Matussek, P., and George, E. I. (1959). An experimental study of schizophrenic thought disorder. *Journal of Mental Science, 105*, 627–652.

Posner, M. I. (1978). *Chronometric explorations of mind*. Hillsdale, NJ: Erlbaum.

Powers, W. F., and Hamlin, R. M. (1955). Relationship between diagnostic categories and deviant verbalizations on the Rorschach. *Journal of Consulting Psychology, 19*, 120–125.

Ragin, A. B., and Oltmanns, T. F. (1986). Lexical cohesion and formal thought disorder during and after psychotic episodes. *Journal of Abnormal Psychology, 95*, 181–183.

Rapaport, D., Gill, M., and Schafer, R. (1968). *Diagnostic psychological Testing*. (Rev. ed., R. R. Holt, Ed.) New York: International Universities Press (originally published in 2 volumes, 1945–1946).

Raye, C. L., and Johnson, M. K. (1980). Reality monitoring vs. discrimination of two external sources. *Bulletin of the Psychonomic Society, 15*, 405–408.

Reilly, F., Harrow, M., Tucker, G., Quinlan, D., and Siegel, A. (1975). Looseness of associations in acute schizophrenia. *British Journal of Psychiatry, 127*, 240–246.

Roberts, G. W., and Crow, T. J. (1987). The neuropathology of schizophrenia — A progress report. *British Medical Bulletin, 43*, 599–615.

Rochester, S. R., and Martin, J. R. (1979). *Crazy talk*. New York: Plenum.

Rochester, S. R., Martin, J. R., and Thurston, S. (1977). Thought-process disorder in schizophrenia: The listener's task. *Brain and Language, 4*, 95–114.

Rosen, J. (1953). *Direct analysis*. New York: Grune & Stratton.

Sacks, M. H., Carpenter, W. T., and Strauss, J. S. (1974). Recovery from delusions: Three phases documented by patient's interpretation of research procedures. *Archives of General Psychiatry, 30*, 117–120.

Schneider, K. (1959). *Clinical psychopathology*. New York: Grune & Stratton.

Schuldberg, D., and Boster, J. S. (1985). Back to Topeka: Two types of distance in Rapaport's original Rorschach thought disorder categories. *Journal of Abnormal Psychology, 94*, 205–215.

Schwartz, S. (1982). Is there a schizophrenic language? *Behavioral and Brain Sciences, 5*, 579–626.

Shimkunas, A. M. (1972). Demand for intimate self-disclosure and pathological verbalizations in schizophrenia. *Journal of Abnormal Psychology, 80*, 197–205.

Singer, M. T., and Wynne, L. C. (1965). Thought disorder and family relations of schizophrenics. III. Methodology using projective techniques. *Archives of General Psychiatry, 12*, 187–212.

Singer, M. T., and Wynne, L. C. (1966a). Principles for scoring communication defects and deviances in parents of schizophrenics: Rorschach and TAT scoring manuals. *Psychiatry, 29*, 260–288.

Singer, M. T., and Wynne, L. C. (1966b). Communication styles in parents of normals, neurotics, and schizophrenics. *Psychiatric Research Reports, 20*, 25–38.

Solovay, M. R., Shenton, M. E., and Holzman, P. S. (1987). Comparative studies of thought disorders. I. Mania and schizophrenia. *Archives of General Psychiatry, 44*, 13–20.

Space, L. G., and Cromwell, R. L. (1978). Personal constructs among schizophrenic patients. In S. Schwartz (Ed.), *Language and cognition in schizophrenia* (pp. 145–191). Hillsdale, NJ: Erlbaum.

Spaulding, W., and Cole, J. (Eds.). (1984). *Nebraska symposium on motivation, vol. 31: Theories of schizophrenia and psychosis*. Lincoln: University of Nebraska Press.

Spaulding, W., Hargrove, D., Crinean, J., and Martin, T. (1981). A micro-computer based laboratory for psychopathology research in rural settings. *Behavior Research Methods and Instrumentation, 13*(4), 616–623.

Spitzer, R. L., Williams, J. B. W., and Skodol, A. E. (1980). DSM-III: The major achievements and an overview. *American Journal of Psychiatry, 137*, 151–164.

Spring, B. (1985). Distractibility as a marker of vulnerability to schizophrenia. *Psychopharmacology Bulletin, 21*, 509–512.

Steffy, R. A., and Waldman, I. (in press). Schizophrenic reaction time: North star or shooting star? In R. L. Cromwell (Ed.), *Schizophrenia: Origins, processes, treatment and outcome*.

Straube, E. R., and Oades, R. D. (1992). *Schizophrenia: Empirical research and findings*. New York: Academic Press.

Strauss, J. S. (1989). Subjective experiences of schizophrenia: Toward a new dynamic psychiatry—II. *Schizophrenia Bulletin, 15*, 179–187.

Strauss, J. S., and Gift, T. E. (1977). Choosing an approach for diagnosing schizophrenia. *Archives of General Psychiatry, 34*, 1248–1253.

Sturm, I. E. (1965). Overinclusion and concreteness among pathological groups. *Journal of Consulting Psychology, 29*, 9–18.

Truscott, I. P. (1970). Contextual constraint and schizophrenic language. *Journal of Consulting and Clinical Psychology, 35*, 189–194.

Tutko, T. A., and Spence, J. T. (1962). The performance of process and reactive schizophrenics and brain injured subjects on a conceptual task. *Journal of Abnormal and Social Psychology, 65*, 387–394.

Venables, P. H. (1984). Cerebral mechanisms, autonomic responsiveness and attention in schizophrenia. In W. Spaulding and J. Cole (Eds.), *Nebraska Symposium on Motivation, Vol. 31: Theories of Schizophrenia and Psychosis*. Lincoln, Nebraska: University of Nebraska Press.

Von Domarus, E. (1944). The specific laws of logic in schizophrenia. In J. S. Kasanin (Ed.), *Language and thought in schizophrenia* (pp. 104–114). Berkeley: University of California Press.

Walker, E. F. (1987). Validating and conceptualizing positive and negative symptoms. In P. D. Harvey and E. F. Walker (Eds.), *Positive and negative symptoms of psychosis* (pp. 30–49). Hillsdale, NJ: Erlbaum.

Walker, E. F. (1991). *Schizophrenia: A life-course developmental perspective*. New York: Academic Press.

Walker, E. and Harvey, P. D. (1986). Positive and negative symptoms in schizophrenia: Attentional performance correlates. *Psychopathology, 19*, 294–302.

Watkins, J. G. and Stauffacher, J. C. (1952). An index of pathological thinking in the Rorschach. *Journal of Projective Techniques, 16*, 276–286.

Wegrocki, H. J. (1940). Generalizing ability in schizophrenia: An inquiry into the disorders of problem thinking in schizophrenia. *Archives of Psychology, 36*.

Weinberger, D. R., and Berman, K. F. (1988). Speculation on the meaning of cerebral metabolic hypofrontality in schizophrenia. *Schizophrenia Bulletin, 14*, 157–168.

Wincze, J. P., Leitenberg, H., and Agras, W. S. (1972). The effects of token reinforcement and feedback on the delusional verbal behavior of chronic paranoid schizophrenics. *Journal of Applied Behavior Analysis, 5*, 247–262.

Winters, K. C., and Neale, J. M. (1983). Delusions and delusional thinking in psychotics: A review of the literature. *Clinical Psychology Review, 3*, 227–253.

World Health Organization. (1973). *The international pilot study of schizophrenia*. Geneva: WHO.

PART III

Integration and Future Directions

Future Trends for Research and Theory in Cognition and Psychopathology

Keith S. Dobson

University of Calgary

Philip C. Kendall

Temple University

As the chapters in this volume attest, there are numerous strategies for examining the role of cognition in psychopathology. Some strategies include self-report methodologies, while others involve procedures adapted from experimental cognitive psychology. One of the goals of this chapter will be to review these methods for measuring cognition in psychopathological states (see also Kendall and Hollon, 1981; Merluzzi *et al.*, 1981; Segal and Cloitre, Ch. 2, this volume).

Research strategies are employed in the service of investigating hypotheses or exploring conceptual models of functioning. Cognitive methodologies are no different, and the previous chapters in this volume reveal that a number of common cognitive constructs are being examined in different research areas. Accordingly, a second goal of this chapter is to examine some of the themes that have emerged across the various domains within which cognitive research in psychopathology has been conducted.

A final goal for this chapter is to abstract from the field trends in theory and research. The chapter will conclude with predictions about future directions in psychopathology research, as well as some challenges for investigators in this field.

475

COMMON CONSTRUCTS IN COGNITIVE RESEARCH

At the outset of this volume, we suggested that cognitive constructs can be conceptualized in terms of structures, processes, contents, and products (Ingram and Kendall, 1986; Kendall, 1985; Kendall and Braswell, 1982; Kendall and Dobson, Ch. 1, this volume). This overall conceptualization was mirrored in many of the chapters, in which specific forms of psychopathology were seen as having their chief elements in one or more of the above areas. Much of the current theory and research in cognitive aspects of psychopathology can be organized around these constructs.

As an example of the convergence in the use of common cognitive constructs, consider cognitive structures in psychopathology: a number of models of psychopathology use constructs that imply dysfunctional cognitive structures. Goldman and Rather (Ch. 8, this volume), for example, discussed the "architecture" of the cognitive structure of persons who suffer from substance use disorders, while Ackermann Engel and De-Rubeis (Ch. 4, this volume) advanced the idea of cognitive schemata in depression. In their discussion of factors that contribute to marital dysfunction, Epstein and Baucom (Ch. 10, this volume) emphasized the role that marital beliefs can play. Such discussions, from our perspective, are mutually compatible with the construct of cognitive structures in that they propose that there are formal, relatively permanent features of the cognitive organization and representation of experience within individuals who suffer from specific types of psychopathology.

It is clear that the content of cognitive structures varies as a function of the type of psychopathology under investigation. Whereas cognitive structures may be relatively similar across different psychopathologies (i.e., the organization of memory and the structure of experience may be relatively immutable), the contents of different forms of psychopathology vary dramatically. In some respects, cognitive contents can be seen as descriptive features of the specific dysfunction being discussed.

Cognitive contents are reflected in the increasing number of methodologies that have been developed to assess cognitions in psychopathology. A number of cognitive contents have been identified, including predictions for future events, recall of past events, explanations, decisions made in lexical tasks, responses to hypothetical situations, and so forth (see Kendall and Hollon, 1981; Merluzzi et al., 1981; Segal and Cloitre, Ch. 2, this volume, and other sources of cognitive assessment for multiple examples).

Although the specific terminology used to refer to cognitive structures varies from disorder to disorder, and although cognitive contents must necessarily be specific to the type of psychopathology being discussed, there appears to be emerging the recognition of the importance of examining the structural principles around which other cognitive processes and products may be organized. Analogous to the emergent theory and research on cognitive structures, it is our contention that some consistent themes around the construct of cognitive processes are beginning to emerge. The literature is replete with discussions of cognitive distortions (Garner *et al.*, 1978; Vitousek and Ewald, 1992; Zotter and Crowter, 1991), dysfunctional attributional processes (Bradbury and Fincham, 1990; Holtzworth-Monroe and Jacobson, 1985; Orvis *et al.*, 1976), catastrophization of experience (Turk, 1985; Weisenberg, 1989), problem-solving deficiencies (Richard and Dodge, 1982), information-processing deficits (Dodge, 1986; Ingram, 1984), and so forth, all of which imply dysfunction at the level of cognitive processing. There is little doubt that the distinction between cognitive deficits and distortions (see Kendall and Dobson, Ch. 1, this volume) has been recognized and examined in many forms of psychopathology, and that the prospects for future developments in this area are manifest. It appears that theorists and researchers within the field of cognition and psychopathology, while employing a wide number of specific constructs and a variety of methodologies, have focused their work around the constructs of structures, processes, and products.

STRATEGIES FOR EXPLORING COGNITION IN PSYCHOPATHOLOGY

One of the emerging achievements of the cognitive trend in psychopathology has been the advancement of strategies for examining cognitive constructs. One of the most consistently used methods for assessing cognitive aspects of psychopathology is self-report assessment. Self-report assessment tools include cognitive checklists, measures that assess the frequency of cognition, measures of the relative strength or intensity of cognition, narrative descriptions of certain situations or memories of situations, incomplete sentences, and others. Self-reports are efficient methods for capturing cognition and, provided that the particular measures were developed using sound test construction methods, can provide important information about cognition in various types of psychopathology.

Despite the wide usage of self-report strategies, one of the debates that has emerged about these assessment strategies is the extent to which their results accurately reflect cognitive structures, processes, contents, or products (e.g., Alloy and Abramson, 1992; Segal and Dobson, 1992). Although there is relative agreement about the fact that self-report strategies must be consistent with the descriptive nature of the particular type of psychopathology being studied, and therefore must have content appropriate to that of the disorder, there is relatively less agreement about the relationship among other cognitive constructs and self-report strategies.

One of the issues that has been discussed is the extent to which self-report measures can measure cognitive structures, processes, and products. It has been argued, for example (Segal, 1988; Segal and Dobson, 1992), that self-report strategies largely reflect cognitive products, in as much as the self-reports are the end product of a potential series of cognitive processes. Consider, for example, attributional measures that respondents to indicate their perception of the likelihood of different potential causes for positive and negative outcomes to hypothetical events. Although it is certainly plausible that individuals naturally provide attributions for events, and so engage in the process of attributing causes, it cannot be assumed that results of attributional self-report measures are more than the result of respondents' evaluating the probability of the different causes provided on the scale and assigning them relative ratings. As such, one cannot infer with certainty that different results on the attribution measures reflect differences in attributional *processes*; it is possible that other unspecified processes lead to differential responses to these self-report strategies.

Another manner in which to restate the above is that while self-report strategies are excellent measures of the topography of cognition in psychopathology, they tell relatively little about the geography of psychopathology, or about the geographical processes that have eventuated in the self-reports themselves. Thus, in an analogous manner, just as topography cannot prove what underlying geology exists, self-report cannot validate causal models of psychopathology. At the same time that self-report cannot prove causal models, self-report data that is inconsistent with causal models can seriously challenge those models.

An alternative methodology from self-report to assessing cognition in psychopathology derives from cognitive psychology (Segal, 1988; Segal and Dobson, 1992). A number of methods have been developed in cognitive psychology to examine cognitive theories, many of which do not rely on self-report and therefore are not subject to the same criticisms about the level of inference potential in self-report methods (MacLeod *et al.*, 1986; Schotte *et al.*, 1990; Segal and Cloitre, Ch. 2, this volume; Walker *et al.*, 1992).

In general, cognitive assessment strategies adapted from cognitive psychology use behavioral measures such as, for example, reaction time, decision time, and rate of responding as an indirect reflection of the organization of cognitive structures and such issues as the efficiency of cognitive processing. One example might help to make this point clear.

MacLeod *et al.* (1986) adapted a lexical decision task for assessing the efficiency of cognitive processing in anxiety patients. Based upon the assumption that subjects who have anxiety disorders will have their attention drawn to anxiety-provoking or threatening stimuli, pairs of stimuli were developed, which included pairs of threatening, pairs of nonthreatening, and pairs of the combination of threatening and nonthreatening words. Patients viewed a computer screen on which these pairs of words were quickly presented. Once the words disappeared, a probe would appear on some trials in the place where one of the words had been. Subjects were instructed to press a response button as soon as they saw a probe (no mention was made of its likely location). It was predicted that subjects who had anxiety problems would be more attentive to threatening words, and that their attention would be draw to these stimuli. As such, it was predicted that anxious subjects would respond to the probes more quickly than nonanxious subjects when the probe appeared in the position in which an anxiety stimulus had been. The results supported this prediction, and therefore provided support for the differential deployment of attention in anxious subjects relative to nonanxious subjects. Theoretically, these results suggest that anxious individuals scan the environment for threats to their security, and attend to these threats when they emerge in a way that can be measured on the lexical decision task.

In addition to the above lexical decision task, a large number of fruitful strategies have been adapted from cognitive psychology to the study of psychopathological groups. One area in which such adaptation has been particularly manifest is that of schizophrenia (Steffy, Ch. 12, this volume). As can be seen, schizophrenia researchers have for some time focused on processes such as memory capacity, short- and long-term delayed recall strategies, and problem-solving tasks in an effort to differentiate the unique types of cognitive deficits represented in those disorders.

Regardless of whether cognitive researchers have utilized self-report or other assessment strategies, their research methods for validating these assessment procedures have been relatively constant. Much of the research in cognition and psychopathology, as this volume demonstrates, consists of work that shows that measures have internal reliability, that cognitive constructs correlate with other related measures (i.e., have concurrent validity) and discriminate appropriate psychopathology groups (i.e., have criterion-related validity), and that measures are appropriate to the constructs to which they are applied (i.e., have construct validity). Researchers will typically develop an assessment strategy with items that appear to measure the cognitive construct in question with the specific form of disorder under investigation; they will then go on to document either that the measure correlates with increasing severity of that disorder or that it discriminates individuals with that disorder from others without that disorder. The vast majority of the research is cross-sectional, examining a particular group of subjects at a single point in time, although there is an increasing trend in psychopathology for more difficult and expensive longitudinal research to also take place.

In summary, although there are a large number of specific self-report and cognitive psychology assessment strategies that have been developed in the cognition research in psychology, the focus of these strategies has been largely on the descriptive features of different aspects of psychological disorders. This work has been integral in delineating the cognitive features of these disorders. It appears that while many psychopathological conditions are now experiencing considerable theoretical development at the level of cognitive processes and structures, these aspects of cognition and psychopathology are relatively less well developed than measures of cognitive contents and products. The development of measures of processes and structures represents an exciting next stage in psychopathology research, and it is likely that developments in one type of psychopathology may help direct researchers in other areas toward the most fruitful strategies for consideration.

FUTURE TRENDS IN COGNITION AND PSYCHOPATHOLOGY

Suggestions about future theory and research in the area of cognition and psychopathology derive from contributions to this volume, as well as other developments within the field of psychopathology in general. From our perspective, there are five critical areas of development: (1) theoretical and technological consistency within and among different forms of psychopathology; (2) issues of covariation and comorbidity; (3) temporal factors in psychopathology; (4) integration with other theoretical models; and (5) advancing the compatibility of theory and treatment models.

Theory and Technology Consistency

Convergence in cognitive theory has revolved around common constructs, and is reflected in the fact that assessment and research strategies show a large degree of commonality across different forms of psychopathology. At the same time, there are technological advances that have been made in some areas of psychopathology that have not been used in other areas. In order for the field of cognition and psychopathology to develop, it is our contention that researchers need to continue to read about advances in other domains of psychopathology, as conceptual and technological advances in one domain may well contribute to advances in other areas. As the field of cognition and psychopathology continues to develop, it is our prediction that theorists and researchers who focus on one particular type of psychopathology must remain abreast of developments with other types of psychopathology. To the extent that different forms of psychopathology share cognitive elements, it is likely that cross-fertilization will be a productive strategy.

Covariation and Comorbidity

A recent theme within psychopathology research has been the examination of the extent to which different forms of psychopathology covary with others (e.g., Kendall and Watson, 1989; Maser and Cloninger, 1990). Although the traditional model of diagnosis makes an assumption that different types of psychopathology are discrete, accumulating data makes such an assumption increasingly tenuous, particularly in some research areas. It has been shown, for example, that anxiety disorders covary with a number of other conditions (Beck and Emery, 1985; Brady and Kendall, 1992; Shaw *et al.*, 1986), as is also true for depression (Beach *et al.*, 1990; Dobson, 1985; Kendall and Watson, 1989; Maser and Cloninger, 1990). In similar fashion, personality disorders have been shown to be present in a number of other different disorders (see the Special Section of the *Journal of Consulting and Clinical Psychology*, December, 1992).

Covariation of various types of psychopathology can be conceptualized in different ways. If a particular form of psychopathology is conceptualized in terms of severity or another dimensional ways, there are a large number of correlational research designs and statistical techniques that exist to examine covariation among constructs (Dobson and Cheung, 1990). In a similar manner, there are numerous methods for examining the issue of comorbidity in psychopathology, when it is conceptualized in a more traditional, discrete fashion (American Psychiatric Association, 1987). A third perspective that is attracting increasing attention is a focus at the symptom level (rather than at the disorder level), in which covariation among symptoms is the focus of research and theory development (e.g., Costello, 1992).

Independent of the particular conceptualization of different types of disorders, and the design and research methodology issues attendant to such conceptualizations, the issue for theorists and researchers is the need to attend to comorbidity and covariation (Kendall and Clarkin, 1992). Cognitive models should be able to account for observed covariation and offer integration across different types of psychopathology. Both disorders with high covariation rates (e.g., anxiety and depression) and those with low covariation rates (e.g., depression and antisocial personality disorder) should be explicable within an integrated model of cognition and psychopathology.

Temporal Aspects of Psychopathology

Although the majority of research in the field of psychopathology is cross-sectional (i.e., occurring at one point in time), the field is increasingly aware of the need to attend to temporal aspects of these disorders. Indeed, there have been a large number of calls for longitudinal research in psychopathology (including several chapters in this volume; see also Segal and Dobson, 1992). Researchers that examine temporal aspects of psychopathology must address a number of issues, in particular, those of onset, maintenance, and recovery.

Onset issues include the original factors associated with different disorders. Research examining onset is perhaps the most difficult to conduct, as these studies often require the identification of an at-risk population, following them for a reasonable period of time until psychopathology could emerge, and then attempting to differentiate those subjects who developed psychopathology from those that did not along cognitive dimensions. Such research implies that the at-risk population can be identified, and that resources to conduct this study are available. As the prevalence rates of many disorders are quite low, it is essential that a large enough number of subjects is included in the sample to ensure that, after attrition, and given the prevalence rates of the particular disorder under investigation, enough subjects remain to make comparisons statistically meaningful. For example, schizophrenia has an approximate 1% prevalence rate. In order to conduct a study of the onset of schizophrenia, in which there are 30 identified schizophrenics to compare with other subjects, an initial sample of more than 3000 subjects is required, given that attrition will lead to the loss of some subjects. Because of the need for large samples and long-term assessments, longitudinal research is often contingent upon large amounts of research funding.

Another temporal aspect of psychopathology is maintenance. For some disorders, it has been suggested that the original onset factors may be different than those that explain the maintenance of these same disorders. In the area of depression, for example, it has been suggested that while structural elements of cognition may be important in the onset of depression, once it has begun to develop, it tends to become more automatic and subject to process-oriented maintenance factors (e.g., Teasdale, 1983). Researchers need to differentiate the developmental variables in psychopathology, as well as determine the types of cognitive constructs (and the related assessment protocols) needed to best describe maintenance of psychopathology.

Recovery from psychological disorders can occur either "spontaneously" (i.e., without direct intervention) or as a result of therapeutic ministrations. Regardless of the form of recovery, however, a comprehensive cognitive model of psychopathology should be able to provide a plausible and empirically supported model for recovery. One of the critical issues that cognitive theorists need to attend to when accounting for recovery is to avoid the logical error of concluding that because cognitive therapies were found to "work," these successes therefore validate the cognitive models of the disorder. Although the efficacy of cognitive therapies provides data that is consistent with cognitive models of psychopathology, one cannot use the treatment results to confirm causal models of psychopathology.

Although not all forms of disorders are recurrent, many are; relapse and recurrence of psychological disorders are developmental processes that need to be accounted for within cognitive models of psychopathology. Similar to the awareness that different processes may be involved in onset and maintenance, it is important for theorists and researchers not to assume that the factors involved in recurrence are the same as those involved in onset. Research strategies must be broad enough to take the possibility of different processes into account.

In summary, there are a number of developmental processes that are involved in the onset, maintenance, recovery, recurrence, and relapse of disorders. Cognitive models of psychopathology must attend to these issues, and must be able to potentially provide plausible and different accounts for each of these developmental aspects of disorder.

Integration with Other Theoretical Models

As was stated in the opening chapter (Kendall and Dobson, Ch. 1, this volume), humans are recognized to be multidimensional, multisystem entities. Normal cognitive functioning of humans (especially those with disorders) involves a complex set of structures, processes, and outcomes. The fact that cognition and psychopathology have been the focus of this volume should not be taken as a tacit endorsement of the primacy of cognition as the cause of these disorders. Although it can be heuristically valuable to delineate cognitive constructs and study these constructs in isolation from other classes of constructs, it is almost certainly the case that any "final" models of psychopathology will involve the integration of cognitive formulations with other theoretical models.

Current research and theory on the integration of cognitive models with other models of psychopathology suggest several primary possible forms of integration. A considerable amount of conjecture has been made concerning the role that early developmental issues, such as trauma, play in the establishment of cognitive structures that might later potentiate psychopathology (e.g., Bowlby, 1980; Ford, 1987; Guidano and Liotti, 1983). Early experience with different parental models, and the internalization of those role models, have been widely discussed as onset variables that might account for some aspects of dysfunction. Thus, early experience has been attended to by a number of theorists as a construct that can help to explain the development of cognitive structures consistent with disorder.

A number of theorists have attempted to delineate the relationship between internal cognitive constructs and external events that might precipitate different disorders. Research on life events has suggested that these events play an important role in the onset of psychopathology; there has been attendant interactional and transactional research that attempts to explore these relationships (Hammen, 1993).

One area of potentially fruitful integration is that of biological and cognitive constructs. To date, such integration has been quite limited, although there is a developing literature in some areas, including childhood disorders (Barkely, 1990), anxiety (Shaw *et al.*, 1986), depression (Gilbert, 1989), and substance use disorders (Goldman and Rather, Ch. 8, this volume). Because of the reemergence of biological models in psychopathology, it is suggested here that theorists and researchers would make an enormous contribution to the literature if they devoted effort to describing the convergent and divergent elements of cognitive and biological models of psychopathology.

Compatibility of Theory and Treatment Models

One development that is not necessarily tied to advances in cognitive theory and research is that of treatment. Although it would be conceptually pleasing (and parsimonious in terms of explanations of change processes) if the same set of cognitive factors were related to both onset and treatment of psychopathology, it is entirely possible that causal, maintenance, and other aspects of psychopathology are different than those variables most appropriately used in treating psychopathology. Understanding the causes of psychopathology may tell us little about the best way to overcome and/or manage a disorder, once it is present.

One specific manner in which cognitive theory may have implications for treatment is in the area of patient matching. If cognitive variables can be shown to correlate with treatment success and failure, it may be possible to create predictors that will enable treatment resources to be directed toward those patients that will maximally benefit. Given that many psychopathologists are also interested in the promotion of human welfare, it is not surprising that a considerable amount of effort is being devoted toward matching patients with treatment programs. Our hope and our hypothesis is that the integration of psychopathology models and treatment models will continue.

REFERENCES

Alloy, L., and Abramson, L. (1992). A consensus report without our consensus. *Psychological Inquiry, 3*, 229–230.

American Psychiatric Association. (1987). *Diagnostic and Statistical Manual-III-Revised.* Washington, D.C.: American Psychiatric Association.

Barkely, R. A. (1990). *Attention deficit hyperactivity disorder: A handbook for diagnosis and treatment.* New York: Guilford Press.

Beach, S. R. H., Sandeen, E. E., and O'Leary, K. D. (1990). *Depression in marriage.* New York: Guilford Press.

Beck, A. T., and Emery, G. (1985). *Anxiety disorders and phobias: A cognitive perspective.* New York: Basic Books.

Beck, A. T., Rush, A. J., Shaw, B. F., and Emery, G. (1979). *Cognitive therapy for depression.* New York: Guilford Press.

Bowlby, J. (1980). *Loss: Sadness and depression (Volume 3 of Attachment and loss).* Harmondsworth, England: Penguin Books.

Bradbury, T. N., and Fincham, F. D. (1990). Attributions in marriage: Review and critique. *Psychological Bulletin, 107*, 3–33.

Brady, E. U., and Kendall, P. C. (1992). Comorbidity of anxiety and depression in children and adolescents. *Psychological Bulletin, 111*, 244–255.

Clark, D. A. (1988). The validity of measures of cognition: A review of the literature. *Cognitive Therapy and Research, 12*, 1–20.

Costello, C. (Ed.). (1992). *Symptoms of depression.* New York: Wiley.

Dobson, K. S. (1985). The relationship between anxiety and depression. *Clinical Psychology Review, 5*, 307–324.

Dobson, K. S., and Cheung, E. (1990). Relationship between anxiety and depression: Conceptual and methodological issues. In J. D. Maser and C. R. Cloninger (Eds.), pp. 611–632. *Comorbidity of mood and anxiety disorders.* Washington, D.C.: American Psychiatric Press.

Dodge, K. A. (1986). A social information processing model of social competence in children. In M. Perlmutter (Ed.), pp. 187–198. *Minnesota symposium on child psychology (Volume 18).* Hillsdale, New Jersey, Erlbaum.

Fincham, F. D., and Bradbury, T. N. (1992). Assessing attributions in marriage: The Relationship Attribution Measure. *Journal of Personality and Social Psychology, 62*, 457–468.

Ford, M. E. (1987). *Humans as self-constructing living systems: A developmental perspective on behavior and personality.* Hillsdale, New Jersey: Erlbaum.

Garner, D. M., Garfinkel, P. E., and Moldofsky, H. (1978). Perceptual experiences in anorexia nervosa and obesity. *Canadian Psychiatric Association Journal, 23*, 249–260.

Gilbert, P. (1989). *Human nature and suffering.* Hove, United Kingdom: L. Erlbaum.

Guidano, V. F., and Liotti, G. (1983). *Cognitive processes and emotional disorders.* New York: Guilford Press.

Hammen, C. (1993). The social context of risks for depression. Paper presented at the 25th annual Banff Conference for Behavioural Sciences, Banff, Alberta, Canada.

Holtzworth-Monroe, A., and Jacobson, N. S. (1985). Causal attributions of married couples: When do they search for causes? What do they conclude when they do? *Journal of Personality and Social Psychology, 48*, 1398–1412.

Ingram, R. E. (1984). Toward an information processing analysis of depression. *Cognitive Therapy and Research, 8*, 443–447.

Ingram, R. E., and Kendall, P. C. (1986). Cognitive clinical psychology: Implications of an information processing perspective. *In* R. E. Ingram (Ed.), pp. 1–21). *Information processing approaches to clinical psychology*. New York: Academic Press.

Kendall, P. C. (1985). Cognitive process and procedure in behavior therapy. In G. T. Wilson, C. M. Franks, P. C. Kendall, and J. Foreyt (Eds.), *Annual review of behavior therapy (Volume 10)*. New York: Guilford Press.

Kendall, P. C., and Braswell, L. (1982). On cognitive–behavioral assessment: Models, measures and madness. In C. D. Spielberger and J. N. Butcher (Eds.), *Advances in personality assessment: Volume 1)*. Hillsdale, New Jersey: Erlbaum.

Kendall, P. C., and Clarkin, J. F. (1992). Introduction to Special Section: Comorbidity and treatment implications. *Journal of Consulting and Clinical Psychology, 60*, 833–835.

Kendall, P. C., and Hollon, S. D. (Eds.). (1981). *Assessment strategies for cognitive–behavioral interventions*. New York: Academic Press.

Kendall, P. C., and Watson, D. (Eds.). (1989). *Anxiety and depression: Distinctive and overlapping features*. New York: Academic Press.

MacLeod, C. M., Mathews, A., and Tata, P. (1986). Attentional bias in emotional disorders. *Journal of Abnormal Psychology, 95*, 15–20.

Maser, J. D., and Cloninger, C. R. (Eds.). (1990). *Comorbidity of mood and anxiety disorders*. Washington, D.C.: American Psychiatric Press.

Merluzzi, T. V., Glass, C. R., and Genest, M. (1981). *Cognitive assessment*. New York: Guilford Press.

Orvis, B. R., Kelley, H. H., and Butler, D. (1976). Attributional conflict in couples. In J. Harvey, W. Ickles, and R. Kidd (Eds.), *New directions in attributional research*. Hillsdale, New Jersey: Erlbaum.

Richard, B. A., and Dodge, K. A. (1982). Social maladjustment and problem solving in school aged children. *Journal of Consulting and Clinical Psychology, 50*, 226–233.

Schotte, D. E., McNally, R. J., and Turner, M. L. (1990). A dichotic listening analysis of body weight concern in bulimia nervosa. *International Journal of Eating Disorders, 9*, 109–113.

Segal, Z. V. (1988). Appraisal of the self-schema construct in cognitive models of depression. *Psychological Bulletin, 103*, 147–162.

Segal, Z. V., and Dobson, K. S. (1992). Cognitive models of depression: Report from a consensus conference. *Psychological Inquiry, 3*, 219–224.

Shaw, B. F., Segal, Z., Vallis, T. M., and Cashman, F. E. (Eds.). (1986). *Anxiety disorders: Psychological and biological perspectives*. New York: Polonium Press.

Teasdale, J. (1983). Negative thinking in depression: Cause, effect, or reciprocal relationship? *Advances in Behaviour Research and Therapy, 5*, 3–25.

Turk, D. C. (1985). Coping with pain: A review of cognitive control techniques. In M. Feuerstein, L. B. Sachs, and I. D. Turkat (Eds.), *Psychological approaches to pain control*. New York: Wiley.

Vitousek, K. B., and Ewald, L. (1992). Self-representation in the eating disorders: The cognitive perspective. In Z. Segal and S. Blatt (Eds.), *Self-representation in emotional disorders: Cognitive and psychodynamic perspectives*. New York: Guilford Press.

Walker, M. K., Ben-Tovim, D. I., Jones, S., and Bachok, N. (1992). Repeated administration of the Adapted Stroop Test: Feasibility for longitudinal study of psychopathology in eating disorders. *International Journal of Eating Disorders, 12*, 103–105.

Weisenberg, M. (1989). Cognitive aspects of pain. In P. D. Wall and R. Melzack (Eds.), *Textbook of pain: II*. Edinburgh: Churchill Livingstone.

Zotter, D. L., and Crowter, J. H. (1991). The role of cognition in bulimia nervosa. *Cognitive Therapy and Research, 15*, 413–426.

Index

List of Previous Volumes

.